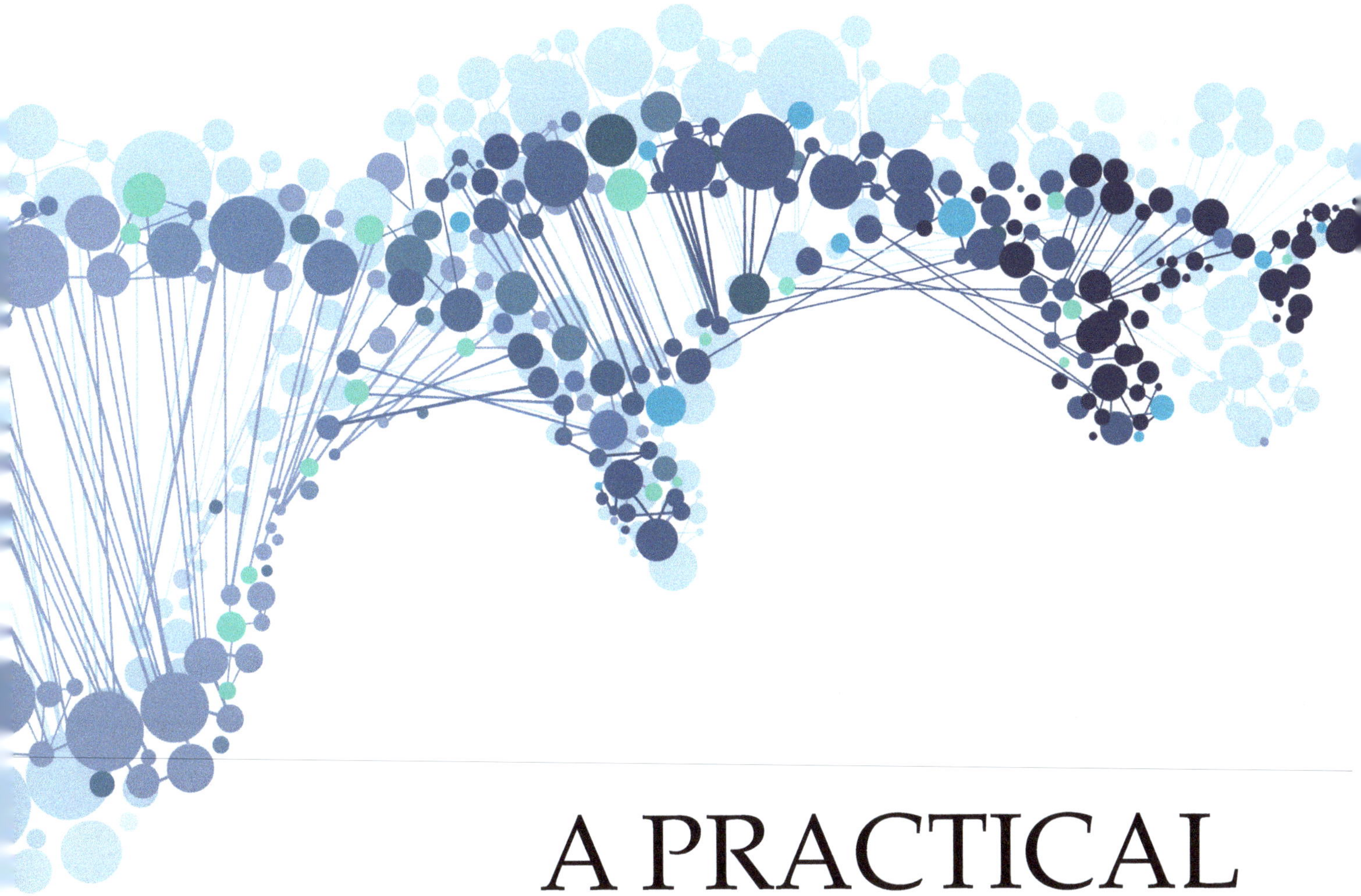

# A PRACTICAL GUIDE TO GLOBAL POINT-OF-CARE TESTING

Editor: Mark Shephard

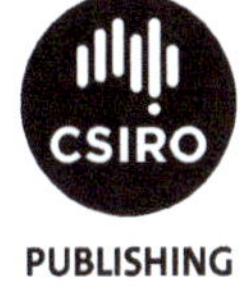


PUBLISHING

National Library of Australia Cataloguing-in-Publication entry

A practical guide to global point-of-care testing / Mark Shephard OAM (editor).

9781486305186 (paperback)
9781486305193 (epdf)
9781486305209 (epub)

Includes bibliographical references and index.

Point-of-care testing.
Medicine, Preventive.
Preventive health services.
Pathology.
Diagnostic services.
Medical technology.

Shephard, Mark, editor.

616.07

Published by

CSIRO Publishing
36 Gardiner Road, Clayton VIC 3168
Private Bag 10, Clayton South VIC 3169
Australia

Telephone: [+613] 9545 8555
Email: csiropublishing@csiro.au
Website: www.publishing.csiro.au

Cover: The artwork on the cover depicts the many linkages that point-of-care testing can facilitate between the patient, the health professional, the health-care service and the community. It was inspired by artwork by Aimee Manion.

Set in 10/13 Minion Pro and ITC Stone Sans
Edited by Peter Storer Editorial Services
Cover design by David Heinrich, Medical Illustration and Media, Flinders Medical Centre, Adelaide
Typeset by Desktop Concepts Pty Ltd, Melbourne
Index by Bruce Gillespie
Printed by Ingram Lightning Source



Feb26_RP_ILS

# Contents

# About the Editor

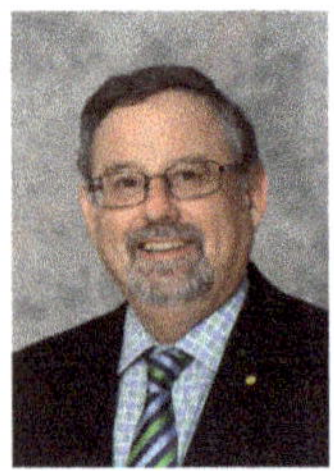

Professor Mark Shephard OAM, BSc (Hons), MSc, MAIMS, MAACB, FFSc (RCPA), PhD is Director of the Flinders University International Centre for Point-of-Care Testing. He has extensive experience in research and management of large point-of-care testing networks across Australia and internationally; including roles as Program Manager of the national Quality Assurance for Aboriginal and Torres Strait Islander Medical Services (QAAMS) Point-of-Care Testing Program for diabetes management; Chair of the Management Committee of the Northern Territory Point-of-Care Testing Program for acute care pathology testing; a Chief Investigator for the TTANGO (Test, Treat and Go) point-of-care testing research program for sexually transmitted infections; and Program Manager of the international ACE (Analytical and Clinical Excellence) Point-of-Care Testing Program for diabetes management operating in seven countries. In regard to teaching, Mark is the Course Coordinator and principal lecturer for the Flinders University's Graduate Certificate in Global Point-of-Care Testing, the first postgraduate academic qualification in the field of point-of-care testing, and Topic Coordinator and principal lecturer for 'Point-of-Care Testing – Application, Management and Effectiveness', taught in the Bachelor of Medical Science degree at Flinders University.

Mark has served as Chair of the Australasian Association of Clinical Biochemists (AACB) Point of Care Testing Working Party (2004–05), Co-Chair of the Australian Institute of Medical Scientists (AIMS) Working Committee on Point-of-Care Testing for Infectious Disease and Drugs of Abuse (2010–2013), and was a member of the Australian Government's National Pathology Accreditation Advisory Council (NPAAC) Point-of-Care Testing Drafting Committee (2013–2015), which developed national guidelines for the conduct of point-of-care testing in Australia.

In 2009, Mark was the recipient of a Distinguished Alumni Award from Flinders University in recognition of his significant contributions to the improvement of Aboriginal health in Australia and his services to the University. In 2011, Mark was elected as a Founding Fellow of the Royal College of Pathologists of Australasia (RCPA) Faculty of Science.

In 2013, Mark was appointed as the inaugural Chair of the WONCA (World Organization of Family Doctors) Special Interest Group on Global Point-of-Care Testing. Since 2014, Mark has been a member of the World Health Organization's Technical Consultation on Point-of-Care Diagnostic Tests for Sexually Transmitted Infections.

Mark has authored more than 100 peer-reviewed published papers and book chapters in the national and international literature.

Mark was the recipient of the Medal of the Order of Australia (OAM) in the 2006 Queen's Birthday Australian Honours list and an Australian of the Year Award in 2004. These awards acknowledged Mark's work in point-of-care testing.

# Contributors

Paul Arbon, PhD, AM, FACN
Matthew Flinders Distinguished Professor
Dean, School of Nursing and Midwifery
Flinders University
Adelaide, South Australia
Australia
Chapter 31

Malcolm Auld, RN, Grad Cert Remote Health Practice
Professional Practice Nurse
Primary Health Care – Remote
Central Australia Health Service
Northern Territory Government
Alice Springs, Northern Territory
Australia
Chapter 36

Jeff Ayton, MBBS, MPH&TM, FACRRM, FRACGP, FACTM, AFFTM, DRANZCOG DA(UK)
Chief Medical Officer
Australian Antarctic Division
Kingston, Tasmania
Australia
Chapter 32

Paul Baum, MD, PhD
Director
Clinical Science
Roche Molecular Systems, Inc
Pleasanton CA, USA
Assistant Adjunct Professor of Medicine
University of California
San Francisco CA, USA
Chapter 20

David Bell, MBBS, MTropHealth, MRCP, FAFPHM, PhD
Director, Global Health Technologies
The Global Good Fund/Intellectual Ventures Laboratory
Bellevue WA, USA
Chapter 22

Susan Best, MAppSci, MASM, MBA
Director
National Serology Reference Laboratory
Fitzroy, Victoria
Australia
Chapter 5

Wilton Braund, MBBS, FRACP
Endocrinologist
Endocrine SA
Tennyson Centre
Kurralta Park, South Australia
Clinical Director
Medical Communications Associates
Blackwood, South Australia
Australia
Chapter 36

Matthew Justin Busbridge, RN, MRemoteIndigHlth, MSc(Adv Pract Nurs), BSc(Nurs), BA(Econ)
Advance Practice Nurse and Remote Area Nurse
Northern Territory
Australia
Chapter 36

Louise Causer, MBBS, MScPH, DTM&H
Lecturer
The Kirby Institute
University of New South Wales
Sydney, New South Wales
Australia
Chapter 17 & 28

Caroline Chartrand, MD, MSc, FRCPC
Associate Professor (Clinics) – Department of Pediatrics
Université de Montréal – CHU Sainte-Justine
Montréal, Québec
Canada
Chapter 21

Damian Conway, MB BCh, MMed, PhD, FAChSHM, MRCGP, DRCOG
Kirby Institute
University of New South Wales
Sydney, New South Wales
Australia
Chapter 19

Jane Cunningham, MD, FRCPC
Technical Officer
Global Malaria Programme
World Health Organization
Geneva

Switzerland
Chapter 22

Wayne Dimech, B App Sci, MASM, MBA, FAIMS, FFSc (RCPA)
General Manager
National Serology Reference Laboratory
Fitzroy, Victoria
Australia
Chapter 5

Ian Farrance, BSc, MCB, FAACB, FRCPath
Associate, RMIT University
Discipline of Laboratory Medicine
School of Health and Biomedical Sciences
Bundoora, Victoria
Australia
Chapter 7

Lauren Foohey, MT ASCP, MPH
Senior Director of Global Marketing
Siemens Healthcare
Point of Care Business Area
Norwood MA, USA
Chapter 36

Professor Hugh Grantham, ASM, MBBS, FRACGP
Professor of Paramedics
Assistant Dean for Student Affairs
Paramedics, School of Medicine
Flinders University
Adelaide, South Australia
Australia
Chapter 30

Andrew Griffin, CSc, FIBMS, CSci
Deputy Section Manager – Clinical and Legal Services
National Association of Testing Authorities
Camberwell, Victoria
Australia
Chapter 7

Rebecca Guy, BAppSc, MAppEpid, PhD
Associate Professor
The Kirby Institute
University of New South Wales
Sydney, New South Wales
Australia
Chapters 17, 19 & 28

Lara Harmans, MSc
Researcher
Saltro Diagnostic Centre
Utrecht
Netherlands
Chapter 25

Heather Halls, BSc (Hons), MSc, MSocSci
Associate Lecturer
Flinders University International Centre for Point-of-Care Testing
Flinders University
Adelaide, South Australia
Australia
Chapter 12 & 16

Volker Harms, Nat Dip Chem Path
Director
Integrated Software Solutions Pty Ltd
Sydney, New South Wales
Australia
Chapter 6

Paul L Harper, MD, MBChB, FRCP, FRACP
Consultant Haematologist
Palmerston North Hospital
Palmerston North
New Zealand
Chapter 13

Geoff Herd, NZCS, Dip MLT, Dip MLS, MAppSci
Point-of-Care Testing Coordinator
Whangarei Hospital
Northland District Health Board
Whangarei
New Zealand
Chapters 29 & 34

Catherine Hogan, MDCM, MSc
Fellow
Infectious Diseases and Medical Microbiology
McGill University
Montreal
Canada
Chapter 23

Rogier Hopstaken, MD, PhD
General Practitioner/POCT specialist
Saltro Diagnostic Centre
Utrecht
Netherlands
Chapter 25

Michael Jong, MBBS, MRCP(UK), CHE, FCFP, FRRMS
Professor
Northern Family Medicine Program
Memorial University of Newfoundland
Labrador Health Centre
Happy Valley-Goose Bay, Newfoundland
Canada
Chapter 35

Phillip Keen, BA
Kirby Institute
University of New South Wales
Sydney, New South Wales
Australia
Chapter 19

James Kiarie, Professor, MBChB, MMed, MPH
Coordinator
Human Reproduction Team
Department of Reproductive Health and Research
World Health Organization
Geneva
Switzerland
Chapter 18

Professor Michael Kidd AM, FAHMS, MBBSHons (Melbourne), MD (Monash), DCCH (Flinders), DipRACOG, FRACGP, FACHI, FACNEM (Hon), FRCGP (Hon) UK, FRNZCGP (Hon) New Zealand, FAFPM (Hon) Malaysia, FHKCFP (Hon) Hong Kong, FCGPSL (Hon) Sri Lanka, MAICD
Executive Dean and Matthew Flinders Distinguished Professor
Faculty of Medicine, Nursing and Health Sciences
Flinders University
Adelaide, South Australia
Australia
President, World Organization of Family Doctors (WONCA)
Chapter 27

Gerald J Kost, MD, PhD, MS, FACB
Emeritus Professor and Director
Point-of-Care Testing Center for Teaching and Research (POCT•CTR™)
School of Medicine, University of California,
Davis CA, USA
President and CEO, Knowledge Optimizationx®
Davis CA, USA
Chapters 24 & 31

Bertil Lindahl, MD, PhD
Professor
Department of Medical Sciences and Uppsala Clinical Research Center
Uppsala University
Uppsala
Sweden
Chapter 16

Robert Luo, MD, MPH
Director
Clinical Science
Roche Molecular Systems, Inc
Adjunct Clinical Faculty
Department of Pathology
School of Medicine
Stanford University
Stanford CA, USA
Chapter 20

Connie Mardis, MEd
POC Value Ambassador
Siemens Healthcare
Point of Care Business Area
Norwood MA, USA
Chapter 36

Cameron Martin, BAppSc (MT), MAppSc (MLS-Haem), MTM
Coordinator, State-Wide Point of Care Testing
Pathology Queensland
Royal Brisbane and Womens Hospital
Herston, Queensland
Australia
Chapter 15

Timothy H Mathew, AM, MBBS, FRACP
Consultant Nephrologist
Kent Town, South Australia
Australia
Chapter 11

Bridgit McAteer, DipAppSc (Nursing), Grad Cert Primary Health Care
Research Scientist
Flinders University International Centre for Point-of-Care Testing
Flinders University
Adelaide, South Australia
Australia
Chapter 6

Tessa McCormack, BMedSc, MPH
Research Scientist
Flinders University International Centre for Point-of-Care Testing
Flinders University
Adelaide, South Australia
Australia
Chapter 8

Lara Motta, BMedSc (Hons)
Research Scientist
Flinders University International Centre for Point-of-Care Testing
Flinders University
Adelaide, South Australia
Australia
Chapter 17

Maurine M. Murtagh, MBA, MPhil, JD
Chief Executive Officer
The International Diagnostics Centre
London School of Hygiene & Tropical Medicine
London, UK
Chapter 18

Samarina MA Musaad, MBBS, FRCPA, MAACB, FAACB, PgDipPH
Chemical Pathologist
Labtests (Healthscope)
Mt Wellington, Auckland
New Zealand
Chapter 29

Lisa Natoli, MPH, PhD
Burnet Institute
Melbourne, Victoria
Australia
Chapter 17

Kevin Norton, BEd (PE) Hons, MA, PhD
Professor of Exercise Science
School of Health Sciences
University of South Australia
Adelaide, South Australia
Australia
Chapter 33

Lynda Norton, RN, Grad Dip Crit Care Nursing, MPH, PhD
Lecturer
Flinders University
Faculty of Medicine, Nursing and Health Sciences
Adelaide, South Australia
Australia
Chapter 33

Madhukar Pai, MD, PhD
Canada Research Chair in Translational Epidemiology and Global Health Professor
Department of Epidemiology and Biostatistics and Occupational Health
McGill University
Montréal, Québec
Canada
Chapter 23

Nitika Pant Pai, MD, MPH, PhD
Associate Professor
Department of Medicine
Division of Clinical Epidemiology
McGill University
Montréal, Québec
Canada
Chapter 20

Michael Parsons, MD, CCFP (EM)
Assistant Program Director
Assistant Professor, Discipline of Emergency Medicine
Cross-appointed, Discipline of Family Medicine
Memorial University of Newfoundland
St. John's, Newfoundland
Canada
Chapter 35

Rosanna W Peeling, PhD
Professor and Chair, Diagnostics Research
Director, International Diagnostics Centre
London School of Hygiene & Tropical Medicine
London, UK
Chapter 18

Timothy Pointon, BSc (Hons), GradCertClinEd, MPA
Lecturer in Paramedics
Paramedics, School of Medicine
Flinders University
Adelaide, South Australia
Australia
Chapter 30

Julie Ratcliffe, PhD, MSc, BA (Hons)
Professor
Flinders Health Economics Group
School of Medicine
Flinders University

Adelaide, South Australia
Australia
Chapter 8

Tia Renouf, MD, CCFP (EM), FCFP
Associate Professor and Chair
Discipline of Emergency Medicine
Memorial University of Newfoundland
St. John's, Newfoundland
Canada
Chapter 35

Christian Renaud, MD, MSc, FRCPC
Assistant Professor (Clinics) – Department of Microbiology, Infectious Diseases, and Immunology
Université de Montréal – CHU Sainte-Justine
Montréal, Québec
Canada
Chapter 21

Jonathan Shaw, MD, FRACP, FRCP (UK), FAAHMS
Associate Professor
Domain Head, Cardiometabolic Risk
Baker IDI Heart and Diabetes Institute
Melbourne, Victoria
Australia
Chapters 9 & 10

Anne Shephard, BSc (Hons)
Research Associate
Assistant Manager, QAAMS Program
Flinders University International Centre for Point-of-Care Testing
Flinders University
Adelaide, South Australia
Australia
Chapters 5, 6 & 12

Mark Shephard, OAM, BSc (Hons), MSc, MAACB, MAIMS, FFSc (RCPA), PhD
Professor and Director
Flinders University International Centre for Point-of-Care Testing
Flinders University
Adelaide, South Australia
Australia
Chapters 1,2,3,4,5,7,8,9,10,11,17,27,28,31,37

Bronwyn Sheppard, Dip Med Lab Tech (NZ)
Business Manager
Roche Diagnostics Asia Pacific
Singapore
Chapter 13

Ken Sikaris, BSc (Hons), MBBS, FRCPA, FAACB, FFSc
Associate Professor
Chemical Pathologist
Melbourne Pathology
Collingwood, Victoria
Australia
Chapter 12

Brooke Spaeth, BMedSc (Hons)
Point-of-Care Coordinator
Northern Territory Point-of-Care Testing Program
Flinders University International Centre for Point-of-Care Testing
Flinders University
Adelaide, South Australia
Australia
Chapters 6, 26 & 36

Igor Toskin, MD, Professor, PhD, DSc
Department of Reproductive Health and Research
World Health Organization
Geneva
Switzerland
Chapter 18

Nicolas Tremblay, MSc
PhD Candidate in Molecular Biology
Centre de Recherche du Centre Hospitalier de l'Université de Montréal (CRCHUM)
Montréal, Québec
Canada
Chapter 21

Santiago Vazquez, PhD, BSc (Hons)
Laboratory Manager
Drug Toxicology Unit
NSW Forensic & Analytical Science Service
Macquarie Hospital
North Ryde, New South Wales
Australia
Chapter 26

Per Venge, MD, PhD
Professor
Department of Medical Sciences
University of Uppsala
Uppsala

Sweden
Chapter 16

Roland Watzl, MBBS, FACRRM
Deputy Chief Medical Officer
Australian Antarctic Division
Kingston, Tasmania
Australia
Chapter 32

Michelle Williamson, BAppSc (MLS)
Technical Services Manager
Alere ANZPI
East Brisbane, Queensland
Australia
Chapter 14

Margo Wilson, MD, CCFP (EM)
Clinical Assistant Professor
Northern Family Medicine Program
Memorial University of Newfoundland
Labrador Health Centre
Happy Valley-Goose Bay, Newfoundland
Canada
Chapter 35

Richard Woodman, BSc (Hons), MMedSci, PhD
Professor and Director for Epidemiology and Biostatistics
School of Medicine
Flinders University
Adelaide, South Australia
Australia
Chapter 8

Paul Zimmett, AO, MD, PhD, FRACP, FRCP, FACE, FACN, FAFPHM, FTSE
Director Emeritus
Victor Smorgon Diabetes Centre
Baker IDI Heart and Diabetes Institute
Adjunct Professor Monash University
Melbourne, Victoria
Australia
Chapter 9 & 10

# Preface

## MY PERSONAL JOURNEY WITH POINT-OF-CARE TESTING

How did my journey in the field of point-of-care testing (POCT) come about? My work in the field of POCT was initially conceived when my interests within and outside my professional career intersected during the mid-1990s.

From the late 1970s to the mid-1990s, I worked as a medical scientist in the clinical biochemistry laboratory at Flinders Medical Centre in Adelaide, the capital city of South Australia. My main areas of scientific work were the development and evaluation of diagnostic methods for pathology tests for the management of diabetes, renal and cardiovascular disease, and the fields of quality assurance and analytical performance standards for pathology tests. In the latter part of this period, I also had responsibility for conducting POCT for haemoglobin A1c (HbA1c), a long-term marker of glycaemic control, using a device called the DCA 2000 device (at the time distributed by Bayer Diagnostics) on patients attending the weekly diabetes clinic at Flinders Medical Centre.

Across the 1980s and 1990s, my wife and I travelled widely across all of Australia's deserts – from the Gibson and Great Sandy, to the Simpson, Strzelecki and Great Victoria Deserts. As a result of our travels, we visited many Aboriginal communities. I felt a strong connection with the community elders who were humble yet passionate about looking after their remote desert lands. At the same time, I observed first-hand the appalling level of poverty and the significant burden of chronic disease in rural and remote Indigenous Australia, which concerned me greatly. Delivery of mainstream health (and laboratory) services to these communities was very poor, the turnaround of laboratory test results was slow, while of most concern was the extreme difficulty in getting chronic disease patients to return for a follow-up visit to enable their doctor to act on laboratory results and mediate treatment.

I wondered whether POCT could have a niche in Indigenous communities, due to its portability, convenience and immediacy of result. I also wondered whether health professionals working in these remote locations, particularly Aboriginal Health Workers – Aboriginal people living and working in the community and skilled in the practice of primary health care – could be trained to conduct POCT in their own health services. Little did I realise that the 'fit' for POCT in this primary care setting would be near perfect and that it would embark me on a career change that has been fulfilling and stimulating.

I left the laboratory at Flinders Medical Centre in 1996 and began my journey with just a series of ideas and a vision in my head. I took a position at the Renal Unit at Flinders Medical Centre and started the 'Umoona Kidney Project' in a remote Aboriginal community, 850 km north of Adelaide. This project was a renal disease prevention and management program, which used POCT for the detection of microalbuminuria as its centrepiece. POCT was very much in its infancy in Australia at this time and the Umoona Kidney Project became the first community-based program to use POCT in an Indigenous setting in this country. This project gave me a solid grounding in how to work with Indigenous people in a culturally safe manner and how to set up a quality-assured and sustainable POCT model in the field.

Two years later, I attended a conference on renal disease in Indigenous peoples at Uluru (Ayers Rock) in the heart of outback Australia's Northern Territory. At the conference dinner I sat next to a delegate named Janet Streatfield, whom I had never met before. I discovered Janet worked with the Australian Government Department of Health and Ageing and her section was responsible for enacting recommendations of the National Diabetes Strategy 1998. One of those recommendations was that a trial of the DCA 2000 POCT device for measuring HbA1c should be conducted in Aboriginal Community Controlled Health Services in Australia. Janet lamented that she wasn't sure how to go about this. I said: 'I think I may be able to help you'. The concept for the 'QAAMS' (Quality Assurance for Aboriginal and Torres Strait Islander Medical Services) Program was seeded at this fateful meeting. A short while later, in July 1999, I became Program Manager of QAAMS, which has now grown to be the largest national POCT field program in Australia and has been continuously funded by the Australian Government to the present day.

POCT has consumed my professional life for the past 20 years and it has been a life-changing experience. I've watched the field mature rapidly on a local, regional and global basis. I've witnessed first-hand the impact POCT can have on the way pathology services are delivered in primary care settings. Most importantly however, I have learnt that POCT is founded upon the people you meet and the partnerships you form. Our Centre recently introduced a POCT service for diabetes at a rural location in Papua New Guinea, through a partnership with the local provincial government and local health services. For the first time, the diabetes specialist at the clinic was able to measure HbA1c on her diabetes patients. She said: 'Point-of-care testing has been an answer to my prayers...'

I've also seen the impact of introducing POCT into the teaching curricula for undergraduate and postgraduate students at Flinders University. Students 'understand' POCT: it's hands-on, it's relevant, it's away from the tedium of the laboratory bench, and it has a clearly defined place in community medicine. These thoughts are echoed by students across disciplines, from those studying medical science, health science, medicine, nursing, paramedics, public health or Indigenous health.

POCT has taken me on an amazing journey in life. I come to work every day, ready to be inspired and challenged by the adventures of a new day. To me, the more challenging the environment for POCT, the more exciting is the task ahead.

## THE PURPOSE OF THIS BOOK ON POINT-OF-CARE TESTING AND ITS INTENDED AUDIENCE

There are now several outstanding books on POCT in the global literature, most notably those written by the distinguished team of Professor Christopher Price and Dr Andrew St John, and those by Professor Gerald Kost – colleagues whom I have known and respected for many years. These works are of the highest academic order.

This book aims to fill a separate and distinctive niche in the book literature on this subject area, by providing a *practically orientated* guide to POCT for a target audience comprising: (i) a range of health professionals working in primary care settings where POCT is needed; and (ii) undergraduate and postgraduate university students from around the world who are studying relevant disciplines such as medicine, medical, health or paramedic sciences, nursing, Indigenous/rural or remote health, and public health. The text is written by the principal author/editor and selected Australian and global experts. It is designed to be easy to read, yet authoritative and of sound academic rigour.

The book is divided into three main themes. The first theme 'sets the scene' for POCT by providing the reader with a solid understanding of the principles and practice of POCT in a primary care setting. The practical orientation of this theme is designed to enable readers to set up and manage their own POCT services safely and sustainably in their own regions and/or countries.

Themes 2 and 3 represent the core of the book and aim to provide an understanding of the global scope, the clinical applications of POCT spanning chronic, acute and infectious diseases, and some of the unique clinical settings in which POCT can be used.

## ACKNOWLEDGEMENTS

The greatest pleasure I have derived from my research work has been the opportunity to work with so many dedicated teams of community health professionals across Australia. The teams of the doctors, nurses, allied health professionals and Aboriginal Health Workers who have all embraced our point-of-care testing models are too numerous to list individually, but I acknowledge that their commitment to conducting point-of-care testing 'at the grassroots' has been a constant source of inspiration to me. I must just mention several colleagues, who have been with me for the majority of this journey together: Malcolm Auld, Glennis Barnes, Tony Burgoyne, Dr David Dunn, Angela Dufek, John Louden, Kay Mundraby and Christopher O'Brien.

A number of senior colleagues have supported and inspired me along my journey, and include: Dr Lindsay Barratt, Dr Kathy Paizis and Dr Tim Matthew AM; Professor Lucie Walters, Professor Jennene Greenhill, Professor Paul Worley and Professor Michael Kidd AM; Dr Ken Sikaris, Associate Professor Rebecca Guy, Associate Professor John Oliver, Janice Gill and Lloyd Penberthy. A special thanks to Professor Callum Fraser also helped shape my early career as a medical scientist.

From industry, I must acknowledge Dean Whiting, Linda Walsh, Lauren Foohey, Yvette Kruger, Patrick Tete, Bronywn Sheppard and (the late) Barry Young OAM. Barry believed in my vision when no-one else would and he provided me with crucial funding support to 'kick-start' my career in point-of-care testing.

My research work would not have been possible without the continuing support of the Australian Government Department of Health and I thank their staff for their assistance and commitment to my point-of-care testing work over many years: Marion Dunlop, Jan Streatfield, Jacquie Millard, Wendy Akers, John Bacon, Jonathan Wraith, Pamela McKittrick, Fifine Cahill and Louis Young.

Heartfelt thanks are also extended to my staff at the Flinders University International Centre for Point-of-Care Testing, who have worked so diligently for me and who have demonstrated unwavering loyalty over many years: Kelly Andrewartha, David Badger, Narelle Brown, Hayden Francis, Heather Halls, Karan Lavender, Bridgit McAteer, Tessa McCormack, Cheryl Marshall, Beryl Mazzachi, Rebeka Milloss, Lara Motta, Nicola Robinson, Pauline Rudevics, Anne Shephard, Claire Simon, Brooke Spaeth, Lori Tietz and Les Watkinson. Particular thanks are extended to Narelle Brown, who tirelessly helped me with the administrative and organisational aspects of the book project, and Pauline Rudevics, who managed the permissions required for the book. David Heinrich and Julie Caddy are also thanked for preparing most of the artwork for the book.

Finally special thanks to my wife Anne for her continuing patience and tolerance with my book writing and my point-of-care testing work over so many years, and to my children Matthew and Emily of whom I am so proud.

Professor Mark Shephard OAM

# 1 An introduction to point-of-care testing and its global scope and application

*Mark Shephard*

**Summary**

Point-of-care testing (POCT) refers to pathology testing performed in a clinical setting at the time of patient consultation, generating a test result that contributes to an immediate informed clinical decision being made and acted upon for patient care. POCT is the fastest growing sector of the diagnostic industry globally. POCT has its origins in the hospital environment but has now devolved to a range of community-based primary care settings. POCT provides innovative opportunities to improve delivery of pathology services for the detection and management of chronic, acute and infectious diseases, and has a particular niche in rural and remote primary health settings globally, including developing countries. The capacity to link POCT devices from rural or remote sites to a central management point has enhanced the ability to develop large-scale POCT networks and streamline the delivery of POCT services.

## SETTING THE SCENE FOR POINT-OF-CARE TESTING

To set the scene for introducing POCT, consider the following three scenarios:

### Health-care setting 1

An elderly patient in an urban nursing home is incapacitated and in a wheelchair. She has long-standing type 2 diabetes and is on insulin. She is required to go to the hospital every 3 months for a blood test to check her diabetes control. This routine task is difficult for the patient due to her immobility, she can't find a carpark easily, there is a lack of access for wheelchairs, and she has to wait 2 h for her appointment and a blood test. A week later, she has to return for a follow-up visit to hospital to get her result and discuss treatment with her doctor.

> *Consider how much easier for the patient it would be if she could have her blood test, get her result within a few minutes, and receive treatment on-site in the nursing home.*

### Health-care setting 2

A male patient on warfarin therapy is required to have regular blood tests to monitor his coagulation status and adjust his dose of warfarin. The patient lives in a remote outback community 500 km from the nearest town (and laboratory). He has to drive 6 h on corrugated outback roads to town every 4 weeks to have his blood tests, stay in town for a day to get his result and then drive 500 km home again.

*Consider how much better it would be for this patient if he could have his blood test, get the result, and have his dose of warfarin adjusted on-site in his own home and community.*

### Health-care setting 3

A patient with a history of heart disease presents at a remote health service at 3 am with crushing chest pain radiating down his arms. Has the patient had a heart attack? The health service has no diagnostic testing available and so the patient is evacuated to the nearest tertiary hospital to have the relevant laboratory tests performed to answer this question. Evacuation is by helicopter at a cost of A$15 000.

*Consider how much better it would be for the patient if the cardiac tests were performed on-site at the remote health centre, where a heart attack could possibly be ruled out, the patient could then be stabilised on-site and the need for the costly retrieval averted.*

In each case, access to POCT could potentially provide the answer to solving these issues.

## WHAT IS POINT-OF-CARE TESTING?

The origins of POCT can be traced to the very beginnings of diagnostic pathology in the 15th century when urine specimens were tested and inspected at the patient's bedside, at their point of care. POCT is therefore not strictly a new discipline of medical science but one that has had a significant re-emergence over the past 20 years.

There have been many different definitions of POCT proposed by numerous authors and professional groups, a representative sample of which are shown in Table 1.1. In addition, a multitude of acronyms have been used to describe this mode of health service delivery. These include terms such as near patient testing (NPT), rapid diagnostic testing (RDT), as well as several historical expressions such as bedside testing, physician office testing, alternate or off-site testing, ancillary testing and decentralised testing.

The variety of definitions and lack of standardisation of a single accepted terminology for POCT reflect the relative youthfulness of this field. For the purpose of this book, which focusses on the use of POCT in the primary care environment, I have developed two working definitions. The first is short and abbreviated and can be used when trying to explain POCT simply and briefly in layman's terms.

*Point-of-care testing is 'pathology testing performed in a clinical setting at the time of patient consultation, generating a rapid test result that enables timely clinical action for patient care.'*

The second is more detailed and deliberately used when I am training health professionals or teaching students about POCT. This definition encompasses all the elements that are essential to the safe conduct of POCT outside the laboratory.

*Point-of-care testing is 'pathology testing that is performed on behalf of the treating medical practitioner by a trained operator in an on-site clinical setting at the time of patient consultation, allowing a test result of desired analytical quality to be generated and to be used to take immediate, informed clinical action that contributes to an improved health outcome for the patient.'*

The various phrases in this more detailed definition can be broken down further to explain POCT more fully (Table 1.2). First, POCT is a pathology investigation: generally a clinical biochemistry, haematology, microbiology or pharmacology test. POCT can generate quantitative results (i.e. generate a number or value) or qualitative results (detecting the presence or absence of a disease or substance).

POCT is most commonly, but not exclusively, performed on small portable *in vitro* medical devices. The term *in vitro* simply means that the fluid to be tested (e.g. blood) is collected from the body, loaded on to the device and tested 'outside the body'. The term 'device' includes benchtop instruments, hand-held devices and test strips.

POCT normally requires a small sample volume (generally ranging from 5 to 50 μL of capillary whole blood, urine or other fluids) to conduct the test, making the sample collection process simple, convenient, less stressful and less invasive for the patient.

The test should only be performed by a POCT operator who has undergone training and certification in performing patient testing and conducting quality testing procedures on the POCT device; these practices ensure that results of acceptable analytical quality (equivalent to

Table 1.1. Representative examples of different definitions of POCT over the past 20 years

| Definition of POCT | Reference source |
|---|---|
| 'Testing at the point of patient care, wherever that medical care is needed' | Kost 1995 |
| 'Those analytical patient testing activities provided within the institution, but performed outside the physical facilities of clinical laboratories …' | College of American Pathologists 1998 |
| 'Any kind of test performed outside the central hospital laboratory, usually at the patient's bedside' | Mor and Waisman 2000 |
| 'Testing that is performed close to the patient' | Hicks *et al.* 2001 |
| 'Any type of testing undertaken close to the patient to enable a decision to be made on the care of that patient' | Price 2001 |
| 'A pathology investigation by or on behalf of the treating medical practitioner on-site, at the time of and for use during consultation' | Guibert *et al.* 2001 |
| 'Any test that is performed at the time at which the test result enables a decision to be made and an action taken that leads to an improved health outcome' | Price and St John 2005 |
| 'Testing that is performed near or at the site of a patient with the result leading to a possible change in the care of the patient' | ISO 2006 |
| 'An investigation carried out in a clinical or non-clinical setting, or in the patient's home, for which the result is available without reference to a laboratory, perhaps rapidly enough to affect immediate patient management' | Dean 2006 |
| '[Rapid diagnostic tests] RDT's are immunoassays that are simple to perform, give results without the need for laboratory equipment, are accurate and can provide on-site (negative) results with a single visit' | Chiu *et al.* 2011 |
| 'A form of testing in which the analysis is performed where healthcare is provided close to or near the patient' | Australian Government 2013 |
| 'Point-of-care testing devices are in-vitro devices that are used for testing outside the laboratory and in the vicinity of patients …' | Musaad and Herd 2013 |
| 'Tests designed to be used at or the site where the patient is located, that do not require permanent dedicated space, and that are performed outside the physical facilities of the clinical laboratories' | College of American Pathologists 2015 |
| 'POC testing is diagnostic testing that will result in a clear and actionable management decision such as when to start treatment or to require a confirmatory test, within the same clinical encounter'. | Pai *et al.* 2015 |

Table 1.2. Dissecting the definition of POCT

| Definition | Context |
|---|---|
| Pathology test | Clinical biochemistry, haematology, microbiological, pharmacological. Quantitative or qualitative. |
| Device | Mainly *in vitro* using small sample volumes (μL) |
| Trained operator | Training and certification of POCT operators is crucial |
| Outside the laboratory | In numerous hospital or community/primary care settings |
| At time of consultation | POCT brings pathology closer to the patient and doctor |
| Analytical quality | Quality of result is paramount. Speed must not compromise quality. |
| Immediate clinical action | POCT result is available in under 10 min generally, but the real impact of POCT comes from implementing effective and timely treatments rather than from the test itself |
| Improved patient outcome | Overarching goal of pathology testing is to maximise health benefit to the patient |

**Table 1.3.** Examples of health-care settings where POCT is now used

| Hospital-based | Community-based | Other settings |
|---|---|---|
| Emergency department | General practice/physician office | Disaster management |
| Adult intensive care unit | Pharmacy | Extreme environments |
| Neonatal intensive care unit | Community health clinic | Military |
| Coronary care unit | Aboriginal medical service | Space research |
| Operating theatre | Retrieval unit | |
| Ward | Workplace | |
| Outpatient clinic | Veterinary clinic | |
| | Leisure facility | |
| | Sports medicine | |
| | Home care | |

that of the laboratory) are generated for patient care. The operator may be one of many health-care professionals including, for example, a doctor, nurse, primary health-care worker, diabetes educator, pharmacist, paramedic and even the patient.

The clinical settings in which POCT can be conducted are numerous, comprising hospital-based, community-based and other diverse locations (Table 1.3).

By conducting POCT on-site at the time of the patient encounter, POCT brings pathology testing closer or 'nearer' to the patient and to the doctor. The speed of the pathology result for the treating medical practitioner is a key feature of POCT. Critically, however, speed must not compromise the analytical quality of the result, which is of paramount importance. Further, as Pai *et al.* (2015) state: 'the impact of a POC test comes from implementing effective treatments rather than from the test itself. Thus, moving rapidly through the test-and-treat cycle in the same clinical encounter is the most important goal for any POC testing program.'

With the development of evidence-based laboratory medicine, an overarching goal of pathology testing, whether POCT or laboratory-based, is to maximise the health outcome benefit for the patient. An underlying theme across evidence-based POCT research is that POCT itself will not deliver improved health outcomes unless it is linked closely to defined clinical pathways and POC test results are actioned clinically within a defined timeframe.

Pai *et al.* (2015) have recently challenged conventional product-oriented definitions of POCT that restrict POCT to a particular class of product (e.g. based on cost, size or where or by whom the test is performed). They argue that the definition of POCT should be goal-oriented, with the rapid initiation of correct treatment the most critical element of any POC test. They contend this approach is more inclusive and more reflective of the diverse spectrum of settings where POCT is used (from hospitals to resource-limited settings) and is 'closer to what all patients want from their care providers'.

## POINT-OF-CARE TESTING 'IN REAL TIME'

With this understanding of what POCT is, how does POCT function 'in real time'? A typical POCT process is summarised and compared with the laboratory testing process in Fig. 1.1.

With POCT, a patient visits his/her primary care clinic in the community, a sample (just of a few microlitres) is taken, loaded on a point-of-care device by a trained POCT device operator, the result is available in just a few minutes, and the patient sees the doctor during their appointment to review the results and have their management/treatment actioned on the spot.

As a general rule, a patient in a community setting whose local doctor has requested laboratory tests will visit a pathology collection centre, have a venous sample drawn from the arm (usually 5–10 mL of blood) and the sample is then transported to the nearest laboratory (which, for a remote community in a country such as Australia, could be several hundred kilometres away and may take several days to reach the laboratory by road courier). Once received by the laboratory, the sample often requires centrifugation to separate the red cells from the serum/plasma, and the serum/plasma is then loaded on to the laboratory analyser by a trained medical scientist or technician. A result is generated, which is then sent back to the requesting doctor (either electronically or in hard copy form; if the latter, then again the return of the result may

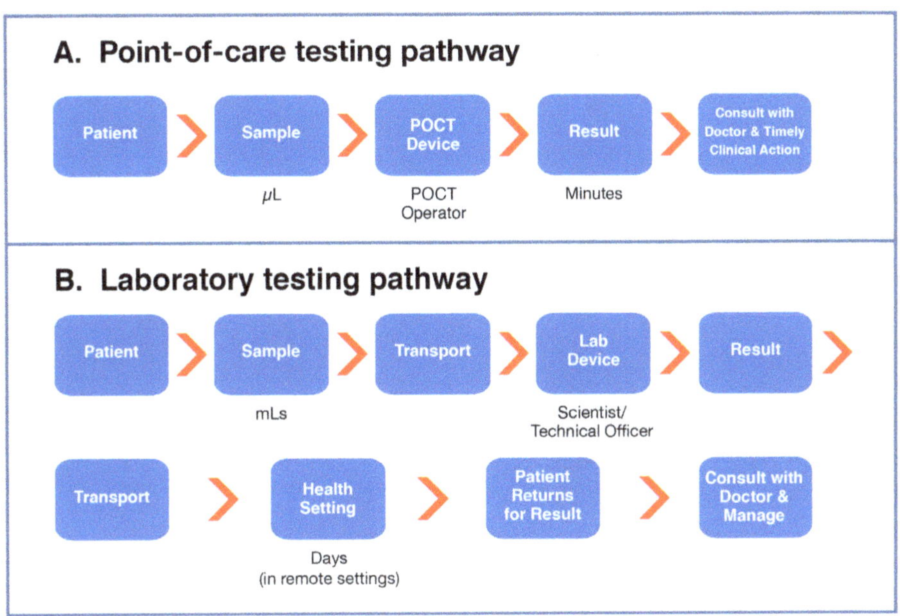


**Fig. 1.1.** Comparing the POC and laboratory test pathways.

take several days in remote locations). The patient is then contacted by the health service and a separate appointment is required for the patient to return to their health service and visit the doctor to discuss the result.

The potential benefits of POCT from a patient, operational and clinical perspective intuitively appear obvious from these simple scenarios, but are they real in practice? The short answer is 'yes' and the evidence base for the benefits (as well as the limitations) of POCT will be explored as a constant point of discussion throughout the book.

## THE INCREASED GLOBAL UPTAKE OF POINT-OF-CARE TESTING

Since the re-emergence of POCT in the late 1980s, the uptake of POCT in the global health sector has burgeoned, mainly in the Western developed world. Globally, the POCT market has been estimated to be worth US$3 billion in 1997, US$5.4 billion in 2002 (Freedman 2002), US$9.6 billion by 2005 (Huckle 2006), and US$15 billion in 2011 (St John and Price 2014). With a compound annual growth rate estimated between 4 and 8%, the global market value is expected to reach US$18 billion by 2016 and US$24 billion by 2017/2018 (St John and Price 2014; Lehr 2013).

St John and Price (2014) note these market sales represent the sum of 'over the counter' or 'non- professional' self-testing products, such as blood glucose and pregnancy tests, and the 'professional market', which includes sales to all major health-care sectors (Table 1.4).

By country/region, the USA dominates the global market share with ~55% of total sales, followed by Europe 30% and Asia around 12% (St John and Price 2014). Fig. 1.2 shows the growth in POCT sales within the European market from 2006 to 2015.

**Table 1.4.** Global market sales of diagnostic products 2011 (Source: adapted from St John and Price 2014)

| Sector | Market sales | Percentage of total diagnostic market sales | Percentage of total POCT market sales |
|---|---|---|---|
| Total IVD diagnostic market sales | US$51 billion | – | – |
| Total POCT market sales | US$15 billion | 29% | – |
| 'Professional' POCT product market sales[a] | US$5.66 billion | 11% | 38% |
| 'Non-professional' POCT product market sales[b] | US$9.34 billion | 18% | 62% |

[a]Hospital and primary care sectors including critical care, chronic disease, infectious disease, coagulation and haematology POCT products
[b]'Over the counter' products for glucose and pregnancy self-testing

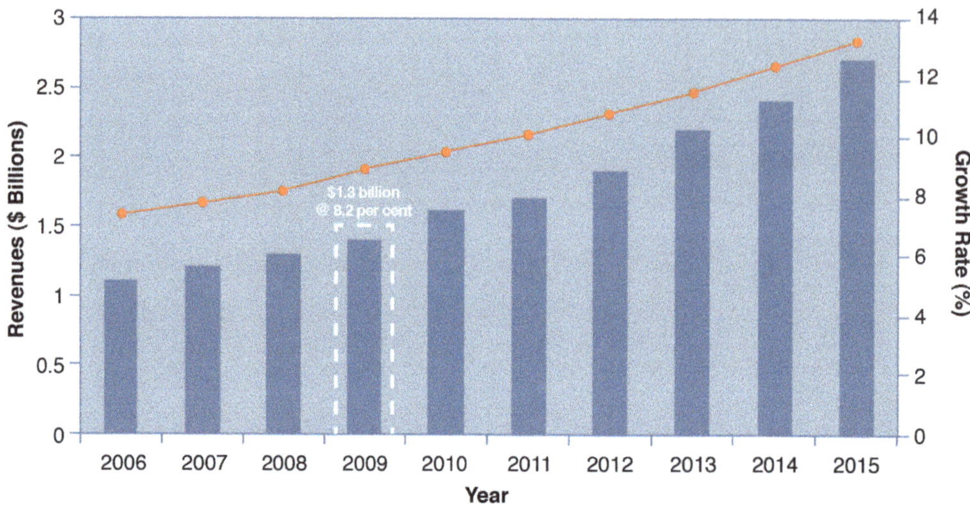


**Fig. 1.2.** Growth in the European POCT market 2006–2015. (Source: Figure from Ramachandran R (2010) used with permission from Frost and Sullivan)

Blood glucose testing represents the largest POCT market sector, followed by pregnancy and critical care testing (St John and Price 2014). Importantly, POCT for infectious diseases is undergoing rapid market development due to the advances in molecular testing technology, and there is likely to be a major surge in sales of these products in the coming years.

## WHAT ARE THE DRIVERS OF THE POINT-OF-CARE TESTING 'REVOLUTION?'

The escalating interest in POCT has been driven by several factors (Table 1.5).

First, there is now greater emphasis on placing the patient at the centre of the health-care process. The patient of the 21st century is more knowledgeable of disease conditions and has higher expectations of the health-care system in terms of quality and convenience of care (Price *et al.* 2004).

Second, care of patients with chronic conditions is being devolved away from the hospital to a range of primary care environments conducive to POCT, including general practice, Indigenous medical services, community health clinics and pharmacies. The way in which laboratory services are provided has also changed. The majority of hospital-based pathology testing is now performed on high throughput, batch-orientated analytical systems in large core laboratories, creating a niche for smaller volume, needs-specific POCT to be undertaken by regional satellite laboratories and primary care settings (Price *et al.* 2004).

**Table 1.5.** Examples of drivers of the POCT revolution in the 21st century

| Driver of POCT |
|---|
| Greater emphasis on patient-focussed care |
| Changes in health-care practices |
| Advances in POCT technology |
| Connectivity of modern POC test systems |

Early critics of POCT argued that the speed of analysis was compromised by lack of quality of the POCT result (Jahn and Van Aken 2003). However, over the last decade, POCT device manufacturers have invested heavily in modern design, new technologies and 'good manufacturing practice' to ensure most modern POCT devices are now analytically sound and 'fit for use' in primary care settings. There have been significant advances in POCT technology including:

- reduction in the size of devices (miniaturisation)
- simplicity of device operation (reflecting the desire of manufacturers to meet the market demand of enabling POCT devices to be used away from the laboratory by non-laboratory-trained health professionals)
- improved reproducibility of manufacturing processes for both devices and reagents (thereby reducing between-batch variability for the latter)
- advances in analytical techniques (including the advent of microfluidics, improved sensor design, and

Table 1.6. Selected examples of POC tests currently available (by medical science discipline). This list is not meant to be exhaustive.

| Discipline | Disease/condition | Examples of POC tests |
|---|---|---|
| Clinical biochemistry | Diabetes | Glucose, HbA1c, lactate |
| | Renal disease | Urea and creatinine, urine albumin:creatinine ratio (ACR) |
| | Cardiovascular disease | Lipids |
| | Acute respiratory and metabolic disorders | Electrolytes and blood gases |
| | Acute cardiac disorders | Troponin I and T, B-type natriuretic peptide (BNP), N-terminal pro B-type natriuretic peptide (NT-proBNP) |
| Haematology | Anaemia | Haemoglobin |
| | Coagulation disorders/ haemostasis | International Normalised Ratio (INR), platelets, activated partial prothrombin time (APTT) |
| | General haematology | Full blood count including red blood cells and related indices, haemoglobin; white blood cells and differential counts |
| Microbiology | Sexually transmitted infections | HIV, syphilis, chlamydia, gonorrhoea, trichomoniasis |
| | Other blood borne viruses | Hepatitis B and C |
| | Vector-mediated | Malaria, dengue fever |
| | Respiratory infection (specific and general) | Influenza, tuberculosis, Group A Streptococcus, C-reactive protein, procalcitonin |
| Pharmacology | Substance abuse | Major drug classes (e.g. amphetamine type substances, benzodiazepines, cannabis and metabolites, cocaine and metabolites, opiates) |

tailoring molecular-based technologies to POCT platforms)
- rapid expansion of the range of tests and test profiles that can be performed by POCT (Table 1.6).
- the ability to conduct specialised tests on small sample volumes of the order of 5–100 μL
- advances in connectivity standards; that is, the ability to electronically capture POC test results and transfer them to a clinical or laboratory patient information system (Mor and Waisman 2000; Price and St John 2005).

Also as a general rule, the applicability of POCT increases with increasing degrees of remoteness due largely to the difficulty of accessing laboratory pathology services in a timely manner. This theme is explored throughout the book and is particularly relevant to Chapter 28.

## ADVANTAGES AND BENEFITS OF POINT-OF-CARE TESTING

The use of POCT in the primary care setting has practical advantages for the patient, the health professional performing POCT, the treating practitioner, the health service and community overall (Table 1.7).

### Patient

Patient satisfaction with the convenience and accessibility of POCT is generally high because pathology testing and consultation with the doctor occurs in the same visit, avoiding the need for a follow-up consultation to obtain pathology results and reducing anxiety levels associated with waiting for a laboratory result (Shephard 2006). Only a small volume of blood or urine (generally <100 μL) is required to perform most POCT and therefore sample collection can be far less stressful and less invasive if, for example, a finger-prick rather than a venepuncture can provide adequate sample volume. With pathology testing being conducted closer to the patient, POCT facilitates a greater sense of ownership of the pathology testing process. The patient can observe his/her own sample being loaded onto the POC device and can see the result displayed on the screen of the device when the test is completed. This can increase levels of patient self-motivation and improve compliance with medication (Gialamas *et al.* 2009).

### POCT device operator

POCT device operators generally enjoy the responsibility of performing POCT, provided they are supported in this

**Table 1.7.** Summary of advantages and benefits of POCT in a primary care setting

| Stakeholder | Advantage | Reference |
|---|---|---|
| Patient | Convenience and accessibility of service (particularly in rural and remote locations) | Shephard *et al.* 2015a |
| | Sample collection generally simple, less stressful and less invasive | Crook 2000 |
| | Speed of result reduces patient anxiety | Dean 2006 |
| | Follow-up visit to obtain result not required/reduced rate of patient loss to follow-up | Keenan *et al.* 2005; Huppert *et al.* 2010 |
| | Improved levels of patient self-motivation/compliance | Gialamas *et al.* 2009; Gaydos *et al.* 2011 |
| | Improved patient–doctor relationship | Shephard 2006 |
| | Improved levels of patient satisfaction | Shephard 2006; Laurence *et al.* 2010 |
| POCT operator | Performing POCT provides increased sense of responsibility/empowerment | Shephard 2006 |
| | Provides opportunities for patient education, awareness and promotion | Ward *et al.* 2012; Natoli *et al.* 2014 |
| | Increased satisfaction with pathology service delivery (by POCT) | Shephard 2006; Shephard *et al.* 2012 |
| Medical practitioner | Immediacy of result facilitates timely clinical decision making | Wood *et al.* 2011 |
| | Improved doctor–patient relationship | Shephard *et al.* 2005 |
| | Improved patient outcomes | WHO 2012; Jani *et al.* 2011; Vassall *et al.* 2011; Boehme *et al.* 2011 |
| Health service | POCT can be performed *in situ* by trained non-laboratory staff | Keenan *et al.* 2005 |
| | POCT does not require expensive ancillary equipment (e.g. centrifuges) | Keenan *et al.* 2005 |
| | Portability of POCT means it can be used for outreach and/or outbreak services | Peeling 2009 |
| | Reduction in over-prescription and unnecessary consumption of medications | Peeling 2009; Thiam *et al.* 2011; Yeboah-Antwi *et al.* 2010 |
| Community engagement | Community empowered to have greater ownership and control of the way their health service is managed | Shephard *et al.* 2015a |
| | Fosters the building of workforce capacity and sustainability of health programs | Shephard *et al.* 2015a |

activity by their health-service managers and clinical staff. In the models managed by the author's Centre and conducted in Indigenous health settings, Indigenous health workers assume a pivotal role as POCT device operators and have consistently stated this role provides them with a strong sense of empowerment (Shephard 2006; Shephard *et al.* 2015b). The time interval while waiting for the POC test result provides opportunity for discussion between patient and device operator around the patient's health, and enables time for health promotion.

### Treating medical practitioner

POCT provides the treating medical practitioner with rapid on-site results that can enhance evidence-based clinical decision making at the time of the patient encounter. There is now a strong evidence base to demonstrate that POCT can be an effective tool in assisting to improve clinical outcomes for patients with chronic, acute and infectious disease. Some examples of outcome measures are summarised in Table 1.8 and these will be described in more detail throughout the book. Treating practitioners have also reported that POCT can improve their relationship with patients (Shephard 2006).

### Health service

POCT can provide a range of operational benefits for the health service. POCT generally does not require ancillary laboratory equipment such as centrifuges to separate serum or plasma from whole blood. Due to their portability, POC devices can be taken into the community and

**Table 1.8.** Selected examples of clinical outcome benefits from accessing POC testing in primary care settings

| Clinical condition | Outcome measure | POC test | Example |
|---|---|---|---|
| Chronic disease | Improved glycaemic control | Haemoglobin A1c | Bubner *et al.* 2009 |
| | Stabilisation of renal function | Creatinine and eGFR | |
| | | Urine albumin:creatinine ratio | Shephard *et al.* 2006 |
| | Stabilisation of patients on warfarin therapy (improved time in therapeutic range) | International normalised ratio | Harper *et al.* 2015 |
| | Reduction in rates of iron deficiency anaemia | Haemoglobin | Ayub 2015 |
| Acute disease | Reduction in cardiac mortality | Troponin I or T | Tideman *et al.* 2014 |
| | Early risk stratification for acute coronary syndrome | | |
| | Rapid stabilisation of patients with severe diarrhoea or vomiting | Potassium | Spaeth 2009 |
| | Negating the need for a medical retrieval (clinical and operational benefit) | Troponin I or T, blood gases, electrolytes | Spaeth 2009 |
| Infectious disease | Increased uptake in testing rates | Malaria | WHO 2012 |
| | Increased rates of initiation of antiretroviral therapy and reduction in time to initiation of treatment | HIV | Jani *et al.* 2011 |
| | Increased rate of case detection and reduction in time to initiate treatment | Tuberculosis | Boehme *et al.* 2011; Vassall *et al.* 2011 |

linked with community outreach events such as health screening days, health promotion activities, and disease awareness programs. Access to, and knowledge about, POCT enables the health service to make a swift response in the event of a disease outbreak or disaster. The judicious use of POCT has been shown to reduce the overprescribing and/or unnecessary consumption of medical products such as peri-operative blood products, antibiotics (Takemura *et al.* 2004) or antimalarial drugs (Thiam *et al.* 2011). The ability to use POCT to make an informed on-site clinical decision on acutely ill patients as to whether they can be stabilised *in situ* or require a medical evacuation to a tertiary hospital has provided significant operational, as well as clinical and cost saving, benefits for the health service and health-care system in general (Shephard *et al.* 2015a).

## COMMUNITY ENGAGEMENT, CAPACITY BUILDING AND RESILIENCE

POCT fosters and builds a strong sense of community engagement by ensuring that the patient is the central focus of the pathology service being delivered and by empowering the health service to have greater ownership and control of the way their pathology service, and resultant health information, is managed.

Access to POCT for chronic conditions, such as diabetes, renal disease and coagulation disorders, enables patients to remain in their communities for treatment and management, meaning they are not dislocated from their family members.

It is imperative to ensure there is an element of progressive knowledge transfer and capacity building with POCT conducted in a community setting so that, as a POCT program is implemented, the community is empowered with the resources to manage and sustain the program long term. The ultimate aim of progressive knowledge transfer is to build a sustainable and resilient community health workforce that has the capacity to undertake routine quality-assured POCT for its intended clinical purpose.

## LIMITATIONS AND BARRIERS FOR POINT-OF-CARE TESTING

While the advantages and benefits of POCT are well documented, there are several challenges, limitations and barriers to the successful implementation and sustainability of a POCT service (Table 1.9).

**Table 1.9.** Summary of limitations and barriers for the implementation of POCT in a primary care setting

| Stakeholder | Advantage | Reference |
|---|---|---|
| Patient | Potentially inaccurate test results due to poor analytical quality | Peeling 2009, 2011 |
| POCT operator | Continuing commitment required for staff training | Shephard 2006 |
| | Time required to conduct and document results of quality testing and basic device maintenance | Laurence *et al.* 2008 |
| | High rates of staff turnover cause disruption and compromise sustainability of POCT (applicable to remote locations in particular) | Shephard *et al.* 2009 |
| | Speed of result can sometimes be a disadvantage for operator when results of a positive/reactive test for HIV, for example, need to be given as part of post-test counselling | Natoli 2015 |
| Medical practitioner | Potential to challenge clinical reasoning, if POCT result does not match clinical signs/symptoms | Wood *et al.* 2011 |
| Health service | POCT may be more expensive than laboratory services due to lack of economy of scale | |
| | Potential for increase in inappropriate testing if/when defined clinical pathways for use of POCT are not followed | Natoli *et al.* 2014 |
| | Lack of industry technical support if device fails or needs repair (applicable to remote locations in particular) | Crook 2000 |
| | Capacity to transport and store reagents/consumables may be compromised (applicable to remote locations in particular) | Jorgensen *et al.* 2006 |
| | Identification of bottlenecks in health service workflow that impede POCT | Peeling 2009 |
| Government | Lack of political will of governments to support changes needing to be implemented to facilitate POCT | Peeling 2009 |
| | Differences between countries regarding guidelines/regulatory frameworks to support POCT | |
| | Lack of government reimbursement to support POCT outside laboratory environments | |

As mentioned, early critics of POCT argued the quality of a result from a POCT device could not match that of the laboratory. This argument generally no longer applies to POC clinical chemistry and haematology tests. However, it is true that many 'first generation' lateral flow rapid immunochromatographic tests for infectious disease lacked the analytical quality of their laboratory counterparts, which held back the widespread uptake of this form of testing in developed countries for many years. In recent years, the adaptation of molecular testing to POCT platforms has changed the landscape for infectious disease POCT, with this technology now of equivalent analytical quality to a laboratory (Gaydos *et al.* 2013).

For the POCT device operator, the continuing time commitments to maintain training and competency standards, conduct quality testing procedures to monitor analytical performance, and perform basic maintenance add to the already heavy workload of working health professionals in busy primary care settings. In remote settings, high rates of staff turnover are a constant problem for the effective delivery of health problems in general and POCT programs specifically. They require flexible solutions for training delivery to ensure POCT services are not disrupted and are sustainable (Shephard *et al.* 2015a). In some specific instances, the speed of result may cause anxiety for the POCT device operator (and the patient); for example, when a reactive POCT result for HIV must be discussed in a post-test counselling session with a concerned patient.

POCT may, in some circumstances, challenge the clinical reasoning of the treating medical officer; for example, if the POCT result is at odds with the clinical presentation or symptoms displayed by the patient (Wood *et al.* 2011). Strategies to deal with the incompatibility of pathology results and clinical judgement need to be incorporated into the design of the POCT system before implementation.

At the health service level, POCT may potentially be more expensive than the equivalent laboratory service due to the economies of scale that large laboratories have with their high throughput pathology testing equipment. POCT is generally conducted as discrete testing – that is, 'one test at a time' – rather than performed in 'large batches' as occurs in a laboratory setting. Potential also exists for an increase in inappropriate levels of POCT simply 'because it is there' (Natoli *et al.* 2014); this is most likely to occur when defined clinical pathways that set out the clinical use and frequency of the POC test are not followed. In remote locations in particular, the provision of technical support from the vendor when a device fails or needs repair is problematic, as is the maintenance of continuous cold chain supply and storage of POCT reagents and consumables (Jorgensen *et al.* 2006). Workflow within a health service may need to be adjusted to accommodate the design and operation of POCT and to ensure that it is accessible and test results are acted upon in real time. In particular, the identification of bottlenecks that may impede the delivery of a streamlined POCT service need to be overcome (Peeling 2009). Jani *et al.* (2011) identified four areas to improve health systems and accommodate POCT: (i) the need for the updating and (global) harmonisation of testing policies/regulations for POCT, which are linked to defined clinical algorithms; (ii) improved operational systems relating to product regulation, supply chain, training and quality management; (iii) systematic steps to streamline and integrate POCT into clinical services with allowance for expanded community-based POCT opportunities; and (iv) strategies to improve the retention of patients before and after POCT.

Finally, there needs to be 'buy in' from governments around the world to support and accommodate POCT as an example of a 'disruptive' technology that can facilitate health system change. In this context, the term 'disruptive' means 'one which makes a radical change that achieves substantially greater benefits primarily by meeting the needs of an unmet market' (Price *et al.* 2010). As Peeling (2009) notes: '… lack of political commitment has resulted in the [POCT] programs not being given a high priority for funding. This is especially true in countries faced with a large number of competing priorities for limited resources.' There is also a lack of consistency among governments of the world as to whether/how they provide reimbursement (fully or in part) for POCT conducted outside of the laboratory system. Lack of a sustainable funding mechanism for POCT impedes its uptake particularly in rural and remote locations, despite a clearly defined clinical need and a strong evidence base for its effectiveness in these settings.

## REFERENCES

Australian Government (2013) *Definitions – Point-of-Care Testing.* Australian Government Department of Health website, Canberra, <http://www.health.gov.au/internet/publications/publishing.nsf/Content/qupp-review~qupp-definitions>.

Ayub R (2015) Point of care testing: An effective approach to develop social responsibility and address iron deficiency anemia in women and children of rural Pakistan. Poster presented at The Towards Unity for Health Conference, Bambanani 2015 Working Together: Education for Change, Gauteng, South Africa, 12–16 September 2015.

Boehme CC, Nicol MP, Nabeta P, Michael JS, Gotuzzo E, Tahirli R, *et al.* (2011) Feasibility, diagnostic accuracy, and effectiveness of decentralised use of the XpertMTB/RIF test for diagnosis of tuberculosis and multidrug resistance: a multicentre implementation study. *Lancet* **377**, 1495–1505. doi:10.1016/S0140- 6736(11)60438-8

Bubner TK, Laurence CO, Gialamas A, Yelland LN, Ryan P, Willson KJ, *et al.* (2009) Effectiveness of point-of-care testing for therapeutic control of chronic conditions: results from the PoCT in General Practice Trial. *The Medical Journal of Australia* **190**, 624–626.

Chiu Y-H, Ong J, Walker S, Kumalawati J, Gartinah T, McPhee D, *et al.* (2011) Photographed rapid HIV test results pilot novel quality assessment and training schemes. *PLoS One* **6**, e18294. doi:10.1371/journal.pone.0018294

College of American Pathologists (1998) *Commission on Laboratory Accreditation. Checklist 30, Point of Care Testing.* College of American Pathologists, Northfield IL, USA.

College of American Pathologists (2015) Point-of-care testing toolkit. College of American Pathologists, Northfield IL, USA, <http://www.cap.org/apps//cap.portal?_nfpb=true&cntvwrPtlt_actionOverride=%2Fportlets%2FcontentViewer%2Fshow&_windowLabel=cntvwrPtlt&cntvwrPtlt%7BactionForm.contentReference%7D=committees%2Fpointofcare%2Fpoc_toolkit_definition.html&_state=maximized&_pageLabel=cntvwr>.

Crook MA (2000) Near patient testing and pathology in the new millennium. *Journal of Clinical Pathology* **53**, 27–30. doi:10.1136/jcp.53.1.27

Dean GL (2006) Near-patient testing will not improve the control of sexually transmitted infections. *Sexually Transmitted Infections* **82**, 509–512. doi:10.1136/sti.2005.017954

Freedman DB (2002) Clinical governance: implications for point-of-care testing. *Annals of Clinical Biochemistry* **37**, 241–243.

Gaydos CA, Hsieh YH, Harvey L, Burah A, Won H, Jett-Goheen M, *et al.* (2011) Will patients "opt in" to perform their own rapid HIV test in the emergency department? *Annals of Emergency Medicine* **58**(1, Supplement 1), S74–S78. doi:10.1016/j.annemergmed. 2011.03.029

Gaydos CA, Van der Pol B, Jett-Goheen M, Barnes M, Quinn N, Daniel G, *et al.* (2013) Performance of the Cepheid CT/NG Xpert Rapid PCR Test for detection of *Chlamydia trachomatis* and *Neisseria gonorrhoeae. Journal of Clinical Microbiology* **51**, 1666–1672. doi:10.1128/JCM.03461-12

Gialamas A, Yelland L, Ryan P, Wilson K, Laurence C, Bubner T, *et al.* (2009) Does point-of-care testing lead to the same or better adherence to medication? A randomised controlled trial: the PoCT in General Practice Trial. *The Medical Journal of Australia* **191**, 487–491.

Guibert R, Schattner P, Sikaris K, Churilov L, Leibowitz R, Matthews M (2001) *Review of the Role and Value of Near Patient Testing in General Practice.* Australia, <http://www.health.gov.au/internet/wcms/Publishing.nsf/Content/health-pathology-poctt-index.htm-copy3>.

Harper P, McMichael I, Griffiths D, Harper J, Hill C (2015) The community pharmacy-based anticoagulation management service achieves a consistently high standard of anticoagulant care. *The New Zealand Medical Journal* **128**, 35–44.

Hicks JM, Haeckel R, Price CP, Lewandrowski K, Wu AHB (2001) Recommendations and opinions for the use of point-of-care testing for hospitals and primary care: summary of a 1999 symposium. *Clinica Chimica Acta* **303**, 1–17. doi:10.1016/S0009-8981(00)00400-9

Huckle D (2006) Point-of-care diagnostics: will the hurdles be overcome this time? *Expert Review of Medical Devices* **3**, 421–426. doi:10.1586/17434440.3.4.421

Huppert J, Hesse E, Gaydos CA (2010) What's the Point? How point of care STI tests can impact infected patients. *Point of Care* **9**, 36–46. doi:10.1097/POC.0b013e3181d2d8cc

ISO (International Organization for Standardization) (2006) *ISO 22870:2006. Point-of-care Testing (POCT) – Requirements for Quality and Competence.* Geneva, Switzerland, <https://www.iso.org/obp/ui/#iso:std:iso:22870:ed-1:v1:en>.

Jahn UR, Van Aken H (2003) Near-patient testing – point-of-care or point of costs and convenience? *British Journal of Anaesthesia* **90**, 425–427.

Jani IV, Sitoe NE, Alfai ER, Chongo PL, Quevedo JI, Rocha BM, *et al.* (2011) Effect of point-of-care CD4 cell count tests on retention of patients and rates of antiretroviral therapy initiation in primary health clinics: an observational cohort study. *Lancet* **378**, 1572–1579. doi:10.1016/S0140-6736(11) 61052-0

Jorgensen P, Chanthap L, Rebueno A, Tsuyuoka R, Bell D (2006) Malaria rapid diagnostic tests in tropical climates: the need for a cool chain. *The American Journal of Tropical Medicine and Hygiene* **74**, 750–754.

Keenan PA, Keenan JM, Branson BM (2005) Rapid HIV testing. Wait time reduced from days to minutes. *Postgraduate Medicine* **117**, 47–52.

Kost GJ (1995) Guidelines for point-of-care testing. Improving patient outcomes. *American Journal of Clinical Pathology* **104**(Supplement 1), S111–S127.

Laurence C, Gialamas A, Yelland L, Bubner T, Glastonbury B, Beilby J, Members of the Evaluation Working Group (2008) *Point of Care Testing in General Practice Trial. Final Report.* Australian Government Department of Health and Ageing, Canberra.

Laurence C, Gialamas A, Bubner T, Yelland L, Willson K, Ryan P, *et al.* (2010) Patient satisfaction with point-of-care testing in general practice. *The British Journal of General Practice* **60**, e98–e104. doi:10.3399/bjgp10X 483508

Lehr P (2013) *Global Markets for Rapid Medical Diagnostic Kits.* BCC Research LLC, Wellesley MA, USA.

Mor M, Waisman Y (2000) Point-of-care testing: a critical review. *Pediatric Emergency Care* **16**, 45–48. doi:10.1097/00006565-200002000-00014

Musaad S, Herd G (2013) Point-of-care testing governance in New Zealand: a national framework. *The New Zealand Medical Journal* **126**, 72–79.

Natoli L (2015) Health service implications of the introduction of STI (sexually transmitted infections) point-of-care testing in Australia. PhD thesis. Kirby Institute, University of New South Wales, Australia.

Natoli L, Maher L, Shephard M, Hengel B, Tangey A, Badman S, *et al.* (2014) Point-of-care testing for chlamydia and gonorrhoea: implications for clinical practice. *PLoS One* **9**, e100518. doi:10.1371/journal.pone. 0100518

Pai M, Ghiasi M, Pai NP (2015) Point-of-care diagnostic testing in global health: what is the point? *Microbe* **10**, 103–107.

Peeling RW (2009) Utilisation of rapid tests for sexually transmitted infections: promises and challenges. *The Open Infectious Diseases Journal* **3**, 156–163. doi:10.2174/1874279301004010156

Peeling RW (2011) Applying new technologies for diagnosing sexually transmitted infections in resource-poor settings. *Sexually Transmitted Infections* **87**(Supplement 2), 28–30. doi:10.1136/sti.2010.047647

Price CP (2001) Point-of-care testing. Impact on medical outcomes. *Clinics in Laboratory Medicine* **21**, 285–303.

Price CP, St John A (2005) Point-of-care testing. In *Textbook of Clinical Chemistry and Molecular Diagnostics.* (Eds C Burtis, E Ashwood and D Bruns) pp. 299-320. AACC Press, Washington DC, USA.

Price CP, St John A, Hicks JM (2004) Point-of-care testing: what, why, when and where? In *Point-of-Care Testing.* 2nd edn. (Eds CP Price, A St John and JM Hicks) pp. 3-9. AACC Press, Washington DC, USA.

Price CP, St John A, Kricka L (2010) Putting point-of-care testing into context: moving beyond innovation to adoption. In *Point-of-Care Testing.* 3rd edn. (Eds C Price, A St John and L Kricka) pp. 1–20. AACC Press, Washington DC, USA.

Ramachandran R (2010) *Point-of-Care Testing: Will the Benefits Overrule the Challenges?* Frost and Sullivan, San Antonio TX, USA, <http://www.shareslide.net/FrostandSullivan/point-of-care-testing-in-europe-will-the-benefits-overrule-the-challenges>.

Shephard MD (2006) Cultural and clinical effectiveness of the 'QAAMS' point-of-care testing model for diabetes management in Australian Aboriginal medical services. *The Clinical Biochemist Reviews* **27**, 161–170.

Shephard MD, Mazzachi BC, Shephard AK, McLaughlin KJ, Denner B, Barnes G (2005) The impact of point of care testing on diabetes services along Victoria's Mallee Track: results of a community-based diabetes risk assessment and management program. *Rural and Remote Health* **5**, 371, <http://www.rrh.org.au/articles/subviewnew.asp?ArticleID=371>.

Shephard M, Allen G, Paizis K, Barbara J, Batterham M, Vanajek A (2006) Results of an Aboriginal community-based renal disease management program incorporating point of care testing for urine albumin:creatinine ratio. *Rural and Remote Health* **6**, 591, <http://www.rrh.org.au/articles/subviewnew.asp?ArticleID=591>.

Shephard M, Mazzachi B, Watkinson L, Shephard A, Laurence A, Gialamas A, *et al.* (2009) Evaluation of a training program for device operators in the Australian Government's Point of Care Testing In General Practice Trial. *Rural and Remote Health* **9**, 1189, <http://www.rrh.org.au/articles/subviewnew.asp?ArticleID=1189>.

Shephard M, Spaeth B, Mazzachi B, Auld M, Schatz S, Loudon J, *et al.* (2012) Design, implementation and initial assessment of the Northern Territory point-of-care testing program. *The Australian Journal of Rural Health* **20**, 16–21. doi:10.1111/j.1440-1584.2011.01243.x

Shephard M, Spaeth B, Motta L, Shephard A (2015a) Point-of-care testing in Australia: Practical advantages and benefits of community resiliency for improving outcomes. In *Global Point-of-Care – Strategies for Disasters, Emergencies, and Public Health Resilience.* (Eds GJ Kost and CM Curtis) pp. 527-535. AACC Press, Washington DC, USA.

Shephard M, O'Brien C, Burgoyne A, Croft J, Garlett T, Barancek K, *et al.* (2015b) A review of the cultural safety of a national Indigenous point-of-care testing program for diabetes management. *Australian Journal of Primary Health* (September). doi:10.1071/PY15050

Spaeth BA (2009) The effectiveness of point-of-care testing in the Northern Territory. BSc (Hons) thesis. Flinders University, Adelaide, Australia.

St John A, Price C (2014) Existing and emerging technologies for point-of-care testing. *The Clinical Biochemist Reviews* **35**, 155–167.

Takemura Y, Kakoi H, Ishida H, Kure H, Tatsuguchi-Harada Y, Sugawara M, *et al.* (2004) Immediate availability of C-reactive protein and leukocyte count data influenced physicians' decisions to prescribe antimicrobial drugs for new outpatients with acute infections. *Clinical Chemistry* **50**, 241–244. doi:10.1373/clinchem.2003.021956

Thiam S, Thior M, Faye B, Ndiop M, Diouf ML, Diouf MB, *et al.* (2011) Major reduction in anti-malarial drug consumption in Senegal after nation-wide introduction of malaria rapid diagnostic tests. *PLoS One* **6**, e18419. doi:10.1371/journal.pone.0018419

Tideman P, Tirimacco R, Senior D, Setchell J, Huynh L, Tavella R, *et al.* (2014) Impact of a regionalised clinical cardiac support network on mortality among rural patients with myocardial infarction. *The Medical Journal of Australia* **200**, 157–160. doi:10.5694/mja13.10645

Vassall A, van Kampen S, Sohn H, Michael JS, John KR, den Boon S, *et al.* (2011) Rapid diagnosis of tuberculosis with the Xpert MTB/RIF assay in high burden countries: a cost effectiveness analysis. *PLoS Medicine* **8**, e1001120. doi:10.1371/journal.pmed.1001120

Ward J, Guy R, Huang RL, Knox J, Couzos S, Scrimgeour D, *et al.* (2012) Rapid point-of-care tests for HIV and sexually transmissible infection control in remote Australia: can they improve Aboriginal people's and Torres Strait Islanders' health. *Sexual Health* **9**, 109–112. doi:10.1071/SH11051

Wood F, Brookes-Howell L, Hood K, Cooper L, Verheij T, Goossens H, *et al.* (2011) A multi-country qualitative study of clinicians' and patients' views on point of care tests for lower respiratory tract infection. *Family Practice* **28**, 661–669. doi:10.1093/fampra/cmr031

WHO (World Health Organization) (2012) *Test. Treat. Track. Scaling Up Diagnostic Testing, Treatment and Surveillance for Malaria.* WHO, Geneva, Switzerland, <http://www.who.int/malaria/test_treat_track/en/index.html>.

Yeboah-Antwi K, Pilingana P, Macleod WB, Semrau K, Siazeele K, Kalesha P, *et al.* (2010) Community case management of fever due to malaria and pneumonia in children under five in Zambia: a cluster randomized controlled trial. *PLoS Medicine* **7**, e1000340. doi:10.1371/journal.pmed.1000340

# THEME 1

# THE MANAGEMENT OF POINT-OF-CARE TESTING SERVICES

# 2 Principles of establishing and managing a point-of-care testing service

*Mark Shephard*

**Summary**

There are many aspects to consider when setting up a routine POCT service and there needs to be a structured approach to the organisation and management of POCT. Multiple guidelines on how to establish and maintain a POCT service have been published by professional societies and expert panels representing many countries and/or regions of the world. Most of these guidelines share common principles that can be applied logically and systematically when establishing and maintaining a POCT service. In wider practice, the key principles recommended for setting up and managing a POCT service must be tailored and adapted to meet local needs and specific clinical settings.

## INTRODUCTION

There is an often mistaken perception among health professionals without a sound understanding of the field of POCT that you can simply buy a POCT device from a vendor 'off the shelf', take it to the location where it is to be used, turn it on and start testing. Importantly, just because a device may look appealing and have many features such as a slim design, a colour display screen or sound alerts, for example, it doesn't necessarily mean that the device can be relied on to produce consistently good quality results for patient care (i.e. it is analytically sound). In reality there are many aspects to consider when setting up a POCT service and there needs to be a logical and systematic approach to its organisation and management.

This chapter will briefly set the scene for the broader regulatory frameworks that support the conduct of POCT regionally and globally and then provide an overview of the key elements that should underpin a POCT service in a primary care setting. Many of these key elements will be described in further detail in subsequent chapters of the book.

## REGULATORY FRAMEWORKS FOR POCT

In a 'perfect' world, POCT should occur in a regulated environment supported by a hierarchical approach that includes:

- a government/regulatory agency overseeing standards and guidelines governing its conduct at the 'local program level'
- an auditing or accreditation process ensuring that the quality processes supporting the POCT program are being met.

Within such a regulatory framework, there is usually a reimbursement method to sustain the POCT program financially. This type of regulated environment is often

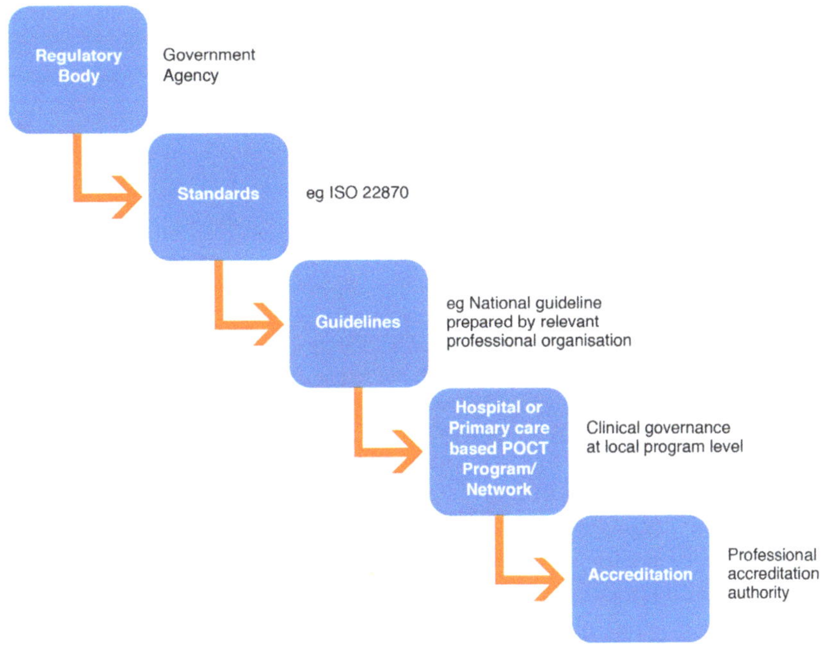


**Fig. 2.1.** An hierarchical approach to the conduct of POCT in a regulated environment.

seen in laboratory-linked, hospital-based POCT settings or large-scale community-based POCT networks (Fig. 2.1).

However, the regulatory frameworks governing POCT are highly variable across countries, and not all countries have this hierarchical structure either wholly or partly in place (Ehrmeyer 2010). At the other extreme, POCT conducted in settings such as home self-testing or POC tests bought over the internet remain largely unregulated and funded by the patient themselves. Across the spectrum of users and settings in which POCT is conducted, the challenge is to ensure that test results remain safe and appropriate for patient care.

## STANDARDS AND GUIDELINES FOR THE CONDUCT OF POINT-OF-CARE TESTING

A decade ago, the International Organization for Standardization (ISO) published a standards document (ISO 22870) that detailed requirements for quality and competence for POCT (ISO 2006). This document stated that these standards could be applied not only to the hospital setting but also to the clinic or health-care organisation providing ambulatory care. However, the standards are written in a highly technical fashion and require constant cross-referencing to a second set of standards (ISO 15189), which provide requirements for quality and competence in medical laboratories. This makes the 2006 ISO standard for POCT difficult to understand, interpret and implement in a practical sense by non-laboratory-trained health professionals and in non-laboratory POCT environments. The ISO standard for POCT is currently being revised as a single stand-alone document that is more applicable and practical to the primary care setting.

In Australia, interim standards for POCT were developed for the conduct of POCT in general practice in Australia as part of a major government-funded trial of POCT in this sector across 2005–2007 (Australian Government 2004; Laurence *et al.* 2008). The standards were based on national quality standards for medical laboratory testing but were tailored to meet the needs of the general practice environment. They aimed to ensure that the quality of POCT conducted in this setting was equivalent to the traditional pathology laboratory and to provide a framework for accreditation of the participating general practices (Tirimacco *et al.* 2011). The standards covered five main areas: clinical governance, analytical requirements, staff training, implementation and performance of POCT, and quality outcomes.

Multiple guidelines on how to establish and maintain a POCT service have also been published by professional societies and expert panels representing many countries and/or regions of the world. The list is ever-increasing and a representative example of guideline documents is provided in Table 2.1.

**Table 2.1.** Examples of international organisations that have published guidelines on establishing and maintaining a POCT service

| Country | Organisation | Title | Year of publication | Reference |
|---|---|---|---|---|
| Australia | National Pathology Accreditation Advisory Council | Guidelines for Point of Care Testing. | 2015 | NPAAC 2015 |
| Canada | Ministry of Health and Long-Term Care | Policies, procedures and quality assurance for point-of-care HIV testing in Ontario. | 2008 | Ministry of Health and Long-Term Care 2008 |
| Germany | German Society for Clinical Chemistry | Recommendations of the German working group on medical laboratory testing (AML) on the introduction and quality assurance procedures for point-of-care testing (POCT) in hospitals. | 1999 | German Society for Clinical Chemistry 1999 |
| Ireland | Joint Committee for POCT in primary care and community care | Guidelines for safe and effective management and use of POCT in primary and community care. | 2009 | Joint Committee for POCT in primary care and community care 2009 |
| Netherlands | Dutch Association of Clinical Chemistry | Point-of-care testing: the views of the working group of the Dutch Association of Clinical Chemistry. | 1999 | Dutch Association of Clinical Chemistry 1999 |
| Spain | Spanish Society of Clinical Biochemistry and Molecular Pathology | Proposed guidelines for point-of-care testing services in Spain. | 2009 | Spanish Society of Clinical Biochemistry and Molecular Pathology 2009 |
| United Kingdom | Medicines and Healthcare Products Regulatory Agency | Management and use of IVD point of care test devices. | 2013 | Medicines and Healthcare Products Regulatory Agency 2013 |
| | British Society for Haematology | Guidelines for point-of-care testing: haematology. | 2008 | British Society for Haematology 2008 |
| United States of America | The National Academy of Clinical Biochemistry | Evidence-based practice for point-of-care testing. | 2007 | National Academy of Clinical Biochemistry 2007 |
| | Department of Health and Human Services Centers for Disease Control and Prevention | Good laboratory practices for waived testing sites. | 2005 | Department of Health and Human Services Centers for Disease Control and Prevention 2005 |

The Clinical and Laboratory Standards Institute (CLSI), based in the USA, has also been particularly proactive in developing a range of guideline documents for POCT over the past decade (http://shop.clsi.org/point-of-care-documents/). Some of these documents are listed in Table 2.2.

The flood of recent activity in the area of POCT guidelines/governance and policy is well exemplified by developments in the Australasian scene. The National Pathology Accreditation Advisory Council (NPAAC), managed by the Australian Government Department of Health, plays a key role in ensuring the quality of Australian pathology services and is responsible for the development and maintenance of standards and guidelines for pathology practice. In 2013, NPAAC established a POCT Drafting Committee, which recently released best practice guidelines for the conduct of POCT in Australia (NPAAC 2015); these guidelines cover governance, specimen and result integrity, staff training, quality systems, and environmental and safety issues, together with an

**Table 2.2.** List of CLSI guideline documents regarding POCT

| Date of publication | Code | Document title |
|---|---|---|
| 01/07/2004 | POCT14-A | Point-of-Care Monitoring of Anticoagulation Therapy; Approved Guideline |
| 28/07/2006 | POCT01-A2 | Point-of-Care Connectivity; Approved Standard: Second Edition |
| 31/08/2006 | POCT04-A2 | Point-of-Care *In vitro* Diagnostic (IVD) Testing; Approved Guideline: Second Edition |
| 27/05/2008 | POCT02-A | Implementation Guide of POCT01 for Health Care Providers; Approved Guideline |
| 15/12/2008 | POCT05-A | Performance Metrics for Continuous Interstitial Glucose Monitoring; Approved Guideline |
| 30/04/2010 | POCT09-A | Selection Criteria for Point-of-Care Testing Devices; Approved Guideline |
| 07/10/2010 | POCT07-A | Quality Management: Approaches to Reducing Errors at the Point of Care; Approved Guideline |
| 03/12/2010 | POCT08-A | Quality Practices in Noninstrumented Point-of-Care Testing: An Instructional Manual and Resources for Health Care Workers; Approved Guideline |
| 28/04/2011 | POCT11-A2 | Pulse Oximetry; Approved Guideline – Second Edition |
| 27/12/2011 | POCT10-A2 | Physician and Nonphysician Provider-Performed Microscopy Testing; Approved Guideline – Second Edition |
| 30/01/2013 | POCT12-A3 | Point-of-Care Blood Glucose Testing in Acute and Chronic Care Facilities; Approved Guideline – Third Edition |
| 29/05/2015 | POCT06-Ed1 | Effects of Different Sample Types on Glucose Measurements – First Edition |
| 18/06/2015 | POCT13-Ed3 | Glucose Monitoring in Settings without Laboratory Support – Third Edition |

appendix that contains checklists to aid the interpretation of these guidelines. They were designed to apply to laboratory as well as primary care users of POCT.

In addition, several Australian professional organisations have developed policies on POCT including the Australasian Association of Clinical Biochemists though their *Point-of-Care Testing Implementation Guide* (AACB 2008) and the Australian Institute of Medical Scientists (AIMS), which made recommendations for the quality-assured conduct of POCT for infectious diseases and drugs of abuse in Australia (Shephard *et al.* 2012). The Royal College of Pathologists of Australasia (RCPA) Quality Assurance Programs Pty Ltd prepared a review of policies, procedures and guidelines for POCT with funds provided by the Australian Government's Quality Use of Pathology Programs (QUPP) (Farrance 2012). The Royal College of Pathologists of Australasia (RCPA) recently published a document concerning elements of a quality framework for POCT (RCPA 2014). The Australasian Society for HIV Medicine (ASHM) developed a position paper on HIV POCT (ASHM 2013) and released a statement concerning HIV oral testing (ASHM 2012). The 2011 National (Australian) HIV Testing Policy, also available on ASHM's testing portal, contains a section (number 13) on POCT for HIV in community settings (ASHM 2013b). The New South Wales Government's Ministry for Health and New South Wales Health Pathology recently released a policy for POCT and a quality manual respectively to support POCT conducted in emergency departments in small public hospitals in that state (NSW Health Pathology 2014; NSW Ministry for Health 2014). In New Zealand, a new national governance framework for POCT is being enacted, with the New Zealand Point-of-Care Testing Advisory Group playing a lead role in driving this change (Musaad and Herd 2013).

Most of the guidelines documents from Australia and around the world share similar underlying key principles that can be applied logically and systematically when establishing and maintaining a POCT service. These principles are shown diagrammatically in Fig. 2.2.

Although many of the early guidelines are focussed on hospital-based POCT applications, more recent guideline documents reflect an understanding of their need to embrace POCT in the wider practice of primary care where these key principles must to be tailored and adapted to meet local needs and specific POCT settings; that is, POCT needs to be 'fit for purpose'. The support and knowledge of the local laboratory or specialist POCT provider is critical in establishing a POCT service in these settings because many of the principles deal with specific analytical and laboratory concepts that are often foreign to the non-laboratory health professional.

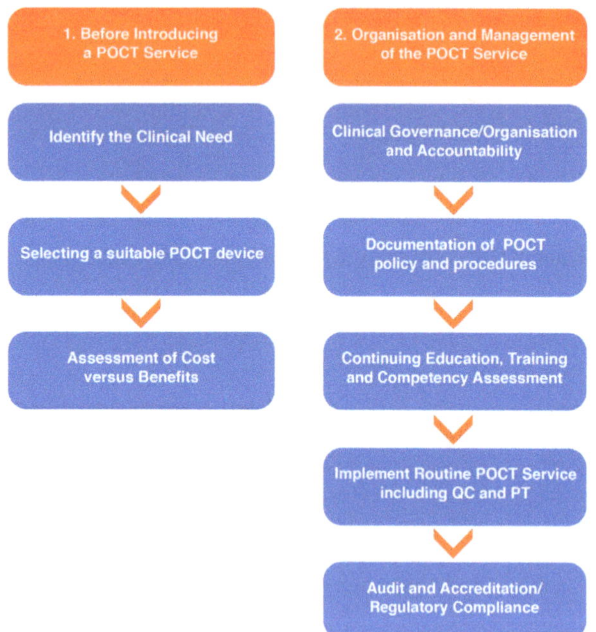


**Fig. 2.2.** Key principles for establishing and managing a POCT service.

## BEFORE SETTING UP A POINT-OF-CARE TESTING SERVICE

### Identify the clinical need for POCT

The key principles for identifying the clinical need for POCT include:

- POCT should be introduced to meet a defined clinical need, with the ultimate goal of providing optimal quality of care for the patient.
- POCT should provide at least an equivalent clinical service to that which is currently available through the laboratory, or
- POCT should provide access to a service that currently does not exist but for which there is an identified clinical need (ISO 2006).

There are many examples of clinical need for a POCT service, which can include screening, risk stratification, diagnosis, case detection or management of existing clinical conditions. For example, a health service may wish to conduct a risk assessment program for their community with a high burden of chronic disease with the aim of detecting patients at high risk for the disease and initiating early preventative measures. Another health service with high rates of chronic disease may choose to introduce a POCT program to better manage patients with established disease and slow the progress of disease complications. There may be a clinical need to introduce a POCT service for cardiac patients that can provide faster risk stratification to identify whether a patient has suffered a myocardial infarction. Another health service with a high burden of a curable sexually transmittable disease among young adults may wish to introduce POCT to identify new cases of the disease with the aim of initiating treatment faster, reducing the risk of onward transmission to partners and decreasing overall disease prevalence in the community.

In summary, the POCT clinical needs assessment should be tailored locally and may be dependent on factors such as population size, age structure, ethnicity and culture, broad community health profile, geographic location and accessibility to a pathology service, and practice infrastructure (current and planned).

### Selecting a suitable POCT device

Having established the need for a POCT service, the next step is to select a suitable POCT device/test system. Key principles include:

- Survey the range of currently available POCT devices that can perform the required tests (being aware the choice may sometimes be very limited).
- Define the analytical expectations of the POCT device/test system.
- Verify the POCT device's performance before its introduction to routine practice.
- Assess the impact of the introduction of POCT on the health service's organisation and infrastructure.

A survey of current POC technology can be undertaken through a peer-reviewed literature search, sourcing product information from the vendor, consultation with the local laboratory or with professional colleagues who have hands-on, practical field experience and knowledge of the candidate POCT system, or through reference to evaluation reports by government agencies (if available) (Pearson 2004).

As a general principle, the POCT device should be able to achieve at least an equivalent level of analytical performance for the required test(s) compared with that of the corresponding laboratory device when used for the same clinical purpose. There are two aspects of analytical performance to consider: first, 'fitness for purpose' of the POC test; and, second, analytical performance standards expected of the device when performing the required test.

The POC test must be fit for the clinical purpose for which it is intended. For example, if a POC test is being used to identify a new case of a sexually transmitted infection that has serious consequences for the patient and their partner if missed, then the test must be able to detect a positive result with as close to 100% certainty as possible. If a seriously ill patient with diabetes is in need of tight glycaemic monitoring, then highly accurate POC test results are required. In contrast, if a test is being used to assess an unconscious patient with diabetes in an emergency situation, then it may be clinically necessary to know only whether the POC test result is very low, normal or very high. If a patient with established diabetes requires regular long-term monitoring of their glycaemic control by serial POCT measurements, then the reproducibility of the test becomes very important.

It is now possible to source detailed information on 'how good pathology tests (including POC tests) should be' because, for most tests (particularly clinical biochemistry and haematology tests), there are well-defined analytical performance standards or 'analytical goals'. These goals have been set according to an internationally recognised, multi-tiered hierarchical approach based on clinical outcome studies, biological variation, opinions of professional groups and data from proficiency testing programs and the general literature (Fraser 2001, 2004; Ricos *et al.* 1999). The renowned clinical chemist James Westgard has devoted an entire website to the topic of analytical goals for common pathology tests: https://www.westgard.com/biodatabase1.htm.

There are also other aspects of analytical performance to consider, such as associated test menu (where appropriate), measuring range, linearity, common interferences, calibration requirements, availability and suitability of quality testing materials, maintenance required for the POC device, level of vendor support for servicing and/or repair, and reference intervals, clinical decision levels and panic values.

Prior to its introduction, the POCT device's performance should be verified to ensure that it meets the analytical (and non-analytical) expectations of the primary care setting. Ideally, verification should take place at the intended site of use by the (trained) operator who would be expected to use it in routine practice, with the support of the laboratory or specialist POCT provider and the vendor.

For a POC test that generates a quantitative result (i.e. a number or value), the key measures of analytical performance are accuracy (closeness of the test result to the true result) and precision (reproducibility/repeatability of the test result when tested multiple times). For a POC test result that delivers a qualitative result (i.e. detects the presence or absence of a disease/marker), the key measures of performance are sensitivity (the proportion of patients with disease who test positive) and specificity (the proportion of patients without disease who test negative).

As a general rule, only select a POCT device that has been scientifically validated by your local laboratory or POCT provider, or a device for which there is a solid evidence base in the published literature that confirms it can meet analytical specifications for its intended use.

Consideration needs to also be given to the impact of the introduction of the POCT service on the organisation and infrastructure of the health service.

Factors to consider include:

- The physical attributes of the POCT device, such as sample type and volume, size and portability of the device, power source (battery, AC or both), degree of device automation and connectivity, and turnaround time for results.
- The user-friendliness of the device, the number of manual steps, complexity and labour intensiveness of device operation, and reagent preparation time.
- Projected future workloads and/or patterns of testing: there needs to be an acceptable level of POCT activity over a defined time period to ensure maintenance of POCT operator skills.
- Adequate space is needed for patient preparation and sample collection, POCT equipment, ancillary equipment such as centrifuges and fridges, and storage of reagents, quality testing kits and consumables. Fridge space may be a crucial element to consider, particularly in rural and remote/low resource settings.
- Health and safety: a safe working environment for both patients and staff is needed for POCT. It should have adequate lighting, power, temperature control, plumbing, waste disposal and infection control.

### Cost–benefit analysis

Key principle:

- An assessment of the costs of introducing the POCT system, and weighing this cost up against the defined benefits of introducing such a system, is an implicit part of the decision-making process for the adoption of POCT (Fig. 2.3).

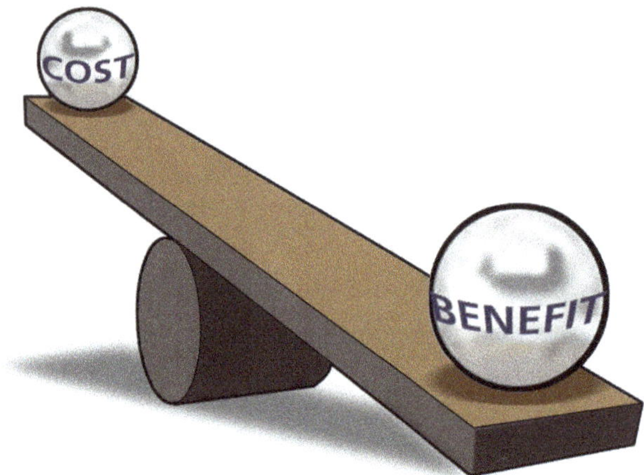


**Fig. 2.3.** Balancing the benefits versus costs of POCT.

There are many hidden costs that need to be taken into account when determining the 'true' or total cost of POCT; these include both fixed and variable costs.

Fixed costs include some/all of the following: the purchase price of the device itself; an annual service contract fee with the vendor; an annual fee for participation in external proficiency testing (PT) programs; fees for accreditation compliance and/or licensing; an external quality management service fee (where a practice may be paying a laboratory or specialist POCT provider to assist in managing their POCT service); and ancillary infrastructure (e.g. site alterations such as new plumbing, power outlets, fridges, centrifuges and computers).

Variable costs (those dependent on workload) include: ongoing reagent supply, with allowance for wastage when actual usage does not meet expected workload or there are high levels of cartridge errors; consumables; quality testing materials; calibrators; staff time (i.e. time required to perform the total testing process [not just the analytical component of testing] and time required for training/retraining and maintenance of professional competency); personal protective equipment (gloves, gowns, eye protection and face masks); waste disposal and infection control.

The initial cost of setting up POCT may be higher than that of the equivalent laboratory service where economies of scale can be factored in due to the laboratory's capacity to use high throughput devices to analyse large batches of pathology samples. Although much more difficult to quantify, the most appropriate assessment of the cost-benefits of POCT needs to take into consideration the 'total episode of care' where the potential longer term benefits of POCT, such as future reduced length of hospital stay, reduced re-admissions and reduced complications of a disease process, are taken into account.

There is little purpose in introducing a POCT service unless there is a defined benefit to be gained. The benefits of introducing POCT are generally classed as: clinical (where a specific improvement in patient outcome can be measured); operational (where benefit relates to improved efficiency in the delivery of patient care); economic (where cost savings in the delivery of care can be made at the patient, health service or societal level); or cultural (when the POCT service involves Indigenous patients).

## ORGANISATION AND MANAGEMENT OF A ROUTINE POINT-OF-CARE TESTING SERVICE

### Clinical governance

The key principles for clinical governance of POCT in a primary care setting include:

- There should be a governance structure in place that: (i) clearly defines the organisation of, and accountability for, the POCT service; and (ii) actively manages the quality and safety risks involved in the delivery of POCT (Freedman 2002, 2004; Pearson 2006).
- The wellbeing, care and rights of individual patients accessing the POCT service should be paramount.

In terms of governance hierarchy, a selected medical practitioner (the 'POCT Director') should ideally have overarching authority and responsibility for POCT and should have an appropriate understanding of the diagnostic and technical applications as well as the limitations of POCT undertaken at their health service (Australian Government 2004). This practitioner is usually the most senior clinical staff member at the health service or a pathologist from the associated laboratory (if they are directly supporting the POCT service).

Under the POCT Director, there is usually a POCT Coordinator – either a senior nurse at the health service or a medical scientist from the supporting laboratory or POCT provider – who is experienced in the practice of POCT. The POCT Coordinator should have overall responsibility for all facets of implementation of the POCT service on a day-to-day basis including, for example, device selection, training of staff, the conduct of patient POCT and all aspects of quality management. (In some more recent guideline documents, the term POCT Coordinator and POCT Supervisor are used interchangeably).

With many POCT services, the POCT Director and Coordinator are supported by a multidisciplinary POCT Management Committee (ISO 2006). This inclusive structure encourages a whole-of-system approach to POCT and ensures all stakeholders feel part of delivering an effective POCT service (Pearson 2006). Members of this committee may vary according to the nature and location of the specific POCT service being implemented but can include, for example, clinical staff, medical scientists, nurses, Indigenous health workers, nurse educators, diabetes educators, IT personnel, pharmacists, finance and planning officers, risk managers and a patient or consumer representative (Price and St John 2005).

A POCT Site Manager (usually a senior nurse) may often act as a link between the POCT Management Committee or POCT Coordinator and the POCT device operator, who represents the person in the organisation who performs POCT at 'the bench level'.

This 'ideal' organisational hierarchy may be impractical or impossible to implement in small services or in rural and remote services with limited staff and should be tailored to suit local needs. Examples of governance structures from a hospital environment (Price and St John 2006) and from a national Australian POCT programs in the primary care environment (Shephard and Gill 2010) are provided in Fig. 2.4.

## Staff training and competency

Training and competency assessment of POCT device operators is a crucial component of a sustainable service. The key principles in delivering a training and competency program are:

- POCT should only be carried out by staff who have undergone appropriate initial training and competency certification, who have their competency levels regularly assessed, and who participate in regular retraining and recertification sessions (ISO 2006).
- POCT training should be organised and delivered by the POCT Coordinator under the direction of the POCT Management Committee.
- A training manual should be provided for all candidate POCT device operators. The content of the training manual should be determined by the nature of the POCT service being implemented and the needs of the organisation undertaking POCT; however, particularly in a non-hospital setting, trainee device operators are unlikely to have had access to previous formal training in laboratory or analytical concepts (including quality testing).
- Training should cover both the theory and practice of conducting POCT.
- At the completion of formal training, the competency of the trained device operator should be determined by written and practical assessment.
- Successful trainees should receive a competency certificate, with a fixed expiry date, at the completion of training.
- Post-training surveillance of competency should be undertaken by regular review of quality control and external PT results.
- Competency should be formally reviewed regularly through retraining and education updates.
- A register of all persons receiving initial and renewed competency certificates should be maintained.

## Documentation of POCT policies and procedures

All services conducting POCT should develop a policy manual that describes all aspects of the quality management system underpinning their POCT service. Key elements of this system should include information on:

- requirements for governance
- location of POCT equipment
- storage of reagents and consumables
- purchasing and inventory procedures
- patient preparation and sample collection procedures
- POC test procedures
- processes for assessing the analytical quality of the testing process (quality control and external PT)
- record keeping/data management (of staff training and competency, as well as patient and quality testing results)
- processes for the timely interpretation and actioning of patient and quality test results
- risk management and procedures for workplace safety, notably infection control.

Each component of the policy manual is often written as a standard operating procedure (SOP) for inclusion in the manual (and with regular updating).

The aim of the policy manual is to provide a benchmark against which the quality of the POCT service can be regularly assessed and improved. The policy manual should be kept in hard copy and electronic form, be centrally located and be accessible to all users of the POCT service.

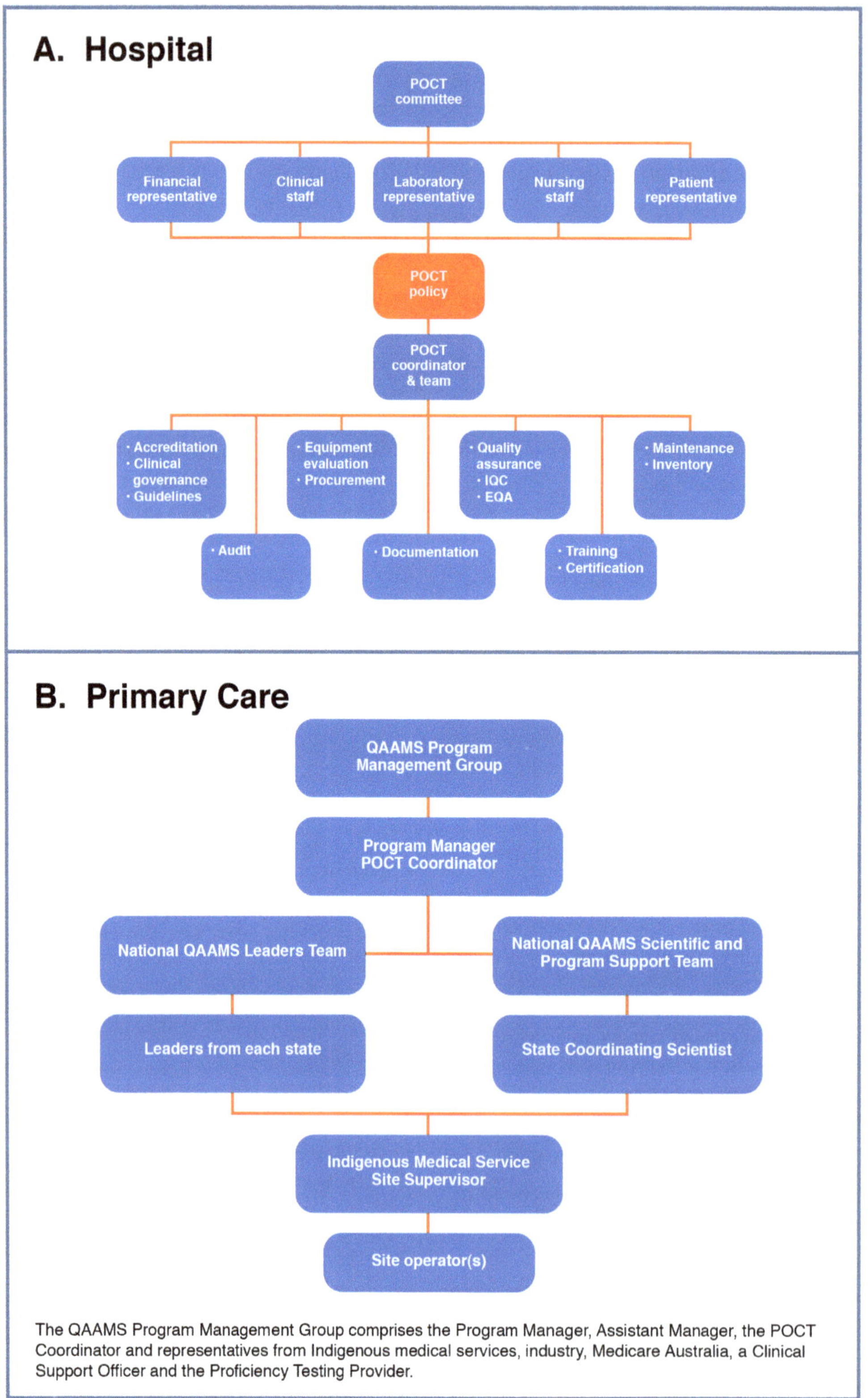


**Fig. 2.4.** (A) Example of a governance structure suitable for POCT conducted in a hospital environment. Modified with permission from the publisher AACC Press (Source: Price and St John A 2006). (B) Example of a governance structure suitable for POCT conducted in an Indigenous primary care setting.

## Implementation of routine point-of-care testing

The conduct of routine POCT should cover all phases of the total testing cycle including:

- pre-analytical (patient preparation and sample collection)
- analytical (the POC testing process on the device)
- post-analytical (turnaround time for the result; and reporting, interpretation and actioning of POC test results).

In practice, most POCT errors are attributable to the pre-analytical phase of testing, rather than to the testing process or to the reporting of results. It is crucial that the patient is prepared and the POCT specimen is collected according to the manufacturer's instructions and with accurate identification. Ideally each specimen should have a minimum of three identifiers recorded on it (name, gender and date of birth); however, this is often not possible if, for example, capillary whole blood is the specimen of choice and the sample is wholly consumed during the testing process. If venous whole blood sample is collected, then it is important that the collection tube contains the correct preservative for that test. Table 2.3 illustrates examples of common errors that can occur in the pre-analytical stage of testing.

Monitoring analytical quality through established practices such as quality control (QC) and external proficiency testing (PT) procedures is an obligatory

**Table 2.3.** Examples of errors that can occur in the pre-analytical stage of testing

| Source of pre-analytical error | Example |
|---|---|
| Patient not fasted | Lipids are requested by the doctor but the patient does not fast. Triglyceride will be falsely elevated. |
| Inadequate identification of a patient POCT sample | Results are reported on the wrong patient. |
| Sample from venous blood tube containing the wrong preservative | If blood for the measurement of potassium and calcium by POCT is collected in a tube containing di-potassium EDTA as preservative, the potassium will be falsely elevated (due to the presence of potassium in the preservative), while the calcium will be falsely lowered (because EDTA binds the calcium in the sample). |
| Finger-prick sampling from unwashed hands | If a patient handles a sugar-containing product such as fruit and does not wash his/her hands before having a finger-prick blood glucose test, then the glucose concentration can be falsely elevated (by 10% or higher). |
| Not sampling from first or second drop of finger-prick blood | For INR testing it is important to use the first drop of blood for analysis as the clotting process commences immediately. For haemoglobin testing, most manufacturers recommend that the first drop of blood is wiped away and the second or third drop of blood is used for this test. It is critical to follow the manufacturer's specification on which drop of finger-prick blood should be used for analysis. |
| The presence of air bubbles in the sample holder | Urine albumin:creatinine ratio (ACR) is a common POC test for early renal disease and is calculated by dividing the urine albumin by the urine creatinine in the sample. If an air bubble is present in the sample holder, which, for example, takes up one quarter of the recommended sample volume space, then both the urine albumin and the urine creatinine values will be falsely low by a factor of one quarter (although the ACR will be reported correctly). If air bubbles or sample under-fill occurs, then a new sample should be collected. |
| Wrong units of measurement set on a POCT analyser | If the POCT device is unintentionally set to a different unit of measurement than the reference interval, then an inappropriate clinical decision could be made. For example, blood glucose units can be reported as either mmol/L or mg/dL (but there is an 18-fold difference in numerical value between the two units). Therefore a glucose result of 2.5 mmol/L (which is a value in the hypoglycaemic range) could be reported as 45 (falsely indicating a result in the hyperglycaemic range) if the unit of measurement on a glucose meter was incorrectly set to mg/dL. |
| Using quality control materials beyond their expiry date | If a quality control sample (once opened) has a shelf-life of 3 months and that material continues to be used beyond the recommended 3 month window, then quality control results are likely to trend lower and drift outside the allowable limits set for acceptable quality. These low quality control results are not due to an inherent analytical fault with the device but rather due to the material being used inappropriately outside the manufacturer's recommendations. |

component of a regulated POCT service in most countries of the world, with government reimbursement for POC testing linked to the health service's regular participation and performance in quality testing programs.

In simplest terms, QC and PT processes generally involve testing artificial blood or biological fluid samples that have a known value for the test being measured. The results for quality testing obtained by POC are compared with the known values in the quality samples to see whether they are close to or agree with the true result in those samples. Quality testing therefore provides a legitimate means of analytical surveillance. Without quality testing to verify the device's performance, how can the operator be confident that their POCT device is working well and that correct patient results have been obtained? QC and PT testing (and the difference between these procedures) will be discussed in Chapter 5.

In terms of post-analytical factors, a POCT device may provide very rapid results but the overall POCT service will be flawed if result reporting and delivery to the doctor does not occur in a timely fashion; that is, does not meet the turnaround time expected by the health service. Importantly, there needs to be a defined policy around what happens in the situation when the POCT result does not fit with the clinical presentation of the patient and/or the initial clinical judgement of the medical practitioner. The capacity to repeat the POC test should always be considered as a first line of troubleshooting and, if clinical doubt remains, then a fresh sample should be collected and sent to the local laboratory.

Poor documentation of manual POCT results was a major source of error and a significant limitation of POCT across the 1990s (Stephens 1999). Nichols *et al.* (2004) reported that patient barcoding, introduced as a means of automating manual data entry, resulted in a significant reduction of error rates for POC tests performed after an initial familiarisation period. In addition, the implementation of a global connectivity standard for POCT in 2001 has facilitated the seamless electronic transfer of test results from POCT devices to clinical/patient management information systems and into the electronic patient record (NCCLS 2001). All modern POCT systems now have connectivity as an integral component of their design, ensuring there is no loss of data and there is a well-defined result audit trail. Plebani (2009) argues connectivity is a tool of prime importance in reducing medical errors at critical steps such as patient identification, results recoding and retrieval.

## Risk minimisation for POCT

Device selection, training of POCT device operators and quality testing procedures are crucial, but often neglected, elements of a POCT service (Kost 2001, 2003). If these elements are not considered appropriately as part of an overall organisational and risk management strategy, then there is increased likelihood that errors will occur in the conduct of POCT. Pearson (2006) reported that major sources of error in conducting POCT included poor selection and maintenance of POCT devices, incorrect storage of consumables, and untrained operators performing POCT. Meier and Jones (2005) identified poor operator skills, non-adherence to test procedures and the use of uncontrolled reagents and equipment by operators as the three main sources of POCT error. Demers (1999) listed the 10 most cited deficiencies in POCT as failure to: follow manufacturer's instructions explicitly; perform quality control testing; document quality control activities and take appropriate corrective action of quality control outliers; perform external proficiency testing; document training and competency; provide continuing education for POCT operators; and have a procedure manual for testing and result reporting. Meier and Jones (2005) describe the need for a 'culture of safety' for POCT by focussing on 'procedural consistency, operator competency, quality control and result integrity, monitoring patient identification, specimen adequacy, and report accuracy.' Plebani (2009) states: 'The probable connection between patient safety and POCT lies at the intersection of technical limitations, rapid availability and the immediate therapeutic implications of this type of test.' Ehrmeyer (2011) argues POCT presents many challenges to quality with its multiple test sites, test menus, testing devices and non-laboratory operators and contends that system planning and management of the entire testing process are essential to reduce errors and improve quality and patient safety.

Failure to recognise and eliminate errors that can occur at each stage of the entire testing process can jeopardise patient results and safety. There is a clear need to ensure that all potential risks to patient safety associated with the use of POCT are appropriately managed.

## Auditing and accreditation of POCT services

It is important to continually audit and document the performance of POCT systems both internally at the health service level and, where required through regulation, externally through an approved accreditation agency. Where findings are below expectations or benchmarks, then continuous quality improvement measures should be implemented.

## REFERENCES


AACB (Australasian Association of Clinical Biochemists) (2008) *Point of Care Testing Implementation Guide.* Mount Lawley, Western Australia, <http://www.aacb.asn.au/documents/item/155>.

ASHM (Australasian Society for HIV, Viral Hepatitis and Sexual Health Medicine) (2012) *FDA's Approval of Over the Counter Home HIV Test – Full Position Statement.* Sydney, <http://www.ashm.org.au/Documents/Position-Papers-Statement-on-PoCT.pdf>.

ASHM (2013a) *ASHM Position Paper – HIV Point of Care Tests/Testing (PoCT).* Sydney, <http://testingportal.ashm.org.au/resources/ASHM_Position_Paper_on_PoCT_05_07_13_FINAL.pdf>.

ASHM (2013b) *National HIV Testing Policy.* Sydney, <http://testingportal.ashm.org.au/hiv>.

Australian Government (2004) *Interim Standards for Point of Care Testing in General Practice incorporating PoCT Trial Guidelines.* Canberra.

British Society for Haematology (2008) Guidelines for point-of-care testing: haematology. *British Journal of Haematology* **142**, 904–915. doi:10.1111/j.1365-2141.2008.07274.x

CLSI (Clinical and Laboratory Standards Institute) (2016) *Point of Care Guidelines.* Wayne, Pennsylvania, <http://shop.clsi.org/point-of-care-documents/>.

Demers LM (1999) Regulatory issues in point-of-care testing. In *Point-of-Care Testing.* (Eds CP Price and JM Hicks) pp. 249-264. AACC Press, Washington DC, USA.

Department of Health and Human Services Centers for Disease Control and Prevention (2005) Good laboratory practices for waived testing sites. *MMWR Morbidity and Mortality Weekly Report* **54** (No. RR-13), DHHSCDCP, Atlanta GA, USA, <http://www.cdc.gov/mmwr/PDF/rr/rr5413.pdf>.

Dutch Association of Clinical Chemistry (1999) Point-of-care testing: the views of the working group of the Dutch Association of Clinical Chemistry. *Clinical Chemistry and Laboratory Medicine* **37**, 675–680.

Ehrmeyer S (2010) Regulatory issues regarding point-of-care testing. In *Point-of-Care Testing.* 3rd edn. (Eds CP Price, A St John and L Kricka) pp. 237-249. AACC Press, Washington DC, USA.

Ehrmeyer S (2011) Plan for quality to improve patient safety at the point of care. *Annals of Saudi Medicine* **31**, 342–346. doi:10.4103/0256-4947.83203

Farrance I (2012) *Policies, Procedures and Guidelines for Point-of-Care Testing.* Australian Government, Canberra, <http://www.aacb.asn.au/documents/item/635>.

Fraser CG (2001) Optimal analytical performance for point of care testing. *Clinica Chimica Acta* **307**, 37–43. doi:10.1016/S0009-8981(01)00429-6

Fraser CG (2004) Analytical performance requirements for point-of-care testing. In *Point-of-Care Testing.* 2nd edn. (Eds CP Price, A St John and JM Hicks) pp. 95-100. AACC Press, Washington DC, USA.

Freedman DB (2002) Clinical governance: implications for point-of-care testing. *Annals of Clinical Biochemistry* **37**, 241–243.

Freedman DB (2004) Clinical governance – the implications for point-of-care testing in hospitals: a UK perspective. In *Point-of-Care Testing.* 2nd edn. (Eds CP Price, A St John and JM Hicks) pp. 171-177. AACC Press, Washington DC, USA.

German Society for Clinical Chemistry (1999) Recommendations of the German working group on medical laboratory testing (AML) on the introduction and quality assurance procedures for point-of-care testing (POCT) in hospitals. *Clinical Chemistry and Laboratory Medicine* **37**, 919–925.

ISO (International Organization for Standardization) (2006) *ISO 22870:2006. Point-of-Care Testing (POCT) – Requirements for Quality and Competence.* Geneva, Switzerland, <https://www.iso.org/obp/ui/#iso:std:iso:22870:ed-1:v1:en>.

Joint Committee for POCT in Primary Care And Community Care (2009) *Guidelines for Safe and Effective Management and Use of POCT in Primary and Community Care.* Ireland, <http://www.acbi.ie/Downloads/Guidelines-for-Point-of-Care-Testing-02.pdf>.

Kost GJ (2001) Preventing medical errors in point-of-care testing: security, validation, safeguards, and connectivity. *Archives of Pathology & Laboratory Medicine* **125**, 1307–1315.

Kost GJ (2003) Preventing problems, medical errors, and biohazards in point-of-care testing. *Point of Care* **2**, 78–88. doi:10.1097/00134384-200306000-00002

Laurence C, Gialamas A, Yelland L, Bubner T, Ryan P, Willson K, *et al.* (2008) A pragmatic cluster randomised controlled trial to evaluate the safety, clinical effectiveness, cost effectiveness and satisfaction with point of care testing in a general practice setting – rationale, design and baseline characteristics. *Trials* **9**, 50–64. doi:10.1186/1745-6215-9-50

Medicines and Healthcare Products Regulatory Agency (2013) *Management and Use of IVD Point of Care Test Devices.* United Kingdom, <http://webarchive.nationalarchives.gov.uk/20141205150130/http://www.mhra.gov.uk/Publications/Safetyguidance/DeviceBulletins/CON071082>.

Meier FA, Jones BA (2005) Point-of-care testing error: sources and amplifiers, taxonomy, prevention strategies, and detection monitors. *Archives of Pathology & Laboratory Medicine* **129**, 1262–1267.

Ministry of Health and Long-Term Care (2008) *Policies, Procedures and Quality Assurance for Point-of-Care HIV Testing in Ontario.* Ministry of Health and Long-Term Care, Canada, <http://www.health.gov.on.ca/english/providers/pub/aids/reports/policies_procedures_quality_assurance.pdf>.

Musaad S, Herd G (2013) Point-of-care testing governance in New Zealand: a national framework. *The New Zealand Medical Journal* **126**, 72–79.

National Academy of Clinical Biochemistry (2007) *Evidence-based Practice for Point-of-Care Testing.* Washington DC, USA, <https://www.aacc.org/~/media/practice-guidelines/point-of-care-testing/poct-entire-lmpg.pdf?la=en>.

NCCLS (National Committee for Clinical Laboratory Standards) (2001) *Point-of-Care Connectivity; Approved Standard. NCCLS Document POCT1-A.* Wayne PA, USA.

NPAAC (National Pathology Accreditation Advisory Council) (2015) *Guidelines for Point of Care Testing.* 1st edn, NPAAC, Canberra, <http://www.health.gov.au/internet/main/publishing.nsf/Content/health-npaac-poctguid>.

NSW Health Pathology (2014) *New South Wales Health Pathology Managed Point of Care Testing (PoCT) Service Quality Manual.* Sydney, <http://www.health.nsw.gov.au/pathology/Documents/Quality-Manual.pdf>.

NSW Ministry for Health (2014) *Policy for Managed Point of Care Testing (PoCT) Service.* New South Wales, Australia, <http://www0.health.nsw.gov.au/policies/pd/2014/pdf/PD2014_003.pdf>.

Nichols JH, Bartholomew C, Brunton M (2004) Reducing medical errors through barcoding at the point of care. *Clinical Leadership Management Reviews* **18**, 328–334.

Pearson JM (2004) Equipment procurement and implementation. In *Point-of-Care Testing.* 2nd edn. (Eds CP Price, A St John and JM Hicks) pp. 127–135. AACC Press, Washington DC, USA.

Pearson J (2006) Point-of-care-testing and clinical governance. *Clinical Chemistry and Laboratory Medicine* **44**, 765–767. doi:10.1515/CCLM.2006.129

Plebani M (2009) Does POCT reduce the risk of error in laboratory testing? *Clinica Chimica Acta* **404**, 59–64. doi:10.1016/j.cca.2009.03.014

Price CP, St John A (2005) Point-of-care testing. In *Tietz Textbook of Clinical Chemistry and Molecular Diagnostics.* (Eds C Burtis, E Ashwood and D Bruns) pp. 299–329. AACC Press, Washington DC, USA.

Price C, St John A (2006) *Point-of-Care Testing for Managers and Policymakers.* AACC Press, Washington DC, USA.

Ricos C, Alvarez V, Cava F, Garcia-Lario JV, Hernandez A, Jimenez CV, *et al.* (1999) Current databases on biological variation: pros, cons and progress. *Scandinavian Journal of Clinical and Laboratory Investigation* **59**, 491–500. doi:10.1080/00365519950185229

RCPA (Royal College of Pathologists of Australasia) (2014) *Point of Care Testing: Elements of a Quality Framework.* RCPA, Sydney, <http://www.rcpa.edu.au/getattachment/26d1e702-f250-4699-a8d2-8044332378e/POCT-Elements-of-a-Quality-Framework.aspx>.

Shephard MDS, Gill J (2010) The National QAAMS Program – a practical example of PoCT working in the community. *The Clinical Biochemist Reviews* **31**, 95–99.

Shephard M, Leibie A, Dimech W, Condie D, Nolan M (2012) Guidelines and recommendations for the quality-assured conduct of point-of-care testing for infectious diseases and drugs of abuse in Australia. *Australian Journal of Medical Science* **33**, 143–154.

Spanish Society of Clinical Biochemistry and Molecular Pathology (2009) Proposed guidelines for point-of-care testing services in Spain. *Point of Care* **8**, 53–55. doi:10.1097/POC.0b013e3181a49777

Stephens EJ (1999) Developing open standards for point-of-care connectivity. *IVD Technology* **10**, 22–25.

Tirimacco R, Glastonbury B, Laurence C, Bubner T, Shephard M, Beilby J (2011) Development of an accreditation program for Point of Care Testing (PoCT) in general practice. *Australian Health Review* **35**, 230–234. doi:10.1071/AH09792

# 3 Selection and evaluation of point-of-care testing devices

*Mark Shephard*

**Summary**

This chapter provides an overview of the different types of point-of-care testing (POCT) devices currently available on the global market. A POCT device should be able to achieve equivalent analytical performance to a corresponding laboratory device. For POC tests where a quantitative result is obtained, there are two main indicators of analytical performance: accuracy and precision. For POC tests where a qualitative result is obtained, the main performance indicators are sensitivity, specificity, negative predicative value and positive predictive value. This chapter provides practical guidance on how to measure these performance indicators in clinical practice.

## AN OVERVIEW OF POCT DEVICES

### 'Ideal' characteristics of a POCT device

As the scope and application of POCT continues to grow, manufacturers face the challenge of designing POCT devices that meet the needs of their consumers and can be adapted to the different clinical settings in which they are used. No single template for the 'ideal' POCT device exists. St John and Price (2014) identified desirable characteristics of POCT devices as: simplicity of use; robust reagents and consumables; results that are concordant with the laboratory; and safe to use.

In 2004, the World Health Organization (WHO) Sexually Transmitted Diseases Diagnostics Initiative (SDI) developed the ASSURED criteria (Table 3.1) to describe the ideal characteristics of POC tests required to tackle the burden of curable bacterial infections (e.g. syphilis, chlamydia and gonorrhoea in the developing world) (Peeling *et al.* 2006; WHO 2004).

These criteria have been well accepted and have provided a framework for guiding research and development and the evaluation of new POC tests and their prototypes (Natoli 2015). The term 'equipment free' originally referred to the use of simple immuno-strip technology, which dominated the POCT market for infectious

**Table 3.1.** The ASSURED criteria for rapid POC tests for sexually transmitted infections

| | | |
|---|---|---|
| A | = | **A**ffordable |
| S | = | **S**ensitive |
| S | = | **S**pecific |
| U | = | **U**ser-friendly (simple to perform in a few steps with minimal training) |
| R | = | **R**obust and rapid (results available in less than 30 min) |
| E | = | **E**quipment-free |
| D | = | **D**eliverable to those who need them |

diseases in the early 2000s; however, recent technological developments have changed the diagnostic landscape.

Simplicity of operation remains a key driver for manufacturers, with the design of an ideal POCT test system incorporating minimal sample and reagent preparation, sample loading that does not require dispensing of an exact sample volume (e.g. using a fixed volumetric pipette) and a minimum number of manual steps that do not require any timed addition of reagents.

## SYNOPSIS OF POCT DEVICES CURRENTLY AVAILABLE

A global compendium a decade ago listed ~200 POCT devices that featured or were likely to feature on the POCT market (Tran and Kost 2006). The number and range of devices on the current POCT market is ever increasing and difficult to track, such is the pace of change and technological innovation.

In broad terms, POCT devices can be grouped according to:

- physical size/portability
- complexity/risk of harm
- whether they provide a qualitative, semiquantitative or quantitative result
- specimen type required for testing
- type of technology (test format)
- method principle.

### Size and portability

In terms of size, most devices can be classed as either 'handheld' or 'bench-top' devices, with the latter ranging in size from small and portable to those that are larger, heavier and more suited to a satellite laboratory (Fig. 3.1).

Common examples of small, portable, hand-held POCT devices include: dipsticks for basic urine chemistry markers; lateral flow immuno-chromatographic test strips for cardiac markers, D-dimer, a range of infectious diseases including HIV and syphilis, for example, and drugs of abuse POC tests; hand-held battery-operated meters for measuring single tests such as glucose and international normalised ratio (INR); and the i-STAT®

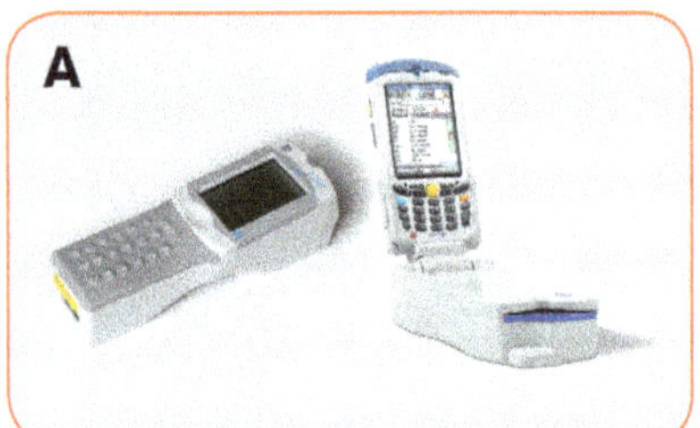


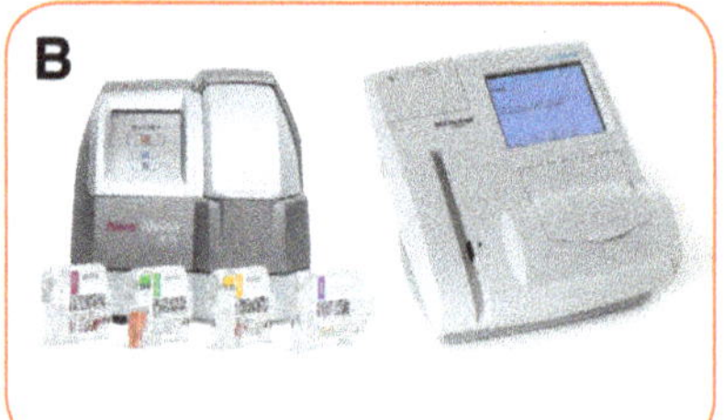


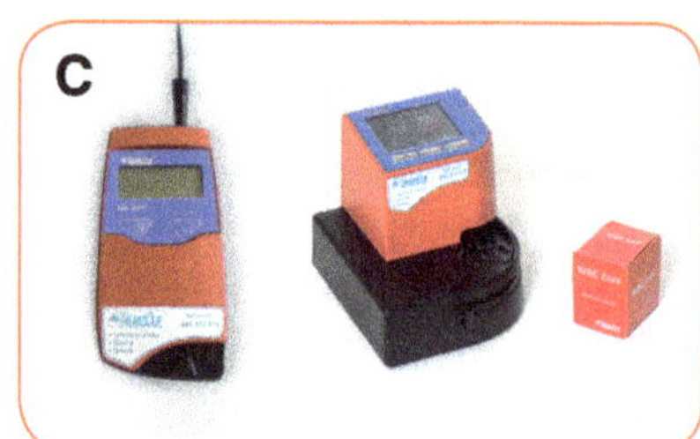


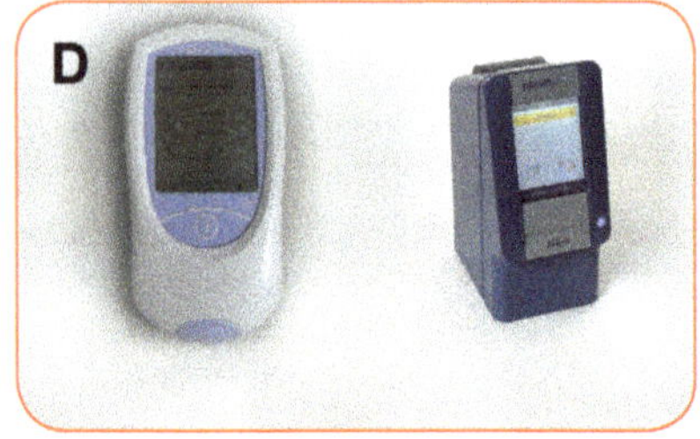


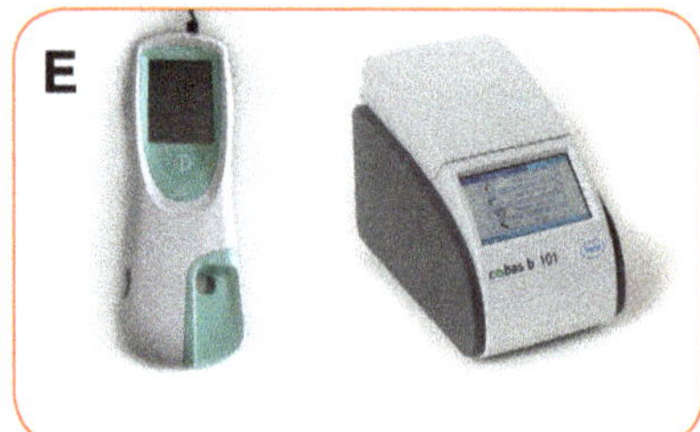


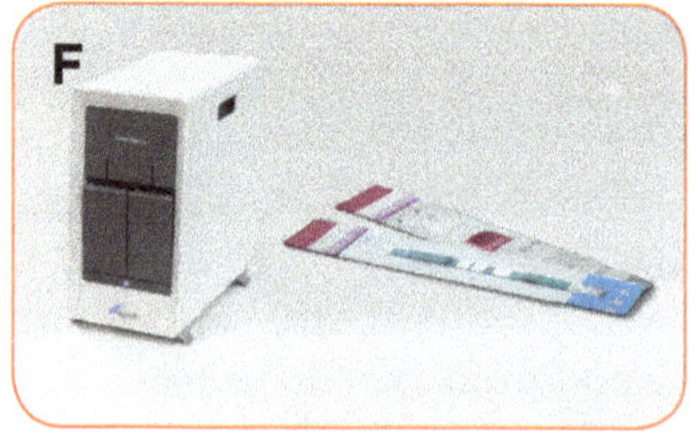


epoc® System and Determine™ HIV Combo strips, supplied courtesy of Alere.

**Fig. 3.1.** Examples of different types of POCT devices and the tests they measure. A: The Abbott i-STAT® and Alere epoc® test systems measure tests such as electrolytes, urea, creatinine, glucose, blood gases and lactate. B: The Alere Afinion™ and Siemens DCA Vantage® measure tests such as haemoglobin A1c and urine albumin:creatinine ratio. C: The Radiometer HemoCue® Hb 201+ and HemoCue® WBC DIFF systems measure haemoglobin and white blood cell count (with 5-part differential) respectively. D: The Roche CoaguChek® XS System measures International Normalised Ratio and the Abaxis Piccolo Xpress® measures electrolytes, lipids, bone and liver function panels. E: The Roche cobas® h 232 measures troponin T and D-dimer and the cobas® b 101 measures haemoglobin A1c and lipids. F: The Cepheid GeneXpert® measures many infectious disease tests including tuberculosis, chlamydia and gonorrhoea and the Alere Determine™ HIV 1/2 Ag/Ab Combo strips measure both HIV-1/2 antibodies and the HIV-1 antigen.

(Abbott Point of Care) or epoc® test systems (Alere), both of which can measure profiles of tests including electrolytes and blood gases and also work from battery power.

Well known examples of small, portable bench-top devices [devices that are lightweight (generally 5 kg or less), have a small footprint (generally around 30 $cm^3$ or less) and sit compactly on a small area of work bench] include:

- the DCA Vantage® (Siemens Ltd), Afinion™ (Alere), cobas® b 101 (Roche), all of which measure HbA1c and variously other chronic disease markers such as urine albumin:creatinine ratio (ACR) and lipids
- the Cholestech LDX® lipid analyser (Alere)
- the Piccolo Xpress® (Abaxis), which has a wide test profile range including electrolyte, bone, liver and lipid function panels
- the LABGEO suite of chemistry and haematology analysers (Samsung)
- the HemoCue® white blood cell differential counter (Radiometer)
- the modular GeneXpert system (Cepheid) for a range of critical infectious diseases and sexually transmitted infections (STIs).

Mid- to large-sized bench-top analysers are generally heavier and lack the portability of the smaller bench-top devices but can be transported to the site where POCT is conducted (e.g. on a hospital trolley). Some would argue that these devices blur the boundaries between a true POCT device and a satellite laboratory device. Examples include:

- blood gas/critical care analysers such as the GEM Premier™ range (Instrumentation Laboratories), ABL Flex range (Radiometer) and RapidPoint® 500 systems (Siemens), which also measure an array of other electrolyte, oximetry and metabolic parameters
- the QBC Star™ Dry Haematology analyser (Drucker Diagnostics), which measures a complete blood count
- the D-10™ (BioRad) device for measuring HbA1c.

## Complexity/risk of harm

In some countries, medical devices (including POCT devices) are classified by government regulation according to the complexity of performing the test and/or the potential risk of harm to the patient or to the general public. In the USA, the *Clinical Laboratory Improvement Amendments (CLIA) Act 1988* classifies tests/test systems as being of low, moderate or high complexity. The list of so-termed 'waived tests' (those performed on devices of low complexity and with low risk) include a large range of handheld and small cartridge-based POCT systems (Washington State Department of Health 2015). Some waived tests do have potential for serious health impacts if performed incorrectly; for example, results from waived tests used to adjust medication dosages, such as INR testing in patients undergoing anticoagulant therapy and glucose monitoring in diabetes patients. In Australia, the Therapeutics Goods Administration (TGA) classifies *in vitro* medical devices (IVD) into four classes (I to IV) based on risk posed to the health of the general public or an individual, with tests for HIV, hepatitis B and C being examples in the high public health risk classification (IV) (Australian Government 2011).

## Qualitative or quantitative result

Most clinical chemistry and haematology POCT devices generate a quantitative result (i.e. provide a number in a specified unit of measurement). Many infectious disease and drugs of abuse POCT devices provide a qualitative result (i.e. determine whether the disease or drug of abuse is present or absent). There are also POCT devices that produce a semiquantitative result, providing a range of concentrations within which the results lay (e.g. a urine ACR result between 3.5 and 30 mg/mmol lies within the microalbuminuria range).

## Specimen type

Many different specimen types can be measured using POCT devices. Capillary (finger prick), venous or arterial whole blood and urine are the most common sample types. Capillary samples (with volumes <50 μL) are the sample of choice with many small handheld devices. Once the sample volume is over 50 μL, then a venous whole blood sample should be collected, because excessive milking of the finger can result in mixing of blood with interstitial fluid. Arterial blood is generally the preferred specimen type for blood gas analysers. Other specimen types such as saliva, semen, sweat or breath, genital, nasal or throat swabs, and faeces are required for some infectious disease POC tests.

## POCT technology design, format and analytical principles

Measurement of POC tests involves recognising the analyte to be tested and detecting the resultant signal. The two most widely available recognition agents (reagents) are chemosensors, which use a chemical indicator or binding molecule, or biosensors, which use an antibody or an enzyme, to recognise the analyte. The two most widely used detection systems are photometric (measurement of light at selected wavelengths) and electrochemical (measurement of electrical energy through the movement of electrons from one element to another, so called 'redox' reactions). Photometric detection systems can be subject to interferences by a range of competing compounds, whereas electrochemical methods are generally highly specific for the test analyte.

POCT devices most commonly employ one of three main testing formats:

- Single-use, qualitative or semiquantitative testing strips or cups; as the name implies, 'single-use' means that only one patient sample can be tested using each strip
- Single-use quantitative testing strips or test receptacles with a reading (or monitoring) device
- Multi-use quantitative testing cartridges with a larger bench-top (reading or monitoring) device; 'multi-use' meaning the cartridges can be used to test multiple patient samples (Price and St John 2008).

The most common qualitative or semiquantitative test strips include urine dipsticks and immuno-chromatographic (lateral flow) test strips. Dipsticks represent the simplest and most basic form of POCT technology. They consist of a series of reagent pads (for up to 10 basic chemistries) on a plastic strip. The pads are immersed in a urine sample and a semiquantitative result for each test is measured by photometry. Manual reading of each pad is time dependent and subjective. Several companies now market automated strip readers (e.g. the Siemens CLINITEK Status®+ range of urinalysis devices).

Test strips employing lateral flow technology are popular for POC tests involving immunological reactions. Lateral flow immunoassay (LFIA) involves the movement of a liquid sample containing the analyte along a thin strip of polymeric material (usually nitrocellulose, nylon or polyethylene). The strips are commonly housed in a plastic holder, in which only the sample application area and the reading window are visible. In a basic lateral flow immunoassay, the major components include:

- a sample application area, where the sample or its extract containing the test analyte is loaded
- a conjugate release pad, containing labelled antigen or labelled antibody as the recognition element. Labels typically include coloured or fluorescent nanoparticles such as colloidal gold, latex or liposomes. The conjugate combines with the sample as its flows towards the detection zone
- the detection zone containing:
  - an immobilised test line, where signal recognition of the analyte occurs
  - a control line, which usually contains an anti-species immunoglobulin G for the purpose of confirming the complete flow of the liquid across the length of the strip
- an absorbent pad attached to the end of the strip, which maintains or 'wicks' the flow of the liquid to the strip's end (Posthuma-Trumpie *et al.* 2009).

There are two main formats for LFIA: competitive LFIA, where the response is negatively correlated with the amount of analyte in the sample; and sandwich LFIA, where the response is directly proportional to the amount of analyte in the sample (Table 3.2).

Although popular for many years, LFIA suffers two main drawbacks: poor sensitivity has been reported for

**Table 3.2.** Examples of different types of lateral flow immunoassay formats

| Format | Number of analyte binding sites in sample | Conjugate (flows with sample) | Test line (immobilised) | Signal |
|---|---|---|---|---|
| Competitive | One epitope | Labelled analyte | Antibody to analyte | Negatively correlated with analyte concentration (more analyte present, less signal) |
| | One epitope | Labelled antibody | Analyte/protein conjugate | |
| Sandwich | Two epitopes | Labelled anti-analyte antibody (secondary) | Anti-analyte antibody (primary) | Signal directly proportional to analyte concentration (free epitope can bind to immobilised antibody at test line) |

many infectious disease POC tests using this format and the capacity to perform more than one POC test at a time (so called 'multiplexing') is limited.

Examples of different types of single-use quantitative test receptacles include the cartridge (with the i-STAT, DCA Vantage and GeneXpert devices, for example), cassette (Cholestech LDX), cuvette (HemoCue haemoglobin and white blood cell differential counter), and rotor (Piccolo and cobas b 101). Along with test strips for glucose and INR, these test receptacles are usually inserted into a reading device where the reaction is monitored and the signal is measured and quantified within a short turnaround time.

In the infectious disease area, a new generation of POCT devices are using nucleic acid amplification technology (NAAT) or 'molecular testing' to measure an ever-widening range of test species. The GeneXpert (Cepheid CA, USA) is one such device. The GeneXpert was recently endorsed by the WHO as being able to support the diagnosis of multi-drug-resistant tuberculosis in high burden, low resource settings (Niemz *et al.* 2011). The GeneXpert employs a fully automated 'sample in/answer out' test system. DNA extraction, amplification using polymerase chain reaction (PCR) and real-time fluorescence detection of the test species occurs in a single cartridge, free of contamination (Fig. 3.2). At this time, the GeneXpert remains expensive and has a long result turnaround time (90–120 min). Cost and turnaround time can be reduced by using other forms of amplification, such as loop-mediated isothermal amplification (where a constant temperature, rather than thermal cycling, is used during amplification) (Mori and Notomi 2009; Parida *et al.* 2008; Tao *et al.* 2011). These molecular testing devices can provide results with sensitivities and specificities approaching 100% and are revolutionising the realm of infectious disease POCT.

Many of the larger critical care bench-top devices now have multi-use quantitative cartridges. Here, re-usable sensors constructed using thick-film technology, together with the required reagents and calibrants, are bundled into a single 'long-life, maintenance-free' cartridge pack. The cartridge pack is inserted into the POCT device and can perform hundreds of analyses. This makes these devices simple to use and cost effective, because the operator only needs to change the disposable pack when it has performed a set number of analyses or after a given time period. The devices also feature automated liquid calibration systems (instead of using gas cylinders) as well as automated QC sampling and QC programs that provide interpretative analysis of results (St John and Price 2014).

There are many new and innovative POCT technologies in the pipeline (St John and Price 2014). 'Lab on a Chip' or 'microchip' technology continues to undergo development and refinement, particularly for use with infectious disease POCT (Daw and Finkelstein 2006). Lab on a Chip technology aims to miniaturise an entire analytical test system for POCT (including separation and analysis using extremely small fluid volumes) onto a small microprocessor chip only a few millimetres to a few square centimetres in size.

Many companies (such as 'Diagnostics for All') are now investing heavily in devices that employ paper as a base material (rather than, for example, nitrocellulose). Paper-based devices are now being developed that use advanced microfluidics and have the potential to perform multiple assays at the same time. Paper is an inexpensive material and can be incinerated following test completion (Yetisen *et al.* 2013), making this technology ideally suited for the developing world. At this time, neither microchip nor paper-based technology has resulted in any commercially available POCT devices.

Table 3.3 compares and contrasts different types of *in vitro* POCT devices currently available. Table 3.4 summarises differences between POC tests for clinical chemistry and haematology and those for infectious diseases and drugs of abuse.

## HOW TO CONDUCT AN ANALYTICAL EVALUATION OF A POINT-OF-CARE TESTING DEVICE – IN PRACTICE

In Chapter 2, factors to consider when selecting the 'right' POCT device for your health service were discussed. The device needs to be fit for purpose and should be able to achieve equivalent analytical performance compared with a laboratory instrument that measures the same test. But how do you evaluate a POCT device's performance in a primary care setting in real terms?

The local accredited laboratory or specialist POCT provider should be consulted to support a health service in setting up an evaluation, as these groups are experienced in this task.

Many global professional organisations and expert groups have provided advice on how to conduct evaluations. For example, the Clinical and Laboratory Standards Institute (CLSI) has published two approved guidelines:

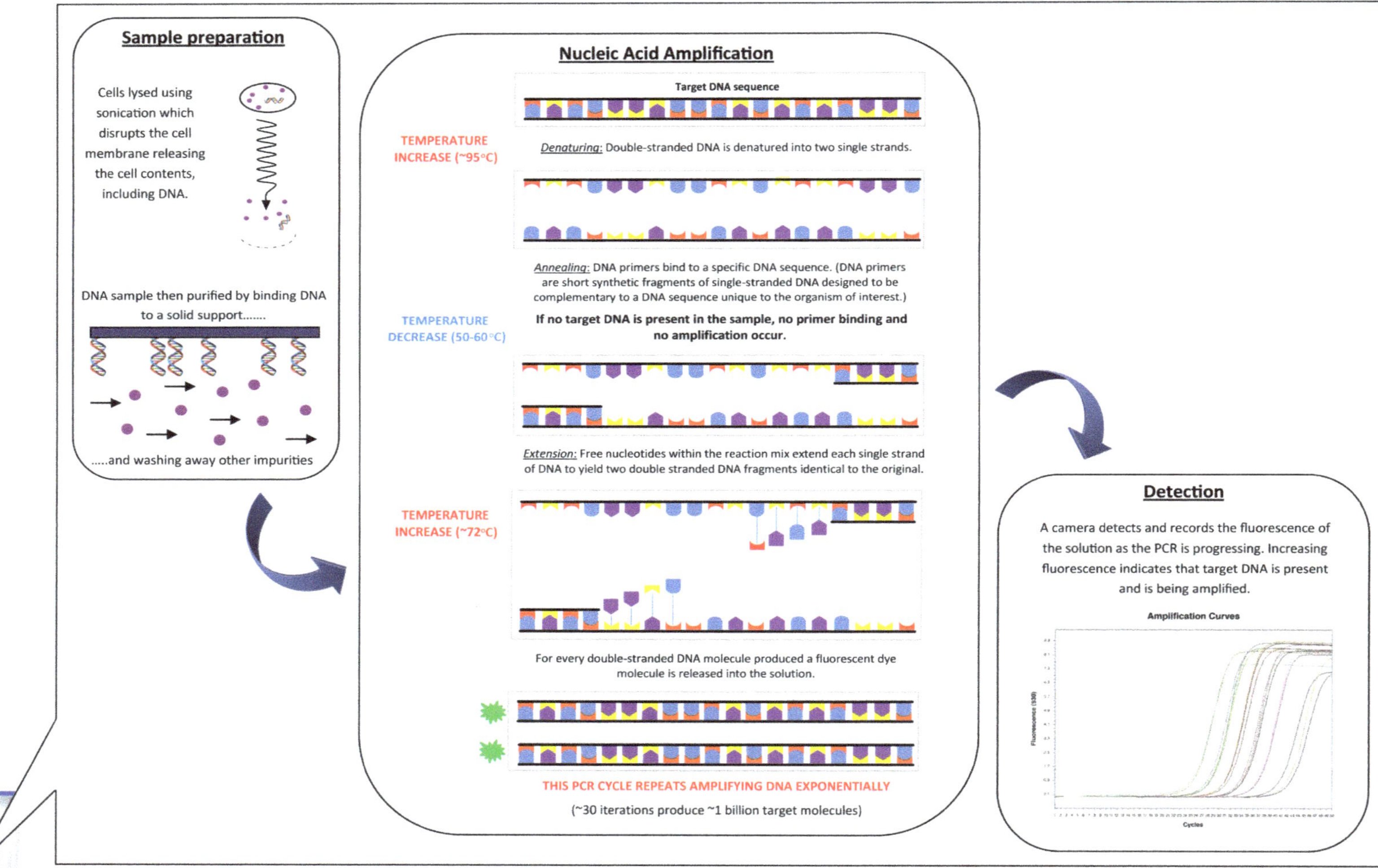


**Fig. 3.2.** Diagrammatic representation of the molecular testing (or NAAT) process, used by the GeneXpert (Cepheid). (Diagram prepared by Claire Simon, Flinders University)

**Table 3.3.** Examples of the range of *in vitro* POCT devices available in today's market

| Device name/ manufacturer | Size | Example of tests measured | Specimen type | Result | Technology | Usage | Analytical principle (recognition/ detection) |
|---|---|---|---|---|---|---|---|
| Urine dipstick (Multistix 10SG)/ Siemens | Hand-held | pH, protein, glucose, ketones, bilirubin, urobilingen, blood, leukocytes, nitrites, specific gravity | Urine | Semiquantitative | Test strip | Single use | Chemical/visual |
| Cardiac Trop T/ Roche | Hand-held | Troponin T | Venous whole blood | Semiquantitative | Test strip in plastic case | Single use | Lateral flow immunoassay/visual |
| CoaguChek S/ Roche | Hand-held | INR | Capillary whole blood | Quantitative | Test strip with reading device | Single use | Enzymatic/ electrochemical |
| i-STAT/Abbott | Hand-held | Electrolytes and blood gases | Venous and arterial whole blood | Quantitative | Cartridge with reading device | Single use | Electrochemical |
| DCA Vantage/ Siemens | Bench-top | HbA1c | Capillary whole blood | Quantitative | Cartridge with reading device | Single use | Immunoassay (inhibition of latex agglutination)/ photometry |
| HemoCue WBC Diff/Radiometer | Bench-top | Total white blood cell count and 5-part differential (lymphocytes, neutrophils, monocytes, eosinophils, basophils) | Capillary whole blood | Quantitative | Micro-cuvette with cell counting device | Single use | Haemolysis with image analysis |
| Piccolo/Abaxis | Bench-top | Lipids | Venous whole blood | Quantitative | Rotor | Single use | Enzymatic/ photometry |
| GeneXpert/ Cepheid | Bench-top | Chlamydia and gonorrhoea | Vaginal swab Urine | Qualitative | Cartridge | Single use | DNA extraction and amplification (NAAT)/ fluorescence |
| QBC Star/Drucker Diagnostics | Mid-sized Bench-top | Complete blood count (9 parameters) | Venous whole blood | Quantitative | Separation tube | Multi use | Centrifugal separation/ optical signal analysis |
| GEM Premier 4000/ Instrumentation Laboratories | Large Bench-top | Blood gases | Arterial whole blood | Quantitative | Cartridge | Multi use | Electrochemical |

**Table 3.4.** Differences between POCT for infectious diseases and drugs of abuse and POCT for clinical chemistry and haematology tests

| Parameter | Infectious disease and drugs of abuse POC testing | Clinical chemistry and haematology POC testing |
|---|---|---|
| Clinical use | Detection | Diagnosis and management |
| Result | Qualitative | Quantitative |
| Analytical performance indicators | Sensitivity and specificity | Accuracy and precision |
| Testing matrices | Multiple fluid types | Mainly blood/urine |

- EP05-A3. Evaluation of precision of quantitative measurement procedures; Approved guideline – 3rd edition (2014)
- EP09-A3. Measurement procedure comparison and bias estimation using patient samples; Approved guideline – 3rd edition (2013).

These two documents are designed for laboratories and, although thorough, their methods are too complex for evaluating a POCT device in a primary care setting.

The UNICEF/UNDP/World Bank/WHO Special Programme for Research and Training in Tropical Diseases (WHO/TFR) Expert Group has published a series of guidelines for the evaluation of rapid diagnostics tests since 2006 (Peeling *et al.* 2006; TDR Diagnostics Evaluation Expert Panel 2010; WHO/TDR Sexually Transmitted Diseases Diagnostics Initiative 2006a,b). In Australia, the Australasian Association of Clinical Biochemists (AACB) and the Australian Institute of Medical Scientists (AIMS) have published information on method evaluations (AACB 2012; Shephard *et al.* 2012).

In 2003, an international expert group of scientists and editors developed the landmark STARD (*Sta*ndards for *R*eporting of *D*iagnostic Accuracy) statement to improve the quality of reporting of studies of diagnostic accuracy (Bossuyt *et al.* 2003). The statement comprised a checklist of 25 items and a flow diagram to ensure that all relevant information is presented when reporting such evaluation studies (www.stard-statement.org; TDR Diagnostics Evaluation Expert Panel 2010).

The remaining section of this chapter provides practical instruction on the principles and practice of how to conduct a basic device evaluation, and attempts to demystify some of the laboratory concepts and terms used in this field. Table 3.5 lists a glossary of key terms relating to the evaluation of quantitative POCT devices.

For POC tests that generate a quantitative result, key analytical performance indicators are accuracy (closeness to the true result) and precision (reproducibility or repeatability of the test result when the same sample is tested multiple times). For POC tests that deliver a qualitative result, key performance indicators are sensitivity (the proportion of patients with disease who test positive) and specificity (the proportion of patients without disease who test negative).

## POCT DEVICE EVALUATION FOR QUANTITATIVE TESTS

All laboratories monitor the accuracy and imprecision of their devices closely, and it is important to do the same with point-of-care devices.

### Explaining the concepts of accuracy and precision

Accuracy refers to how close the POC test result is to the true value in the sample tested (Shephard 2006). For example, if a POC test result for cholesterol is 5.5 mmol/L and the true result on that sample is 5.3 mmol/L, then the POCT device has an inaccuracy or positive bias of 0.2 mmol/L. Small biases are acceptable but it is important that the bias observed with the POCT device is not so great that it can incorrectly change patient management.

Precision refers to 'how much variability there is when a patient sample is tested repeatedly' (Shephard 2006). Intuitively, a health professional may think that all devices (whether laboratory or point-of-care) should give the same result every time, but this is not the case. All medical devices have a degree of random error (or uncertainty) around their ability to consistently measure the same sample. It is important that the degree of imprecision is known and that this level of 'analytical noise' is kept as small as possible. For example, let's assume we have a blood sample in which the true cholesterol value is

**Table 3.5.** Definitions for key terms for evaluation of quantitative POCT devices

| Term | Definition |
|---|---|
| Accuracy | The closeness of the agreement between the measured value and the true value of an analyte. |
| Analytical goal | The level of performance required to ensure that a pathology test fulfils its stated or implied purpose. The terms analytical goals, analytical quality specifications, and allowable limits of performance are used interchangeably. |
| Analyte | The pathology test that is being measured. |
| Bias (or inaccuracy) | The numerical difference between the measured value and the true value of an analyte. |
| Coefficient of variation (CV%) | A statistical measure of imprecision, calculated as the standard deviation divided by the mean of replicate measurements and expressed as a percentage. Thus CV% = (s.d./mean) × 100. |
| Imprecision (or analytical imprecision) | The standard deviation or coefficient of variation of the results in a set of replicate measurements of an analyte. |
| Precision | The closeness of agreement between replicate measurements on the same analyte under specified conditions; precision is also often referred to as the reproducibility, repeatability or scatter of a set of replicate measurements. |
| Standard deviation | A statistical measure of imprecision (or the dispersion of replicate measurements on the same analyte), calculated as the square root of the sum of the squares of the difference between each data point and the mean divided by the total number of data points minus one. |
| Total (analytical) error | The sum of the bias and imprecision, usually defined by the formula TE = [bias] + 1.65 × imprecision; where bias does not have a sign. |
| Total allowable error | The analytical goal or quality specification for total error. |

7.5 mmol/L. If that sample is tested 5-times (on either a laboratory or POC device), the result may be, for example, 7.4 mmol/L the first time the sample is measured, 7.7 the next time, 7.6 the third time, then 7.5 and 7.3. The average of the 5 results is 7.5 mmol/L but there is a degree of variability or dispersion around that mean result – and that degree of variability is what is termed the imprecision of the device.

The sum of the bias and imprecision is called the total error of measurement (usually defined by the formula TE = [bias] + 1.65 × imprecision, where the bias does not have a sign).

The analogy of a golfer putting a golf ball towards the hole can be used to further explain the difference between accuracy and precision (Fig. 3.3). Ideally, the golfer is trying to hit the golf ball into the hole or as close to it as possible; if the golfer does, then his putting will be both accurate (because his putts are close to the target – the hole), and precise (because the golf balls are tightly bunched). But consider when his putts miss the hole by a long distance but are tightly bunched together. Here, his putting is precise (because there is not much variability in his putts) but they are not accurate (because they have missed the hole, or target). Finally, consider when his putts are widely scattered and away from the hole (and therefore the putts are neither precise nor accurate). As with the golf analogy, our POCT device should ideally produce results that are both accurate and precise. Precision is about getting the 'same result' when a sample is tested multiple times, while accuracy is about getting the 'right result'.

## Why do we need precise and accurate results?

With a POC test such as HbA1c or cholesterol, where a patient is having repeated tests across time for their diabetes management, the results will change across these serial measurements. It's important the treating doctor is confident that these changes truly reflect a clinically significant change in the patient and are not masked by the analytical imprecision or 'noise' of the test method (i.e. any analytical imprecision needs to be as small as possible to see those clinically significant changes).

Also, for tests such as HbA1c and cholesterol, there are targets or optimal management goals for the diabetes patient: for example, 53 mmol/mol (7%) for HbA1c and 4.0 mmol/L for cholesterol. It's therefore important that the POCT device can measure these targets accurately.

In a network of POCT devices measuring HbA1c or cholesterol, for example, it's vital that all devices in the

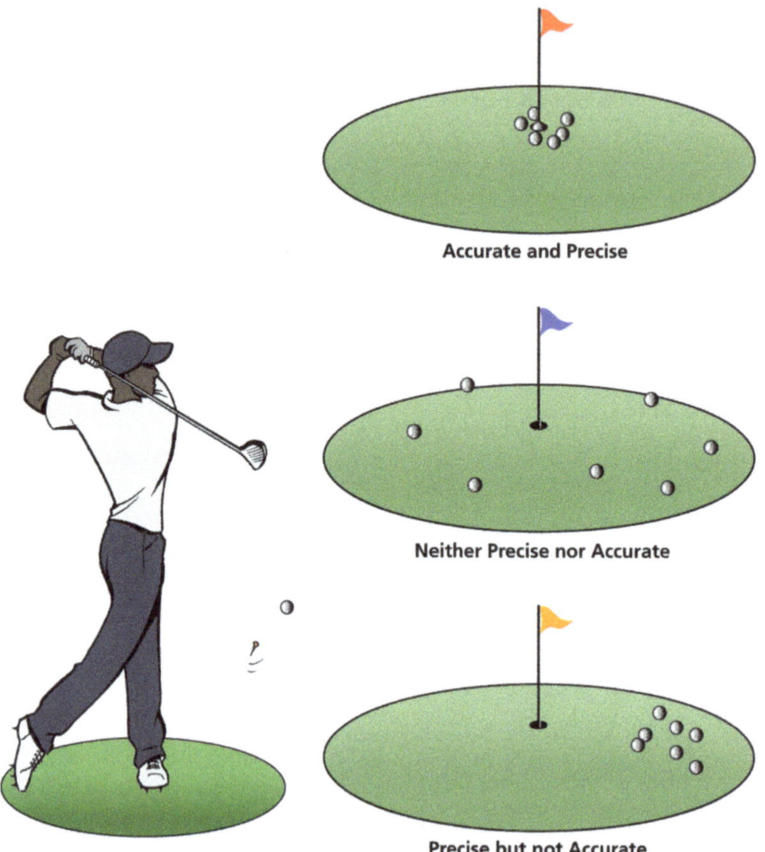


**Fig. 3.3.** Explaining the concepts of accuracy and precision.

network are performing well analytically and giving close to the same results for these tests. If, for example, a patient from one community moves to a different community for his/her POC testing; there needs to be transferability of quality between health facilities conducting POCT.

## How then is an evaluation of a POCT device performed in practice?

### Accuracy

To determine how well a POCT device performs in terms of accuracy, a patient comparison study is performed whereby a selected number of patient samples are tested by both the POCT and the laboratory devices. As a minimum requirement, 40 samples (ideally 100) with a wide range of concentrations should be tested by both devices.

#### *Passing and Bablock (linear) regression*

Passing and Bablock linear regression is used explicitly for method comparison studies (Bablock *et al.* 1988). Unlike least-squares (LS) linear regression, Passing and Bablock regression assumes there is measurement error in the independent variable. Passing and Bablock regression also allows for the assessment of both fixed and proportional bias. Using the Passing and Bablock method, results obtained by both the POCT (y) and the laboratory methods (x) are plotted against each other and the following parameters can be calculated:

- slope (m) – the closer the slope is to 1.00, the better the performance of the POCT method
- intercept (c) – the closer the intercept is to zero, the better the performance of the POCT method.

Fig. 3.4 shows examples of Passing and Bablock regression analysis for a POCT device with good (A) and poorer accuracy (B, C). Even visually, it is possible to see in plot A that the results obtained by POCT (*y*-axis) for each patient sample are very close to those results obtained by the laboratory (*x*-axis), the slope is close to 1 (actual slope 1.02) and the intercept coefficient is close to zero (actual –0.1).

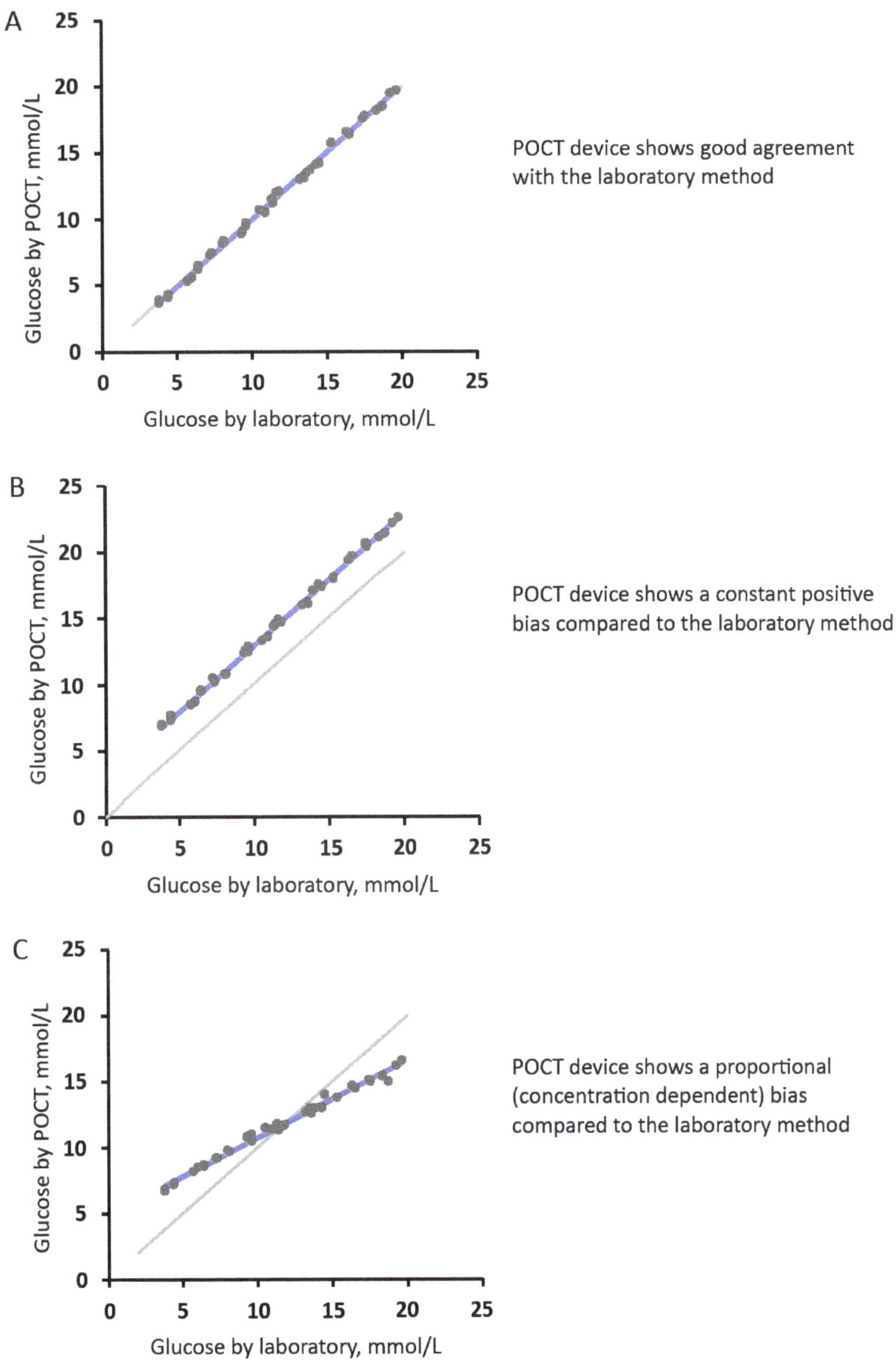


**Fig. 3.4.** Passing and Bablock linear regression analyses showing a POCT device with good (A) and poorer accuracy (B, C).

In contrast, plots B and C in Fig. 3.4 show examples of a POCT device with poorer accuracy. Plot B indicates that the POCT results are always higher than the laboratory method's results; that is; the POCT device has a constant positive bias. Here the slope is 1.00 but the intercept is 3.0. POCT results in plot C show a proportional bias; that is, the bias of the POCT device is concentration dependent with a positive bias observed at low concentrations and a negative bias at higher concentrations (actual slope 0.59 and intercept 4.9).

*Bland-Altman difference plots*

Results of a patient comparison can be examined in another way; this time the difference between the POC test result and the laboratory result (POCT result – laboratory result) is plotted on the *y*-axis versus the mean concentration of the test results (POC result + laboratory result/2) on the *x*-axis. This is called a Bland-Altman difference plot (Bland and Altman 1999). Here it is possible to calculate the average (mean) bias of the POCT device relative to the laboratory, and the limits of agreement (LOA) (i.e. the limits within which 95% of the differences fall). These parameters provide a sound indication of 'how good' a POCT method is in terms of its accuracy. Obviously the closer the mean bias is to zero the more accurate is the method, while the limits of agreement should not be too wide; that is, the absolute values for both the upper and lower limits should be within clinically acceptable differences. Using this type of plot, it is also possible to see if the bias is constant or proportional.

Fig. 3.5 displays a Bland-Altman plot for two POCT lipid analysers versus the same laboratory instrument. The mean bias for cholesterol was –0.08 (LOA –0.63 to +0.48 mmol/L) for device 1 (plot A), but was +0.58 mmol/L (–0.75 to +1.93 mmol/L) for device 2 (plot B). Even visually, it is possible to see that POCT device 1 has almost zero bias compared with the laboratory method and the limits of agreement are much tighter than that seen with POCT device 2 (which has a positive bias of ~0.6 mmol/L and wider limits of agreement). Similar trends are evident for triglyceride estimation on device 1 (plot C) and device 2 (plot D).

*Concordance*

As another measure of accuracy, the ability of the POCT device to correctly classify results as being within or outside therapeutic targets compared with the laboratory device can be determined. For example, tests such as HbA1c and lipids have defined therapeutic targets for diabetes patients, with an HbA1c of 53 mmol/mol (7%) and a cholesterol of 4 mmol/L being targets for optimal control. Results are concordant if both POCT and laboratory devices classify the patient as being within (or outside) the range, and discordant if the POCT and laboratory results classify patients differently (Gialamas *et al.* 2010). Concordance/discordance can be expressed as a number or percentage. Ideally, the degree of discordance should be small (e.g. <10%) for POCT methods with sound accuracy.

**Precision**

Imprecision, expressed as a coefficient of variation [CV%], is calculated using the formula:

$$CV\% = \frac{s.d.}{\overline{X}} \times 100\%$$

where s.d. = standard deviation and $\overline{X}$ = mean of all results.

As a general rule, the lower the imprecision, the better the performance of the device.

Imprecision can be assessed in several ways.

The samples used in the patient comparison can be tested in duplicate on the POCT device, with the imprecision estimated as follows: take the differences between the duplicates, square each difference, add up all the squares, divide by twice the number of pairs of results and take the square root (Fraser 1986). The full formula is:

$$s.d. = \sqrt{\frac{\sum (difference\ between\ pairs)^2}{2\,x\,number\ of\ pairs}}$$

This s.d. and the mean $\overline{X}$ concentration is used to calculate the CV%.

Table 3.6 shows how to construct a template to calculate the imprecision using POCT samples analysed in duplicate.

Alternatively, two, or ideally three, patient samples with different concentrations can be tested once per day for a minimum of 10 days. The mean, s.d. and CV% can be calculated for each concentration level to give an estimate of the between-day imprecision. If patient samples are not available, then two or three levels of quality control testing material can be used instead. If the test being measured is not stable for up to 10 days, then the 10 repeat measurements can be performed on the same day to give an estimate of within-day imprecision. There are other

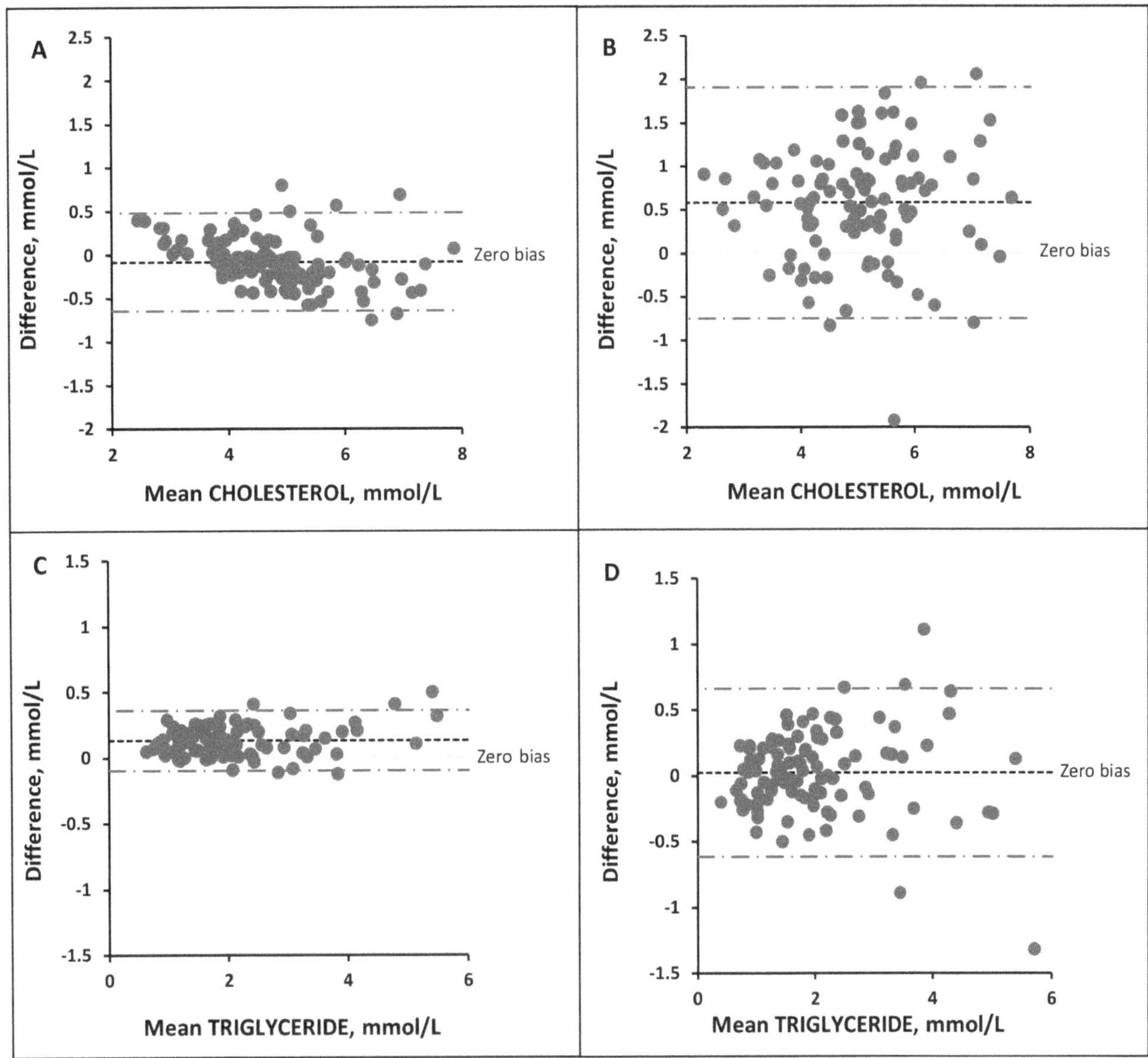


**Fig. 3.5.** Bland Altman plot showing a lipid POCT device with good (A and C) and poorer accuracy (B and D) for total cholesterol and triglyceride.

ways of reporting imprecision depending on how the evaluation is constructed; these can include for example:

- between-batch imprecision to see if there are differences in imprecision between different lot numbers of the same reagent when testing the same samples
- between-device imprecision, when one or more devices are used to test the same samples in the patient comparison
- between-operator imprecision to see if there is any difference in imprecision recorded between two or more device operators when testing the same samples.

Table 3.7 illustrates how to record data from a basic imprecision study where three patient samples with different levels of HbA1c were tested daily for 10 days.

### Analytical goals

Having determined the accuracy and precision of a POCT device, how is it possible to know whether the observed performance is 'good enough'; that is; meets analytical standards expected for the test? For most laboratory analytes, published analytical performance standards or 'analytical goals' provide the benchmark against which

**Table 3.6.** An example of a template for conducting an imprecision study using paired patient samples

| Patient | POCT result 1 (HbA1c mmol/mol) | POCT result 2 (HbA1c mmol/mol) | Difference between result (d) | Difference squared ($d^2$) |
|---|---|---|---|---|
| 1 | 53 | 58 | 5 | 25 |
| 2 | 87 | 84 | –3 | 9 |
| 3 | 110 | 117 | 7 | 49 |
| 4 | 77 | 73 | –4 | 16 |
| 5 | 95 | 97 | 2 | 4 |
| | Mean concentration of all 10 POCT HbA1c results = 85.2 mmol/mol | | | Sum of squares = 103 |

Sum of squares = 103
Divide by twice the number of pairs = 2 × 5 pairs = 10; 103/10 = 10.3; take the square root = 3.2 = s.d.
CV = (3.2/mean concentration of 10 HbA1c POCT results = 85.2) ×100
CV% from duplicate pairs = 3.8%

performance for bias, imprecision and total allowable error can be assessed (Westgard 2014). Using the premise that POC tests should be of equivalent standard to the laboratory, these laboratory-derived goals can also be used to assess POCT performance (Fraser 2001).

In Table 3.8, the results of an evaluation of two POCT devices for cholesterol are compared with the analytical goals for imprecision, inaccuracy and total error for cholesterol set by the National Cholesterol Education Program (NCEP) (Warnick *et al.* 2002). Device 1 met all the NCEP goals for cholesterol, while Device 2 did not meet the NCEP goals and showed significant bias and total error well outside the recommended goals.

**Table 3.7.** An example of a template for conducting a between-day imprecision study using patients with different analyte concentrations

| Day | Patient 1 (HbA1c 7.0%) | Patient 2 (HbA1c 9.0%) | Patient 3 (HbA1c 11.0%) |
|---|---|---|---|
| 1 | 6.9 | 9.4 | 11.1 |
| 2 | 6.7 | 9.1 | 10.7 |
| 3 | 7.1 | 9.1 | 11.2 |
| 4 | 7.1 | 9.0 | 10.9 |
| 5 | 6.9 | 8.9 | 10.8 |
| 6 | 7.1 | 9.3 | 11.4 |
| 7 | 7.2 | 9.1 | 10.7 |
| 8 | 6.7 | 9.2 | 11.2 |
| 9 | 6.9 | 8.8 | 11.3 |
| 10 | 6.8 | 8.9 | 11.1 |
| Mean | 6.94 | 9.08 | 11.06 |
| s.d. | 0.18 | 0.19 | 0.23 |
| CV% | 2.6% | 2.1% | 2.3% |

Different levels of analytical goals (minimum, desirable and optimal) have also been published for many common tests, based on fractions of within- and between-subject biological variation data, expert opinion or data from external proficiency testing programs (Westgard 2014; Shephard 2006). The minimum goal provides a measure of the widest allowable standard of analytical performance that a device/method should be able to achieve for a particular test; the desirable goal represents the standard of performance generally achievable by most devices/methods for a particular test; while the optimal goal is the standard of performance that only the very best methods can achieve for a particular test (Shephard *et al.* 2009). In practice, these analytical goals equate approximately to the standard of performance that the top 75%, top 50% (median) or top 20% of laboratories, respectively, can achieve in proficiency testing programs.

Table 3.9 shows the results of an HbA1c imprecision study conducted using three patient samples on two different POCT devices. POCT device 1 met the desirable (<3%) and minimum (<4%) analytical goals for HbA1c and compared closely with the performance of the laboratory HbA1c analyser. POCT device 2 could not meet the minimum imprecision goals at any level of patient HbA1c tested. Which POCT device would you choose?

## POCT DEVICE EVALUATION FOR QUALITATIVE TESTS

The two main performance indicators used to assess the performance of a qualitative POCT device are sensitivity and specificity.

Sensitivity is defined as the proportion of patients with the disease who test positive (i.e. the number of true

**Table 3.8.** Performance of two different POCT devices for cholesterol compared with the analytical goals recommended by the National Cholesterol Education Program

| Analyte | POCT device | Observed imprecision (CV%) | NCEP goal for imprecision (%) | Observed bias (%) | NCEP goal for bias (%) | Observed total error (%) | NCEP goal for total error (%) |
|---|---|---|---|---|---|---|---|
| Cholesterol | Device 1 | 3.0 | 3 | 1.7 | 3 | 6.7 | 9 |
| | Device 2 | 4.4 | | 12.1 | | 19.3 | |

**Table 3.9.** Comparison of imprecision (CV%) of two POCT devices for HbA1c versus the laboratory device and the analytical goals for HbA1c (minimum goal 4%, desirable goal 3% and optimal goal 2%) (Source: Shephard 2006)

| | Between-day imprecision (CV%) | | |
|---|---|---|---|
| **Device** | **Patient 1 (HbA1c 5.5%)** | **Patient 2 (HbA1c 7%)** | **Patient 3 (HbA1c 10%)** |
| Laboratory | 2.3 | 2.2 | 1.9 |
| POCT device 1 | 2.5 | 2.1 | 2.2 |
| POCT device 2 | 7.0 | 5.8 | 6.1 |

positive results divided by the number of true positive results plus the number of false negative results, expressed as a percentage). Specificity is the proportion of people without the disease who test negative (i.e. the number of true negative results divided by the number of true negative results plus the number of false positive results, expressed as a percentage).

Two other measures of performance are positive predictive value (PPV) and negative predicative value (NPV). The positive predictive value is the proportion of positive test results that are true positives (i.e. the number of true positive results divided by the number of true positive plus false positive results, expressed as a percentage). The negative predictive value is the proportion of negative test results that are true negatives (i.e. the number of true negative results divided by the number of true negative plus false negative results, expressed as a percentage).

Fig. 3.6 shows how the calculation of these performance indicators occurs in practice.

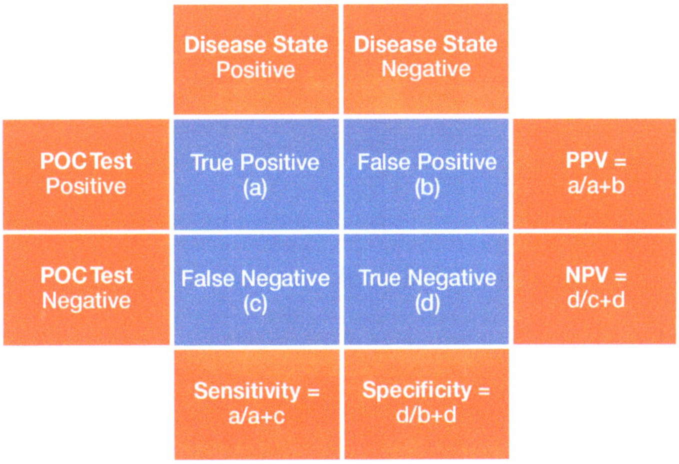

| | Disease State Positive | Disease State Negative | |
|---|---|---|---|
| POC Test Positive | True Positive (a) | False Positive (b) | PPV = a/a+b |
| POC Test Negative | False Negative (c) | True Negative (d) | NPV = d/c+d |
| | Sensitivity = a/a+c | Specificity = d/b+d | |

**Fig. 3.6.** Template for the calculation of sensitivity, specificity, positive predictive value and negative predictive value (when a POC test method is compared against a reference standard laboratory method that has determined the subject's clinical status)
Sensitivity = the proportion of those subjects with disease who test positive = a/(a + c)
Specificity = the proportion of those subjects without disease who test negative = d/(b + d)
PPV = the proportion of positive test results that are true positives = a/(a + b)
NPV = the proportion of negative test results that are true negatives = d/(c + d)
Prevalence = the proportion of subjects in a population who have the disease = a + c/(a + b + c + d)

Although the analytical goal for qualitative POC testing is to have 100% sensitivity and 100% specificity, all devices (both laboratory and POCT) will report some false positive and some false negative test results. As the percentage of false positive results increases, the percentage of false negative results decreases, meaning there is usually a trade-off between sensitivity and specificity.

Performance goals also relate to the intended use of the POC test (or fitness for clinical purpose). A POC test with high sensitivity is usually selected to screen a selected population for the presence of an infectious disease, because this will limit the number of false negative results (those with the disease who test negative) being reported. A POC test with poor sensitivity will result in many people being falsely informed they have a negative test result, which could contribute to wider exposure to an STI for example.

It is also important to have a test with high specificity, because this will limit the number of false positive results (those without disease who test positive) being detected. With most POC tests where the results can have serious health ramifications, such as HIV, all patients with POC test results that are initially reactive (positive) are generally referred for confirmatory testing to a laboratory. It is important that the confirmatory laboratory test does not share common false reactivity with the POC test, because it is then more likely that a false positive result will be reported. Unfortunately, a false initially reactive result can cause great anxiety for the individual while awaiting laboratory confirmation (especially with STIs, or when employment status is tied to the results of a workplace drug screen for example). There is also stigma associated with the consequence of a (false) positive result for STI, which can potentially lead to relationship issues. A test with poor specificity (high rates of false positives) can cause unnecessary overtreatment, potentially leading to antibiotic resistance with, for example, gonorrhoeal or tuberculosis infections (Peeling *et al.* 2006).

In countries where confirmatory testing of initially reactive samples by a laboratory is unavailable or not feasible, POC testing algorithms may be employed (Motta *et al.* 2013). These algorithms involve the use of a combination of POC tests, either serially or in parallel, to achieve predictive values close to 100%. Such an algorithm for HIV testing is currently being implemented in the Pacific Islands (Dick *et al.* 2010).

It is important to note that prevalence will affect the PPV and NPV of a test but does not affect sensitivity or specificity.

It should also be noted that use of the terms sensitivity and specificity (as well as PPV and NPV) assumes that the POC test/device under evaluation is being compared against a reference (or 'gold') standard laboratory method. The term reference standard is usually established by evidence-based opinion and practice within the medical, laboratory and regulatory fraternity. If a non-reference standard method is used for such studies, then sensitivity, specificity (and PPV and NPV) calculations will produce biased estimates of these parameters because the non-reference standard does not as reliably produce the correct results. In this case, the terms positive percent agreement (PPA) and negative percent agreement (NPA) can be substituted for sensitivity and specificity respectively, using the same numerical calculations:

PPA = the proportion of non-reference standard positive subjects in whom the POC test is positive = $a/(a + c) \times 100)$

NPA = the proportion of non-reference standard negative subjects in whom the POC test is negative = $d/(b + d) \times 100$

The overall percentage agreement is a measure of the proportion of subjects in whom the non-reference test and the POC test give the same outcome = $(a + d)/(a + b + c + d) \times 100$.

In essence, these terms reflect that estimates made are not strictly of accuracy but rather of the agreement of the POC test with the non-reference standard.

## REFERENCES

AACB (Australasian Association of Clinical Biochemists) (2012) Guidelines for the evaluation of PoCT instruments, Sydney, <http://www.aacb.asn.au/documents/item.244>.

Australian Government (2011) *Classification of IVD Medical Devices*. Canberra, <http://www.tga.gov.au/publication/classification-ivd-medical-devices>.

Bablok W, Passing H, Bender R, Schneider B (1988) A general regression procedure for method transformation. Application of linear regression procedures for method comparison studies in clinical chemistry, Part III. *Journal of Clinical Chemistry and Clinical Biochemistry* **26**, 783–790.

Bland J, Altman D (1999) Measuring agreement in method comparison studies. *Statistical Methods in Medical Research* **8**, 135–160. doi:10.1191/096228099673819272

Bossuyt PM, Reitsma JB, Bruns DE, Gatsonis C, Glasziou PP, Irwig LM, *et al.* (2003) The STARD statement for reporting studies of diagnostic accuracy: explanation and elaboration. *Clinical Chemistry* **49**, 7–18. doi:10.1373/49.1.7

Daw R, Finkelstein J (2006) Lab on a chip. *Nature Insight* **442**, 367. doi:10.1038/442367a

Dick S, Best S, Wilson K, Garvez AM, Duffy GM, Blair DH (2010) Validation of a rapid testing algorithm for confirming HIV infection in the Pacific region. In *22nd Annual Conference of the Australasian Society for HIV Medicine*. 20–22 October, Sydney.

Fraser CG (1986) *Interpretation of Clinical Chemistry Laboratory Data*. Blackwell Scientific Publications, Melbourne.

Fraser CG (2001) Optimal analytical performance for point of care testing. *Clinica Chimica Acta* **307**, 37–43. doi:10.1016/S0009-8981(01)00429-6

Gialamas A, Laurence CO, Yelland LN, Tideman P, Worley P, Shephard MD, *et al.* (2010) Assessing agreement between point of care and laboratory results for lipid testing from a clinical perspective. *Clinical Biochemistry* **43**, 515–518. doi:10.1016/j.clinbiochem.2009.11.014

Mori Y, Notomi T (2009) Loop-mediated isothermal amplification (LAMP): a rapid, accurate, and cost-effective diagnostic method for infectious diseases. *Journal of Infection and Chemotherapy* **15**, 62–69. doi:10.1007/s10156-009-0669-9

Motta LA, Shephard MDS, Keen P (2013) A review of the use of rapid HIV testing in community settings, with specific reference to Australia. *Point of Care* **12**, 27–32. doi:10.1097/POC.0b013e318265f7b3

Natoli L (2015) Health service implications of the introduction of STI (sexually transmitted infections) point-of-care testing in Australia. PhD thesis. Kirby Institute, University of New South Wales, Sydney.

Niemz A, Ferguson TM, Boyle DS (2011) Point-of-care nucleic acid testing for infectious diseases. *Trends in Biotechnology* **29**, 240–250. doi:10.1016/j.tibtech.2011.01.007

Parida M, Sannarangaiah S, Dash PK, Rao PVL, Morita K (2008) Loop mediated isothermal amplification (LAMP): a new generation of innovative gene amplification technique; perspectives in clinical diagnosis of infectious diseases. *Reviews in Medical Virology* **18**, 407–421. doi:10.1002/rmv.593

Peeling RW, Holmes KK, Mabey D, Ronald A (2006) Rapid tests for sexually transmitted infections (STIs): the way forward. *Sexually Transmitted Infections* **82**(Supplement 5), v1–v6. doi:10.1136/sti.2006.024265

Posthuma-Trumpie GA, Korf J, Amerongen AV (2009) Lateral flow (immuno)assay: its strengths, weaknesses, opportunities and threats. A literature survey. *Analytical and Bioanalytical Chemistry* **393**, 569–582. doi:10.1007/s00216-008-2287-2

Price CP, St John A (2008) Point-of-care testing. In *Tietz Fundamentals of Clinical Chemistry*. (Eds CA Burtis, ER Ashwood and DE Burns) pp. 188-200. Saunders Elsevier, St Louis MI, USA.

Shephard M (2006) Analytical goals for point-of-care testing used for diabetes management in Australian health care settings outside the laboratory. *Point of Care* **5**, 177–185.

Shephard M, Shephard A, Watkinson L, Mazzachi B, Worley P (2009) Design, implementation and results of the quality control program for the Australian government's point of care testing in general practice trial. *Annals of Clinical Biochemistry* **46**, 413–419. doi:10.1258/acb.2009.009045

Shephard M, Leibie A, Dimech W, Condie D, Nolan M (2012) Guidelines and recommendations for the quality-assured conduct of point-of-care testing for infectious diseases and drugs of abuse in Australia. *Australian Journal of Medical Science* **33**, 143–154.

St John A, Price C (2014) Existing and emerging technologies for point-of-care testing. *The Clinical Biochemist Reviews* **35**, 155–167.

Tao Z-Y, Zhou H-Y, Xia H, Xu S, Zhu H-W, Culleton RL, *et al.* (2011) Adaptation of a visualised loop-mediated isothermal amplification technique for field detection of *Plasmodium vivax* infection. *Parasites & Vectors* **4**, 115. doi:10.1186/1756-3305-4-115

TDR Diagnostics Evaluation Expert Panel (2010) Evaluation of diagnostic tests for infectious diseases: general principles. *Nature Reviews. Microbiology* **8**, S17–S29.

Tran NK, Kost GJ (2006) Worldwide point-of-care testing. Compendiums of POCT for mobile, emergency, critical, and primary care and of infectious diseases tests. *Point of Care* **5**, 84–92. doi:10.1097/00134384-200606000-00010

Warnick GR, Myers GL, Cooper GR, Rifai N (2002) Impact of the third cholesterol report from the adult treatment panel of the National Cholesterol Education Program on the clinical laboratory. *Clinical Chemistry* **48**, 11–17.

Washington State Department of Health (2015) *Waived Tests and CPT Codes*. Washington DC, <http://www.doh.wa.gov/portals/1/Documents/Pubs/681018.pdf>.

Westgard J (2014) *Desirable Specifications for Total Error, Imprecision and Bias, Derived from Biological Variation*, <www.westgard.com/guest17.htm>.

WHO (World Health Organization) (2004) *Mapping The Landscape of Diagnostics for Sexually Transmitted Infections: Key Findings and Recommendations*. WHO, Geneva, Switzerland.

WHO/TDR Sexually Transmitted Diseases Diagnostics Initiative (2006a) Evaluation of rapid diagnostic tests: syphilis. *Nature Reviews. Microbiology* **4**, S33–S40. doi:10.1038/nrmicro1563

WHO/TDR Sexually Transmitted Diseases Diagnostics Initiative (2006b) Evaluation of rapid diagnostic tests: chlamydia and gonorrhoea. *Nature Reviews. Microbiology* **4**, S41–S48. doi:10.1038/nrmicro1562

Yetisen AK, Akram MS, Lowe CR (2013) Paper-based microfluidic point-of-care diagnostic devices. *Lab on a Chip* **13**, 2210. doi:10.1039/c3lc50169h

# 4 Training and competency assessment for device operators

*Mark Shephard*

**Summary**

Point-of-care testing (POCT) should only be performed by health professionals who have undergone initial training and competency certification, who have their competency levels regularly assessed, and who participate in regular recertification. Training should be organised and delivered by a POCT Coordinator, who is usually a medical scientist or a senior nurse with wide experience in POCT. The content of the training manual will be determined by the nature of the POCT service being implemented and the needs of the organisation undertaking POCT. In a primary care setting, device operators are unlikely to have any previous training in laboratory medicine and therefore it is important to translate scientific and analytical concepts into images and messages that can be readily understood. Training should cover both the theory and practice of conducting POCT. At the completion of training, trainee competency should be assessed by written and practical means. Successful trainees should receive a competency certificate. Post-training surveillance of competency should be undertaken by regular review of quality control and proficiency testing results and through re-training and education updates. A register of all personnel receiving competency certificates should be maintained.

## INTRODUCTION

As described in Chapter 2, there are a multitude of guidelines from governments and professional bodies that describe the principles of how to set up and manage a POCT service. These guidelines stress the need for a systematic approach to the governance, implementation and delivery of POCT. All of the guidelines also emphasise that a sound training program is critical to underpinning a sustainable and quality-assured POCT service.

This chapter describes the key principles for developing and delivering a POCT training program and for monitoring the competency of the 'on-site' device operators who are at the front-line of conducting routine POCT. These principles will be illustrated, where appropriate, by practical examples from POCT field networks in Australia and internationally.

## DEVELOPMENT AND DELIVERY OF A TRAINING PROGRAM

There are now a wide variety of health professionals who can perform routine POCT in both hospital and specialised primary care environments; these include (but are not limited to) medical scientists, nurses, Indigenous and community health workers, diabetes educators, sexual health workers, paramedics, pharmacists and, in some cases, administrative or security staff.

As an overarching principle, POCT should only be carried out by health professional staff who have undergone appropriate initial training and competency certification, who have their competency levels regularly assessed, and who participate in regular recertification sessions (ISO 2006).

## Organisation and delivery of training

Training programs for POCT are most commonly delivered by a recognised training organisation, course or program. The World Health Organization (WHO) has prepared several excellent training packages for HIV and malaria (WHO 2005, 2006, 2009), while the London School of Hygiene & Tropical Medicine recently developed a toolkit for rapid syphilis testing (London School of Hygiene & Tropical Medicine 2011). The Australasian Society for HIV Medicine has also developed a training program for device operators involved in HIV POCT in community settings, which has been endorsed by New South Wales Health (New South Wales Ministry of Health 2015). The Flinders University International Centre for Point-of-Care Testing delivers a range of training and education programs for chronic, acute and infectious diseases across its national and international POCT networks (Chapter 28). The Australasian Association of Clinical Biochemists provides education opportunities for POCT through the Australian Point of Care Practitioner's Network (www.appn.net.au).

At the individual POCT program or network level, the POCT Coordinator is usually responsible for the organisation and delivery of training under the direction of a POCT Management Committee. The training program should be targeted to the specific clinical need and setting where POCT is undertaken. The POCT Coordinator is most commonly a medical scientist from an accredited pathology laboratory or a specialist POCT provider with a formal supervisory link to the program, or a senior nurse who is skilled and experienced in the practice of POCT and in the delivery of training.

However, it is not just a matter of assigning *any* scientist or nurse to the role of POCT Coordinator; the selection of the appropriate person needs to be considered carefully, with the following essential qualities required:

- a strong interest in POCT
- a strong interest in staff training
- good communication skills
- good people skills
- patience
- respect for other health professionals.

It is often advantageous for the POCT Coordinator to be supported by a training team comprising other scientific or nursing staff from the local program and/or regional or mobile trainers from a network. Representative(s) from the device manufacturer can also assist in training, because they know their POCT devices well and are generally keen to be an active participant in training.

Some personal rules learnt through years of training experience include: never use words or phrases such as 'no' or 'that's wrong'; never discourage the trainee if they make a mistake while learning; try not to be too formal and authoritarian; speak with an encouraging voice; be a good listener; and try to make training as engaging as possible.

## Flexible modes of training delivery

Training should be offered using as many flexible modes of training delivery as possible (Table 4.1). It is important to acknowledge and recognise that different individuals learn at a different pace and respond differently to various teaching styles.

Face-to-face training conducted in a small group setting is generally the best mode of training delivery. This forum enables the audience to engage closely with the POCT Coordinator and allows trainees to learn in an interactive and collegiate environment, as well as being able to experience using the POCT device in a 'hands-on' sense and gain confidence as a device operator. Face-to-face training can be conducted: locally (and on-site) at individual health services; regionally, where several services from a common geographic location meet centrally

**Table 4.1.** Examples of modes of training delivery for POCT

| Modes of training delivery |
|---|
| Face-to-face (e.g. at individual services, regional or annual training workshops) |
| Self-directed or e-learning (e.g. web-streamed videos) |
| DVD |
| Teleconference |
| Videoconference |
| Skype |

for a training workshop; or nationally, where an annual training workshop is held in a capital city and as many of the network's device operators as possible attend this event. The annual workshop provides an exceptional medium for networking and sharing experiences. It also fosters an environment where the often-isolated device operator no longer feels 'alone' but rather can experience the cooperative and collaborative nature, as well as a sense of group ownership, of the program or network.

Organisation of face-to-face training sessions for health professional staff from remote communities can be very challenging. Due to the competing time demands on staff in remote health services, not all staff are able to attend on-site training sessions; conversely, the cost of flying remote staff to a central location for training may be prohibitive and health service administrators are often reluctant to allow staff the additional time away from the service. Staff turnover rates in remote health centres are also high (Dade-Smith 2007; Shephard *et al.* 2009, 2015a) and it is often difficult to maintain continuity of routine POCT during periods when services are understaffed or when there are no trained operators available at remote services. Hard copies of training resources are often misplaced when staff leave, resulting in the new device operator being without key training reference material. The ability of the POCT Coordinator to deliver immediate on-site training sessions when new staff arrive may also be compromised by the demands of distance and time.

Training for large networks now often includes a range of flexible e-learning or self-directed learning options, which aim to reduce the travel and time demands on the POCT Coordinator as well as provide a more sustainable means for the delivery of training for participating sites.

In the national 'QAAMS' POCT network for diabetes management in Indigenous communities managed by the Flinders University International Centre for Point-of-Care Testing (ICPOCT), web-streamed videos of training are available through a password-protected 'Participant Only' section of the network's website (www.qaams.org.au). These videos take the participant systematically through the principles and practice of POCT for this program. The full training resource package (training manual, poster sets, training aids for the interpretation of patient POC test results, quality control result sheets, reagent and consumable order forms, quarterly newsletters, contact details for the POCT Coordinator, POCT Management Committee and scientific and technical support) are also all available for direct electronic downloading from the website. Web-based training has many advantages: it enables trainees to learn at their own pace, the videos can be paused and repeated to facilitate reinforcement of key messages or content and they can be viewed at any time that is convenient for the trainee (24 h a day/7 days a week). Some remote services in this network experience difficulties with internet service provision and are unable to effectively access the web resources. For this reason, all participating services are also provided with a DVD containing all the training information available on the website.

As additional options, training can be conducted using teleconference, videoconference or Skype meeting systems. These are ideal for regular small group training of health professional staff from participating communities. Some teleconference formats allow the POCT Coordinator and participants to dial in to a training session and for participants to view a PowerPoint presentation of training over the internet while listening to the Coordinator deliver the presentation. This latter format has proven popular and is now used to conduct weekly training sessions for remote health centres participating in the Northern Territory Point-of-Care Testing Program, with multiple centres being able to link in to a single training session (Shephard *et al.* 2015b).

### Essential components of training delivery and a training resource package

Key elements of a good training program include: (i) instruction on both the theory and practice of POCT; and (ii) access to a comprehensive, user-friendly training resource package. The content of the resource package should be tailored to the specific POCT application and to the target audience. For Indigenous POCT programs, it is critical that the training resources are culturally safe (Shephard 2006; Shephard *et al.* 2015b).

With POCT networks managed by ICPOCT, a standard resource package includes a training manual, posters, a PowerPoint presentation (all of which are available in hard copy and electronic formats) and a DVD containing all resources (Table 4.2).

The training manual should systematically guide the trainee device operators through the principles and practice of POCT. This manual should be user-friendly, intuitive, and not require specialised technical knowledge. Table 4.3 lists examples of major themes/headings that could be included in the content of the training manual.

The development of a training manual provides significant opportunities for the POCT Coordinator to be

Table 4.2. Examples of components of a training resource package for POCT

| Components of a training resource package |
|---|
| Training manual |
| Posters (step-by-step guide to patient, QC and PT testing) |
| DVD |
| Power-point presentation |
| Training aids (e.g. how to interpret patient or quality test results) |
| Standard Operating procedures (if not incorporated into training manual) |
| Training checklist |
| Competency assessment questions (written) |
| Template for competency certificate |

creative and resourceful. In primary care settings, trainee operators are unlikely to have had previous formal training in laboratory medicine and therefore it is important for the Coordinator to translate medical, scientific and analytical concepts into messages or images that can be readily understood. Fig. 4.1 shows selected images from the training manual used in the national QAAMS Program for diabetes management in Indigenous medical services. These figures depict the mechanism of action of insulin and how concepts of accuracy and precision are explained using the analogy of an Indigenous footballer having shots for goal in Australia's national football code (AFL).

Fig. 4.2 also shows an interpretation aid used in QAAMS to describe diabetes-induced damage to the kidney's glomerulus, which normally acts as a filter or 'web' to prevent protein leakage into the urine. This aid was conceived by a QAAMS participant, Adeline Drogemuller from a remote Northern Territory community.

In the networks managed by ICPOCT, the jewel in the crown of the resource package is the poster, which is intended to sit next to or near the POCT device and describes for the operator in a simple step-by-step manner how to perform a patient test and a quality test. Posters are generally prepared in laminated A3 format, are highly visual and use colour images. These posters have been well received by all health professional groups in these networks, as shown in Table 4.4, where ratings for posters were 9.3 or higher (out of a 10) for device operators from urban, rural and remote general practices participating in the Point-of-Care Testing in General Practice Trial (Shephard *et al.* 2009).

For the practical side of training, the POCT Coordinator should perform a complete, hands-on demonstration that includes the items shown in Table 4.5. Once this demonstration has been completed, all trainees should participate in a hands-on practice session in their own time and at their own pace, under the supervision of the Coordinator.

Table 4.3. Training manual content

| Major themes/headings for content of a POCT training manual |
|---|
| Setting the clinical scene (prevalence, disease process and pathophysiology) |
| A description of the clinical significance of the test |
| Analytical performance characteristics and technical specifications of the POCT device, as well as limitations of the POCT device |
| Validated sample types (consistent with the manufacturer's specifications) |
| Patient preparation and specimen collection requirements (including pre-test discussion and gaining informed consent) |
| Conditions for reagent preparation and storage |
| How to perform the patient test on the POCT device, following the manufacturer's instructions |
| Documentation, interpretation, reporting and traceability of patient results |
| Action required on patient POCT results (with particular reference to those relating to potentially life-threatening or life-changing conditions, for example troponin and acute coronary syndrome, and initially reactive POCT results for HIV along with associated post-test discussion) |
| Principles and practice of quality management (including quality control and external proficiency testing) |
| Interpretation, documentation, reporting and actioning of quality testing results |
| Maintenance and common troubleshooting (if appropriate) |
| Occupational health and safety issues including infection control practices |
| Statement of compliance with national standards, policy documents or accreditation requirements (when required or available). |

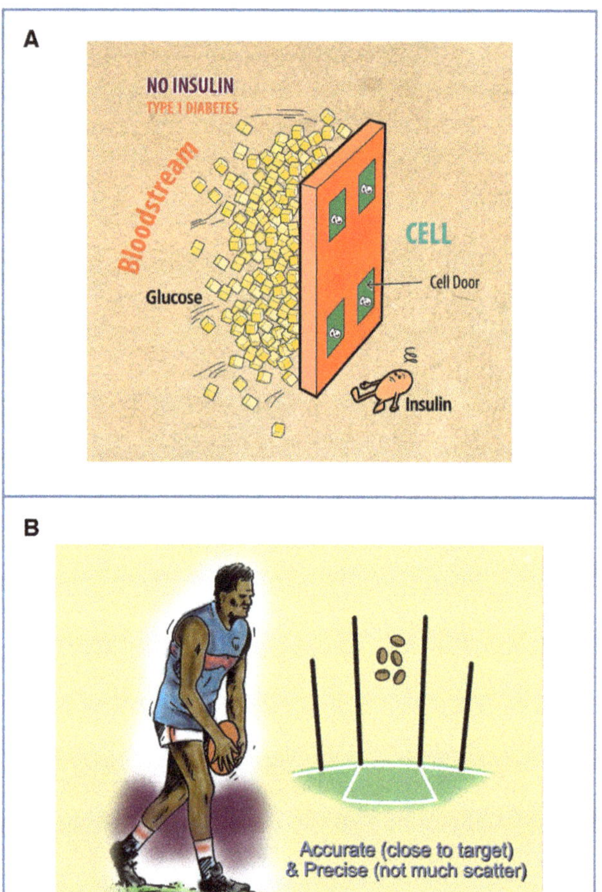


**Fig. 4.1.** Visual images from the QAAMS Training Manual showing: (A) the mechanism of action of insulin and (B) how concepts of accuracy and precision are explained.

Photographs of rapid test results, either on paper or via the internet, have also been used to assess the trainee's ability to read and interpret results of qualitative HIV POC assays (Chang *et al.* 2006; Chiu *et al.* 2011; Learmonth *et al.* 2008). This practice has potential to complement operator training programs, but should not substitute for the need and requirement for operators to undertake practical training.

Ideally, a checklist can be prepared that details every aspect of training (including theory and practice) that the trainee should complete.

An important, but often overlooked, aspect of training is to continually evaluate, review and critically reflect on the delivery of your training sessions. Consideration should be given to provide a questionnaire for trainees to provide feedback on the completed session. Shephard *et al.* (2009) describe examples from the Point-of-Care Testing in General Practice Trial, looking at the quality and appropriateness of training resources from multiple training sessions.

## COMPETENCY ASSESSMENT AND CERTIFICATION

Competency assessment and maintenance of a competency register is an important adjunct to training and another pivotal role of the POCT Coordinator.

### Competency assessment

Following training, competency should be assessed in a structured manner that includes completion of a written and a practical assessment. The written assessment

**Table 4.4.** Satisfaction of device operators with training and training resources provided in the Australian Point-of-Care Testing in General Practice Trial (split by geographic region). The higher the score (out of 10), the greater the level of satisfaction among the operators. Table reproduced with permission of Rural and Remote Health (Source: Shephard *et al.* 2009).

| Characteristic | Urban | Rural | Remote |
|---|---|---|---|
| | *n* = 13 | *n* = 19 | *n* = 23 |
| Quality of training was satisfactory: median (IQ[a] range) | 8.5 (7.7–9.5) | 8.2 (6.4–9.0) | 8.6 (7.4–9.3) |
| Usefulness of POCT Training Manual for POCT devices: median (IQ range) | 8.2 (6.8–9.6) | 8.5 (7.2–9.5) | 8.6 (7.0–9.5) |
| Usefulness of posters for POCT devices: median (IQ range) | 9.6 (8.6–9.8) | 9.4 (6.1–9.8) | 9.3 (8.3–9.8) |
| I am competent in the use of POCT devices: median (IQ range) | 9.4 (8.1–9.6) | 8.2 (7.2–9.7) | 9.0 (7.7–9.6) |
| POCT devices were easy to use: median (IQ range) | 8.3 (7.0–9.5) | 8.5 (7.2–9.7) | 9.1 (8.3–9.5) |
| POCT devices were easy to maintain: median (IQ range) | 9.0 (8.8–9.4) | 9.1 (7.9–9.8) | 8.9 (8.2–9.2) |
| Confident in accuracy of POCT results: median (IQ range) | 8.4 (7.2–8.5) | 7.3 (5.8–8.3) | 8.5 (7.7–9.2) |
| Prefer POCT to conventional pathology testing: median (IQ range) | 7.9 (6.2–9.2) | 8.5 (7.3–9.2) | 8.8 (7.4–9.6) |

[a]IQ = interquartile range

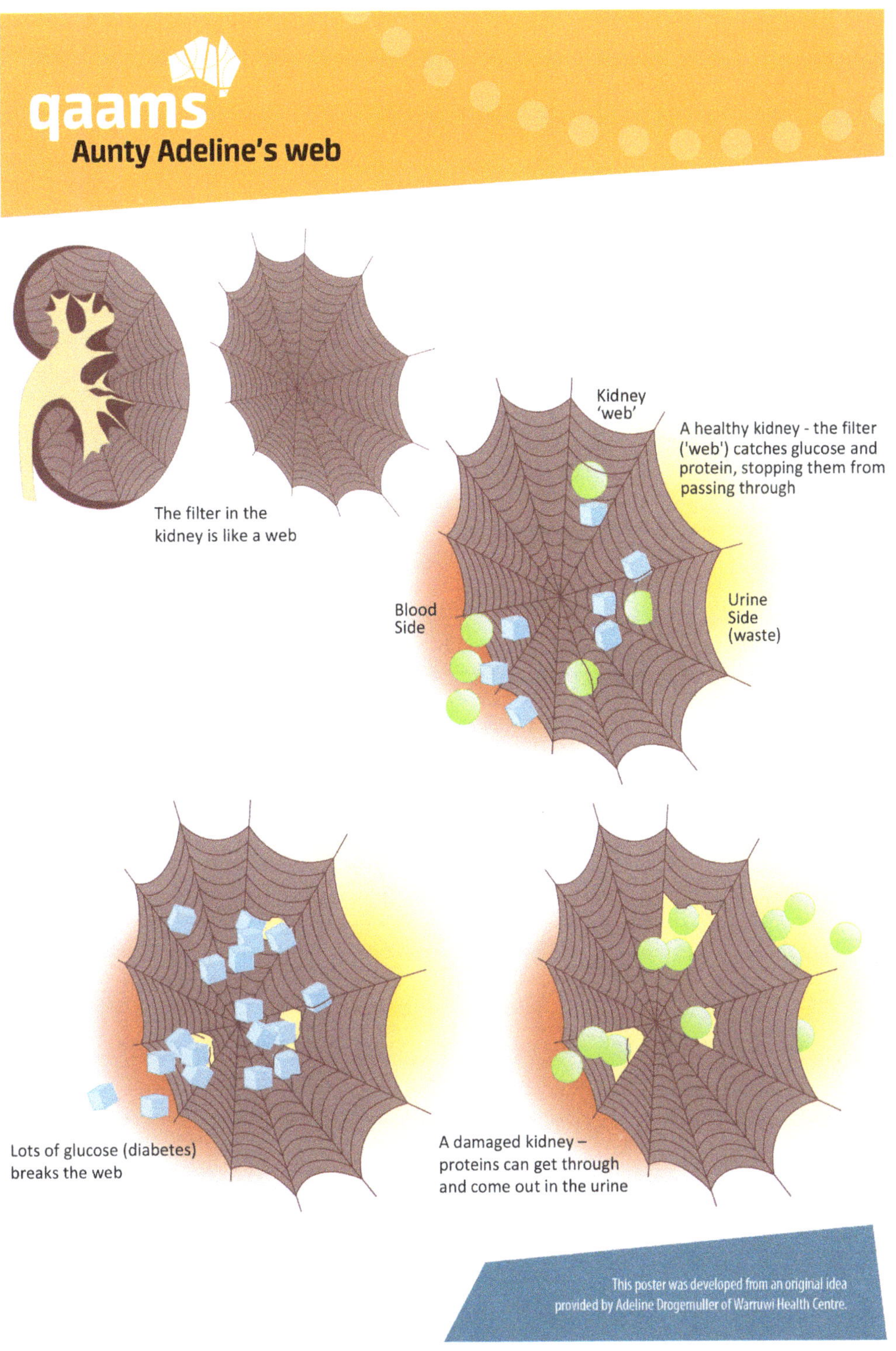


**Fig. 4.2.** 'Aunty Adelines web': a culturally safe resource to depict kidney damage, and resultant protein loss into the urine, caused by diabetes. (Source: Figure used with permission from Adeline Drogemuller)

**Table 4.5.** Items to include in a practical demonstration of training

| Items for a practical demonstration of training |
|---|
| Main features of the device |
| How to collect a sample for testing |
| How to prepare the required reagents |
| How to perform a patient test following the manufacturer's instructions closely |
| How to conduct quality testing |
| How to record (and action) patient and quality testing results |
| How to perform basic maintenance procedures |

generally consists of a series of multiple-choice questions that assess whether the trainee has grasped key concepts and facts required to perform the test. The practical assessment usually involves the trainee completing a patient and/or a quality test (and obtaining acceptable results for that test) in the presence of the POCT Coordinator or a member of the training team. In many POCT networks, written competency assessment can be undertaken online with automatic/electronic marking of the assessment.

### Competency certification

All trainees who successfully complete their written and practical assessment should be issued with a competency certificate, which should ideally feature the following minimal information:

- a certificate number (which can also be used as an operator identification number for accessing the specific POCT device for which competency has been obtained)
- the name of the successful trainee
- a summary of the competency skills obtained for the POC test(s) and device
- a fixed expiry date (after which competency should be renewed, with most programs recommending that competency should be reassessed after a period not shorter than 12 months and not longer than 2 years)
- the signature of the POCT Coordinator and date issued.

### Post-training surveillance of competency

Post-training surveillance of competency should be undertaken by regular review of quality control and external proficiency testing results.

Competency should be reviewed regularly through re-training and education updates. Attendance at re-training sessions is considered compulsory in many POCT networks, especially those subject to regulation/accreditation. These sessions may be conducted on-site, at regional workshops, at annual workshops or possibly by videoconference if the organisation is geographically isolated. If a POCT operator fails a competency review (e.g. because their QC/PT performance has been poor, their level of testing activity has fallen below minimum requirements, or they exhibit a high rate of analytical errors with their testing), then they should be re-trained before being re-issued with a new competency certificate.

A register of all staff receiving initial and renewed competency certificates should be maintained as part of the service's quality management system and may also be required by government or accreditation agencies.

## REFERENCES

Chang D, Learmonth K, Dax EM (2006) HIV testing in 2006: issues and methods. *Expert Review of Anti-Infective Therapy* **4**, 565–582. doi:10.1586/14787210.4.4.565

Chiu YHC, Ong J, Walker S, Kumalawati J, Gartinah T, McPhee DA, Dax EM (2011) Photographed rapid HIV test results pilot novel quality assessment and training schemes. *PLoS One* **6**, 1–7. doi:10.1371/journal.pone.0018294

Dade-Smith J (2007) *Australia's Rural and Remote Health. A Social Justice Perspective.* Tertiary Press, Melbourne.

ISO (International Organization for Standardization) (2006) *ISO 22870:2006. Point-of-care Testing (POCT) – Requirements for Quality and Competence.* Geneva, Switzerland, <https://www.iso.org/obp/ui/#iso:std:iso:22870:ed-1:v1:en>.

Learmonth KM, McPhee DA, Jardine DK, Walker SK, Aye T, Dax EM (2008) Assessing proficiency of interpretation of rapid human immunodeficiency virus assays in non-laboratory settings: ensuring quality of testing. *Journal of Clinical Microbiology* **46**, 1692–1697. doi:10.1128/JCM.01761-07

London School of Hygiene & Tropical Medicine (2011) *Rapid Syphilis Test Toolkit*, <http://www.lshtm.ac.uk/itd/crd/research/rapidsyphilistoolkit/>.

New South Wales Ministry of Health (2015) *Framework and Standard Operating Procedure for the Provision of Point of Care Testing for HIV in Clinical and Non-clinical Settings*, <www.health.nsw.gov.au/policies/gl/2015/pdf/GL2015_003.pdf>.

Shephard MD (2006) Clinical and cultural effectiveness of the 'QAAMS' point-of-care testing model for diabetes management in Australian Aboriginal medical services. *The Clinical Biochemist Reviews* **27**, 161–170.

Shephard MD, Mazzachi B, Watkinson L, Shephard A, Laurence A, Gialamas A, *et al.* (2009) Evaluation of a training program for device operators in the Australian Government's Point of Care Testing In General Practice Trial. *Rural and Remote Health* **9**, 1189, <http://www.rrh.org.au/articles/showarticlenew.asp?ArticleID=1189>.

Shephard MDS, Spaeth B, Motta LA, Shephard A (2015a) Point-of-care testing in Australia: Practical advantages and benefits of community resiliency for improving outcomes. In *Global Point of Care. Strategies for Disasters, Emergencies and Public Health Resilience.* (Eds GJ Kost and CM Curtis) pp. 527-535. AACC Press, Washington DC, USA.

Shephard M, O'Brien C, Burgoyne A, Croft J, Garlett T, Barancek K, *et al.* (2015b) A review of the cultural safety of a national Indigenous point-of-care testing program for diabetes management. *Australian Journal of Primary Health* Published online 2 September 2015. doi:10.1071/PY15050

WHO (World Health Organization) (2005) *HIV Rapid Test Training Package.* WHO, Geneva, Switzerland, <http://www.who.int/diagnostics_laboratory/documents/guidance/rt_training/en/index.html>.

WHO (2006) *The Use of Malaria Rapid Diagnostic Tests.* 2nd edn. Geneva, Switzerland, <http://www.wpro.who.int/publications/PUB_9290612045/en/>.

WHO (2009) *How to Use Rapid Diagnostic Tests (RDT): a Guide for Training at a Village and Clinic Level.* Geneva, Switzerland, <http://www.wpro.who.int/malaria/NR/rdonlyres/23DD7DCB-48C4-4CFF-BD45-332F0BE3DCC7/0/generic_PfPan_training_manual_web.pdf>.

# 5 Quality management of point-of-care testing devices

*Mark Shephard, Anne Shephard, Wayne Dimech and Susan Best*

**Summary**

Quality control (QC) testing and proficiency testing (PT) are integral components of a quality system to monitor analytical performance in the laboratory and at the point of care. These two processes check the quality of a device's performance by comparing observed results of QC testing or PT with a target with pre-set specifications. QC testing provides an immediate check of quality, while PT provides a delayed, peer-reviewed, external assessment of quality. However, many modern POCT devices now feature sophisticated in-built quality checks within their single use, disposable testing units. A tailored, flexible and balanced approach to quality surveillance is therefore required, taking into account the degree of the device's technological sophistication, practicality, cost of QC/PT and size/scope of POCT networks.

## INTRODUCTION

In the laboratory setting, analytical quality is usually monitored by two equally important and complementary processes called quality control (QC) and external proficiency testing (PT). PT has a wide variety of synonyms that are used by different professional bodies and providers of PT programs around the world, including external quality assurance (EQA) and external quality assessment schemes or programs (EQAS). Table 5.1 provides working definitions of terms related to quality and quality systems.

The aim of conducting QC and PT testing is to monitor an analytical measurement system and to alert the operator when a change to the system has occurred that

**Table 5.1.** Distinction between terms used to describe quality (Source: adapted with permission from Shephard *et al.* 2012)

| Term | Definition |
|---|---|
| Quality management system (QMS) | A systematic approach to document the quality principles used by a POCT facility. |
| Quality assurance (QA) | An over-arching term to describe all activities to improve or maintain quality of POC tests and testing. |
| Quality control (QC) | The routine testing of sample(s) with known concentrations or reactivity to ensure the POC test device is performing to analytical expectations. |
| Proficiency testing (PT); also known as external quality assessment scheme (EQAS) or external quality assurance (EQA) | The periodic testing of a panel of samples containing a range of concentrations or infectious loads. The test results of the samples are unknown to the tester and the results obtained are submitted to the PT provider for peer assessment. |

may compromise the integrity of the patient result and potentially lead to a medically important error (Ehrmeyer and Laessig 2001).

These two processes check the quality of a device's performance by comparing observed results of testing samples with differing concentrations or infectious loads to a target with pre-set specifications. Although the underlying principle of these two forms of testing is the same, there are some fundamental differences between QC and PT.

For QC testing, samples (often in a kit form) are usually provided by manufacturer of the device, but can also be supplied by a third-party provider or be produced in-house by the laboratory. One to three levels of QC are generally provided for testing, with the manufacturer or the POCT Coordinator setting the 'target' values (and the limits for acceptable performance) for these QC materials. These values are known at the time of QC testing and therefore an immediate assessment of the quality of the device's performance can be made. QC testing is often termed 'internal' QC testing.

PT samples (for laboratory and POCT programs) are provided by recognised and, preferably accredited, proficiency testing providers. Selected examples of PT providers from Australia, USA and the UK are listed in Table 5.2. These providers support a range of specific POCT programs (and linked laboratory-based PT programs) that can assess the quality of testing on POCT devices.

PT samples have multiple levels of test concentrations or infectious loads, with accurate target values and acceptable limits (because the PT material is manufactured to tight specifications set by the PT provider). With PT samples, the true result is not known at the time of testing and the operator sends the result to the PT provider. The PT provider returns a report that documents how close the observed result for that sample was to the target value and how the results from that testing facility (laboratory or POCT) compare with all other (de-identified) facilities in the program.

**Table 5.2.** Examples of external PT program providers to support POCT

| PT provider | Website |
|---|---|
| National Serology Reference Laboratory (NRL) | www.nrl.gov.au |
| RCPA Quality Assurance Programs | www.rcpaqap.com.au/poct |
| College of American Pathologists | www.cap.org |
| Wisconsin State Laboratory of Hygiene | www.slh.wisc.edu/proficiency |
| American Proficiency Institute | www.api-pt.com |
| United Kingdom National External Quality Assessment Service (UKNEQAS) | www.ukneqas.org.uk |
| Wales External Quality Assessment Scheme (WEQAS) | www.weqas.com |

Thus QC provides an immediate check of quality, while PT provides a delayed, peer-reviewed, external assessment of quality. Table 5.3 summarises the main differences between QC and PT testing.

For analytes with quantifiable concentrations, repeated testing of QC and PT samples at defined time intervals enables statistical measures of the accuracy and imprecision (reproducibility) of testing to be calculated, which determine whether the testing device is performing to acceptable analytical standards. QC is generally used for monitoring the imprecision of a device's performance, because that same QC material is tested repeatedly across time and therefore the variability of those repeated measurements can be calculated. Testing of QC samples can also be used to monitor accuracy, although the target values set by the manufacturer are generally not as tightly assigned as the targets set by the PT provider. PT therefore delivers a more robust measure of accuracy, while PT samples can also monitor imprecision if the same samples are provided and measured several times across a testing period.

Ideally, sample matrices for QC and PT material should be the same as that of the patient sample being tested. In practice, this is often not the case, because the quality samples need to have long stability across their intended period of use (often 1 or 2 years). PT materials are often provided as freeze-dried (lyophilised) human blood or urine that requires reconstitution, as clear liquids, or as swabs coated with dried, inert bacteria or virus. Consideration of the sample matrix and the type of patient sample being routinely tested is required when choosing an appropriate QC or PT material for a laboratory or POC testing program (Shephard *et al.* 2012).

## MONITORING THE ANALYTICAL QUALITY OF POC TEST SYSTEMS

QC and PT provide a formal means of monitoring the analytical quality of a device. Without quality testing:

Table 5.3. Main differences between quality control testing and proficiency testing

| Parameter | Quality control testing | Proficiency testing |
|---|---|---|
| Assessment and reporting | Internal, immediate | External, delayed, peer-reviewed |
| Supplier | Manufacturer or third party | Accredited PT provider |
| Samples tested | Usually one to three levels | Multiple levels |
| Target values | Known by operator when tested | Not known by operator when tested |
| Testing frequency | Frequently: checks quality over time | Periodic: checks quality at a set point in time |
| Performance indicator assessed (quantitative tests) | Reproducibility (Precision) | Accuracy and precision |
| Interpretation | Assesses performance of 'your' device only | Compares performance of 'your' device with other participants using the same device |

- How can an operator know that their device is working well?
- How can the operator know with any confidence that the test has been performed correctly?
- How can the operator know that a patient's test results are appropriate and safe for their clinical care?

Although these quality processes have served the laboratory well and are available to support POCT programs, a key issue that continues to be debated worldwide is: 'Are these traditional QC and PT processes relevant, transferable, practical and cost-effective for monitoring analytical quality on POCT devices?' (Bullock 2004; Gill and Shephard 2010; Martin 2008). There is no simple answer or solution to this question. In attempting to consider the issue, it is necessary to:

- understand the total patient testing process
- understand the difference between laboratory and POCT systems
- assess the degree of technological sophistication that individual POC devices/test systems have, particularly their 'in-built' quality checks
- find the appropriate balance between ensuring safety and analytical quality of POCT and implementing a quality framework that is practical, achievable and cost-effective in a primary care setting.

## THE TOTAL PATIENT TESTING PROCESS

The total testing process includes pre-analytical, analytical and post-analytical phases.

The pre-analytical phase of testing generally includes patient sample collection, labelling and handling. Pre-analytical steps are the most difficult to control, and errors in sample collection can lead to grossly misleading results. Training and competency assessment for device operators is perhaps the best form of 'control' of pre-analytical errors, where it is crucial that operators fully understand the errors that will occur if the sample is collected improperly.

Analytical steps generally involve calibration, sample delivery, reagent delivery, reaction between sample and reagent, and measurement of a signal and conversion to an analyte concentration.

The post-analytical phase of testing involves manual transcription or electronic transmission of the result into the patient record.

A sound quality management system should incorporate procedures to check all steps of the total testing process (Fig. 5.1).

## DIFFERENCES BETWEEN LABORATORY AND POCT DEVICES

Most laboratory instruments are closed or self-contained and have the ability to measure large numbers of samples in batches throughout the day. For these types of analysers, the testing of multi-level QC throughout the day combined with monthly PT testing and regular maintenance is considered standard practice.

In contrast, many POC test systems comprise a disposable single-use testing unit with or without a reading device (NCCLS 2002; Phillips 2004). For qualitative tests, the sample is added to the testing unit, the analyte is measured and a negative or positive result is generated. For quantitative tests, the reaction process takes place in the testing unit and the reader converts the signal generated into a numeric result.

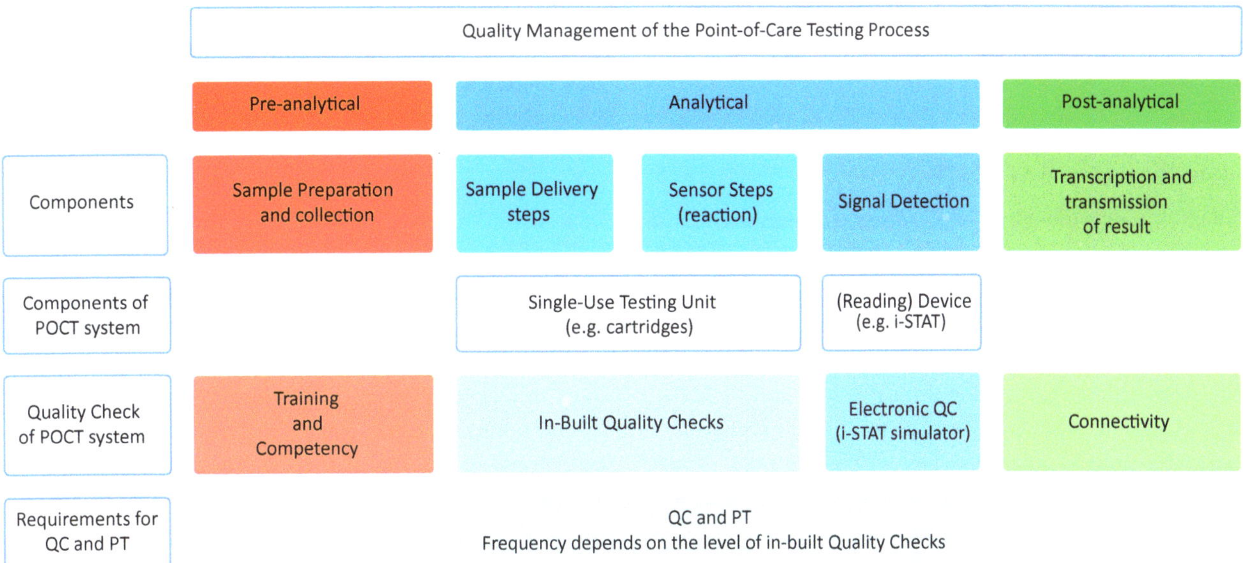


**Fig. 5.1.** Schematic representation comparing aspects of quality management using POCT-based single-use testing systems.

An argument can be mounted that traditional QC and PT processes are not necessarily applicable to these types of POC test systems because each testing unit is discrete and disposable, and checking the performance of a single testing unit does not guarantee with any certainty the quality of the next testing unit. How then have manufacturers of such systems approached the problem of quality management?

## QUALITY CHECKS FOR POC TEST SYSTEMS

With most modern POCT devices, there has been significant technological investment by manufacturers in the development of sophisticated in-built quality checks within the testing unit itself (these checks have been described variously as 'on-board QC', 'intelligent QC' and 'internal checks'). Manufacturers have recognised that the main consumers of POCT in the future will be health professionals from a non-laboratory background and they have tried to make the devices as simple as possible for the operator and well controlled internally.

The Abbott i-STAT® cartridge has a calibration solution contained in a pouch in every cartridge and performs a calibration before each sample is tested. In-built checks of the calibration fluid include that it is free of bubbles, has not burst in the handling process and is present at the correct concentration. Every Roche CoaguChek XS® test strip has in-built control checks for strip deterioration due to exposure to excessive temperature and humidity. The Abaxis Piccolo® rotor quantifies interferents such as haemolysis, lipaemia and icterus and suppresses results when interference limits are exceeded. It also validates the composition and delivery of all reagents, confirms correct sample and diluent volumes have been delivered and verifies the presence of diluted sample in all reaction cuvettes. The Cepheid GeneXpert® performs a 'sample adequacy control', which is designed to detect the presence of a single copy human gene per cell to ensure that the sample contains human cells and that the cells are adequately lysed to extract nucleic acids. A negative sample adequacy control indicates that no human cells are present in the sample due to insufficient mixing, inadequate sampling or inefficient lysis. The GeneXpert® system also performs a 'sample processing control' and a 'probe check control'.

Manufacturers of qualitative rapid POC tests based on lateral flow technology often state that their devices include an in-built 'quality control' check. What in fact they mean is that there is simply a check of the flow of liquid from the sample application area to the strip's end.

Many POCT devices incorporate quality checks by which signal generation is monitored. These are known as electronic QC checks (Westgard 2001). The Abbott i-STAT® has an electronic simulator that specifically measures electrical signal generation and ensures that these signals are within tight specification limits. Electronic QC should not be considered a surrogate for traditional QC because this only checks signal generation and does not monitor the analytical reaction process (Fig. 5.1).

The best single-use POCT systems are those with the highest degree of in-built quality checks to monitor the analytical steps.

## FINDING THE BALANCE

Given this level of technological sophistication with most POCT devices today, the role of traditional QC and PT has come under question in some quarters. A training manual for a widely used POCT device recently contained the following statement: 'Quality control and system checks using control test solutions that you may be familiar with from other systems are no longer required …' Certainly this is not the view of the authors. There unquestionably remains a continuing place for traditional QC and PT as an independent check of the quality of POCT systems, but one needs to tailor the degree of technical sophistication of the device with a QC/PT frequency regimen that is cost-effective and practical.

There is no 'one size fits all' policy that can be applied universally across all POC test systems in terms of frequency of QC/PT testing. Ideally QC samples should be tested with each group of patient tests performed, but this may be impractical. As a minimum requirement, QC testing should be conducted once a month, when a new delivery of reagents is received, when there is change in reagent lot number, when a patient result does not fit the clinical presentation, or following a major maintenance or repair procedure for a POCT device (Gill and Watkinson 2010). Beyond these scenarios, frequency of QC testing in particular should take into account the actual volume and nature of patient testing conducted in the field. Many clinical chemistry and haematology PT programs provide samples for testing on a monthly or bi-monthly basis, while infectious disease PT programs provide panels of samples to be tested at selected testing events or 'challenges' two to four times per year.

The cost of purchasing QC and PT materials is of relevance for small primary care settings with limited financial budgets for conducting POCT and for large POCT networks where costs of conducting QC and PT at every site can potentially become a large percentage of the consumable budget.

An alternative to traditional PT testing is 'parallel' or 'split' patient sample testing, in which the same patient sample is tested by a POCT site and by the laboratory and then results are compared. Potential advantages of parallel patient sample testing are: like PT, it provides a delayed external check of quality; testing uses a sample of identical matrix (e.g. whole blood) to that of the routine patient samples rather than a lyophilised or liquid PT material; with samples equivalent to routine specimens, parallel patient testing can check the pre-analytical component of testing; and parallel patient testing can be a cost-effective external assessment of quality. Potential drawbacks include: this mode of external assessment only tests a limited range of concentrations compared with PT, which can assess an analytical method across a wide range of concentrations; parallel patient testing does not involve peer comparison; there is a need to define appropriate acceptability criteria that recognise measurement uncertainty; and there can be problems associated with the transport and delivery of patient samples to the laboratory from geographically isolated rural and remote locations.

In terms of practicality in the field, we should never lose sight of the complexities faced by a POCT operator performing QC and PT in a non-laboratory environment. Operators in primary care facilities may be required to conduct POCT on multiple levels of QC and PT samples each month and work with a range of different sealed vials, liquid solutions and pipetting equipment to fulfil their quality testing requirements. The realities of busy health professionals who are not familiar with laboratory practice, but are required to conduct POCT in the field, are often overlooked or misunderstood (Fig. 5.2).

## AN EXAMPLE OF QUALITY TESTING IN PRACTICE

The next section provides a brief practical example of the quality testing system employed by the national QAAMS HbA1c POCT program for diabetes management operating in Indigenous medical services in Australia (Shephard *et al.* 2015; Shephard and Gill 2005, 2006, 2010). This example illustrates how this quality program operates in practical terms; one that has now been successfully translated across different primary care settings, different countries and different clinical scenarios (Motta and Shephard 2015; Shephard *et al.* 2009, 2014).

### Quality control testing in the QAAMS program

In the QAAMS program, device operators are required to test one set of QC materials, comprising two levels of HbA1c (reflective of a patient with optimal and poor glycaemic control) every month across the calendar year.

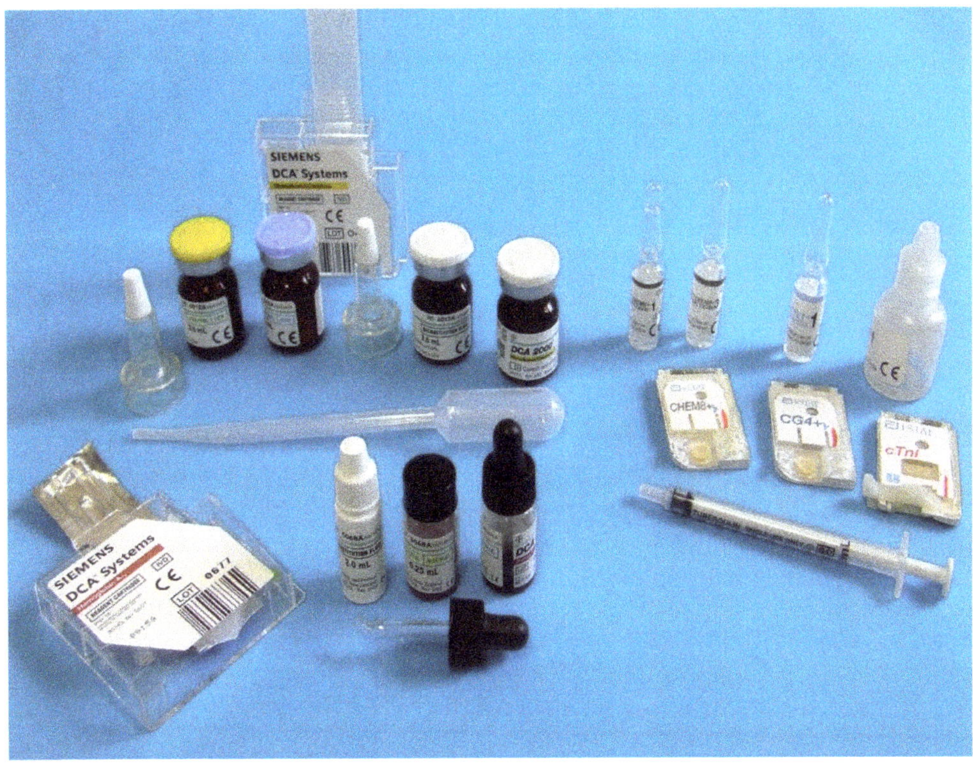


**Fig. 5.2.** An array of different quality control solutions and associated consumables for use with the DCA Vantage and i-STAT devices, exemplifying the realities of conducting QC testing in the field.

With the support of the manufacturer, an annual batch of QC kits with the same lot number is ordered and stored specifically for use by the participating QAAMS health services (which now number 190). The use of a single lot number of QC enables the program management team to monitor the imprecision of QC testing more efficiently than if there were multiple lot numbers.

Device operators are provided with a colour-coded QC result sheet on which to record their monthly QC results. The colour codes are designed to mimic a 'traffic light' system (i.e. a QC result in the green zone means 'go', orange means 'proceed with caution' and red means 'stop'); this system provides device operators with a practical and user-friendly method of interpreting their QC results on-site and making an informed decision to accept the QC results and proceed with patient testing or reject the QC results and cease testing patients until the reason for unacceptable performance has been investigated and corrected (with the assistance of the POCT Coordinator).

QC results can be entered electronically by the operator into the 'QC Results' section of the QAAMS website, where the site's imprecision is automatically updated and results can be reviewed by the POCT Coordinator.

## Proficiency testing in the QAAMS Program

At the beginning of each calendar year, the QAAMS PT provider (the Royal College of Pathologists of Australasia's Quality Assurance Programs Pty Ltd) sends a PT kit containing 24 lyophilised PT samples (each numbered and dated for the next year of the program), together with vials of reconstitution fluid and a Quality Testing Calendar, to each participating service. Two samples per month are made up and tested by the participants (according to the calendar) across two 6-monthly testing cycles per year (January–June and July–December). Each sample has a target value and a limit for acceptable performance set by the PT organisers. The material provided (and acceptable performance limits set for QAAMS) are identical to those used by the PT provider for their HbA1c program for Australasian laboratories, which enables direct comparison between the two programs. The samples for each cycle comprise six paired and linearly related levels of analyte across a range of HbA1c values from 5 to 14% (31 to 130 mmol/mol). The use of paired samples enables calculation of imprecision for PT testing on the POCT device for both individual services and the group as a whole.

The HbA1c results obtained for the two PT samples tested for that month can be entered electronically onto the PT section of the QAAMS website. Within a week after the due date for the return of results for that month, the PT provider sends a report to each participating service.

Monthly scientific meetings between the QAAMS POCT Coordinator and a scientist from the PT provider are held to discuss and review all QC and PT results returned by services for that month. These QC/PT review meetings enable poor analytical performance and/or non-compliance with QC and/or PT testing schedules to be actioned and fixed in a timely fashion.

As discussed later in the book, this quality framework has been robust and sustainable for more than 16 years, with the long-term analytical performance for both QC and PT testing in the QAAMS POCT program consistently meeting analytical benchmarks for quality recommended by the Australian Government and expected of Australasian laboratories.

## ENSURING QUALITY FOR INFECTIOUS DISEASE POINT-OF-CARE TESTING

Testing for infectious diseases is prone to variation, whether the test is laboratory-based or a POC test. Some of the sources of variation experienced in each setting are the same, but there are sources of variation unique to the POCT setting. Even though POC tests are designed to be robust and easy to use, testing errors still occur (Wolpaw *et al.* 2010). Although the sensitivity and specificity of POC tests for HIV antibodies have been reported as being as high as 100% under well-controlled evaluations (Motta *et al.* 2013), evidence indicates that the performance in the field is often much poorer (Bloch *et al.* 2014; Learmonth *et al.* 2008; Plate *et al.* 2007; Wolpaw *et al.* 2010). Therefore, it is important that facilities using POC tests for infectious diseases participate in well-designed and ongoing quality testing processes to ensure test results are accurate. Knowledge of the sources of variation is beneficial when designing and implementing quality materials for infectious disease POC tests because each variable can be targeted and so minimise the potential effect it has on patient test results.

### Sources of variation in infectious disease POC tests

Many health professionals using infectious disease POC tests are not necessarily expected to have strong scientific or technical knowledge and may be unaware of the influences that sources of variation may have on the test results (Constantine *et al.* 2005). These variables may include: environmental changes, reagents, equipment and processes, as discussed in the following sections.

#### Environmental changes

POCT kits are usually transported and stored refrigerated or at room temperature. However, environmental conditions such as extreme temperature and/or humidity may have an adverse effect on performance (WHO 2005a). If stored refrigerated, results from a test that is undertaken before the reagents can equilibrate to room temperature may be incorrect. Test kits or reagents that are stored refrigerated need to have their storage conditions monitored. Any unidentified, intermittent changes in refrigeration temperatures may adversely affect the performance of the test kit. Some nucleic acid tests (NAT) used at the point of care or in remote facilities require reagents to be stored frozen. If stored in an automatic defrost freezer, the reagents may undergo inadvertent and damaging freeze–thaw cycles.

#### Reagents

Test kits sold into countries with *in-vitro* diagnostic device (IVD) regulations such as Australia are manufactured under strict conditions. In some regulated countries, each new lot of test kits is tested to ensure the quality of its performance (lot release testing). However, reagent lots will occasionally display sub-optimal performance when used to test patient specimens in testing facilities if issues are not detected in lot release testing. Some POC tests require reagents not provided in the test kit. Even basic reagents such as water may be contaminated or at a grade unsuitable for use.

#### Equipment

Many infectious disease POC tests require little or no equipment or have equipment such as disposable plastic pipettes provided in the test kit. Other more sophisticated POC tests may require readers or even, in the case of NAT POC tests, small-scale instrumentation. Failure of equipment or instrumentation may affect results. For example, plastic pipettes that dispense incorrect volumes of samples or devices that fail to allow the flow of sample may report incorrect results.

#### Processes

Each POC test is provided with instructions for use. These instructions guide the user through the testing process and highlight critical steps, such as time to reading the results after the addition of the patient specimen. POC test instructions are usually simple and user friendly; however, some steps are critical and must be adhered to. If manufacturer instructions at critical steps are not followed, false positive or negative results may be reported.

## Quality management systems for infectious disease POC tests

The results of POC tests can have a significant impact on a patient's wellbeing, especially when testing for infectious diseases such as HIV or syphilis (WHO 2015). A false positive result will cause unnecessary further testing, counselling and anxiety for the patient as they await confirmation of the result and lead to a lack of confidence in the testing. A false negative result may give a patient a false sense of security, delay treatment and expose the community to the spread of disease. The testing facility should minimise the risk of false results by developing and adhering to strict procedures and employing quality management measures that are designed to detect unexpected changes in the testing process (Constantine *et al.* 2005; Yao *et al.* 2010). These include quality control and proficiency testing.

## Proficiency testing for infectious disease POC tests

PT is a quality management service where testing facilities are provided with a panel of samples periodically throughout the year. The reactivity of the samples is unknown to the facility participating in the program. The participant tests the samples as they would a patient specimen and reports the results and any associated data (e.g. test kit name, lot number and expiry dating) to the PT provider. The PT provider analyses the results, usually by comparing the submitted results with a reference result, and writes a report, which is sent back to the testing facility. A distribution of samples is often defined as a 'challenge'. The purpose of PT is to monitor the test system from the receipt of the sample to the reporting of results.

Testing facilities can use PT results as objective and independent evidence of the quality of testing. PT can be used to periodically assess the competency of the user and identify training needs. The results allow the monitoring and comparison of the performance of testing facilities and the test kits used. Any errors or anomalies arising from PT participation must be investigated. The root source of the problem should be determined, actions to remove that source of variation implemented and resolution of the problem confirmed. In this way, a continual improvement cycle can be put into effect.

Participation in a PT program for all medical testing, including POCT, is mandatory in most developed countries (Valenti 2003). When selecting a PT provider, it is important to take several issues into account. The PT provider should be compliant with ISO 17043: 2010, General Requirements for Proficiency Testing – an international standard for PT providers. Accreditation to this standard provides evidence that the PT provider has robust sample preparation, shipping, analysis and reporting processes and has undertaken extensive testing to prove the PT samples are homogeneous and stable (Shephard *et al.* 2012).

A PT provider should supply sufficient samples to maximise the chance of detecting testing errors. Ideally, each person performing a test on a patient specimen should participate in at least one PT challenge per year. If too few samples are sent to participating facilities, errors inherent in the testing process may not be detected (Constantine *et al.* 2005). NRL recommends that PT challenges have at least five samples and that there are at least three challenges per year. The PT samples provided should reflect, as closely as possible, patient samples (Shephard *et al.* 2012). Where possible, the PT samples should also occasionally challenge the POCT with well characterised but rare genotypes/serotypes or other samples that may be encountered in a testing facility. PT also assesses the administration processes in the testing facility, with a view to emphasising the importance of these processes in ensuring that the correct test is performed on the correct sample and reported on the correct patient. The PT challenge should be designed to ask a question.

The analysis of PT results relies on reviewing results from peer groups; that is, testing facilities that test the panel samples using the same brand of POC test kit. Maximising the number of participants in peer groups allows the PT provider to employ more powerful statistical methods and have greater confidence in the conclusions drawn.

The PT provider should report the results of the analysis back to the participants quickly so that errors detected can be investigated expeditiously. An extensively delayed report may allow testing facilities to continue using poor testing procedures or reagents. The reporting process can be facilitated by the use of internet-based software, which allows the participant to enter test results directly into the database. The automatic analysis and reporting of PT results allows the PT provider to issue reports to participants quickly.

#### Alternatives to traditional PT

Sometimes it is impractical to conduct PT using real samples due to sample stability, importation difficulties or geographical challenges. Although less valuable, alternative methods of monitoring parts of the testing process may be substituted in these situations. However, it is not recommended that alternative PT methods are used if traditional PT is available.

*Laboratory-based PT for infectious disease POCT*

There are numerous providers that offer PT for laboratory-based infectious disease testing. These schemes usually provide plasma or serum-based samples in liquid, frozen or freeze-dried (lyophilised) form. If a whole-blood PT product is unavailable, these PT programs may be a suitable alternative. A small selection of laboratory-based infectious disease PT providers is presented in Table 5.2.

*Photography*

Some infectious disease PT providers have reported using photographs of patient's POC test results and asked that the participants read the result from the photograph (Chiu *et al.* 2011; Learmonth *et al.* 2008). This method has the advantages in that all participants receive exactly the same photographs and therefore their results can be meaningfully compared. Photographs are easily provided via email or the internet, thereby removing importation or shipping barriers. However, this PT method does not assess the pre-analytical or the analytical stages of the POCT process: only the ability of a participant to read and interpret the test result. The ability of the participant to accurately read the result is dependent on the resolution of the photograph. The PT program must also be POCT device-specific.

Alternatively, an assessment of a facility's staff to read results accurately may be assessed by the facility referring photographs of patient results to a third party for a 'second read'. This may be useful in providing oversight of a remote facility, but it will only assess the ability to read the result rather than the complete test process.

*Sample re-test*

Some infectious disease networks or facilities employ a re-test protocol where a defined percentage of patients, often 5–10%, have an additional sample taken and referred to a centralised reference laboratory. The reference laboratory re-tests the sample and compares the result with the original POCT result. This system has limitations (WHO 2005a). It is labour intensive, creates delays and, in low volume testing facilities, a very large percentage of POC tests would need to be re-tested in order to detect errors. This method of PT is not suited to developed countries, and its utility in resource-limited countries is questionable.

### Quality control testing for infectious disease POC tests

Whereas PT assesses the performance of the POC test and the processes of a testing facility several times per year, QC provides ongoing and frequent monitoring (Shephard *et al.* 2012). QC for infectious diseases involves the testing of the same sample with known reactivity on a frequent (e.g. daily) basis or every time testing is performed. As mentioned previously, the purposes of PT and QC are different, but complementary. Whereas participation in PT is mandatory in most regulated jurisdictions, the use of QC is highly recommended.

#### In-built control checks

Most POC tests for infectious diseases employ a method of test validation through the use of an in-built control. Generally, this is in the form of a control band or spot built into the device (WHO 2005b). In some POC tests, the in-built control changes colour with the addition of any human sample, indicating that the sample has flowed past the control line. Other POC tests, however, change colour with the addition of any fluid, even water. Either type of in-built control of flow has little value because they are non-specific and monitor the mechanical aspect of the device rather than the analytical performance.

#### 'Third party' quality controls

Some infectious disease POCT manufacturers provide a positive and negative quality control but most do not. Manufacturer-provided QC material should be tested as specified by the instructions for use.

Irrespective, it is beneficial to test a 'low positive' QC sample from a third party (non-manufacturer) to monitor test performance because this QC can often be used over a long period of time (Shephard *et al.* 2012). Running a 'negative' third-party control is also recommended (WHO 2015). A well-designed third-party QC program will provide access to sufficient QC sample vials so that the same QC lot can be used over an extended period of time (e.g. 6–12 months). In this way, the facility can monitor variation that may be attributed to changes in test kit lots (Shephard *et al.* 2012).

Like PT, the QC sample type should preferably reflect the sample type being tested. Infectious disease POC tests may be validated for several different sample types such as serum, plasma, whole blood and/or saliva (CDC 2003, 2007; North Carolina HIV Prevention Program 2015). Generally, commercial third-party QC samples are made of plasma. To date, there are no whole blood QC samples for infectious disease POC tests. A plasma-based QC sample will monitor the performance of the POC test and the testing processes used, and is generally appropriate for the purpose. Sometimes the procedures for testing plasma and capillary blood are different; this needs to be considered when testing a QC sample.

At a minimum, a 'low positive' third-party QC should be tested in the following circumstances (CDC 2003, 2007; WHO 2005a) before testing patient samples:

- by a new user to assess competency
- when a new test kit lot is opened
- when a new shipment of test kits is delivered
- when storage conditions fluctuate outside specified limits.

The NRL suggests that a third-party QC is tested daily if patient testing is performed daily. If patient testing is performed infrequently, the third-party QC should be tested on each day that patient testing is performed. WHO recommends testing a QC sample at least once per week (WHO 2005a). The frequency of testing should be determined by the facility manager.

It is important to ensure third-party QC samples are stored and used as described in the instructions for use. Commercial third-party QC samples may be considered prohibitively expensive or be unavailable for certain analytes. In these situations, an in-house or locally made QC sample may suffice (WHO 2005b). The development of an appropriate in-house QC sample for infectious disease POCT requires significant expertise. Variability inherent in a QC sample may mask variability in the test kit, or be misinterpreted as poor performance of the test kit. An in-house QC sample must also be proven to be homogeneous and stable over time. The storage conditions must be validated and instructions for use developed. Long-term storage at –20°C may be effective to maintain stability but repeated freeze–thaw cycles should be avoided. If being provided beyond one's own facility, the QC sample must be validated on all POC tests it is being used to monitor. In countries with stringent regulatory systems, the use of commercial QC sample is recommended if available.

Because infectious disease POC tests are generally qualitative – that is, provide positive or negative results – it is not possible to plot QC results on a graph. However, QC test results should be recorded in a systematic manner, each time detailing the date of test, person testing, test name and kit lot number, identification of any critical equipment or instrumentation if applicable along with the QC test results (CDC 2007). The use of a –, +/–, +, ++, +++ system of recoding results may be useful, but it is important to assure standardisation of interpretation between operators (Shephard *et al.* 2012). These records should include any QC test results that fail, because this will aid in determining the frequency of failures and in troubleshooting. All failures of QC should be brought to the attention of the POCT Coordinator or POCT site supervisor. In the case of QC failures, remedial action will need to be determined and whether it is safe to test patients using the test kit in which the QC sample failed.

**Table 5.4.** Suggested checks that can be implemented in the case of unexpected proficiency test (PT) or quality control (QC) results for infectious disease POC tests

| Proficiency testing | Quality control |
|---|---|
| Check the results sent to the PT provider for errors in transcription. | Check the expiry date of the POCT reagent kit used to test the QC sample. |
| Check the expiry date of the POCT reagent used to test the PT samples. | Re-test the QC sample using the same and a different operator to rule out operator error. |
| Re-test the PT samples if possible; the PT provider may be able to supply additional samples. | Review the storage conditions of the POC test and the QC. |
| Check the instructions for use for the POC test to ensure the test has been performed correctly. | Repeat the QC test using a new lot of QC and a new lot number of reagent. |
| Check the PT report from the provider to determine whether other facilities using the same POC test also obtained an incorrect result. | Check the instructions for use for the POC test to ensure the test has been performed correctly. |
| Review the PT provider's instructions. | |
| Review the storage conditions of the POC test kits and the PT samples. | |
| Check for a change in critical reagents. | |

The recording of QC test results should be documented with a written procedure that includes the processes employed when QC failures occur.

### Corrective action

Participation in PT and QC programs provides facilities with mechanisms to detect error or deviation in infectious disease POC testing systems. The records of PT and QC should be reviewed periodically (e.g. monthly) by the POCT Coordinator or POCT site supervisor. The reviewer should sign and date the reviewed documents as evidence of oversight. When errors or deviations are identified, corrective action should be implemented (CDC 2007; Constantine *et al.* 2005; WHO 1996).

A documented action plan will assist site operators when corrective action is warranted. A flow chart is a convenient way of displaying required troubleshooting actions. The facility should be responsible for drafting the plan. Without being exhaustive, some considerations for each of PT and QC are presented in Table 5.4.

Ideally, the source of the incorrect test result should be determined and rectified. In the case of QC, the investigation should be undertaken and a valid QC test result obtained before testing patient samples.

## REFERENCES


Bloch EM, Shah A, Kaidarova Z, Laperche S, Lefrere JJ, van Hasselt J, *et al.* for the Anglophone Africa Transfusion Research Group (2014) A pilot external quality assurance study of transfusion screening for HIV, HCV and HBsAg in 12 African countries. *Vox Sanguinis* **107**, 333–342. doi:10.1111/vox.12182

Bullock DG (2004) Quality control and quality assurance in point-of-care testing. In *Point-of-Care Testing.* 2nd edn. (Eds CP Price, A St John and JM Hicks) pp. 137-145. AACC Press, Washington DC, USA.

CDC (Centers for Disease Control and Prevention) (2003) *Quality Assurance Guidelines for Testing Using the OraQuick® Rapid HIV-1 Antibody Test,* <ftp://ftp.cdc.gov/pub/CLIAC_meeting_presentations/pdf/Addenda/cliac0903/C_GuidlinesOraQk.pdf>.

CDC (2007) *Quality Assurance Guidelines for Testing Using Rapid HIV Antibody Tests Waived Under the Clinical Laboratory Improvement Amendments of 1988,* <http://www.cdc.gov/hiv/pdf/testing_qa_guidlines.pdf>.

Chiu YH, Ong J, Walker S, Kumalawati J, Gartinah T, McPhee DA, *et al.* (2011) Photographed rapid HIV test results pilot novel quality assessment and training schemes. *PLoS One* **6**, e18294. doi:10.1371/journal.pone.0018294

Constantine NT, Saville RD, Dax EM (2005) *Retroviral Testing and Quality Assurance: Essentials for Laboratory Diagnosis.* MedMira Laboratories, Halifax, Canada.

Ehrmeyer SS, Laessig RH (2001) Electronic "Quality Control" (EQC): is it just for unit use devices? *Clinica Chimica Acta* **307**, 95–99. doi:10.1016/S0009-8981(01)00438-7

Gill J, Shephard M (2010) The conduct of quality control and quality assurance testing for PoCT outside the laboratory. *The Clinical Biochemist Reviews* **31**, 81–84.

Gill J, Watkinson L (2010) Quality control and quality assurance in point-of-care testing. In *Point-of-Care Testing.* 3rd edn. (Eds CP Price, A St John and LL Kricka) pp. 225-236. AACC Press, Washington DC, USA.

Learmonth KM, McPhee DA, Jardine DK, Walker SK, Aye TT, Dax EMJ (2008) Assessing proficiency of interpretation of rapid human immunodeficiency virus assays in non-laboratory settings: ensuring quality of testing. *Clinical Microbiology* **46**, 1692–1697.

Martin C (2008) Quality control issues in point of care testing. *The Clinical Biochemist Reviews* **29**, S79–S82.

Motta L, Shephard M (2015) The international Analytical and Clinical Excellence program: point-of-care testing for diabetes management. *Point of Care* **14**, 76–80. doi:10.1097/POC.0000000000000053

Motta LA, Shephard MDS, Keen PBA (2013) A review of the use of rapid HIV testing in community settings with specific reference to Australia. *Point of Care* **12**, 27–32. doi:10.1097/POC.0b013e318265f7b3

NCCLS (National Committee for Clinical Laboratory Standards) (2002) *Quality Management for Unit-Use Testing; Approved Guideline.* NCCLS document EP18-A. Wayne PA, USA.

North Carolina HIV Prevention Program (2015) *Quality Assurance Protocol for State Purchased Rapid HIV Testing Kits.* Raleigh NC, USA, <http://epi.publichealth.nc.gov/cd/stds/docs/Rapid_Testing_Quality_Assurance_Protocols.pdf>.

Phillips DL (2004) Unit-use quality control. In *Point-of-Care Testing.* 2nd edn. (Eds CP Price, A St John and JM Hicks) pp. 147-154. AACC Press, Washington DC, USA.

Plate DK, Rapid HIV Test Evaluation Working Group (2007) Evaluation and implementation of rapid HIV tests: the experience in 11 African countries. *AIDS Research and Human Retroviruses* **23**, 1491–1498. doi:10.1089/aid.2007.0020

Shephard MDS, Gill JP (2005) An innovative Australian point-of-care model for urine albumin:creatinine ratio testing that supports diabetes management in indigenous medical services and has international application. *Annals of Clinical Biochemistry* **42**, 208–215. doi:10.1258/0004563053857806

Shephard MDS, Gill JP (2006) The analytical quality of point-of-care testing in the 'QAAMS' model for diabetes management in Australian Aboriginal medical services. *The Clinical Biochemist Reviews* **27**, 185–190.

Shephard M, Shephard A, Watkinson L, Mazzachi B, Worley P (2009) Design, implementation and results of the Quality Control program for the Australian Government's Point of Care Testing in General Practice Trial. *Annals of Clinical Biochemistry* **46**, 413–419.

Shephard MDS, Gill JP (2010) The National QAAMS program. *The Clinical Biochemist Reviews* **31**, 95–99.

Shephard M, Leibie A, Dimech W, Condie D, Nolan M (2012) Guidelines and recommendations for the quality-assured conduct of point-of-care testing for infectious diseases and drugs of abuse in Australia. *Australian Journal of Medical Science* **33**, 143–154.

Shephard MDS, Spaeth B, Mazzachi B, Auld M, Schatz S, Lingwood A, *et al.* (2014) Towards sustainable point-of-care testing in remote Australia – the Northern Territory i-STAT point-of-care testing program. *Point of Care* **13**, 6–11. doi:10.1097/POC.0000000000000009

Shephard MDS, Spaeth B, Motta LA, Shephard A (2015) Point-of-Care Testing in Australia: Practical advantages and benefits of community resiliency for improving outcomes. In *Global Point-of-Care – Strategies for Disasters, Emergencies and Public Health Resilience.* (Eds GJ Kost and CM Curtis) pp. 527-535. AACC Press, Washington DC, USA.

Valenti WM (2003) Rapid HIV testing and quality assurance. *The AIDS Reader* **13**, 520–522, 526–527.

Westgard JO (2001) Electronic quality control, the total testing process, and the total quality control system. *Clinica Chimica Acta* **307**, 45–48. doi:10.1016/S0009-8981(01)00430-2

WHO (World Health Organization) (1996) *Guidelines for Organizing National External Quality Assessment Schemes for HIV Serological Testing (UNAIDS/96.5).* WHO, Geneva, Switzerland, <http://www.who.int/diagnostics_laboratory/publications/quality/en/>.

WHO (2005a) *Guidelines for Assuring the Accuracy and Reliability of HIV Rapid Testing: Applying a Quality System Approach.* U.S. Department of Health and Human Services Centers for Disease Control and Prevention USA and WHO, Geneva, Switzerland, <http://www.who.int/diagnostics_laboratory/publications/HIVRapidsGuide.pdf>.

WHO (2005b) *Module 12: Quality Control Participant Manual.* WHO, Geneva, <http://www.who.int/diagnostics_laboratory/documents/guidance/module12_quality_control.pdf>.

WHO (2015) *WHO Recommendations to Assure HIV Testing Quality.* WHO, Geneva, <http://apps.who.int/iris/bitstream/10665/179521/1/WHO_HIV_2015.15_eng.pdf?ua=1.>.

Wolpaw BJ, Mathews C, Chopra M, Hardie D, de Azevedo V, Jennings K, *et al.* (2010) The failure of routine rapid HIV testing: a case study of improving low sensitivity in the field. *BMC Health Services Research* **10**, 73. doi:10.1186/1472-6963-10-73

Yao K, Wafula W, Bile EC, Cheignsong R, Howard S, Demby A, *et al.* (2010) Ensuring the quality of HIV rapid testing in resource-poor countries using a systematic approach to training. *American Journal of Clinical Pathology* **134**, 568–572. doi:10.1309/AJCPOPXR8MNTZ5PY

# 6 Use of connectivity for managing point-of-care testing results

*Bridgit McAteer, Brooke Spaeth, Volker Harms and Anne Shephard*

**Summary**

Connectivity encompasses the electronic capture of test results from a POCT device and the transfer of those results to a local computer, systems databases or electronic medical records. The introduction of an international connectivity standard in 2002 helped to provide the framework for engineers to design devices and work station interfaces that allowed multiple types of POCT devices to communicate bidirectionally with data management systems or laboratory information systems. For connectivity to be successful, the set-up process must be seamless, reliable and involve both clinical and technical professional staff. Attributes of a connectivity solution should allow control and management of all aspects of remote POCT, from quality control, calibration and maintenance protocols through to result validation, and include training records for all certified operators, POCT site accounts and workload statistics, a complete audit trail and traceability of testing pathways for individual POCT sites.

## INTRODUCTION

In general terms, connectivity refers to the ability of electronic devices to link to, and communicate with, other computer systems, electronic devices, software or the internet. In the point-of-care testing (POCT) environment, connectivity 'encompasses the electronic capture of test results within a POCT device and transfer of those results to other computer systems, databases, or electronic medical records' (College of American Pathologists 2015).

Most POCT devices now have connectivity, enabling immediate availability of test results for viewing by clinicians and facilitating prompt clinical management (DuBois 2013). Connectivity has many benefits and, with innovative technological advancements being developed at an extraordinary rate, there seems to be limitless boundaries for the future of POCT with connectivity.

The first POCT or near-patient testing devices began to emerge in the 1980s and were designed for clinicians to use in general practices or, as they are known in the US, physician office laboratories (POLs). These devices were stand-alone, had manual data recording procedures and had little or no data output capability (DuBois 2013). The first POCT device to feature connectivity in the mid-1980s was a small, desktop chemistry instrument, the Kodak DT60, which was interfaced to a microcomputer at a POL. This device formed the foundation for understanding the operational and technical requirements for POCT connectivity (Jones 2010).

Initial attempts at connectivity were predominantly undertaken through proprietary firmware and software with scripted interfaces (DuBois 2010). Auto-scripting (automatically running a script) for POCT connectivity was established in 1991 for the then new i-STAT® POCT device (Abbott Laboratories, Abbott Park, Illinois PA, USA), which was developed for testing basic blood chemistry. Connectivity trials of this device began at the Geisinger Medical Centre in Pennsylvania, where as part of their trauma protocol, they serially connected i-STAT devices to their laboratory information system (LIS). Connectivity proved beneficial because it reduced both administration time and turnaround time (TAT) for results (Jones 2008). As the benefits of connectivity became clearer, additional POCT devices were connected. It was not until the late 1990s that POCT connectivity became established in the marketplace. However, by the year 2000, there were still only around 20% of POCT devices connected (Jones 2010).

Early POCT devices were developed with manufacturer-specific data management interfaces, meaning there was little or no standardisation of these interfaces. Health organisations, information technology (IT) departments and data management system vendors were consequently left to deal with the challenges of different communication systems (wiring, computer, software) for each device.

## STANDARDISATION

With so many different manufacturer-specific interfaces on the market and with each requiring different communication systems, it was evident there was a need for standardisation. In 1999, the Clinical and Laboratory Standards Institute Area Committee on Automation received a proposal for POCT Connectivity Standardisation. The Point of Care Industry Connectivity Consortium was established at the same time and the two groups collaborated to develop the first POCT Connectivity Standard: POCT1-A, which was published in 2002 by the National Committee for Clinical Laboratory Standards (NCCLS), now known as the Clinical and Laboratory Standards Institute (CLSI). The introduction of standardisation helped provide the framework for engineers to design devices and workstation interfaces that allowed multiple types of POCT devices to communicate bidirectionally with access points and data management system (middleware) databases (POCT Consultative Group 2007). A newer, modified standard, POCT01-A2 (CLSI 2006), has since been released, which has further improved connectivity by reducing the complexity of technical terms and incorporating a simpler, universal language, thereby making the guideline more user friendly and communication simpler (Bogner 2010). POCT01-A2 has also evolved to incorporate guidelines on wireless communication (DuBois 2010).

In principle, standardisation has benefitted both manufacturers and users by reducing the cost of product manufacture and decreasing the complexity of installation. Data management systems have become streamlined and more cost effective and network infrastructure and hardware (access points) are now re-usable. Standardisation has meant the selection of POCT devices can now be focussed on the functionality and effectiveness of the device, rather than the constraints of connectivity.

## CONNECTIVITY OF POCT DEVICES

Connected POCT devices can send results to an intermediate data management system or a laboratory information system; from there results may be sent to an electronic medical record, or clinical information system (Fig. 6.1). Many POCT devices are 'intelligent' and have bidirectional interfaces that can send to and receive information from the POCT data management system. Other devices are unidirectional and can only send results to a data management system (Table 6.1).

Connectivity between the analyser and POCT data management system should be 'plug and play'. Access to the device settings required to set up the POCT device for connectivity may vary from manufacturer to manufacturer. Some device manufacturers will have a menu item on the device providing access to the parameter fields, while others supply software that needs to be installed on a computer before connecting to the analyser via a USB cable to configure the connectivity parameters. Manufacturers can also use a pre-configured USB stick to allow the upload of connectivity parameters to the analyser. These connectivity parameters are supplied by the IT department that controls the network where the analysers are installed. Once an analyser has been configured on the network, via the parameters set up on the analyser, the analyser should connect to the POCT data management system seamlessly.

Data management system (middleware or connectivity) software can be provided by a specialised vendor or the device manufacturer. Some current suppliers (vendor and non-vendor specific) of data management software include:

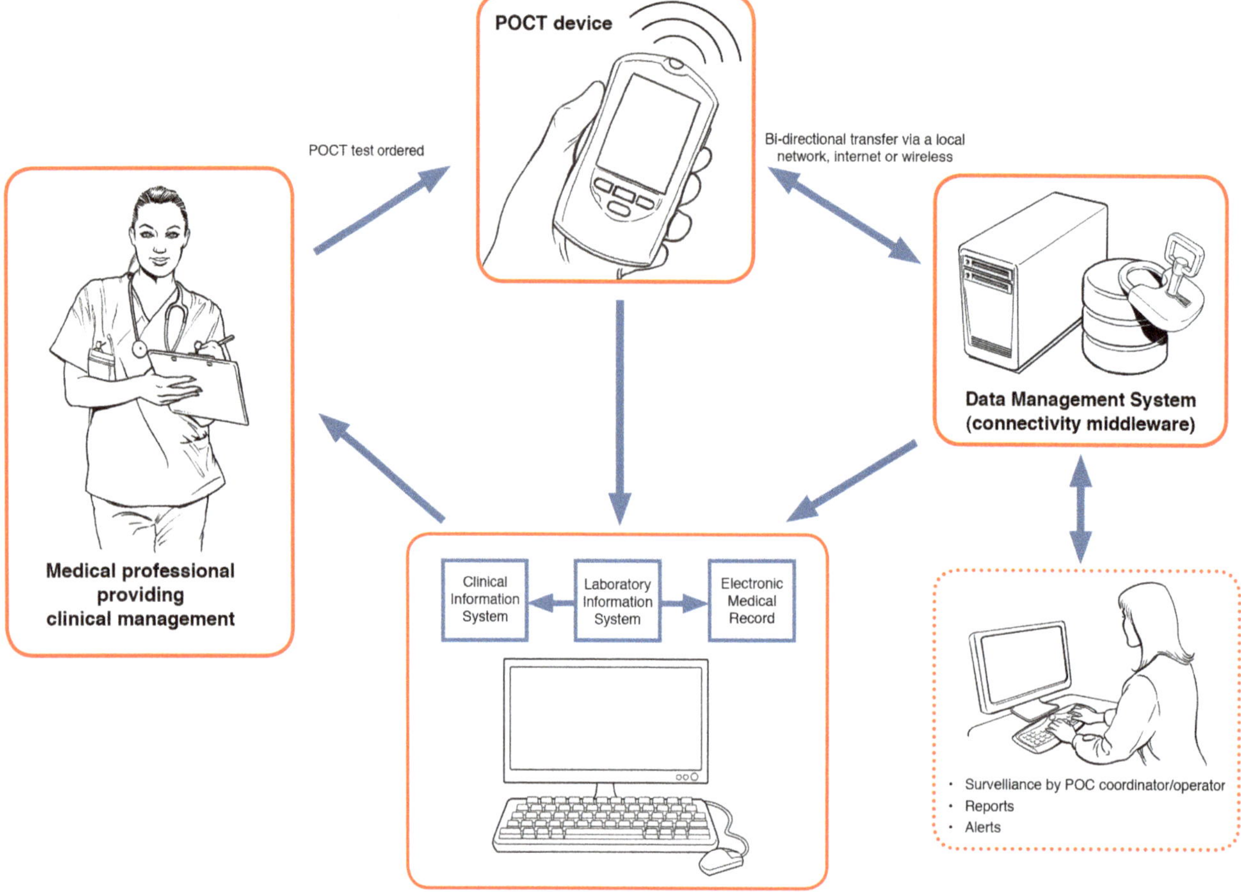


**Fig. 6.1.** Schematic diagram of POCT connectivity.

- Integrated Software Solutions Ltd, (Winchester, Hampshire, UK) *v-Lab*
- Medical Communications Associates (Adelaide, SA, Australia) *ONDAS and POC2Doc*
- Abbott Laboratories, (Abbott Park, Illinois PA, USA) *Central Data Station System; Info HQ*
- Alere™ (Waltham MA, USA) *RALS® systems*
- Radiometer (Copenhagen, Denmark) *Aqure*
- Conworx Technology GmbH (Berlin, Germany) *POCcelerator™*
- Roche (Basel, Switzerland) *IT 1000*
- TELCOR (Lincoln NE, USA) *QML®*

POCT data management systems must be able to interface to analysers using the following message protocols: HL7, ASTM, POCT01-A2, proprietary messages and ODBC type connections. A new protocol, Audio16, is being finalised by the Clinical and Laboratory Standards Institute and will be available in the near future, enabling a much more standardised approach to the interfacing of instruments.

## BENEFITS OF CONNECTIVITY

### Flow of information to and from the POCT device

A major benefit of connectivity is its ability to improve the flow and management of information to and from POCT devices, enabling faster, more informed and coordinated clinical decisions to be made. Seamless transfer of data reduces the amount of time spent on clerical transcription while reducing the possibility of clerical error and loss of results. Devices that have the option of bidirectionality allow information, such as alerts and software upgrades, to be relayed back to the point-of-care device. Additionally, where customised clinical reference ranges have been set and where test results fall outside the acceptable range, connectivity can allow a warning to be

Table 6.1. Examples of devices that offer connectivity (Source: adapted with permission from McClintock 2014)

| Point of care device | Manufacturer |
|---|---|
| ACCU-CHEK® Inform and Inform II via Cobas® IT 1000 | Roche Diagnostics |
| Afinion™ AS100 Analyser System | Alere |
| CLINITEK 500® Urine Chemistry Analyser | Siemens Healthcare |
| [a]CLINITEK Advantus® Urine Chemistry Analyser | Siemens Healthcare |
| [a]CLINITEK Status® Urine Chemistry Analyser | Siemens Healthcare |
| [b]CoaguChek® XS Plus | Roche Diagnostics |
| [b]Cobas® b 221 and b 123 | Roche Diagnostics |
| [b]DCA Vantage® Analyser | Siemens Healthcare |
| epoc® | Alere |
| [b]Gem Premier® 3000, 3500, 4000 | Instrumentation Laboratory |
| [a]HemoCue® Hb 201 DM System | Radiometer |
| [a]In2it™ A1c | Bio-Rad Laboratories |
| IRMA TruPoint® | LifeHealth |
| [a,b]i-STAT® via CDS5 | Abbott Point of Care |
| [a]Piccolo® xpress | Abbott Point of Care |
| Radiometer ABL700 Series | Radiometer |
| StatSensor® Creatinine | Nova |
| [b]StatStrip® Glucose | Nova |
| [a,b]Triage® Meter | Alere |

[a]Requires serial to network adaptor
[b]Bidirectional

sent to a clinical expert who can take action if required (Travanty 2011). Some devices have a laser scanner, which can scan the patient's bar code to assist the direct uploading of results into the patient's medical record. This further reduces data entry error and administration time. To reduce the possibility of results being sent to the wrong medical record, second and third unique identifiers confirm the patient's ID before data is uploaded. Typically, results with invalid patient identifiers will not enter patient records until reviewed, corrected and re-sent (Travanty 2011).

From the data management system, data can be stored, transformed if required, organised and backed up. Reports can be generated and may include external quality assurance (EQA), quality control (QC), operator competency and individual and cohort patient reports. Some systems can automate data analysis and prepare and distribute reports automatically (POCT Consultative Group 2007). Data collection using connectivity allows for audit controls, logs, accountability and can be used to inform consumable orders. In addition, when POCT data is uploaded to a LIS, the results can be integrated with other laboratory results to enable the provision of coordinated care. Connectivity can also enable automated billing with the benefit of streamlining the financial administration process (Yu *et al.* 2010).

The functionality of the data management system can be limited by the POCT device itself; for example, how the incoming data is organised will depend on the labels associated with that incoming data. The label attached to the incoming results may, for example, be an operator identifier (ID), unique patient identifier(s) or a quality control lot number. Labelling of incoming data allows for easy identification of the type of test and for differentiation between incoming patient test results, quality testing results or errors.

### Treatment and medication compliance

Connectivity was shown to support medication compliance in a network of 10 anticoagulation clinics using connected POCT devices for international normalised ratio (INR) at the Giesinger Health System, Pennsylvania. Connectivity facilitated a more streamlined, or 'lean', patient workflow, which in turn assisted in improving compliance rates and avoided adverse clinical events (Jones 2010). POC test results were immediately uploaded to the LIS and reviewed by clinic pharmacists who made changes to medication dose based on the current test result as well as a comparison with previous results (Jones 2010).

POCT connectivity has also been linked to reducing turnaround time for patient results, leading to earlier medication intervention and improving the ability to be able to flag, track and follow-up test results (Dabkowski 2009; Kost 2001). Not only can connectivity help reduce turnaround time but patient results can be shared instantaneously with all members of a medical team to facilitate coordinated care.

POCT connectivity also permits faster clinical decision making in life threatening situations such as disaster management, where the bidirectional exchange of diagnostic data between device and medical personnel permits real-time, evidence-based treatment and disaster response coordination (Yu *et al.* 2010).

### Operator competence and lockout

To ensure appropriate clinical decisions are being made, compliance with regulations is met and the possibility of technical errors reduced, POCT operators should be trained and competent in both test performance and data entry procedures for each POCT device (POCT Consultative Group 2007; Travanty 2011). Assigning a unique operator ID when a POCT device is connected allows the benefit of traceability and accountability and enables maintenance of operator competency records. Reports on operator competency (certification date and date of certification expiry) can be regularly reviewed by POCT Coordinators. A bidirectional interface can include a lockout system that prohibits an operator with expired competency or an unauthorised operator from using a device. Operator compliance has been shown to be improved with operator lockout functions (Salka and Kiechle 2003). Lockouts can additionally discourage fraudulent use including tampering and theft (Kost 2001).

### Monitoring of quality testing and reagents

For there to be confidence in the accuracy and precision of test results, the POCT device must be properly configured, should be in sound working order and meet the manufacturer's specifications and recommendations (POCT Consultative Group 2007). Connectivity can be used to monitor, track and record the performance of quality testing of each POCT device (Kost 2001). POCT Coordinators and/or medical staff can remotely monitor EQA and QC results to be certain the device conforms to acceptable analytical standards (Gramz *et al.* 2013; Travanty 2011).

Connectivity can also be used to monitor reagent and control lot numbers, as well as expiry dates, and if reagents are out of date or have incorrect lot number, lockouts can be applied.

## CHALLENGES FOR CONNECTIVITY

### Information technology

POCT with connectivity represents a departure from traditional laboratory medicine, especially with results potentially by-passing the laboratory and being accessed in real-time by clinical decision makers. For connectivity to be implemented successfully, the set-up process must be seamless, reliable and involve both clinical and technical professionals.

One of the first challenges to operating a connected POCT program is the time, cost and effort associated in selecting a device that is analytically sound, meets the organisation's clinical and operational needs, and has interface compatibilities with the organisation's IT infrastructure (Gramz *et al.* 2013).

Transfer of data requires an internet connection (wireless or cabled) via a network to a secure server, where the data management system holds the data, which is made accessible to authorised personnel only. In order for data to be held on the database and accessed, there must be a well-planned, systematic approach involving collaboration between multiple stakeholders, including device manufacturers, health service managers, POCT Coordinators, IT personnel, internet service providers and data management system vendors.

Importantly, the IT department must be skilled enough to manage the device connections, information system and the network operations. They must be able to ensure security over the network and be able to support device operators and data management system vendors as required. The IT department will need to supply and/or install ports and network cabling for devices and be able to configure networks for wireless devices. Not all POCT devices share the same functionality, so the IT department may need to interface multiple devices with the one information system. There must also be consideration and preplanning for growth in the number of devices and the addition of new and different devices as the POCT network expands (Moorman 2010).

The data management system vendor must have the architecture in place to store, organise and manipulate auditable data. To ensure patient confidentiality, the system must have the ability to restrict access to include authorised personnel only. The data management system must be able to meet the required specifications of the device in order for it to be able to accept the data. It must also have the capacity to regularly back up data and allow ready access to that data.

Finally, for the seamless transfer of data, internet access should be available, reliable and be able to deliver data in real-time so that clinical decisions can be made immediately. Where internet connection has been lost, the health service should expect timely notification, reconnection and the recovery of any missing data (Gramz *et al.* 2013).

### Operator

A major challenge to maintain the viability/accuracy of data is correct data entry. Data entry errors in relation to patient identifiers by device operators (particularly if the data entry is performed manually) can result in risk to patients and loss of information. Operator training and competence is the key to good data entry and therefore valid and viable data. POCT Coordinators are likely to have responsibility for performing software updates and will also be undertaking the day-to-day troubleshooting. Consequently, selecting suitable and proficient device operators and POCT Coordinators is vital (Gramz *et al.* 2013).

### Cost

The initial cost of setting up a connected POCT program can be expensive. The ongoing maintenance and system upgrades can also be costly in both time and money and may interrupt patient care (Travanty 2011).

The unavoidable push for cheaper, faster, smaller devices by consumers also presents a challenge to the success of connectivity. Manufacturers should not compromise accuracy and reliability but bear in mind the desired outcome of connected POCT devices is to improve the flow and management of information to and from devices to enable faster, more coordinated clinical management and to improve patient outcomes (Travanty 2011).

## THE FUTURE FOR CONNECTIVITY

Recently, POCT devices capable of transmitting data wirelessly have been adopted at a fast rate. Wireless technologies enable devices to be more portable and patients more mobile. In a hospital setting, vital signs, blood pressure, electrocardiogram and temperature can be continuously monitored, allowing patient mobility (McClintock 2014).

Wireless POCT devices are also available for home monitoring, minimising patient trips to general practices or hospitals and saving time and expense. For instance, the Nova StatStrip® (Nova Biomedical, Waltham MA, USA) blood glucose meter has a docking station allowing POC results to be uploaded, either by wireless modem or Ethernet connectivity directly to a data management system. The Accu-Chek Inform II® glucose meter (Roche, Basel, Switzerland) can send POC test results to the data management system immediately and automatically without the need to even be docked. The new i-STAT 1 Wireless Analyser® (distinguished from the original i-STAT by its blue cover) is portable and results can be transferred to the data management system via the docking station either wirelessly through a wide-area network (WAN), by using a 3–4G wireless telephone network or by Ethernet cable (Francis and Martin 2010). This seamless, immediate transfer of test results facilitates patient self-monitoring and/or external monitoring by a clinician (McClintock 2014). Some examples of wireless POCT devices are shown in Fig. 6.2.

Heart rate and blood pressure are also frequently monitored wirelessly in the home by patients receiving cardiac care (Francis and Martin 2010). Data can be sent to a general practice for review using a software application installed on a computer, smartphone or tablet in the patient's home.

Recently, implantable glucose monitors have been developed that continuously transmit results to a networked computer at the patient's home with the results being able to be accessed and monitored remotely by health professionals (GlySens Inc 2015). Even critical life-sustaining devices, such as pacemakers, can now be checked by doctors using wireless technology. Wireless technology enables configuration updates to be sent

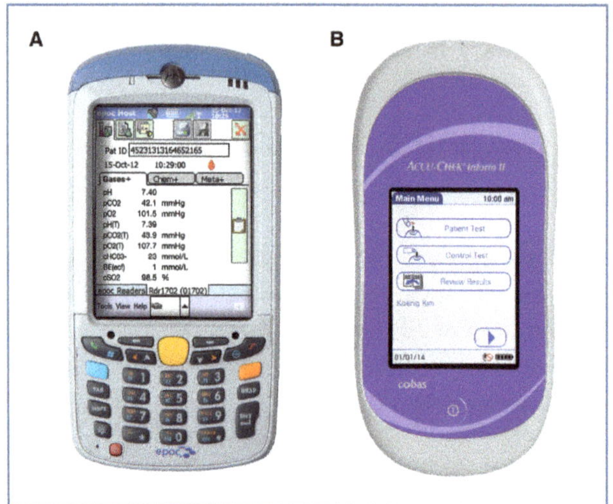


Fig. 6.2. Example of wireless POCT devices currently available: (A) epoc® blood analysis system; (B) Roche ACCU-CHEK® Inform II (reproduced with permission from Roche Diagnostics Pty Ltd and Alere™ ©2015 Alere).

directly to devices and has been associated with better availability, easier use, lower costs and easier access to patient data for health professionals while allowing timely critical care decisions to be made (DuBois 2010).

Bluetooth is the most recent wireless protocol in POCT devices (Velez and Shanblatt 2011), where mobile phone networks are used to immediately transfer data to a mobile phone, computer or information system from where the data can be monitored. Examples of Bluetooth POCT devices include the Accu-Chek Aviva Connect® wireless glucose monitor (Roche, Basel, Switzerland), the VivaChek®Smart glucose meter (Wilmington DE, USA) and the epoc® (Alere, Waltham MA, USA), which is a handheld, wireless device used for testing gases, electrolytes and metabolites.

Remotely monitoring patients using wireless technology can be used to identify trends and send bidirectional alerts when necessary. It allows health professionals to intervene early and potentially prevents hospital admissions. Remote monitoring allows regular communication between clinician and patient and facilitates coordinated care and improved self-management. It helps reduce travel time and costs for patients and can reduce the number of home visits, as well as prevent admissions to aged care facilities by helping keep elderly patients in their homes longer (RACGP 2015).

The rapid growth of wireless connectivity allows instantaneous bidirectional transfer of information. However, not all wireless networks are of the same standard; there can be dead spots, connection issues, and downtime and bandwidth limitations. Wireless technology, at this stage, is not as reliable as hard-wired systems; however, its benefits may outweigh the limitations (McClintock 2014). Additionally, patients may be reluctant to use this new technology because they may feel more at ease visiting a health professional face to face. They may also experience anxiety with having some responsibility for monitoring their own treatment and medications (RACGP 2015).

## ROLE OF THE POCT COORDINATOR IN CONNECTIVITY

### Surveillance of incoming data

A POCT Coordinator has the responsibility of overseeing a network of POCT devices, ensuring those devices are being used in the manner for which they were intended and are producing results of the required analytical quality to ensure patient safety. This role may include surveillance of incoming patient data to ensure there are no errors in measurement or any gross abnormalities in pathology results. If such errors or abnormalities are found, this information can then be reported back to the health service manager or discussed with the POCT operator (if an operator ID is included in the data label). The frequency of surveying incoming POCT data by the POCT Coordinator will depend on the size of the network and the coordinator's designated responsibilities. For example, the POCT Coordinator may survey the incoming data daily to check for a pattern of errors from a particular operator ID to inform if more education or training is needed, or weekly to check for error patterns on a particular POCT device to determine if maintenance is required.

Surveillance of incoming data can be enhanced if the data storage system has an alert system built-in, which can be customised to notify the POCT Coordinator (via phone SMS or email) if an incoming result is within or outside a particular range. The customisation of an alert system may also include the timing of the alert, which may be instantaneous for critical errors so they can be followed up immediately, or daily, for results within a particular target range of interest. As an example, the POCT Coordinator may set up an immediate alert system if a grossly high potassium (>8.0 mmol/L) result is recorded, because this result may be caused by incorrect

**Table 6.2.** Example of a feedback report for an individual health service

| Health service name - POCT device name - Month | | | | |
|---|---|---|---|---|
| **Total tests** | **Cartridge A** | **Cartridge B** | **Cartridge C** | **Cartridge D** |
| 48 | 22 | 13 | 8 | 5 |
| **Patient tests** | | | | |
| 35 | 15 | 9 | 8 | 3 |
| **Quality tests** | | | | |
| 9 | 4 | 3 | 0 | 2 |
| **Errors** | | | | |
| 4 | 3 | 1 | 0 | 0 |

| Tests by operator | Total tests | Patient tests | Quality tests | Total errors (%) |
|---|---|---|---|---|
| Operator 1 | 25 | 24 | 1 | 0 (0%) |
| Operator 2 | 13 | 8 | 4 | 1 (8%) |
| Operator 3 | 10 | 3 | 4 | 3 (30%) |
| **Total** | **48** | **35** | **9** | **4 (8.3%)** |

| Errors by type | Number of errors | Comment |
|---|---|---|
| Overfilled cartridge | 1 | Operator 2 |
| Underfilled cartridge | 1 | Operator 3 |
| Interference between cartridge and device | 2 | Error caused by operator 3, device requires cleaning |

| Quality testing | Cartridge A | Cartridge B | Cartridge C | Cartridge D |
|---|---|---|---|---|
| Quality Control (2 required for each cartridge) | 2 | 1 | 0 | 1 |
| Quality Assurance (2 required for each cartridge) | 2 | 2 | 0 | 1 |

| | Summary of recommendations to Health Service Manager |
|---|---|
| 1 | Operator 3 has produced a high error rate (30%); however, 2 of these errors relate the maintenance requirements for the POCT device; please perform cleaning procedure |
| 2 | Discuss correct cartridge filling procedure with operators 2 and 3 |
| 3 | Quality testing was not performed on cartridge C; perform QC and QA checks immediately to ensure patient safety |

**Table 6.3.** Example of a monthly management statistics report for a POCT network

| Health service name | Total tests | Total errors | Error rate (%) | Cartridge A | Cartridge B | Cartridge C | Cartridge D |
|---|---|---|---|---|---|---|---|
| Site 1 | 48 | 3 | 6.2 | 21 | 16 | 8 | 3 |
| Site 2 | 56 | 2 | 3.6 | 10 | 25 | 6 | 15 |
| Site 3 | 20 | 8 | 40.0 | 5 | 4 | 9 | 2 |
| Site 4 | 88 | 2 | 2.5 | 41 | 32 | 7 | 8 |
| Site 5 | 33 | 0 | 0 | 5 | 3 | 4 | 21 |
| TOTAL | **245** | **15** | **6.1** | **82** | **80** | **34** | **49** |

sampling technique – for example, the blood was collected into the wrong preservative tube (containing di-potassium EDTA) – or the blood sample was grossly haemolysed. A less critical daily alert system may include all incoming results without a valid patient identifier so these results can be followed up with the operator who performed the test and the correct information entered.

### Reporting on incoming data

As part of continuing quality management processes, the POCT Coordinator may be required to provide a feedback summary of the incoming data to key stakeholders within a POCT network. Considerations for reporting this data include:

- what data are to be reported
- to whom the feedback report will be provided (e.g. the medical director, health service manager or multidisciplinary POCT management committee)
- an appropriate frequency to provide feedback (e.g. daily, weekly, monthly or annually).

The types of information that the feedback report may include are:

- total number of patient tests
- total number or percentage of errors produced
- common or re-occurring errors
- individual POCT operator usage (for the health centre manager or individual to inform if further training/education is required)
- total number of individual test cartridges/strips performed (to inform ordering processes)
- number and type of quality tests performed on each POCT device (to monitor the rate of participation in quality testing procedures)
- individual patient report (based on a unique patient ID) (for the treating medical professional).

Table 6.2 provides an example of an individual health centre feedback report used in the Northern Territory Point-of-Care Testing Program in Australia (Shephard *et al.* 2014). These individual health centre feedback reports are a useful means of providing information to senior management at participating health services about the real-time field use of their POCT device in this program.

Table 6.3 provides an example of a monthly summary report of the total number of tests performed in a POCT network for management committee personnel. This type of report is useful to provide the total cartridge usage by site, as well as monitoring high error rates for individual services.

## CONCLUSION

Information technology is the single most rapidly advancing industry in the world. Every day new technologies are developed, while old technologies are retired or improved. This too will be the case for POCT devices and their connectivity capabilities. Already there has been dramatic change over the past 30 years and no doubt there will be more. POCT is becoming more mobile, sophisticated and accurate. Costs of devices and tests are reducing and, with this, demand will continue to increase at a dramatic rate. Providers, manufacturers and regulators should look 5–10 years in the future and work together to plan for new and novel technologies, connectivity systems and processes (DuBois 2010). Manufacturers, alongside independent IT vendors, need to continue evolving data management solutions to better support all aspects of POCT because the new generation of products will need to incorporate new and evolving communication and information technologies. The ideal POCT data management system is a comprehensive and powerful single-platform system for POCT connectivity that is a truly open (non-vendor specific) platform and able to interface with all types of analysers, irrespective of manufacturer. Such POCT data management systems must be web-based and can be learnt quickly and relatively easily. Attributes of a connectivity solution should allow control and management of all aspects of remote POCT, from quality control, calibration and maintenance protocols through to result validation, including training records for all certified operators, POCT site accounts and workload statistics, a complete audit trail and traceability of testing pathways for individual POCT sites.

## REFERENCES


Bogner D (2010) Connectivity Industry Consortium and point-of-care. *Point of Care* **9**, 171. doi:10.1097/POC.0b013e3181fc76aa

CLSI (Clinical and Laboratory Standards Institute) (2006) POCT01-A2: *Point-of-Care Connectivity; Approved Standard.* 2nd edn. Wayne PA, USA, <http://shop.clsi.org/point-of-care-documents/POCT01.html>.

College of American Pathologists (2015) *Point of Care Testing Toolkit.* Northfield IL, USA, <http://www.cap.org>.

Dabkowski B (2009) *Aiming for Lab-Like Accuracy at the Point of Care. CAP TODAY,* College of American Pathologists, Northfield IL, USA, <http://www.captodayonline.com/Archives/0409/0409g_aiming_for_lab_like_accuracy.htm>.

DuBois JA (2010) Point of care testing connectivity: past present and future. *Point of Care* **9**, 196–198. doi:10.1097/POC.0b013e3181fc7486

DuBois JA (2013) The role of POCT and rapid testing. *Medical Laboratory Observer* **45**, 18–22.

Francis AJ, Martin CL (2010) A practical example of POCT working in the community. *The Clinical Biochemist Reviews* **31**, 93–97.

GlySens Inc (2015) Company website. San Diego CA, USA, <http://glysens.com>.

Gramz J, Joerte P, Stein D (2013) Managing the challenges in point-of-care testing. *Point of Care* **12**, 76–79. doi:10.1097/POC.0b013e3182685e33

Jones JB (2008) Improving economic outcome with POCT: the "LEAN" perspective. *Point of Care* **7**, 127. doi:10.1097/01.POC.0000335832.77121.67

Jones JB (2010) The point-of-care testing connectivity continuum. *Point of Care* **9**, 158–161. doi:10.1097/POC.0b013e3181ecc9f6

Kost JK (2001) Preventing medical errors in point of care testing. *Archives of Pathology & Laboratory Medicine* **125**, 1307–1315.

McClintock D (2014) *Point of Care Testing and Informatics: How to Prepare for the POCT explosion.* Pathology Informatics Summit 2014, Pittsburgh PA, USA.

Moorman B (2010) *Medical Device Interoperability: Standards Overview.* Personal Connected Health Alliance, Beaverton OR, USA, <http://www.continuaalliance.org/sites/default/files/132-138_IT_WorldMA2010.pdf>.

POCT Consultative Group (2007) *Guidelines for Safe and Effective Management and Use of Point of Care Testing.* Royal College of Physicians of Ireland, Ireland.

RACGP (Royal Australian College of General Practitioners) (2015) *Using Technology to Deliver Healthcare: Remote Monitoring Devices,* RACGP, Melbourne, <http://www.racgp.org.au/digital-business-kit/remote-monitoring-devices/>.

Salka L, Kiechle F (2003) Connectivity for point-of-care glucose reduces error and increases compliance. *Point of Care* **2**, 114–118. doi:10.1097/00134384-200306000-00007

Shephard M, Spaeth B, Mazzachi B, Auld M, Schatz S, Lingwood A, *et al.* (2014) Toward sustainable point-of-care testing in remote Australia – the Northern Territory i-STAT point-of-care testing program. *Point of Care* **13**, 6–11. doi:10.1097/POC.0000000000000009

Travanty A (2011) Connectivity aids compliance. *Advance Healthcare Network for Laboratory* **20**, 18–19.

Velez D, Shanblatt M (2011) Taxonomy of current medical devices for POCT applications and potential acceptance of Bluetooth technology for secure interoperable applications. In *13th International Conference on e-Health Networking, Applications and Services.* 13–15 June, Columbia, Missouri. Pp. 288–295. Institute of Electrical and Electronics Engineers, Piscataway NJ, USA.

Yu JN, Brock TK, Mecozzi DM, Tran NK, Kost JK (2010) Future connectivity for disaster and emergency point of care. *Point of Care* **9**, 185–192. doi:10.1097/POC.0b013e3181fc95ee

# 7 Regulation and accreditation of point-of-care testing services

*Ian Farrance, Andrew Griffin and Mark Shephard*

**Summary**

This chapter summarises existing policies, procedures or guidelines that govern the use of point-of-care testing (POCT), and in particular any mandatory requirements and accreditation issues. In most countries, including Australia, there are no specific regulations preventing the use of POCT if used in the manner or for the purpose specified by the manufacturer. In a hospital or primary care setting, however, the operation of POCT devices should be implemented using a quality management approach with some form of accreditation strongly recommended. An international model for accreditation is described, which is directly applicable to POCT and includes three basic elements: regulation, standards and accreditation or audit by an independent authority.

## INTERNATIONAL STANDARDS FOR POCT

In many countries, it is a mandatory policy requirement for medical testing laboratories to show compliance with designated standards. These standards have components that incorporate both quality management and technical competence. In general, the manner in which this compliance is demonstrated is through an *accreditation system* provided by an independent third-party organisation. The defined standards may be locally derived, based on recognised professional guidelines or those produced, for example, by the International Organization for Standardization (ISO) or the Clinical Laboratory Standards Institute (CLSI) in the USA.

The term *standard* is itself defined by ISO as a document describing 'a set of rules that control how people develop and manage materials, products, services, technologies, processes, and systems.' ISO standards are developed by technical committees whose members represent many countries and professional groups and generally have very broad international support. In addition, ISO has provided a specific definition of the term accreditation for use within their various standards. This ISO definition of a 'procedure by which an authoritative body gives formal recognition that a body or person is competent to carry out specific tasks' varies slightly from the usual dictionary definition of accreditation, but is certainly appropriate for medical testing laboratories and primary care settings conducting POCT (ISO/IEC 2004).

The international standard for POCT is ISO 22870, *Point-of-Care Testing – Requirements For Quality and Competence* (ISO 2006). This standard gives specific requirements applicable to POCT and is intended to be used in conjunction with the more comprehensive ISO 15189, *Medical Laboratories – Particular Requirements for*

*Quality and Competence* (ISO 2012). The requirements of ISO 22870 'apply when POCT is carried out in a hospital, a clinic, or healthcare organisation providing ambulatory care.' Patient self-testing is excluded from ISO 22870, but is covered specifically in related documents such as ISO 15197 *In Vitro Diagnostic Test Systems – Requirements for Blood Glucose Monitoring Systems for Self-Testing in Managing Diabetes Mellitus* (ISO 2013), and ISO 17593 *Clinical Laboratory Testing and In Vitro Medical Devices – Requirements for In Vitro Monitoring Systems for Self-Testing of Oral Anticoagulant Therapy* (ISO 2007).

## NATIONAL OR JURISDICTIONAL STANDARDS AND PROFESSIONAL GUIDELINES FOR POCT

In addition to ISO standards, there are many other sources of standards, guidelines and recommendations for POCT, as described in Chapter 2. In some jurisdictions, specific national standards may be mandated or professional guidelines used in association with ISO or national standards. Previous concerns over the quality of POCT have resulted in a hierarchy of regulations in the USA and other countries in order to maximise patient benefit and minimise testing errors.

In addition to the many pathology and medical colleges and associations that provide guidelines for POCT, there are also many examples of national or health department policies that mandate accreditation or attainment of a specified standard in order to provide POCT services. A common theme through all these standards and guidelines prescribes the quality of patient care as the highest priority. As such, POCT should not be regarded as a special case exempt from the quality standards of laboratory practice. From an operational perspective, all such standards and guidelines for POCT require adherence to the principles of best practice, the performance of internal quality control (QC), participation in a proficiency testing (PT) or external quality assurance/assessment program, and adherence to quality management procedures with recording of test results in patients' medical records. Collectively, these principles indicate technical competence to perform testing.

## ACCREDITATION OF POCT

Even though there are professional recommendations and guidelines that cover all forms of POCT, it is probably unrealistic to expect devices used exclusively for home testing (personal use) to be covered by an accreditation system. Under these circumstances, device quality and reliability is dependent on the manufacturer providing a safe, user-friendly, robust testing device that includes built-in quality checks, with the various national agencies that regulate medical devices or therapeutic goods providing an assurance that compliance with a defined quality standard has been achieved for the given device.

In a hospital, primary care or community setting (e.g. a general practice, a community pharmacy, a community clinic or health centre, an industrial medical centre, an anticoagulation clinic or diabetes clinic), operation of POCT devices should be implemented using a quality management approach with formal accreditation strongly recommended (ACBI 2009; Lord Carter of Coles 2008; NACB 2006). In most countries, including Australia, there are no specific regulations preventing the use of POCT if used in the manner or for the purpose intended by the manufacturer. In Australia, the use of any commercial *in vitro* diagnostic device (IVD) that is used outside of the manufacturer's intended purpose is considered as 'off label' use. In this situation, additional Therapeutic Goods regulations then apply and accreditation is required as described below. When used according to the manufacturer's instructions, however, the main impediment to the widespread use of POCT is often related to funding. In countries where health-care funding is provided by government or by a private health insurer, some form of regulation is usually required, which governs the manner in which POCT may be implemented.

In many countries, reimbursement of testing costs is used to ensure compliance with the required standard or guideline; that is, reimbursement for testing is only provided under specified circumstances and only if defined guidelines or quality management procedures are being used. Formal accreditation or some form of licensure is often the process through which these quality procedures are recognised. Reimbursement arrangements with respect to POCT only appear problematical when performed outside of a formal accreditation system. Even though some POCT is available as waived tests in the USA, basic quality control is still required as specified by the manufacturer. In general, it would appear that when POCT is performed within an approved accreditation system, government or health insurer reimbursement is often available. In Australia, for example, government reimbursement of testing fees associated with a blood gas analyser – principally operated by nursing and medical staff in a critical care setting – would be governed by a quality management program with full accreditation based on the National Pathology Accreditation Advisory Council (NPAAC) and ISO 15189 standards. A table summarising reimbursement arrangements for several countries (Australia, France, Germany, Italy, Spain, United Kingdom and United States) is provided by Wittels *et al.* (2010).

## MINIMUM OR APPROPRIATE QUALITY STANDARDS?

Professionally developed ISO standards are designed to provide a high degree of confidence in testing facilities to which the relevant standard applies. However, the term *minimum standard* is often used to describe the least permissible condition or procedure required to demonstrate a basic level of performance (or provision of test results in the current context). In circumstances where quality is not considered a necessary objective, *minimum* usually becomes synonymous with *actual*. When discussing any testing situation where quality is an important component of the expected outcome, appropriate standard(s) provide the desired level of quality management and measurement uncertainty (the latter term refers to the reliability of the measurement as characterised by statistics such as accuracy and precision, which then provide a range of measurement values within which the true value may lie).

For POCT and quantitative pathology testing in general, appropriate analytical tolerance levels are defined by quality goals based on biological variation or internationally recognised clinical decision values. The desirable analytical variability required to ensure that a test is fit for purpose is fully discussed by Fraser (1999, 2001), Fraser and Scott (2010) and White and Farrance (2004). Failure to meet *appropriate standards* and failure to demonstrate that quality once attained is also maintained may jeopardise patient safety and contribute to a poor health outcome. Incorrect or misleading test results that initiate inappropriate treatment may cause more harm than no results at all.

Appropriate standards that support quality testing should be the desired approach, not minimum standards that provide the opportunity for quality failures. This view is supported by Burnett (2015) with regard to medical laboratory testing, where the question is asked 'Do you want to risk patient safety by running a laboratory that does not operate in compliance with the minimum requirements for quality and competence set out in ISO 15189?' The same principle applies to POCT in the primary care setting.

## QUALITY MANAGEMENT, INTERNAL QUALITY CONTROL AND EXTERNAL PROFICIENCY TESTING

The various standards and guidelines that have been developed for POCT are designed to assist with the implementation, management, operation and ongoing quality assessment of the selected technology. As stated in the introduction to ISO 22870 'Advances in technology have resulted in compact, easy-to-use *in vitro* diagnostic medical devices that make it possible to carry out some examinations at, or close to, the location of the patient. POCT or 'near patient testing' may benefit the patient as well as health-care facilities. Risk to the patient and to the facility can be managed by a well-designed, fully implemented quality management system that facilitates:

- evaluation of new or alternate POCT instruments and systems
- evaluation and approval of end-user proposals and protocols
- purchase and installation of equipment
- maintenance of consumable supplies and reagents
- training, certification and recertification of POCT systems operators
- quality control and quality assurance.' (ISO 2006)

When discussing the introduction of a quality management system, a question often asked is 'how much will it cost?' However, the real question to be asked is 'how much is poor quality going to cost (or how much is poor quality costing now)?' The principal issue here, particularly when discussing health economics and POCT, is the influence of cost shifting. In the current context of laboratory or community-based POCT, poor quality in one sector of the health system adds costs to another sector as increased resource requirements. Poor quality in laboratory or community-based POCT often results in increased doctor visits, additional unnecessary test procedures, inappropriately changed medication or additional unnecessary medication, and/or hospitalisation. The real cost of not identifying poor quality testing is often hidden until a quality system has been implemented. In quality management texts, this is usually described as the 1-10-100 rule:

that is, $1 of prevention is better than $10 of corrective action (or of appraisal costs or re-testing costs), which is better than the $100 required to recover from a quality failure.

If meeting patient needs in a timely manner is the true motivation for the introduction of POCT, then using quality management principles with quality control (QC) and proficiency testing (PT) is the best way to achieve this objective. This will be true even if a service or entrepreneurial goal is more important to the organisation, because it is good business to also practise good medicine. There are many articles in the reviewed medical and scientific literature demonstrating the requirement for all testing to be performed under a quality management system, with internal QC and PT (Gill and Shephard 2010; Goldsmith and Porter 2005; Okorodudu 2012; Portogallo and Barlow 2010). The topics of quality management, quality control and proficiency testing are also covered in Chapter 5.

As discussed previously, the Australian Government Point-of-Care Testing in General Practice Trial (Laurence *et al.* 2009) has also provided confirmation that quality management practices are required for POCT. The particular quality management procedures used in the trial were:

- device operator training and certification
- internal quality control and participation in an external quality assurance (PT) program
- an accreditation program based on the (interim) standards for POCT in general practice.

For POCT to provide value in the general practice situation '... an effective quality management system is essential. Clinicians need reassurance that their decisions are based on reliable, accurate and precise results to ensure that patient safety is not compromised.' (Laurence *et al.* 2009).

The basic principle for requiring QC and PT for all medical testing, including POCT, is to demonstrate that a defined standard of testing has been achieved and is able to be maintained. This testing standard will depend on the clinical requirements of the test results or their fitness for purpose (as described below). There are many excellent articles that describe the implementation and conduct of QC and PT for POCT (Gill and Shephard 2010; Gill and Watkinson 2010), including specific guidelines provided by professional organisations such as the Australasian Association of Clinical Biochemists (AACB 2010).

## FITNESS FOR PURPOSE

The role of both medical laboratory and POCT is to produce results that are fit for their intended clinical purpose. This essentially means that the analytical performance of the measurement device must produce results that are appropriate for their intended use. Fitness for purpose should thus be an essential criterion in the choice of any POCT device. This may be achieved by evaluating the usual analytical parameters of imprecision (precision) and bias (systematic error), or by adopting quality specifications based on biological variation or clinical requirements (Fraser 2001; Fraser and Scott 2010). Some methods have internationally agreed analytical goals (e.g. cholesterol and haemoglobin A1c), but in their absence various approaches have been used to set relevant goals for imprecision and bias. A widely used and internationally recommended concept is to define the upper acceptable limit for imprecision as a proportion of the intra-individual biological variation of the particular analyte. With correct choice of the proportionality factor, analytical imprecision should not contribute significant additional variation to the test result when compared with the natural variation of the analyte being determined.

The determination of imprecision is relatively straightforward, but the range of procedures that have been used to report the findings from bias studies may provide additional complications if not carefully considered. For example, one clinical trial evaluating the performance of two glucose meters used in an intensive care unit showed satisfactory results when compared with a laboratory blood gas analyser using linear regression and error grid analysis, but both devices failed to provide the accuracy required for tight glucose control when evaluated using a Bland-Altman difference plot and specialist statistical procedures (Van Vlasselaers *et al.* 2008).

## THE INTERNATIONAL ACCREDITATION MODEL

An international model for accreditation that is directly applicable to POCT has been described by Burnett (2002, 2015). The model has three basic elements:

- The standards – with which the facility must comply in order to gain accreditation
- The accreditation authority – which oversees the assessment and compliance with the required standard(s). Qualified laboratory personnel may also

form part of the assessment team under the guidance of the accreditation authority.

- Regulation by government or a designated regulator – mandates accreditation to the chosen standard(s). The accreditation authority may then inform the designated regulator as to the accreditation status of the laboratory or primary care site and provide evidence of compliance with the regulatory requirement.

These three elements are the basic tenets that underlie accreditation. In the case of POCT, there may be 'standards', there may be 'regulation', but without a formal audit and assessment system to assure compliance, an ISO style accreditation system does not apply. This appears to be the situation in many jurisdictions; that is, the formal audit and assessment component is missing. As a consequence, when discussing accreditation for POCT, there is a strong reliance on the standard and regulatory components and the assumption that these have been correctly implemented. The absence of a formal audit component is also unfortunate for a less legalistic reason, because audit can provide significant education and training assistance. This educational focus provided by skilled assessors would be invaluable to many POCT operators.

As the term accreditation has a very specific ISO definition, internationally recognised accreditation bodies or authorities with membership of the International Laboratory Accreditation Cooperation (ILAC) are required to accredit to the relevant ISO standard. For medical testing laboratories this is ISO 15189. This standard may be considered too rigid or too impractical for many POCT applications, even if there is a requirement to demonstrate good management practices with QC and satisfactory participation in PT. As a consequence, some jurisdictions have developed their own policies, regulations or guidelines to which a POCT service must comply. Under these circumstances, the POCT service is technically not 'accredited', but may be appropriately 'licenced' or 'credentialed' to perform testing. In whatever manner the local jurisdiction chooses to describe this approval, however, a common theme remains with regard to quality management, performance of QC and participation in PT, as outlined previously. In Australia, for example, the NPAAC guidelines for POCT (NPAAC 2015) provide a good basic framework for managing a POCT service and provide some assurance that patient safety has not been compromised.

In addition, the Australian-based NPAAC guidelines for POCT also make a specific comment with regard to 'off label' use; that is, the use of any commercial *in vitro* device (IVD) that is used outside of the manufacturer's intended purpose or in a manner not compliant with the manufacturer's instructions. In such cases, 'off label use' includes using the device for a clinical purpose other than that originally specified or intended. In these circumstances, the POCT device is considered an 'in-house' IVD and must then comply with much stricter regulations such as those of the Therapeutic Goods Administration (TGA) IVD medical device regulations (NPAAC 2014; TGA 2015).

## ACCREDITATION OF PATHOLOGY SERVICES IN AUSTRALIA

The format for regulated Medicare funded pathology and POCT in Australia follows the general principles as described by Burnett (as above). These have been mandated since 1986 when the pathology accreditation scheme was linked to pathology funding under the *Health Insurance Act 1986*. Under this scheme:

- Designated regulator: The Australian Government Department of Health is responsible for mandating the use of the accreditation scheme (Department of Health 2015).
- Standards for accreditation: The National Pathology Accreditation Advisory Council is responsible for the development and maintenance of standards and guidelines for pathology laboratories. NPAAC is a government-appointed Council comprising laboratory professional and health department representatives (see http://www.health.gov.au/npaac). Its principal functions are to 'advise the Commonwealth, state and territory health ministers on matters relating to the accreditation of pathology laboratories, and for the development and maintenance of standards and guidelines which help define the quality procedures for the practice of pathology.' As well as mandated NPAAC standards, the principal standard used for pathology laboratory accreditation by the National Association of Testing Authorities Australia (NATA) is ISO 15189. ISO 22870 is not used as part of the accreditation requirements. In addition, advisory guidelines that relate to specific applications within pathology and POCT have been developed by NPAAC.

These NPAAC documents are updated regularly and current listings are available on the internet (NPAAC publications).

- Accreditation authority: Pathology services (including POCT services that claim Medicare funding) are assessed (audited) against NPAAC and ISO standards by NATA (see http://www.nata.com.au/nata/). NATA assessment reports are considered by the Commonwealth Department of Human Services who oversee the Medicare Benefits Scheme, to determine the accreditation status of a pathology service and its eligibility for payment. NATA is an internationally recognised accreditation authority and a member of the International Laboratory Accreditation Cooperation (ILAC) (see http://ilac.org/).

In addition to NPAAC, professional colleges and associations involved with the practice of pathology and POCT have developed specific purpose standards and guidelines for defined applications. The Australian Government 'Point-of-care Testing in General Practice Trial', discussed previously, provided a strong evidence base in support of the requirements for a quality management system to underpin the use of POCT procedures (Laurence *et al.* 2009). The POCT in General Practice Trial also implemented an interim accreditation framework designed to provide a possible future base for accreditation of POCT in this sector (Tirimacco *et al.* 2011). This accreditation framework included the three basis elements as discussed above: the development of (interim) standards; the requirement to adhere to these standards; and an inspection and audit system to assure compliance and to provide education and training.

Recently, the New South Wales (NSW) state government established a POCT network across emergency departments within small country hospitals that did not have the support of a 24/7 on-site laboratory (NSW Health 2015). NSW Health Pathology has been responsible for a systematic approach to the assessment of needs and the implementation of a quality framework to support POCT devices within the network. The initial POC test profile included electrolytes, urea, creatinine, blood gases, lactate, haemoglobin, troponin and INR/PT. Part of this network has recently been accredited by NATA.

In addition to hospitals, POCT is now routinely practiced in many primary care and community facilities in Australia (as well as in Canada, the UK and USA). For example, Australian POCT networks and facilities perform: (i) a range of acute care and cardiac biomarker testing including troponin for assessment of myocardial infarction (Shephard *et al.* 2014a,b, 2012; Tideman *et al.* 2010; Tirimacco *et al.* 2009); (ii) tests for diabetes and renal disease (Francis and Martin 2010; Shephard *et al.* 2009; Shephard and Gill 2010) and anticoagulation therapy (Martin 2010); (iii) workplace drugs of abuse testing; (iv) sexual health clinics perform infectious disease testing; and (v) primary care facilities perform glucose and INR testing and oversee coagulation and diabetes management programs. Most of these networks/facilities have defined regulatory requirements and/or defined operational and quality procedures and/or an accreditation component.

## ACCREDITATION FOR POCT IN COUNTRIES OTHER THAN AUSTRALIA

A summary of international policies, procedures and guidelines for POCT as they appeared in 2012 is available on the internet (Farrance 2012). The following summary provides some examples of accreditation or regulation of POCT in New Zealand, the United Kingdom (UK) and the United States of America (USA).

### New Zealand

The health system in New Zealand in many ways is similar to Australia's. District Health Board (DHB) contracts for medical laboratory testing require accreditation to ISO 15189, but may exclude some forms of POCT from the contract. Laboratories that perform POCT under a DHB contract must be accredited to ISO 22870. There are no regulations governing POCT in general medical practice or in a community setting, but also no government reimbursement or testing fee. A summary of POCT in New Zealand has been provided by Sheppard *et al.* (2013).

District Health Boards, however, may directly fund defined POCT projects. Such a DHB-funded project has been described in the rural hospital of Rawene in New Zealand's North (Blattner *et al.* 2010). This report describes the changes in clinical practice and patient disposition following the introduction of POCT in a rural hospital without immediate laboratory support. In addition to improved patient care, the report shows a saving of approximately NZ$360 000 within the global DBH budget.

As described in Chapters 13 and 34, community pharmacy-based POCT INR testing is now available in New Zealand through the Community Pharmacy

Anti-coagulation Management Service (or CPAMS) program. This program is well governed and well regulated, using local best practice standards for POCT and a quality framework consistent with ISO 22870.

## United Kingdom

Different operational health-care policies may apply to England, Scotland, Northern Ireland and Wales. The National Health Service (NHS) is the name commonly used to refer to the four single-payer publicly funded health-care systems in the UK (collectively or individually), although only the health service in England uses the name National Health Service without further qualification. In addition, much of the decision making is made through local *trusts,* which provide policy and guidance for health-care providers within their jurisdiction.

Various agencies within the UK Department of Health provide a plethora of guidelines and recommendations on health-related issues, including POCT. These guidelines are used by local trusts and health-care providers as recommendations or policy statements. For example, the Medicines and Healthcare Products Regulatory Agency (MHRA), previously the Medical Devices Agency (MDA), provides the recently updated guideline *Management and Use of IVD Point-of-Care Test Devices* (MHRA 2013).

A review of the NHS in England chaired by Lord Carter of Coles defines a clear path for the reorganisation of pathology services. This report states that quality management procedures and an upgraded accreditation system should be mandatory for all pathology service providers, including providers of POCT (Lord Carter of Coles 2008). In particular, recommendation 12 states '... that all pathology service providers should be subject to mandatory accreditation by an organisation independent of the providers and the professions. Mandatory accreditation (including point-of-care testing) gives members of the public and other NHS staff the confidence that the quality of the service has been independently verified as meeting objective service standards.' In addition to recommendation 12, recommendation 14 states '... that all providers of pathology services (including providers of point-of-care testing) should be required to participate in clinical audit and other clinical governance activities, as a further means of underpinning quality; and that all staff involved in the delivery of pathology services, including technical and support staff, participate in relevant continuous professional development as part of maintaining their competence.' An outline of the modernisation of pathology services and the role of POCT in the UK is provided by Beastall (2008), while Holloway (2015) describes the increased use of POCT in secondary and tertiary care facilities with improved clinical governance and accreditation.

Many of the NHS health trusts have long-standing policy statements with regard to POCT. Most (if not all) of these policy statements follow a similar template and provide similar information. All include specific reference to QC and PT, which are obligatory procedures for POCT operators. Many of these policies still apply, with local audit to assess compliance. However, with the advent of POCT accreditation through Clinical Pathology Accreditation (UK) Ltd (CPA 2015) and the development of *Additional Standards for Point-of-Care Testing (POCT) Facilities* (CPA 2010), with policy recommendations by the MHRA in their document *Management and Use of IVD Point-of-Care Test Devices* (MHRA 2013), local audit using CPA standards or full CPA accreditation is becoming the preferred procedure. In situations where the POCT service is under the jurisdiction of an accredited pathology laboratory, however, POCT accreditation procedures (i.e. the inspection and approval by CPA) are already part of laboratory accreditation.

In a similar manner to England, health care in Northern Ireland is provided by five regional trusts (see http://www.nidirect.gov.uk/health-and-social-care-trusts). POCT is managed under this regional framework with CPA accreditation standards and MHRA guidelines. The South Eastern Health and Social Care Trust (2010, 2014) provides a good example of POCT policy, which applies to secondary care settings, with strong recommendations for primary care.

In 2010, the Scottish Medical and Scientific Advisory Committee (SMASAC) determined there was a lack of overall standards for the performance of POCT within the Scottish NHS. As a consequence, up-to-date guidelines were developed as part of a review of the use of POCT in primary and secondary care in Scotland (SMASAC 2011). Annex E of this report provides an example of what should be implemented more widely: the Greater Glasgow and Clyde Point of Care Testing Policy, which states 'Any site providing a POCT service should undergo a relevant accreditation procedure and if the service is under the auspices of the local laboratory this will happen as part of their ongoing accreditation process by CPA (UK) Ltd'.

In Wales, the Welsh Scientific Advisory Committee (WSAC) directly advises the Welsh Assembly Government on professional scientific and technological matters related to health issues. Policy documents such as *Welsh Health Circular – Point of Care Testing* (WAG 2004) and *The Future Delivery of Pathology Services in Wales* (WAG 2008) have clearly defined requirements regarding quality and governance. Primary care sites should have a close liaison with an accredited pathology laboratory and 'The accredited laboratory will take responsibility for providing advice on the purchase of devices, training, maintaining and monitoring the quality of these services.'

Even though many of the compliance audits currently undertaken within NHS trusts in England, Northern Ireland, Scotland and Wales may not conform to the rigorous accreditation requirements of a central pathology laboratory, mandatory requirements, which are based on (or aligned with) CPA POCT standards, are being implemented. An outline of the issues in quality assurance and accreditation for POCT is provided by Thomas (2008).

As an example of community based POCT, the National Health Service Community Pharmacy Contractual Framework (CPCF) was introduced in April 2005. The CPCF includes the provision for pharmacies in England to be commissioned to perform public health services and be defined as 'enhanced services'. NHS England on behalf of local authorities or Public Health England can commission pharmacies to perform anticoagulation monitoring in a POCT setting.

### United States of America

In 1988, the USA Government passed the *Clinical Laboratory Improvement Amendments Act* (CLIA 88 or CLIA), which specified regulations and standards for all facilities in the USA that perform laboratory testing on human specimens for health assessment or the diagnosis, prevention, or treatment of disease (CLIA 1988; e-CFR 2015). CLIA classifies tests by a complexity model rather than testing location or intended use and tests are defined as waived, of moderate complexity or high complexity. Waived tests include test systems cleared by the Food and Drug Administration (FDA) for home use and those tests approved for waiver under the CLIA criteria. The only criteria for non-accredited laboratories to perform waived tests are for the device to have been cleared by the FDA, for operators to follow manufacturer's instructions as a minimum requirement (including the performance of QC at the frequency defined in the manufacturer's package insert) and to allow random inspection of the testing facility to establish compliance. Of note, however, is that all laboratories that perform testing on human samples (with the exception of defined research laboratories and personal home use testing) are required to be certified (registered) by the Centers for Medicare and Medicaid Services (CMMS) in order to perform any testing procedure. In this regard, a 'laboratory' is essentially any site where testing occurs; this includes a hospital ward, a doctor's office, a community testing facility or ambulatory testing service.

The CLIA requirements are administered through the CMMS, which regulate all laboratory testing (except research) performed on humans. A 20 year review of CLIA regulations with comments from the principal agencies involved with laboratory regulation and accreditation is provided as a summary report from the Clinical Laboratory Improvement Advisory Committee (CLIAC) *Recognising 20 years of CLIA* (CLIAC 2008). An overview of the categorisation of laboratory tests (waived, moderate and high complexity) and accreditation procedures in the USA is provided by Sautter and Lipford (2007) and by Ehrmeyer (2011).

The original list of waived tests was relatively small and consisted mainly of 'dipstick' tests for urine and some monitoring devices cleared by the FDA for home-use (e.g. blood glucose). However, the list of waived tests has grown considerably and now includes a large number of analytes, including many which can be performed at the point of care (FDA 2015). Tests that remain in the moderate complexity category (and thus require full accreditation) include blood gas instruments and activated clotting time tests. In addition, a waived POC test, which is used in a manner that differs from the manufacturer's instructions, automatically becomes a high complexity test and requires full accreditation. This is similar to the 'off label' use as described above with regard to the Australian NPAAC guidelines. An overview of the procedures for implementing the CLIA regulations is provided by the Centers for Disease Control and Prevention (CDC 1992).

With the increased use of waived tests beyond the accredited laboratory, there has also been increasing concern as to the quality of results and the potential harm to patients. The identification of quality issues in waived testing sites has been compiled from on-site inspection reports obtained by CMMS during the period 1999 to 2003 and summarised by the CDC in their report and recommendations paper *Good Laboratory Practices for Waived Testing Sites* (Hoverton *et al.* 2005). In addition to a review of quality failures, the report provides recommendations for improving the quality of waived tests. Issues with regard to the quality of waived tests were also discussed during the CLIAC meeting of February 2008 (CLIAC 2008).

As the principal provider of standards to US pathology and associated diagnostic industry, the Clinical and Laboratory Standards Institute (CLSI) provide a range of standards and guidelines to assist laboratories (including POCT facilities) with the accreditation process (CLSI 2015). Even though CLSI is the principal provider of pathology standards in the US, ISO 15189 is used by some diagnostic laboratories as their accreditation standard. Although CLIA defines the minimum requirements for all testing, many POCT facilities may decide to undertake professional accreditation through one of the approved accreditation agencies. An overview of the US regulations for POCT and the requirements for the three complexity categories of test methods (waived, moderate complexity and high complexity) has been provided by Ehrmeyer (2011).

## ACKNOWLEDGEMENT

The authors wish to acknowledge that selected material provided in this chapter is based on a report commissioned by RCPA Quality Assurance Programs Pty Ltd (QAP), and funded by the Australian Government Department of Health through the Quality Use of Pathology Program. The full report is available at http://www.aacb.asn.au/documents/item/635. Permission to use this report has been given by the QAP.

## REFERENCES

AACB (Australasian Association of Clinical Biochemists) (2010) *Guidelines for Conduct of Quality Control and External Quality Assurance for PoCT.* AACB, Sydney, <http://www.aacb.asn.au/documents/item/243>.

ACBI (Association of Clinical Biochemists in Ireland) (2009) *Point of Care Testing in Primary and Community Care.* ACBI, <http://www.acbi.ie/Articles.asp?id=1>.

Beastall GH (2008) The modernisation of pathology laboratory medicine in the UK: networking into the future. *The Clinical Biochemist Reviews* **29**, 3–9.

Blattner K, Nixon G, Dovey S, Jaye C, Wigglesworth J (2010) Changes in clinical practice and patient disposition following the introduction of point-of-care testing in a rural hospital. *Health Policy (Amsterdam)* **96**, 7–12. doi:10.1016/j.healthpol.2009.12.002

Burnett D (2002) *A Practical Guide to Accreditation.* ACB Venture Publications, London, UK.

Burnett D (2015) ISO standards for pathology – a step too far? *Annals of Clinical Biochemistry* **52**, 712–714. doi:10.1177/0004563215589792

CDC (Centers for Disease Control and Prevention) (1992) *Regulations for Implementing the Clinical Laboratory Improvement Amendments of 1988: a Summary.* CDCP, <http://www.cdc.gov/mmwr/preview/mmwrhtml/00016177.htm>.

CLIA (Clinical Laboratory Improvement Amendments Act) (1988) *Public Law 100–578, October 31.* United States Government, <https://www.gpo.gov/fdsys/pkg/STATUTE-102/pdf/STATUTE-102-Pg2903.pdf>.

CLIAC (Clinical Laboratory Improvement Advisory Committee) (2008) *Recognising 20 years of CLIA. Summary report of meeting February 2008.* CLIAC, <http://wwwn.cdc.gov/cliac/pdf/CLIAC0208.pdf>.

CLSI (Clinical and Laboratory Standards Institute) (2015) POCT documents, CLSI, <http://shop.clsi.org/Point-of-Care-Testing>.

CPA (Clinical Pathology Accreditation (UK) Ltd) (2010) *Additional Standards for Point-of-Care Testing (POCT) Facilities. CPA,* <https://www.ukas.com/download/CPA/Additional%20Standards%20for%20Point_of_Care%20Testing_POCT_Facilities.pdf>.

CPA (2015) *Point of Care Testing Accreditation.* CPA, <https://www.ukas.com/download/brochures/B23%2009_2015%20POCT%20Leaflet.pdf>.

Department of Health (2015) *Pathology Accreditation.* Australian Government Department of Health, <http://www.health.gov.au/npaac>.

e-CFR (2015) *Electronic code of Federal Regulations, December 10.* US Government Publishing Office, <http://www.ecfr.gov/cgi-bin/ECFR?page=browse>.

Ehrmeyer SS (2011) The US regulatory requirements for point-of-care testing. *Point of Care* **10**, 59–62. doi:10.1097/POC.0b013e31821bd6af

Farrance I (2012) *Review: Policies, Procedures and Guidelines for Point-of-Care Testing.* Royal College of Pathologists of Australasia (RCPA) Quality Assurance Programs Pty Ltd, <http://www.aacb.asn.au/documents/item/635>.

FDA (US Food and Drug Administration) (2015) *CLIA – Clinical Laboratory Improvement Amendments – Currently Waived Analytes.* US Food and Drug Administration, <http://www.accessdata.fda.gov/scripts/cdrh/cfdocs/cfClia/analyteswaived.cfm>.

Francis AJ, Martin CL (2010) A practical example of PoCT working in the community. *The Clinical Biochemist Reviews* **31**, 93–97.

Fraser CG (1999) General strategies to set quality specifications for reliability performance characteristics. *Scandinavian Journal of Clinical and Laboratory Investigation* **59**, 487–490. doi:10.1080/00365519950185210

Fraser CG (2001) Optimal analytical performance for point of care testing. *Clinica Chimica Acta* **307**, 37–43. doi:10.1016/S0009-8981(01)00429-6

Fraser CG, Scott MG (2010) Analytical performance requirements for point-of-care testing: glucose as an example. In

*Point-of-Care Testing. Needs, Opportunities, and Innovation.* (Eds CP Price, A St John and LL Kricka) pp. 145–156. AACC Press, Washington DC, USA.

Gill JP, Shephard MDS (2010) The conduct of quality control and quality assurance testing for PoCT outside of the laboratory. *The Clinical Biochemist Reviews* **31**, 81–84.

Gill JP, Watkinson L (2010) Quality control and quality assurance in point-of-care testing. In *Point-of-Care Testing. Needs, Opportunities, and Innovation.* (Eds CP Price, A St John and LL Kricka) pp. 225–236. AACC Press, Washington DC.

Goldsmith BM, Porter E (2005) Ensuring quality in a multihospital POC program. *Point of Care* **4**, 167–173. doi:10.1097/01.poc.0000191405.34822.d9

Holloway PAH (2015) Point-of-care testing in the United Kingdom. *Point of Care* **14**, 121–123. doi:10.1097/POC.0000000000000075

Hoverton D, Anderson N, Bosse D, Granade S, Westbrook G (2005) *Good Laboratory Practice for Wavered Testing Sites.* Centers for Disease Control and Prevention (CDC), <http://www.cdc.gov/mmwr/preview/mmwrhtml/rr5413a1.htm>.

ISO (International Organization for Standardization) (2006) *ISO 22870:2006. Point-of-Care Testing (POCT) – Requirements for Quality and Competence.* International Organization for Standardization, Geneva, Switzerland, <https://www.iso.org/obp/ui/#iso:std:iso:22870:ed-1:v1:en>.

ISO (2007) *ISO 17593:2007. Clinical Laboratory Testing and in Vitro Medical Devices –Requirements for in vitro Monitoring Systems For Self-Testing of Oral Anticoagulant Therapy.* International Organization for Standardization, Geneva, Switzerland, <http://www.iso.org/iso/home.html>.

ISO (2012) *ISO15189:2012. Medical Laboratories –Requirements for Quality and Competence.* International Organization for Standardization, Geneva, Switzerland, <http://www.iso.org/iso/home.html>.

ISO (2013) *ISO15197:2013. In Vitro Diagnostic Test Systems – Requirements For Blood Glucose Monitoring Systems for Self-Testing in Managing Diabetes Mellitus.* International Organization for Standardization, Geneva, Switzerland, <http://www.iso.org/iso/home.html>.

ISO/IEC (International Electrotechnical Commission) (2004) *Guide 2: Standardization and Related Activities – General Vocabulary.* International Organization for Standardization, Geneva, Switzerland, <http://www.iso.org/iso/home.html>.

Laurence C, Gialamas A, Yelland L, Bubner T, Glastonbury B, Beilby J, *et al.* (2009) *Point of Care Testing in General Practice Trial. Final Report January 2009.* Australian Government Department of Health, Canberra, <http://www.appn.net.au/Data/Sites/1/SharedFiles/Publications/200901-poct-finalreport27jan09amended5feb09.pdf>.

Lord Carter of Coles (2008) *Report of the Second Phase of the Review of NHS Pathology Services in England,* <http://webarchive.nationalarchives.gov.uk/20130107105354/http://www.dh.gov.uk/en/Publicationsandstatistics/Publications/PublicationsPolicyAndGuidance/DH_091985>.

Martin CL (2010) iSTAT – combining chemistry and haematology in PoCT. *The Clinical Biochemist Reviews* **31**, 81–84.

MHRA (Medicines and Healthcare Products Regulatory Agency) (2013) *Management and Use of IVD Point-of-Care Test Devices,* <https://www.gov.uk/government/uploads/system/uploads/attachment_data/file/371800/In_vitro_diagnostic_point-of-care_test_devices.pdf>.

NACB (National Academy of Clinical Biochemistry) (2006) Evidence based practice for point-of-care testing. AACC Press, Washington DC, USA, <https://www.aacc.org/~/media/practice-guidelines/point-of-care-testing/poct-entire-lmpg.pdf?la=en>.

NPAAC (National Pathology Accreditation Advisory Council) (2014) Requirements for the development and use of in-house *in vitro* diagnostic medical devices. 3rd edn. NPAAC, Canberra, <http://www.health.gov.au/internet/main/publishing.nsf/Content/health-npaac-dhaivd.htm>.

NPAAC (2015) *Guidelines for Point of Care Testing.* 1st edn, NPAAC, Canberra, <http://www.health.gov.au/internet/main/publishing.nsf/Content/health-npaac-poctguid>. NPAAC functions, <http://www.health.gov.au/internet/main/publishing.nsf/Content/health-npaac-function.htm>. NPAAC home page, <http://www.health.gov.au/npaac>. NPAAC publications, <http://www.health.gov.au/internet/main/publishing.nsf/Content/health-npaac-publication.htm>.

NSW Health (2015) *NSW POCT Policy.* New South Wales Government, Ministry of Health, Sydney, <http://www.health.nsw.gov.au/policies/pd/2015/pdf/PD2015_028.pdf>.

Okorodudu AO (2012) Optimizing accuracy and precision for point-of-care testing. *Point of Care* **11**, 26–29. doi:10.1097/POC.0b013e318246a675

Portogallo C, Barlow I (2010) Implementing a quality assurance system for point-of-care blood glucose monitoring. *Journal of Diabetes Nursing* **14**, 63–67.

Sautter RL, Lipford EH (2007) Point-of-care testing: guidelines and challenges. *North Carolina Medical Journal* **68**, 132–135.

Shephard MDS, Gill JP (2010) The national QAAMS program – a practical example of PoCT working in the community. *The Clinical Biochemist Reviews* **31**, 95–99.

Shephard M, Shephard A, Watkinson L, Mazzachi B, Worley P (2009) Design, implementation and results of the quality control program for the Australian government's point of care testing in general practice trial. *Annals of Clinical Biochemistry* **46**, 413–419. doi:10.1258/acb.2009.009045

Shephard M, Spaeth B, Mazzachi B, Auld M, Schatz S, Loudon J *et al.* (2012) Design, implementation and initial assessment of the Northern Territory Point-of-Care Testing Program. *The Australian Journal of Rural Health* **20**, 16–21. doi:10.1111/j.1440-1584.2011.01243.x

Shephard M, Spaeth B, Motta L, Shephard A (2014a) Point-of-care testing in Australia: practical advantages and benefits of community resiliency for improving outcomes. In: *Global Point-of-Care – Strategies for Disasters, Emergencies, and*

*Public Health Resilience*. (Eds GJ Kost and CM Curtis) pp. 527–535. AACC Press, Washington DC, USA.

Shephard M, Spaeth B, Auld M, Schatz M, Lingwood A, Loudon J, *et al.* (2014b) Towards sustainable point-of-care testing in remote Australia – the Northern Territory i-STAT Point-of-Care Testing Program. *Point of Care* **13**, 6–11. doi: 10.1097/POC.0000000000000009

Sheppard BI, Smith KA, Horman JE (2013) Health system operations and point-of-care coordination, a national survey with implications for standardization in New Zealand. *Point of Care* **12**, 46–51. doi:10.1097/POC.0b013e3182677720

SMASAC (Scottish Medical and Scientific Advisory Committee) (2011) Review of the use of point of care testing in primary and secondary care in Scotland, <http://www.biochemscotland.org.uk/ESW/Files/9-5_DSG_(12)_10a_-_SMASAC_POCT_Report.doc>.

South Eastern Health and Social Care Trust (2010) *Point of Care Testing Policy*, <http://www.southerntrust.hscni.net/pdf/PointOfCareTestingPolicy.pdf>.

South Eastern Health and Social Care Trust (2014) *Point of Care Testing Policy*, <http://www.setrust.hscni.net/pdf/POCT_Policy.pdf>.

TGA (Therapeutic Goods Administration) (2015) *IVD Medical Device Regulations*. TGA, <https://www.tga.gov.au/ivd-medical-devices-regulation-basics>.

Thomas MA (2008) Quality assurance and accreditation in point-of-care testing. *Point of Care* **7**, 227–232. doi:10.1097/POC.0b013e3181885e8f

Tideman P, Simpson P, Tirimacco R (2010) Integrating PoCT into clinical care. *The Clinical Biochemist Reviews* **31**, 99–104.

Tirimacco R, Tideman P, Simpson P (2009) Design, implementation, and outcomes for point-of-care pathological testing in a cardiac clinical network. *Point of Care* **8**, 56–60. doi:10.1097/POC.0b013e3181a4b3c2

Tirimacco R, Glastonbury B, Laurence CO, Bubner TK, Shephard MD, Beilby JJ (2011) Development of an accreditation program for point of care testing (PoCT) in general practice. *Australian Health Review* **35**, 230–234. doi:10.1071/AH09792

Van Vlasselaers D, Van Herpe T, Milants I, Eerdekens M, Wouters PJ, De Moor B, *et al.* (2008) Blood glucose measurements in arterial blood of intensive care unit patients submitted to tight glycaemic control: agreement between bedside tests. *Journal of Diabetes Science and Technology* **2**, 932–938. doi:10.1177/193229680800200603

WAG (Welsh Assembly Government) (2004) *Point of Care Testing*. National Health Service, Cardiff, UK, <http://www.wales.nhs.uk/documents/whc-2004-005-e.pdf>.

WAG (2008) *The Future Delivery of Pathology Services in Wales*. National Health Service, Cardiff, UK, <http://www.wales.nhs.uk/sitesplus/documents/829/Future%20Delivery%20Pathology.pdf>.

White GH, Farrance I (2004) Uncertainty of measurement in quantitative medical testing. A laboratory implementation guide. *The Clinical Biochemist Reviews* **25**(Supplement 2), S1–S24.

Wittels P, Charny MC, Jordan M, Seeger T, St John A, Dettwyler WK (2010) Reimbursement of point-of-care testing. In *Point-of-Care Testing. Needs, Opportunities, and Innovation*. (Eds CP Price, A St John and LL Kricka) pp. 181–195. AACC Press, Washington DC, USA.

# 8 How to evaluate the effectiveness of point-of-care testing

*Richard Woodman, Tessa McCormack, Julie Ratcliffe and Mark Shephard*

**Summary**

This chapter describes the key issues to consider when designing and analysing a study to evaluate the effectiveness of point-of-care testing (POCT). To date, the quality of information relating to the effectiveness measures for POCT studies has been relatively poor; the purpose of this chapter is therefore to provide the reader with a systematic overview of how to frame a research study, select an appropriate study design and to collect and describe data to evaluate the effectiveness of POCT, using the appropriate statistical techniques.

## INTRODUCTION

The effectiveness of POCT is most commonly investigated from a clinical, operational and cost perspective using a range of different outcome measures (see Chapter 1). The first major section of this chapter explores designing a study and analysing the data produced using quantitative research methods that generally focus on clinical effectiveness of POCT. The second section focusses mainly on qualitative research methods commonly used for evaluating operational effectiveness of POCT. The chapter concludes with a discussion of the key principles of cost-effectiveness studies.

## DIFFERENT TYPES OF RESEARCH METHODS

### Quantitative and qualitative research methods

There are two main methods of health research: quantitative and qualitative research. Quantitative research methods, traditionally used in clinical sciences and epidemiology, use numerical data that can be analysed statistically to give conclusions that are highly applicable to researching clinical conditions, disease states and epidemiology. Quantitative methods primarily aim to answer the questions 'how many', 'how much' and 'how often' (Green and Thorogood 2004). Quantitative methods can be observational (e.g. cross-sectional, case-control and cohort studies) or experimental (randomised-controlled trials).

Qualitative research, traditionally associated with social and behavioural sciences, has become popular in epidemiology. Typically, research is focussed on one key concept or phenomenon, and the researchers ask broad, general questions about the topic. Analysis is based on the interpretation of data by the researcher, and therefore conclusions drawn from the data are subjective. Qualitative methods focus on questions of 'what', 'why' and 'how' (Green and Thorogood 2004). Typical qualitative research methods include qualitative surveys, interviews, focus groups, participatory observation and document analysis.

### Mixed methods study design

Mixed-methods research combines quantitative and qualitative methods to provide breadth and depth of understanding about a particular issue. The weaknesses of one method can be outweighed by the strengths of another method, producing more rigorous data and providing an improved understanding of the topic. Integrating results of qualitative and quantitative approaches enables blending of structured and semi-structured data into findings that enhance understanding. This approach also means that methodological triangulation can be used to overcome bias that might occur when a single data collection method is used (Williams *et al.* 2005).

## QUANTITATIVE RESEARCH

### Generating a research hypothesis

Before embarking on a study and collecting data, it is important to consider the research question carefully to ensure that it is answerable using the collected data, and that the results apply to an appropriate population.

### Forming a testable research question

Forming a testable research question involves framing a research hypothesis so that it can be tested using appropriate statistical methods. Essentially, this means forming the research question so that it can be translated into a 'null' hypothesis ($H_0$). For example:

$H_0$: Self-monitoring of blood glucose (SMBG) by POCT for 12 weeks in patients with type 2 diabetes does not improve glycaemic control, or

$H_0$: $\Delta$ Glycaemic control = 0

*where $\Delta$ means change

Here, $H_0$ is testable statistically and is also very specific about the proposed intervention (SMBG), the duration of the intervention (12 weeks), the study population (patients with type 2 diabetes) and the outcome to be measured (glycaemic control). If the null hypothesis is rejected then the *alternative hypothesis* ($H_A$), which is the opposite of $H_0$, can be accepted (i.e. there will be a change in glycaemic control).

### Generalisability of the findings of a study

Researchers should consider to what extent their findings apply to other individuals. In the example that assesses the effect of SMBG on glycaemic control, the findings are unlikely to apply to individuals who don't have diabetes since they will not be included in the study population. The specific study inclusion criteria will also influence the generalisability of the findings to the wider population with diabetes. For example, if all study subjects have *well-controlled* diabetes, the effectiveness of the intervention may not apply to individuals with *poorly controlled* diabetes.

### Designing a quantitative study

The choice of study design will partly relate to the type of research question being considered, such as the effectiveness of treatment, prevalence of disease, incidence of adverse events/complications, or diagnostic accuracy of POCT. Other factors affecting the choice of study design include:

- ethical issues
- does available data on the outcomes of interest already exist?
- is collecting additional data feasible?
- the ease of recruiting subjects or patients.

As a consequence, it is impossible to be prescriptive about the 'best' type of study to perform. Here we focus on several main quantitative study designs that are relevant to POCT. As described above, these include observational study designs (such as cross-sectional, case-control or longitudinal cohort studies) and intervention studies (such as randomised controlled trials).

Fig. 8.1 illustrates the differences between these study designs using a common model involving a study population (100 patients with type 2 diabetes), an exposure (did the study group have access to POCT for blood glucose self-monitoring?) and an outcome measure (the development of retinopathy, as a complication of diabetes). The model is adaptable for other clinical conditions of interest to POCT; for example, the study group could be patients on warfarin therapy, the exposure could be access to INR POCT (or not), and the outcome could be percentage of time in therapeutic range (%TTR) or the study group could be patients presenting with chest pain, the exposure access to troponin POCT and the outcome myocardial infarction.

#### The cross-sectional study design

Cross-sectional (or prevalence) studies are designed to provide a snapshot of the health of a group of subjects at one point in time rather than over a period of time. They are descriptive studies that simultaneously collect

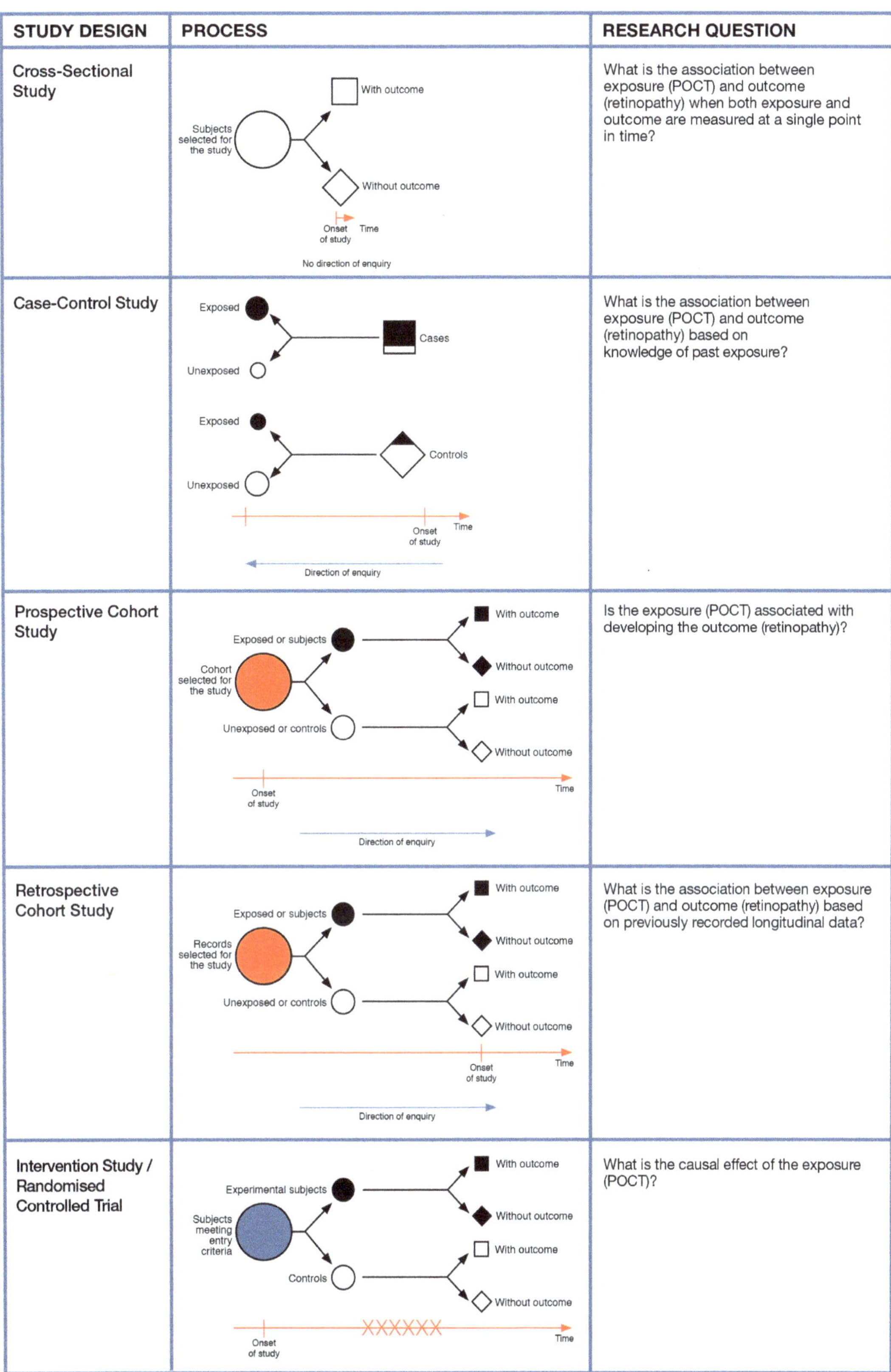

| STUDY DESIGN | PROCESS | RESEARCH QUESTION |
|---|---|---|
| Cross-Sectional Study | Subjects selected for the study<br>With outcome<br>Without outcome<br>Onset of study<br>Time<br>No direction of enquiry | What is the association between exposure (POCT) and outcome (retinopathy) when both exposure and outcome are measured at a single point in time? |
| Case-Control Study | Exposed<br>Unexposed<br>Cases<br>Exposed<br>Unexposed<br>Controls<br>Onset of study<br>Time<br>Direction of enquiry | What is the association between exposure (POCT) and outcome (retinopathy) based on knowledge of past exposure? |
| Prospective Cohort Study | Cohort selected for the study<br>Exposed or subjects<br>Unexposed or controls<br>With outcome<br>Without outcome<br>With outcome<br>Without outcome<br>Onset of study<br>Time<br>Direction of enquiry | Is the exposure (POCT) associated with developing the outcome (retinopathy)? |
| Retrospective Cohort Study | Records selected for the study<br>Exposed or subjects<br>Unexposed or controls<br>With outcome<br>Without outcome<br>With outcome<br>Without outcome<br>Onset of study<br>Time<br>Direction of enquiry | What is the association between exposure (POCT) and outcome (retinopathy) based on previously recorded longitudinal data? |
| Intervention Study / Randomised Controlled Trial | Subjects meeting entry criteria<br>Experimental subjects<br>Controls<br>With outcome<br>Without outcome<br>With outcome<br>Without outcome<br>Onset of study<br>Time | What is the causal effect of the exposure (POCT)? |

**Fig. 8.1.** Examples of different study designs using a common clinical scenario: Study participants = 100 subjects with type 2 diabetes; Exposure = Point-of-care testing for blood glucose; Outcome measure = Development of retinopathy
Key: Shaded = exposed (blood glucose tested by POCT); Unshaded = unexposed (blood glucose not tested by POCT – e.g. tested by laboratory); Squares = with outcome (retinopathy); Diamonds = without outcome (no retinopathy).

information on exposure and outcomes and ask the question: 'What is the association between exposure and outcome when both exposure and outcome are measured at a single point in time?' (Fig. 8.1). Subjects selected for the study are categorised according their current exposure status (e.g. using POCT or not using POCT at the time they are assessed for retinopathy).

The two primary aims of cross-sectional studies are:

- to describe the populations in terms of clinical characteristics, demographics and use of POCT
- to examine associations between participant characteristics (e.g. whether or not individuals had access to POCT) and the prevalence of outcomes (e.g. whether or not the outcome of interest was observed). These are commonly expressed using odds ratios or prevalence ratios.

### The case-control study design

The case-control study is designed for efficiency in terms of both time and cost. Case-control studies look at a group of people who have the disease of interest (e.g. those with retinopathy) and compare them with a group of people without the disease (those without retinopathy). The histories and exposures of the two groups (e.g. POCT or not) are then compared to identify possible links between exposures and the disease of interest (Fig. 8.1). In the case-control study, the nature of the inquiry looks back in time and aims to answer the question: 'What is the association between exposure and outcome based on knowledge of past exposure?' For example, after identifying subjects with and without retinopathy, details are obtained using case records and/or interviews to determine whether each individual had been using POCT for blood glucose on a regular basis in the past (this will be a period before when the retinopathy cases developed retinopathy, and should cover the same period of time for both controls and cases).

The case-control study provides stronger evidence for the causal effects of an exposure compared with cross-sectional study designs where it cannot be determined whether exposure to treatment preceded the condition, and therefore the causal direction of the association is less certain.

### The prospective cohort study design

The cohort study is another major type of observational design. The term 'cohort' is used to describe a group of individuals who share similar characteristics (e.g. having type 2 diabetes or having a particular risk factor for disease).

In the prospective cohort study, all subjects within the cohort do *not* have the outcome (retinopathy) when the study begins. However, exposure (using POCT or not using POCT) is known. The subjects, both exposed and unexposed, are followed over a certain time period to observe whether they develop retinopathy. Any association that is then established between POCT and retinopathy at the end of the study is more likely to have a causal nature since there was no evidence of retinopathy when exposure status was assessed. The direction of the study is forward in time, hence the term 'prospective' (Fig. 8.1). It asks the question: 'Is the exposure (POCT) associated with the development of the outcome (retinopathy)?'

*Advantages and disadvantages of prospective cohort studies*

Advantages:

- allows for the estimation of multiple different outcomes (e.g. different causes of mortality) with the same measure of exposure (e.g. POCT or not)
- useful for new exposures for which the beneficial health effects are not known
- minimises the risk of selection bias since outcome status is not known at the start.

Disadvantages:

- generally time consuming and expensive if active follow-up of subjects is required
- outcomes need to be relatively common because rare outcomes would require extremely large studies
- there is an increased risk of bias as a result of loss to follow-up (subjects withdrawing from the study or becoming non-contactable), which may especially occur with very long duration follow-ups.
- possible bias due to what is known as 'reverse causation'; for example, in the Fig. 8.1 example, those that eventually develop retinopathy (and who had poorer glycaemic control) may have deliberately chosen to have (or not have) POCT based on their glucose measures at the start of or during the study.

### The retrospective cohort design

This study design is identical to the prospective cohort study except that in a retrospective cohort study both the exposure (POCT) and the outcome (retinopathy) are known when the study starts (Fig. 8.1). Here, researchers can examine previously recorded longitudinal data (e.g. hospital admission records, GP records) on exposure and outcome and analyse their associations. A cohort is first established based on known exposure status (e.g. individuals with type 2 diabetes who have documented use of POCT) and then outcome data is obtained from the same database (or another, linked database). As the researcher examines existing data rather than collecting new data, the term 'retrospective' is used for the design name. It asks the question 'What is the association between the exposure (POCT) and the outcome (retinopathy) based on previously recorded longitudinal data?'

*Advantages and disadvantages of a retrospective cohort study*
Advantages:

- The retrospective cohort study is generally much quicker and cheaper than a prospective study since all relevant outcome events have already occurred when the study begins.

Disadvantages:

- Reliance on exposure information is possibly recorded much earlier, and for the purposes of administration rather than research. This may mean either missing or inaccurate data.
- Information on potential confounders such as diet, smoking and other lifestyle characteristics that would be recorded in a prospective study are unlikely to be available from administrative databases/records.
- Definitions of disease may have changed over time and information may not be comparable across all subjects.
- There is a potential for bias because outcome status is known at the start of the study and may potentially influence researchers as to whether or not the individual is recorded as being exposed (or not).

### The intervention study/randomised controlled trial

This is the strongest of all epidemiological study designs in terms of establishing whether or not an association between an exposure (POCT) and an outcome (retinopathy) is causal in nature. Intervention trials differ from observational studies in that the subjects meeting the entry criteria are randomly assigned into two different groups: one receives the intervention (i.e. exposure) (the intervention group) and the other does not (the control group) (Fig. 8.1). The intervention is administered by the investigator, who has control over the nature of the exposure (e.g. POCT for blood glucose) and who can closely monitor the effects or outcomes (e.g. retinopathy). An intervention study with both a control group and intervention group and random allocation to one or the other is often called a randomised controlled trial (RCT). In a blinded RCT, subjects do not know if they have been allocated to the control group or the intervention group. In a double-blinded RCT, the investigator is also unaware which subjects have been assigned to which groups, which helps to minimise bias. Randomly allocating the subjects into two groups also makes them as representative of the wider population as possible, and reduces potential for bias due to confounding. The intervention trial is an *experimental* study rather than an *observational* study.

*Advantages and disadvantages of an intervention study*
Advantages:

- Because the exposure (POCT) occurred before the development of the outcome, this satisfies the requirement of temporality that is necessary for defining whether or not the exposure had a causal effect.
- Because subjects are randomised to either receiving or not receiving the POCT, a major advantage of such trials is that they balance both known and unknown confounders between treatment groups.

Disadvantages:

- Intervention studies take longer and cost more.
- Ethical implications – is it appropriate to perform the trial in the way the investigators need to in order to answer their research question?
- Ethical implications – POCT should not be withheld from any potential subjects if it has already been shown to be effective in previous trials.

### Meta-analyses

The results from separate studies (observational or RCTs) are often combined in order to synthesise available evidence. Results are weighted towards larger (and therefore more reliable) studies. The so-called summary estimates that are reported provide the overall (weighted) mean of the separate studies, and a smaller 95% confidence interval than the individual trials (due to the larger number of subjects).

## Analysis of data – data types and distributions

The type and distribution of data will influence the type of statistical analysis that you perform.

**Table 8.1.** Measures of central tendency and dispersion for different types of quantitative data

| Type of data | Measure of central tendency | Measure of dispersion/ 95% confidence interval |
|---|---|---|
| Normal interval or ratio, $x$ | Mean, $\bar{x}$ | Standard deviation (s.d.)<br>95% confidence interval = $\bar{x} \pm 1.96 \times$ s.d. |
| Skewed interval or ratio, $x$ | Median, $M$ | Inter-quartile range (25th to 75th percentile)<br>95% confidence interval = $\bar{x} \pm 1.96 \times$ s.d. |
| Binary (0 or 1) | Proportion, $p$ | Standard error (SE) = $\frac{p(1-p)}{\sqrt{n}}$<br>95% confidence interval = $p \pm 1.96 \times$ SE |
| Count, $C$ | Mean count, $\bar{C}$ | Standard error (SE) = $\sqrt{C}$<br>95% confidence interval = $\bar{C} \pm 1.96 \times$ SE |

The various *types* of quantitative data normally encountered in POCT studies can be described as being:

- *nominal data:* for example, gender (male/female/other) or place of residence (urban/rural/remote)
- *ordinal data:* for example, 1 = Very difficult 2 = Difficult 3 = OK 4 = Easy 5 = Very easy
- *binary data:* nominal data with *two categories only* (e.g. male/female)
- *interval data:* continuous data that has order. Differences between each value are the same on all parts of the scale, and the data can take on both negative and positive values; for example, temperature of reagent storage.
- *ratio data:* continuous data with an absolute zero. For example, weight, cholesterol and glucose concentrations cannot go below zero.
- *count data:* discrete ratio data. It can take any integer values from zero; for example, number of POCT blood glucose measurements performed in a day by an individual, number of exercise sessions performed in one week by an individual.
- *rates:* counts that are *adjusted for the level of exposure.* They have a numerator (the count) and a denominator (the exposure). The exposure might be measured by *persons* or *time*; for example, the number of days in which the study was conducted.

#### Parametric data

Quantitative data can often be characterised by well-known statistical distributions. For example, continuous data that follows a normal (or 'Gaussian') distribution can be summarised using the mean and standard deviation of the data. Such data follows a bell-shaped distribution of values.

#### Non-parametric data

Continuous data that cannot be described using well-defined statistical distributions or their associated parameters is known as non-parametrically distributed data. For example, continuous data might follow a skewed distribution that requires different summary statistics to describe the central tendency and spread of the data (e.g. the distribution of urine ACR POCT results from a group of type 2 diabetes patients).

Statistical measures of central tendency and dispersion for both parametric and non-parametric data are summarised in Table 8.1.

### What analysis should I use?

Given that the mean change (Δ) in the outcome being measured is very unlikely to be *exactly* zero, statistical testing takes into account the variability in the change that occurs between subjects. Statistical software is used to create a 95% confidence interval (95% CI) for the mean change and to assess if it includes zero.

Examples of different statistical approaches that can be used to analyse quantitative data are summarised in Table 8.2.

### Adjusting for confounding

When evaluating the observed associations between an exposure (POCT) and health outcomes, the roles of chance and bias may partly explain any observed association. Chance (or random) variation may occur via the random differences in the selected subjects and the random differences in their health outcomes. Bias may be introduced either before or during the study by the investigator. For example, if subjects with higher levels of blood glucose are selected for POCT than those not selected,

**Table 8.2.** Different statistical approaches to be applied depending on type of data and study design

| Research hypothesis/study design | Data distribution | Unpaired data | Paired data |
|---|---|---|---|
| Compare two groups at one time point | Binary | Chi-square ($\chi^2$) test of association | |
| | Normal continuous | Independent *t*-test | |
| | Non-parametric | Mann–Whitney U test | |
| | Count | Poisson regression | |
| Compare more than two groups at one time point | | One-way ANOVA | |
| Compare pre- and post-measurements from the same group | Binary | | McNemar's test |
| | Normal continuous | | Paired *t*-test |
| | Non-parametric | Mann–Whitney U test | Sign-rank test |
| | Count | | Poisson regression with adjustment for baseline values |
| Compare two groups or more across three or more time points | Normal continuous or Non-parametric | | Repeated-measures ANOVA Multilevel models Generalised estimating equations (GEE) |
| Test for an association between an outcome (dependent variable) and an exposure (independent variable) | Normal continuous | Simple linear regression | |
| Test for an association between an outcome and several independent variables | Normal continuous | Multivariate linear regression | |
| Test for an association between an outcome and several independent variables across time | | | Repeated-measures ANOVA Multilevel models Generalised estimating equations (GEE) |

this would introduce a selection bias that may affect the results. Alternatively, there may be measurement bias if the investigator knows which group the subject is in when recording or analysing the results. A third alternative explanation for any observed association between exposure and outcome is confounding.

Confounding is a form of bias that occurs when measuring the relationship between an exposure and outcome. There is a mixing of the effect of the exposure on the outcome with that of a third variable. If at least part of the exposure–outcome relationship is due to this third variable then it is known as a confounder. For example, age may confound the exposure–outcome relationship between POCT creatinine levels and staging of chronic kidney disease (CKD) risk (Fig. 8.2); because creatinine levels increase with age and an elderly subject may be classified as having stage 3 CKD (a point where treatment options are usually considered) when in fact the patient's renal function is appropriate for a person of that age (see Chapter 11).

A study can control for potential confounders either at the design stage or the analysis stage of the study. In the design stage, it is possible to use the following options:

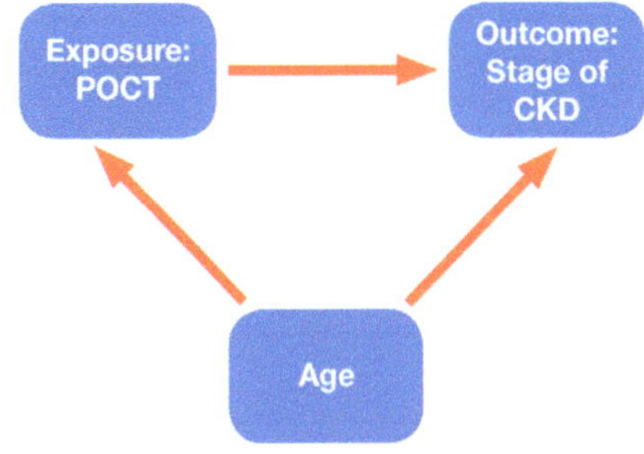


**Fig. 8.2.** Age may confound the exposure–outcome relationship between POCT creatinine concentration and staging of chronic kidney disease levels.

- randomisation of subjects
- restriction of subjects into the study (e.g. only non-smokers or only younger subjects)
- matching (matching individuals between groups by potential confounders, such as age and gender).

In the analysis stage, options to control confounders include:

- stratification (e.g. analysing smokers and non-smokers separately)
- adjusted multivariate regression analysis (with exposure and confounders included as the independent variables).

### Interpreting data and reporting results

Following analysis, results should be appropriately described and interpreted. It is often helpful to start by preparing the tables that will accompany the text of your paper/report. Table 8.3 typically describes the subjects within the study and Table 8.4 reports the main results of the hypothesis tests.

The highlights within each table should also be described in the text. For example, what were the significant differences in subject characteristics (if any) between the groups, was the study population generally healthy, and which outcomes were significantly different between study groups?

## QUALITATIVE RESEARCH

### Introduction

Qualitative research methods are commonly used to assess aspects of the operational effectiveness of a health intervention. In the context of POCT, operational effectiveness generally refers to how well the device and program are integrated into routine practice without causing adverse disruption to regular work patterns and patient flow. Evaluating operational effectiveness of POCT can mean:

- understanding how the POCT program fits into allocated appointment times
- defining the role of POCT operators and how they communicate with patients and other clinicians
- assessing how well the POC devices and tests are accepted by the staff and patients
- ensuring that trained POCT operators are competent and feel comfortable using the device.

Cultural effectiveness is a specific and distinct category of operational effectiveness, relevant to POCT programs involving Indigenous and/or ethnic groups. Cultural effectiveness refers to the appropriateness and acceptability of a POCT program for the Indigenous/ethnic community in which it is being used. Cultural acceptability is crucial for program longevity and translation into routine practice in an Indigenous setting.

The following section describes designing and implementing a study using qualitative research methods and outlines the principles of qualitative data analysis, using operational effectiveness of POCT as a working example.

### Designing a qualitative study

A clearly defined research question is required to identify the most appropriate qualitative study design. Qualitative methods often produce transcripts and recordings that need to be coded and organised into themes for analysis. Qualitative data provides depth of understanding of a

**Table 8.3.** Participant characteristics ($n$ = 80)

| Parameter | Females ($n$ = 38) Mean ± s.d. | Males ($n$ = 42) Mean ± s.d. | P-value[a] |
|---|---|---|---|
| Age (years) | 53.6 ± 10.5 | 59.2 ± 11.1 | 0.02 |
| Glucose (mmol/L) | 5.0 ± 0.9 | 4.7 ± 0.9 | 0.21 |
| Systolic blood pressure (mm/Hg) | 126.4 ± 16.6 | 129.3 ± 14.3 | 0.41 |
| HDL-cholesterol (mmol/L) | 0.95 ± 0.05 | 0.96 ± 0.04 | 0.58 |
| Socioeconomic status | **n (%)** | **n (%)** | |
| Level 1 | 7 (18) | 6 (14) | |
| Level 5 | 2 (5) | 8 (19) | 0.21 |

[a]Using a $t$-test for continuous variables and a $\chi^2$ test of association for categorical variables (socioeconomic status). A $p$-value <0.05 indicates statistical significance.

**Table 8.4.** Predictors of fasting glucose (mmol/L) amongst individuals using SMBG at home

| Parameter | β[a] | 95% CI | *p*-value[b] |
|---|---|---|---|
| Age (years) | 0.1 | (–0.2, 0.21) | <0.05 |
| Gender (*F* = 0, M = 1) | 0.6 | (0.4, 0.8) | <0.05 |
| Regular home SMBG | –0.5 | (–0.6, –0.4) | <0.05 |
| Systolic blood pressure (mm/Hg) | 0.05 | (–0.01, 0.11) | 0.46 |
| Physical activity/week (1000 kJ) | –0.8 | (–1.4, –0.2) | <0.05 |
| Education | | | |
| Left school 16 | 0.5 | (0.3, 0.7) | <0.05 |
| Completed year 12 | 0.3 | (0.1, 0.5) | |
| Trade certificate or Diploma | 0.2 | (0.1, 0.3) | |

[a]β (pronounced beta) is known as a regression coefficient, and is obtained from a multivariate regression analysis. It indicates the independent effect of a one unit (or one-category) increase in each variable included in the regression model on fasting glucose.
[b]Using multivariate linear regression. A *p*-value <0.05 indicates statistical significance.

particular topic, usually from a small number of participants. This gives greater insight into the research topic but results are less generalisable across the population. This may not be an issue, especially if the purpose of the research is to assess the operational effectiveness of POCT in a specific health service.

#### Interviews

*Purpose*

Interviews can help the researcher gain an in-depth understanding about a particular issue, and how subjects perceive, understand and feel about the issue under investigation.

*Methods/principles*

Interviews used in qualitative health research are generally unstructured or semi-structured. The interviewer uses an inductive approach to questioning, and the direction, length and pace of the interview is determined by the responses of the participant. In preparation for the interviews, the interviewer will generate topics of discussion informed by the main research question, and use these as prompts throughout the interview.

Interviewers use open-ended questions, usually beginning with a general question that does not purposefully inform or direct the respondent's answer (Low 2013). In a POCT study, this may simply be 'tell me about the POCT program in your health service.' Any subsequent questions are informed by the responses given. Consequently, each interview that is conducted will differ from the next, and will provide different perspectives on the same issue.

*Things to consider*

The interviewer should be knowledgeable about the research topic, and ideally be a part of the research team. Other important qualities of an interviewer (depending on the study population) are:

- suitable language skills
- appropriate age, gender and culture
- empathy, patience and respect (Baum 2008).

Creating an environment where the respondent feels safe and respected is important to ensure the study follows ethical guidelines and to guarantee researchers maximise the quality of the information collected. This is particularly relevant to research conducted with Indigenous people.

*Data produced*

Dialogue can be recorded by hand or with a voice recorder and be later transcribed. The respondent must give permission for the use of audio recording devices (part of signed informed consent).

*Advantages and disadvantages of interviews*

Advantages:

- provide in-depth descriptions of how individuals experience and explain 'their world' (Baum 2008)
- flexible – the direction is determined by the respondent and the data is not influenced by leading questions or assumptions from the interviewer.

Disadvantages:

- time consuming (for researchers and participants)
- costly in terms of labour.

*Example involving POCT*

Prost *et al.* (2009) used semi-structured interviews to explore the feasibility and acceptability of offering rapid HIV tests to patients attending a general practice for a new patient health check. They offered patients a rapid HIV test and the opportunity to be interviewed. In total, 20 patients agreed to be interviewed and, of these, 17 had accepted the rapid HIV test and three declined. Purposive sampling (selecting participants based on certain characteristics or descriptions) was used to ensure that interviewees were from diverse ethnic backgrounds. Interviews were conducted in the clinic at the time of the patient consultation, and were recorded and transcribed verbatim. Issues explored in the interview included:

- reasons for choosing to/choosing not to have a rapid HIV test
- the accessibility of HIV testing in general practices compared with sexual health clinics
- potential lack of support for people with a reactive test result.

**Focus groups**

Focus groups (also called group interviews) use group discussions to generate research data (Barbour 2010). They serve a different purpose to one-on-one interviews because they highlight differing viewpoints and opinions and provide a basis for comparison of group/stakeholder perspectives. Unlike interviews, they do not provide substantial insight into individual experience. When facilitating a focus group, researchers should obtain data that provides rich explanation of the research topic, rather than simple description. Focus groups provide an opportunity for representative stakeholders to help the researcher gain an understanding of the research topic from different perspectives. They are particularly useful for research relating to new systems or procedures (i.e. introduction of POCT) (Barbour 2010).

**Questionnaires**

*Purpose*

Surveys are multi-purpose tools that are widely used in public health research and epidemiology and have broad applicability to POCT. They combine quantitative and qualitative lines of questioning and can be used to ask questions of a descriptive or analytical nature. They are often useful when trying to collect data from a large number of participants.

*Methods/principles*

Survey methods (notably the questionnaire) can evaluate the operational (including cultural) effectiveness of POCT. The questionnaire can be written or verbal and can be conducted by a researcher or be self-completed. Questionnaires can be conducted by post, telephone, face-to-face or online.

Questionnaires will normally contain a combination of different questions including census or demographic questions, yes/no questions, questions regarding satisfaction, attitude or understanding, and open-ended questions.

Likert scales are used in public health research to assess people's attitudes, opinions or beliefs. A Likert scale is an ordered scale allowing the respondent to state their level of agreement with particular statements. They are a useful tool when conducting POCT program evaluations, needs assessments and policy research. Table 8.5 shows the use of a 5-point Likert scale, giving the participant equal opportunity to either agree or disagree with the statement.

*Things to consider*

Survey and question design need to be optimised to prevent introducing bias. This means avoiding leading questions that steer the responder towards a specific answer, and eliminating ambiguity in the questions (Baum 2008). Tips for writing clear questions and reducing bias include:

- Use plain language.
- Avoid leading questions such as 'Do you avoid getting tested for HIV because you are scared of getting a positive result?' A better question would be 'which of the following reasons make it less likely for you to have an HIV test?' (Conway *et al.* 2015).
- Pay attention to wording and ask direct questions. For example, if the researcher wants to know if the

**Table 8.5.** Example of a 5-point Likert scale to assess Indigenous patient satisfaction with POCT (Source: Shephard 2006)

| Statement | Strongly disagree | Disagree | Unsure | Agree | Strongly agree |
|---|---|---|---|---|---|
| I understand what POCT machines are used for | 1 | 2 | 3 | 4 | 5 |
| I am happy to receive my results immediately | 1 | 2 | 3 | 4 | 5 |
| The educational resources are useful and culturally safe | 1 | 2 | 3 | 4 | 5 |

participant currently has type 2 diabetes, they could ask:

- Do you have diabetes? Please circle 'yes' or 'no'
  This question will not yield accurate data because it does not give the participant enough information to answer the question. Individuals may select 'yes' if they have type 1 diabetes or gestational diabetes, confounding the data. A better way to ask the question is:
  Do you currently have type 2 diabetes? Please circle 'yes' or 'no'.

Before it is used as a study tool, a new questionnaire should always be tested using friends and colleagues, or with a group of people similar to the study population (Baum 2008).

*Data produced*

Questionnaires, depending on the design, often yield numerical and textual data. Numerical data is most likely to be ordinal data collected from questions using Likert scales.

*Advantages and disadvantages of questionnaires*

Advantages:

- simple administration – relatively cheap and easy to collect data
- participants may find them less demanding than participating in an interview or focus group
- more feasible to survey large numbers of people than it is to interview them, so data will be more generalisable
- analysis of the data will be less time-consuming.

Disadvantages:

- Surveys do not capture the same depth of understanding as other methods. There is less exploration into meaning, perception and context than with interviews and focus groups.
- Recruitment and engagement can be difficult. Generally, a large number of responses are needed to yield data that is reliable, valid and can be generalised. Response rates are typically poor, and it can be hard to motivate people to complete the surveys wholly and properly (particularly open-ended questions).

*Example*

Shephard *et al.* (2015) used an online questionnaire to assess the cultural effectiveness of a POCT program for diabetes management in Australian Indigenous medical services. The survey was sent to 470 POCT operators (104 responses). The researchers used online survey software to design the survey, monitor responses and analyse results. Some optional open-ended, qualitative questions were included:

- How do you use the waiting time for a POCT result to engage with your client?
- What are the main issues for you and your service in maintaining POCT for your diabetes clients in the long term?

### Ethics and consent

Ethics review and approval is a core component of any (qualitative or quantitative) research project. It is the researcher's responsibility to ensure the research proposal has been reviewed and approved by the relevant ethics committee. This may be the ethics committee of the workplace or institution, or, depending on the nature of the research and the source of the funding, the proposal may require approval from other jurisdictional committees. If the research involves specific cultural or minority groups, there may be additional ethics procedures to complete.

Ethics applications and reviews can take considerable time, so early planning is the key – particularly if the study needs to be completed in a given time period. Ethics approval demonstrates that the research plan will uphold the principles of bioethics, ensuring participants in the study are treated respectfully, fairly and equally. It also shows the outcomes of the research have potential benefit, and that the study will be conducted with integrity (NHMRC 2007).

The ethics process should ensure that every participant recruited:

- is participating on a voluntary basis, has made their own choice to participate and knows that they can choose *not* to participate at any time
- understands their role in the study
- understands the purpose of the research
- understands how the results of the research will be used and/or published
- gives their informed consent to participate in the study, which can be withdrawn at any time.

Preparing an information sheet is an efficient way of ensuring potential participants receive all the information needed to decide if they will participate. This should include a brief description of the study, an explanation of the rights and responsibilities of the participant (as listed above), and a statement about how their privacy and confidentiality will be maintained (Baum 2008). This sheet

**Table 8.6.** Examples of categories of data that can be coded

| | |
|---|---|
| Context | Definitions |
| Feelings | Perspectives |
| Ways of thinking | Processes |
| Activities | Strategies |
| Relationships | Meanings |
| Actions | Events |
| Conditions | Consequences |

should be given to the participant along with an informed consent form to be signed before the study commences.

## Analysis of textual data

Qualitative research yields textual data that may be directly written or transcribed from an audio recording of an interview, focus group or other documents. A large amount of unstructured data generally needs to be analysed to identify emerging themes and patterns (Baum 2008). Finding meaning in the data helps transform raw data into results that answer the research question.

Reducing subjectivity and potential bias requires data analysis to be thorough, methodical, systematic and comprehensive and ensures rigour in reporting and validity of the results.

Qualitative data analysis should begin during the data collection phase, allowing the researcher to identify saturation of data. Data saturation is achieved when no new themes are emerging in the data. Starting analysis early helps identify questions or techniques that could be improved or changed. Qualitative data analysis is time consuming – the process of transcribing 1 h of audio recording from an interview can take up to 6 h (Bryman 2012).

### Coding

Coding can be simply defined as 'marking sections of data and giving them labels or names' (Holloway and Wheeler 2010). Examples of categories of data that can be coded are listed in Table 8.6.

The first step in coding and analysing data is reading the text without making any notes (Liamputtong 2013). Then the researcher should read the text again and start to make notes on the page, as shown in Table 8.7.

Themes start to emerge in the data as analysis progresses – some will become prominent and these should be focussed on for interpreting and reporting. Keeping a list of all the codes that are created is useful for quick referral during further data analysis and when creating themes.

### Thematic analysis

Thematic analysis is 'a method for identifying, analysing and reporting patterns within data' (Braun and Clarke 2006). After coding, the codes can be organised into themes and sub-themes. A theme that could be identified from the data in Table 8.7 is 'good patient outcomes', and the sub-themes could include 'reduced TAT', 'motivational tool' and 'empowerment'. Names should be given

**Table 8.7.** Example of an excerpt from a focus group discussion about the operational effectiveness of a POCT program for diabetes management

| Speaker | Quotation | Code |
|---|---|---|
| KM | I like using the machine for diabetes patients, I think they like coming in and getting their results straight away. It makes them want to take better control of their health. It's good that we can do the testing because we had training and that's part of our job now. | Turnaround time (TAT)<br>Empowerment<br>Motivational tool<br>Training<br>Responsibility |
| GJ | It can be hard getting the doctors on board with the device. They didn't do the training to use it like we did so maybe they don't really understand what it's all about, or how good it can be for the patients. | Resistance from doctors<br>Lack of understanding<br>Training |
| KM | I know what you mean, it can be hard when the doctors don't encourage you to use it, but I can see the difference it makes for my patients so I always just go ahead and do it anyway. | Affecting change<br>Proactive<br>Good patient outcomes |
| GJ | Maybe the doctors should do the training too, then we might be able to use it more. I feel scared to do the test myself if the doctor thinks it should be done at the laboratory. | Training<br>Fear<br>Resistance from doctors |

to themes and these should be continually developed during data analysis, because new themes may emerge and others may become less important. Ideally, themes emerging in the data will relate to the research question. These themes can also be systematically categorised according to age, gender, occupation and experience, if this is relevant to the study outcomes.

### Interpreting data and reporting results

Once thorough data analysis has been conducted, the researcher should then interpret the meaning in the data and relate this back to the research question to see if it can be answered. There is no single correct way in which to convey the information – interpretation is subjective, but made as objective as possible via the process of thematic analysis. Quotes from specific individuals can be added to the summary if they encapsulate the findings of the thematic analysis. These findings can then be reported as a journal article, poster, report or other publication, as well as distributed to stakeholders.

## EVALUATING COST-EFFECTIVENESS

Economic evaluation is the comparative assessment of the cost and benefits of alternative health-care interventions, such as POCT (Drummond *et al.* 2005). There are five main types of economic evaluation that can be used in the context of the evaluation of POCT (Table 8.8) (Drummond *et al.* 2005; St John and Price 2013). The key feature that distinguishes the different types of economic evaluation is the unit for measuring the benefits of health care.

In a recent review of economic evidence and POCT, St John and Price (2013) note that the evidence base for the cost-effectiveness of POCT services is limited. They suggest the main reason for this could be that reimbursement strategies traditionally used in laboratory medicine in Australia and overseas provide funding for tests based on their complexity and on a fee-for-service basis. Cost-minimisation analysis is therefore reflective of the way that tests are currently funded or reimbursed in most health systems.

Gray *et al.* (2000) assessed the cost-effectiveness of using POCT for an intensive blood glucose control policy (relative to conventional blood glucose control) in patients with type 2 diabetes. The main outcome measure was the incremental cost per event-free year gained within the trial period. Events were defined according to the diabetes related end-points measured in the trial (myocardial infarction, congestive heart failure, stroke, renal replacement therapy, amputation, cataract extraction, vitreous haemorrhage or death from any cause). Although intensive blood glucose control in patients with type 2 diabetes significantly increased treatment costs, it was associated with a reduction in the incidence and cost of complications and increased time free of complications.

Cost-utility analysis has been very rarely employed to date in POCT economic studies despite representing the

**Table 8.8.** Types of economic evaluation and their units of measurement

| Type of economic evaluation | How it measures health benefits |
|---|---|
| Cost-minimisation analysis | Assumes that the health outcomes associated with the technologies being compared are equivalent. |
| Cost-effectiveness analysis | Determines the best method of achieving a given outcome, usually measured in clinical or 'natural' units, and presents results in terms of cost per unit of effect (e.g. cost per symptom free day, cost per one unit improvement in systolic blood pressure). |
| Cost-utility analysis | Compares the costs of alternative health-care programs with their utility, usually measured in terms of quality adjusted life years (QALYs). The QALY combines quality of life and length of life into a single index of utility or value on a '0' to '1' scale, where '0' is defined as a state equivalent to being dead and '1' is defined as a state equivalent to full health (Brazier *et al.* 2007). |
| Cost-benefit analysis | Compares the benefits of a health-care program with the cost. All benefits are valued in monetary terms, including health improvement. |
| Cost-consequence analysis | The results of a cost-consequence analysis are presented in table form, where all the relevant factors are presented, but are not collapsed into a single number to enable a unique and complete ranking of different treatment options (as would be the case with results presented in terms of cost per QALY estimates). |

most prevalent form of economic evaluation conducted internationally. A rare example is a study undertaken alongside a randomised controlled trial to evaluate the introduction of POC cardiac markers in the emergency department (Goodacre *et al.* 2011).

There are several examples of cost-consequence analyses of POCT interventions in the literature, including:

- a study to assess the economic impact of telemedicine and self-monitoring of blood glucose in patients with type 2 diabetes (Kesavadev *et al.* 2012)
- a study to assess the acceptance of POC INR testing in a hospital based anticoagulation clinic (Kong *et al.* 2008)
- a study to assess the implementation of a multi-parameter POCT blood analyser in very low birthweight infants (Mahieu *et al.* 2012).

Although some experts argue that the presentation of findings from a cost-consequence analysis are less robust than those obtained from cost-utility analysis, others state this approach may be more informative for providing economic evidence for POCT (St John and Price 2013). Cost–consequence analysis may more closely meet the needs of decision makers and has the additional benefit of being easily understood and thus more likely to influence decision making in practice (Coast 2004).

In summary, economic evaluations of POCT remain rare. Economic evidence relating to the value for money of new innovations in POCT should seek to provide a comprehensive, systematic and robust assessment of costs and outcomes, including consideration not only of testing accuracy but ultimately the impact that any new innovations in POCT have upon patients' health and quality of life.

## REFERENCES


Barbour RS (2010) Focus groups. In *The SAGE Handbook of Qualitative Methods in Health Research.* (Eds I Bourgeault, R Dingwall and R de Vries) pp. 327–352. Sage, London, UK.

Baum F (2008) *The New Public Health.* Oxford University Press, South Melbourne.

Braun V, Clarke V (2006) Using thematic analysis in psychology. *Qualitative Research in Psychology* **3**, 77–101. doi:10.1191/1478088706qp063oa

Brazier J, Ratcliffe J, Salomon J, Tsuchiya A (2007) *Measuring and Valuing Health Benefits for Economic Evaluation.* Oxford University Press, Oxford, UK.

Bryman A (2012) *Social Research Methods,* Oxford University Press, Oxford, UK.

Coast J (2004) Is economic evaluation in touch with society's health values? *British Medical Journal* **329**, 1233–1236. doi:10.1136/bmj.329.7476.1233

Conway DP, Guy R, Davies SC, Couldwell DL, McNulty A, Smith DE, *et al.* (2015) Rapid HIV testing is highly acceptable and preferred among high risk gay and bisexual men after implementation in Sydney sexual health clinics. *PLoS One* **10**, e0123814. doi:10.1371/journal.pone.0123814

Drummond M, Sculpher M, Torrance G, O'Brien B, Stoddart G (2005) *Methods for the Economic Evaluation of Health Care Programmes.* 3rd edn. Oxford University Press, Oxford, UK.

Goodacre SW, Bradburn M, Cross E, Collinson P, Gray A, Hall AS; RATPAC Research Team (2011) The randomised assessment of treatment using panel assay of cardiac markers (RATPAC) trial: a randomised controlled trial of point-of-care cardiac markers in the emergency department. *Heart (British Cardiac Society)* **97**, 190–196. doi:10.1136/hrt.2010.203166

Gray A, Raikou M, McGuire A, Fenn P, Stevens R, Cull C, *et al.* (2000) Cost effectiveness of an intensive blood glucose control policy in patients with type 2 diabetes: economic analysis alongside randomized controlled trial (UKPDS 41). *British Medical Journal* **320**, 1373–1378. doi:10.1136/bmj.320. 7246.1373

Green J, Thorogood N (2004) *Qualitative Methods for Health Research.* Sage, London, UK.

Holloway I, Wheeler S (2010) *Qualitative Research in Nursing and Healthcare.* Wiley-Blackwell, Chichester, UK.

Kesavadev J, Shankar A, Pillai PB, Krishnan G, Jothydev S (2012) Cost-effective use of telemedicine and self-monitoring of blood glucose via Diabetes Tele Management System (DTMS) to achieve target glycosylated hemoglobin values without serious symptomatic hypoglycemia in 1,000 subjects with type 2 diabetes mellitus – a retrospective study. *Diabetes Technology & Therapeutics* **14**, 772–776. doi:10.1089/dia.2012.0088

Kong MC, Lim TG, Ng HJ, Chan YH, Lee LH (2008) Feasibility, cost-effectiveness and patients' acceptance of point-of-care INR testing in a hospital-based anticoagulation clinic. *Annals of Hematology* **87**, 905–910. doi:10.1007/s00277-008-0530-8

Liamputtong P (2013) *Qualitative Research Methods,* Oxford University Press, South Melbourne.

Low J (2013) Unstructured and semi-structured interviews in health research. In *Researching Health: Qualitative, Quantitative and Mixed Methods.* (Eds M Saks and J Allsop) pp. 87–105. Sage, London, UK.

Mahieu L, Marien A, De Dooy J, Mahieu M, Mahieu H, Van Hoof V (2012) Implementation of a multi-parameter point-of-care-blood test analyzer reduces central laboratory testing and need for blood transfusions in very low birth weight infants. *Clinica Chimica Acta* **413**, 325–330. doi:10.1016/j.cca.2011.10.027

NHMRC (National Health and Medical Research Council) (2007) *National Statement on Ethical Conduct in Human Research.* NHMRC, Canberra.

Prost A, Griffiths CJ, Anderson J, Wight D, Hart GJ (2009) Feasibility and acceptability of offering rapid HIV tests to patients registering with primary care in London (UK): a pilot study. *Sexually Transmitted Infections* **85**, 326–329. doi:10.1136/sti.2008.033233

Shephard M (2006) Cultural and clinical effectiveness of the 'QAAMS' point-of-care testing model for diabetes management in Australian Aboriginal medical services. *The Clinical Biochemist Reviews* **27**, 161–170.

Shephard M, O'Brien C, Burgoyne A, Croft J, Garlett T, Barancek K, *et al.* (2015) Review of the cultural safety of a national Indigenous point-of-care testing program for diabetes management. *Australian Journal of Primary Health* (Online September). doi:10.1071/PY15050

St John A, Price C (2013) Economic evidence and point-of-care testing. *The Clinical Biochemist Reviews* **34**, 61–74.

Williams CL, Rittman MR, Boylstein C, Faircloth C, Haijing Q (2005) Qualitative and quantitative measurement of depression in veterans recovering from stroke. *Journal of Rehabilitation Research and Development* **42**, 277–290. doi:10.1682/JRRD.2004.02.0017

# THEME 2

# A GLOBAL PERSPECTIVE ON THE CLINICAL USE OF POINT-OF-CARE TESTING

# 9 Point-of-care testing for diabetes: glucose

*Mark Shephard, Jonathan Shaw and Paul Zimmet*

**Summary**

Over the past several decades, significant changes in human behaviour, lifestyle and the environment have led to a rapid escalation in the prevalence of diabetes worldwide. The global burden of diabetes exceeded 150 million adults in the year 2000 and is predicted to reach 642 million by 2040. The prevention of diabetes and its micro- and macro-vascular complications should now be regarded as an essential component of public health strategies for all nations globally. Blood glucose monitoring by point-of-care testing (POCT) represents more than half of the global market sales of POCT products. There is a myriad of blood glucose meters available in today's market. But how analytically sound are blood glucose meters and has the widespread global practice of blood glucose monitoring translated into improved outcomes for diabetes patients?

## INTRODUCTION

### Global, regional and local burden of diabetes

Diabetes mellitus is a global health priority and represents one of the most challenging contemporary health problems. There have been numerous publications over the past 20 years estimating the number of people with diabetes worldwide, including reports from the World Health Organization and the International Diabetes Federation (Amos *et al.* 1997; King *et al.* 1998; Shaw *et al.* 2010; Wild *et al.* 2004; Zimmet *et al.* 2001). The most recent International Diabetes Federation (IDF) *Diabetes Atlas* (IDF 2015) describes a 'diabetes pandemic' sweeping the world, a statement supported by a compelling array of facts and figures including:

- There were estimated to be 415 million adults living with diabetes worldwide in 2015, of whom 193 million (46.5%) were undiagnosed (Fig. 9.1).
- The number of adults living with diabetes is expected to increase to 642 million by 2040.
- By region, the Western Pacific had 153 million adults with diabetes in 2015, substantially more than any other IDF region; however, the North America and Caribbean region had the highest prevalence per capita, with one in every eight adults having diabetes.
- By country, China and India lead the way with 109.6 and 69.2 million adults with diabetes in 2015, respectively, followed by the USA (35.1 million).

Showing other alarming trends, the IDF Diabetes Atlas made the following estimates:

- The number of children with type 1 diabetes exceeded half a million for the first time in 2015.

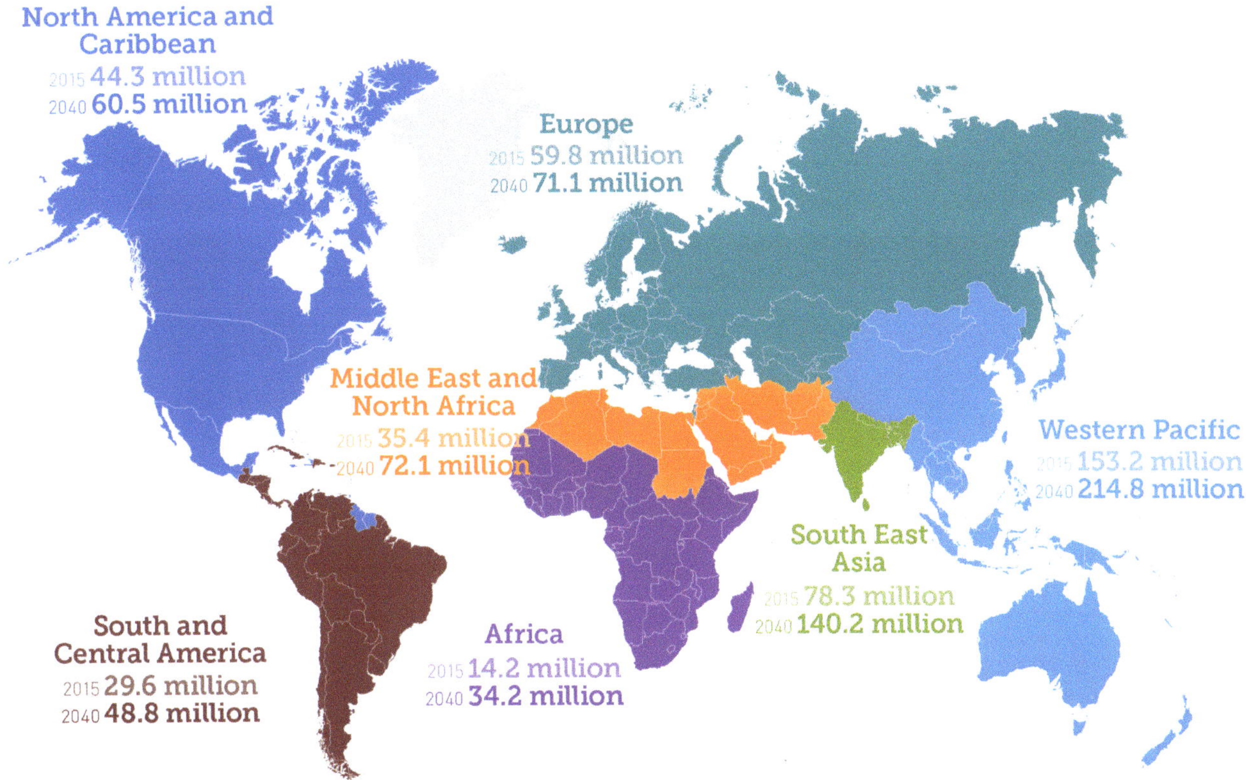


**Fig. 9.1.** Estimated number of people with diabetes worldwide and per region in 2015 and 2040 (20–79 years). (Source: Reproduced with permission from IDF 2015)

- There is an ever-increasing trend towards younger people developing type 2 diabetes.
- One in seven births is affected by gestational diabetes.
- More than 318 million people worldwide (6.7% of adults) are at high risk of diabetes (with impaired glucose tolerance or pre-diabetes).
- Indigenous people remain extremely vulnerable to diabetes, with an approximate 40% prevalence in some North American native Indian populations and 30% in Australian Aboriginal people (Minges *et al.* 2011).

The escalating human toll and financial burden of diabetes are also staggering (Zhang *et al.* 2010). In 2013, there were 5.1 million deaths due to diabetes (equating to one death every 6 seconds). Global health spending to treat diabetes and prevent complications in 2015 was conservatively estimated to be US$673 billion (equating to 11.6% of the total health budget worldwide) (IDF 2015).

## Pathophysiology

In a healthy person, blood glucose is maintained within tight limits by the actions of two main pancreatic hormones: insulin and glucagon. Insulin is synthesised in and secreted from the β cells of the pancreas in response to raised blood glucose (e.g. following a meal). Insulin reduces blood glucose by promoting the uptake of glucose into cells, with some glucose used to satisfy energy requirements through the glycolysis pathway and any excess glucose stored as glycogen in liver or muscle cells (glycogenesis) or as fat (triglyceride) in adipose tissue (lipogenesis). Insulin also inhibits the production of glucose from non-carbohydrate sources.

Glucagon is synthesised in and released from the α cells of the pancreas in response to reduced blood glucose. Glucagon is an insulin antagonist, increasing hepatic production of glucose from glycogen (glycogenolysis) as well as increasing the production of glucose from non-carbohydrate sources (gluconeogenesis).

Three other hormones, cortisol and adrenalin (synthesised in the adrenal gland), and growth hormone (secreted from the anterior pituitary) also increase blood glucose in response to reduced blood glucose and/or stress.

The continuous opposing effects of insulin and glucagon (as well as cortisol, adrenalin and growth hormone) maintain the blood glucose within normal limits (Fig. 9.2).

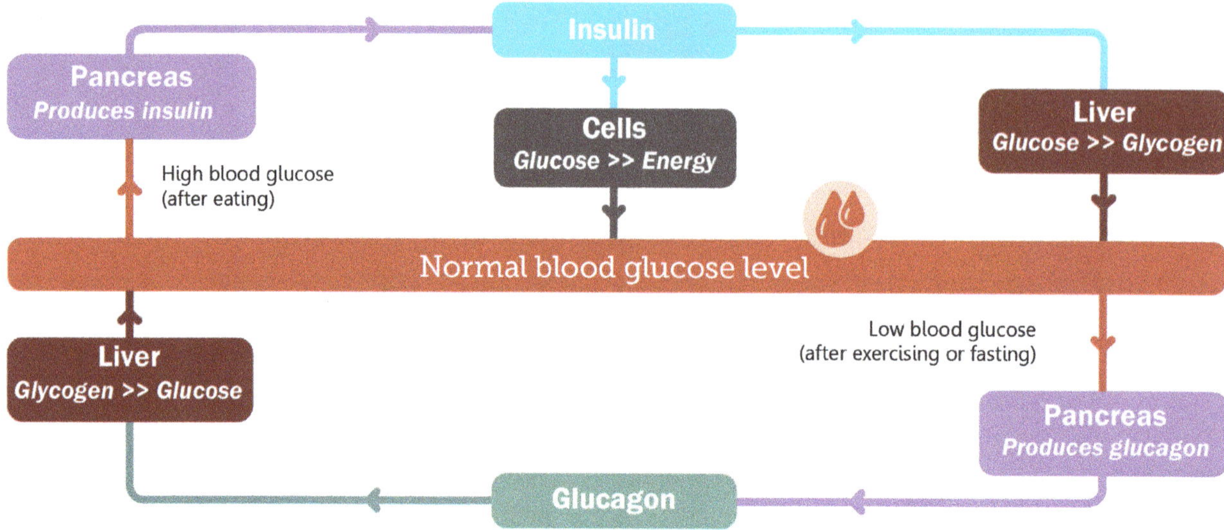


**Fig. 9.2.** Insulin production and action. (Source: Reproduced with permission from IDF 2015)

## Classification of diabetes

Diabetes mellitus is a group of common metabolic disorders that are characterised by chronic hyperglycaemia resulting from defects in insulin secretion, insulin action or both (ADA 2012a).

There are two main types of diabetes:

- *Type 1 diabetes* (previously known as insulin dependent diabetes or juvenile-onset diabetes) results from the autoimmune destruction of β cells of the pancreas, leading to an absolute insulin deficiency. Type 1 diabetes accounts for ~5–10% of patients with diabetes (ADA 2015). Type 1 diabetes patients need to take multiple insulin injections each day or receive continuously administered insulin through an insulin pump.
- *Type 2 diabetes* (previously known as non-insulin dependent diabetes or adult-onset diabetes) is in most cases a (preventable) chronic progressive condition. With type 2 diabetes, patients are able to produce insulin but the body cannot respond adequately to its effects (insulin resistance) and/or it is produced in insufficient quantities to meet the person's needs.

Type 2 diabetes is the most common form of diabetes (Sacks *et al.* 2011). The perception that type 2 diabetes only afflicts people aged 40 or over no longer holds true, with many cases of type 2 diabetes now being diagnosed in younger people and adolescents. Patients with type 2 diabetes can often manage their condition with a healthy diet, weight loss and an active lifestyle, although most patients ultimately require support with oral glucose-lowering medications, while some may need insulin if they are unable to control their blood glucose levels well.

In 2015, the IDF estimated that 20.9 million (16.2% of) live births had some form of hyperglycaemia in pregnancy (IDF 2015). More than 85% of these cases were due to gestational diabetes mellitus (GDM) where pregnant women develop a resistance to the action of insulin during the second or third trimester of pregnancy (Sacks *et al.* 2011). GDM usually disappears after birth, but women with GDM are at high risk of developing gestational diabetes in further pregnancies and of developing type 2 diabetes later in life. Uncontrolled GDM can lead to a significantly larger baby, and to obstetric and neonatal problems. It is also important to recognise that the offspring of a pregnancy complicated by GDM are at higher risk of obesity and type 2 diabetes in later life (IDF 2015).

There are several, relatively uncommon, specific types of diabetes due to other causes; these include (but are not limited to):

- monogenic diabetes syndromes, which are caused by genetic defects of β cell function
- diseases of the exocrine pancreas
- endocrinopathies, where excess amounts of hormones that antagonise the action of insulin are produced
- drug- or chemical-induced diabetes (ADA 2012a, 2015).

## Risk factors for diabetes

Both genetic and environmental factors appear to be important for the development of type 1 diabetes, but the precise role and nature of each remains inadequately understood. Risk factors for type 2 diabetes include: obesity (notably central, or 'apple-shaped' obesity), poor diet, lack of physical exercise and a sedentary existence, increasing age (due to declining β cell function), ethnicity (with Indigenous, Pacific Islanders, south Indian and Hispanic people being the most susceptible to diabetes) (Chen *et al.* 2012), impaired glucose tolerance, and history of gestational diabetes. Type 2 diabetes in particular is being driven by an ageing population and by environments that favour poor lifestyle choices (Shaw *et al.* 2010). Fortunately many of the risk factors are modifiable with lifestyle adjustments, while education and support for self-management or empowerment provide opportunities to prevent or delay the progression of the disease.

Different electronic tools to assess an individual's risk of diabetes have been developed. For example, the Australian Type 2 Diabetes Risk Assessment tool or AUSDRISK (www.bakeridi.edu.au/aus_diabetes_risk) was established in 2007 and approved as the country's national diabetes risk assessment tool by state and federal governments (RACGP and DA 2014) (Fig. 9.3). The Finnish Diabetes Risk Score (FINDRISC) was developed for use in Finland (Saaristo *et al.* 2005) and has been modified for use in several countries including Canada, where the Canadian Diabetes Risk Questionnaire (CANRISK) was created by the Public Health Agency of Canada (http://guidelines.diabetes.ca/CDACPG_resources/CANRISK_eng.pdf). These screening tools are designed to be simple and rapid means of identifying individuals at high risk of diabetes.

## Complications of diabetes

Persons with long-standing poorly controlled diabetes are at significant risk of developing a range of micro- and macro-vascular complications of diabetes, all of which are debilitating and some of which are life-threatening. Diabetes affects many parts of the body. Cardiovascular disease (CVD) is the major cause of morbidity and mortality for people with diabetes. Cardiovascular and cerebrovascular diseases associated with diabetes include myocardial infarction, congestive heart failure, peripheral artery disease and stroke. The combination of type 2 diabetes, high blood pressure and dyslipidaemia is a potent cocktail of risk factors for CVD. Eye disease (retinopathy) and kidney disease (nephropathy) are common sequelae of diabetes. They are caused by damage/blockage to small blood vessels supplying the retina and the glomerulus and can result in blindness and end-stage renal disease, respectively. Damage to the peripheral nerves (neuropathy) and the peripheral vascular system caused by diabetes can result in erectile dysfunction in men and may lead to serious infection or ulceration to the feet or limbs, which may in turn require amputation.

## Pathology tests to diagnose and manage diabetes

Pathology testing has an important role in the diagnosis and management of diabetes. The World Health Organization (WHO 2006, 2011) now recommends the following options for diagnosing diabetes:

- a fasting plasma glucose of ≥7.0 mmol/L (126 mg/dL)
- a 2-h plasma glucose ≥11.1 mmol/L (200 mg/dL) performed as part of an oral glucose tolerance test (OGTT)
- haemoglobin A1c (HbA1c) ≥6.5% (48 mmol/mol). (Currently there are two units of measurement for HbA1c. The rationale for this will be discussed in Chapter 10.)

If the patient shows classical symptoms of diabetes, then diagnosis can be made on a single test meeting any one of the criteria above. However, in the absence of this, any abnormal test needs to be confirmed on a separate day before making the diagnosis of diabetes (IDF Guideline Development Group 2014). HbA1c is not an appropriate diagnostic test for suspected type 1 diabetes or GDM, because these two conditions can have too rapid an onset to be reflected in HbA1c.

The WHO defines individuals with both a fasting plasma glucose of <7.0 mmol/L (126 mg/dL) and a 2-h plasma glucose between 7.8 (140 mg/dL) and 11.1 mmol/L (200 mg/dL) with the OGTT as having impaired glucose tolerance (IGT), while those with both a fasting glucose of between 6.1 (110 mg/dL) and 6.9 mmol/L (125 mg/dL) and a 2-h plasma glucose (if measured) of <7.8 mmol/L (140 mg/dL) as having impaired fasting glucose (IFG). The American Diabetes Association (ADA) has a slightly different classification for IFG (fasting plasma glucose of 5.6 [100 mg/dL] to 6.9 mmol/L [125 mg/dL]). The ADA also classify individuals with IGT or IFG or those with an HbA1c between 5.7 and 6.4% (39 and 46 mmol/mol) as

# The Australian Type 2 Diabetes Risk Assessment Tool (AUSDRISK)

1. Your age group

| | | |
|---|---|---|
| Under 35 years | ☐ | 0 points |
| 35 – 44 years | ☐ | 2 points |
| 45 – 54 years | ☐ | 4 points |
| 55 – 64 years | ☐ | 6 points |
| 65 years or over | ☐ | 8 points |

2. Your gender

| | | |
|---|---|---|
| Female | ☐ | 0 points |
| Male | ☐ | 3 points |

3. Your ethnicity/country of birth:

3a. Are you of Aboriginal, Torres Strait Islander, Pacific Islander or Maori descent?

| | | |
|---|---|---|
| No | ☐ | 0 points |
| Yes | ☐ | 2 points |

3b. Where were you born?

| | | |
|---|---|---|
| Australia | ☐ | 0 points |
| Asia (including the Indian sub-continent), Middle East, North Africa, Southern Europe | ☐ | 2 points |
| Other | ☐ | 0 points |

4. Have either of your parents, or any of your brothers or sisters been diagnosed with diabetes (type 1 or type 2)?

| | | |
|---|---|---|
| No | ☐ | 0 points |
| Yes | ☐ | 3 points |

5. Have you ever been found to have high blood glucose (sugar) (for example, in a health examination, during an illness, during pregnancy)?

| | | |
|---|---|---|
| No | ☐ | 0 points |
| Yes | ☐ | 6 points |

6. Are you currently taking medication for high blood pressure?

| | | |
|---|---|---|
| No | ☐ | 0 points |
| Yes | ☐ | 2 points |

7. Do you currently smoke cigarettes or any other tobacco products on a daily basis?

| | | |
|---|---|---|
| No | ☐ | 0 points |
| Yes | ☐ | 2 points |

**If you scored 6-11 points in the AUSDRISK you may be at increased risk of type 2 diabetes.** Discuss your score and your individual risk with your doctor. Improving your lifestyle may help reduce your risk of developing type 2 diabetes.

8. How often do you eat vegetables or fruit?

| | | |
|---|---|---|
| Every day | ☐ | 0 points |
| Not every day | ☐ | 1 point |

9. On average, would you say you do at least 2.5 hours of physical activity per week (for example, 30 minutes a day on 5 or more days a week)?

| | | |
|---|---|---|
| Yes | ☐ | 0 points |
| No | ☐ | 2 points |

10. Your waist measurement taken below the ribs (usually at the level of the navel, and while standing)

Waist measurement (cm) ☐

**For those of Asian or Aboriginal or Torres Strait Islander descent:**

| Men | Women | | |
|---|---|---|---|
| Less than 90 cm | Less than 80 cm | ☐ | 0 points |
| 90 – 100 cm | 80 – 90 cm | ☐ | 4 points |
| More than 100 cm | More than 90 cm | ☐ | 7 points |

**For all others:**

| Men | Women | | |
|---|---|---|---|
| Less than 102 cm | Less than 88 cm | ☐ | 0 points |
| 102 – 110 cm | 88 – 100 cm | ☐ | 4 points |
| More than 110 cm | More than 100 cm | ☐ | 7 points |

Add up your points ☐

Your risk of developing type 2 diabetes within 5 years*:

☐ *5 or less: Low risk*
Approximately one person in every 100 will develop diabetes.

☐ *6-11: Intermediate risk*
For scores of 6-8, approximately one person in every 50 will develop diabetes. For scores of 9-11, approximately one person in every 30 will develop diabetes.

☐ *12 or more: High risk*
For scores of 12-15, approximately one person in every 14 will develop diabetes. For scores of 16-19, approximately one person in every 7 will develop diabetes. For scores of 20 and above, approximately one person in every 3 will develop diabetes.

*The overall score may overestimate the risk of diabetes in those aged less than 25 years.

**If you scored 12 points or more in the AUSDRISK you may have undiagnosed type 2 diabetes or be at high risk of developing the disease.** See your doctor about having a fasting blood glucose test. Act now to prevent type 2 diabetes.

**Fig. 9.3.** The AUSDRISK Tool (Source: ©2010 Commonwealth of Australia. Reproduced with permission from the Department of Health). The AUSDRISK Tool was designed for the Australian population, with risk scores calculated and validated based upon the results of the participants in the Australian Diabetes, Obesity and Lifestyle Study (AusDiab). Consequently the AUSDRISK Tool is not reliable or suitable for use in non-Australian populations.

having prediabetes, although the HbA1c range for prediabetes varies between countries (ADA 2012b).

For management of patients with diabetes, HbA1c is well established as the 'gold standard' pathology test for monitoring long-term glycaemic control. The higher the level of HbA1c, the poorer is the recent glycaemic control and the greater is the risk of developing complications.

Self-monitoring of blood glucose (SMBG) levels is widely used to support patients with type 1 and type 2 diabetes, but, as the ADA recommends, SMBG 'should only be performed by people with diabetes who have the knowledge, skills and willingness to use the information obtained to actively adjust treatment, enhance understanding of diabetes and assess the effectiveness of their management plan on glycaemic control' (ADA 2015).

Both glucose and HbA1c are common tests measured by laboratories throughout the world, but both tests can also now be conveniently performed at the point-of-care. Blood glucose POCT will be discussed in detail in this chapter, while HbA1c and its measurement by POCT will be described in Chapter 10. These two analytes have been given significant coverage in the book because POC glucose testing accounts for more than 50% of the market sales of POCT products globally, while POC HbA1c testing is one of the most topical, widely debated and researched subjects in the contemporary POCT arena.

There are several other pathology tests that are clinically useful in the management of diabetes and that form part of the annual cycle of diabetes care and/or emergency diabetes care; these include: lipids; urea and creatinine; urinalysis and urine albumin:creatinine ratio (ACR); liver function tests; lactate and ketones; C-peptide and autoantibodies (e.g. autoantibodies to glutamate decarboxylase [anti-GAD]). Most of these tests can also be performed by POCT and most will be described in other chapters of the book.

## GLUCOSE

### Introduction

Blood glucose testing is a long-standing and widely used application of POCT globally; as mentioned previously, blood glucose self-monitoring dominates the POCT market, representing 55–60% of global sales and is a multi-billion dollar industry (Huckle 2006; St John and Price 2014).

There are now a multitude of POCT glucose meter systems available globally. It is almost impossible to know just how many there are, but the ADA's consumer magazine *Diabetes Forecast* recently listed 84 different glucose meters from 22 diagnostic companies (Diabetes Forecast 2013). An earlier report from the UK's National Health Service Purchasing and Supply Agency reported 29 meters on the market in that country in 2008 (NHS 2008).

There are now multiple clinical settings and applications where POC glucose testing is regularly performed, including hospitals, primary care settings and the home (Table 9.1). Glucose meters are also an integral part of continuous glucose monitoring systems used by a small percentage of diabetes patients to monitor their glycaemia.

The Clinical and Laboratory Standards Institute (CLSI) has recently published comprehensive guidelines on POC blood glucose testing conducted (i) in acute and chronic care (hospital) settings where laboratory support is available (CLSI 2013) and (ii) in settings without laboratory support (CLSI 2015).

### POCT glucose meter technology

The general principle by which most glucose meters work is as follows:

- a drop of capillary whole blood is applied onto a glucose test strip
- red blood cells are then removed
- glucose is measured in the plasma phase following enzymatic digestion using either glucose oxidase (GO) or glucose dehydrogenase (GDH), coupling with an indicator reaction, and measurement of the resultant signal by photometry or electrochemistry (Sluss 2006). In GDH-based systems, the indicator reaction may involve nicotinamide adenine dinucleotide (NAD), flavin adeninine dinucleotide (FAD) or pyrroloquinolinequinone (PQQ), with the importance of the latter being discussed below.

Today's glucose meters are markedly improved compared with older devices; for example:

**Table 9.1.** Clinical settings and applications for POC blood glucose testing

| Setting | Example(s) | Clinical use |
|---|---|---|
| Hospital | Diabetes wards and clinics | Diabetes patients having their therapy managed |
| | Operating theatres and recovery suites | Intraoperative and perioperative management of blood glucose may be needed in surgical patients |
| | Emergency departments | Rapid detection of extreme blood glucose concentrations may be needed in patients whose symptoms suggest hypo- or hyperglycaemia or in patients who are unconscious without an identifiable cause |
| | Maternity wards | Monitoring of mothers with diabetes (in the peri-partum period) and their infants |
| | Neonatal and intensive care units | Patient's glycaemic control may need to be closely monitored (under tight glycaemic control) to limit hypo- and hyperglycaemic episodes |
| Primary care settings | General practices, Indigenous medical services, community clinics, pharmacies, occupational health facilities, residential care communities, schools, and student related facilities, day care centres, and prisons | Blood glucose monitoring is required to manage therapy for patients with diabetes<br>Note: Most recommendations state that POC blood glucose testing should not be used for screening patients at high risk for diabetes |
| Home use | Patient self-testing | Type 1 and type 2 diabetes patients conduct their own glucose testing as part of a tailored self-monitoring regimen |

- Sample volumes are now very small.
- The time for a test result is now very short (~5 s with some meters).
- Most meters can store hundreds of test results, which can be downloaded to a computer or clinical information system. Results can also be graphed or analysed statistically by other software, once downloaded from the meter.
- Operators can be locked out from performing a patient test if QC testing has not been performed within the required interval.
- Some glucose meters feature audio prompts.

The specifications of four different glucose meters that have been used widely in Australia in recent years are compared and contrasted in Table 9.2. All are lightweight, require a small sample volume, provide a rapid result (except the HemoCue), and have wide measuring ranges. Calibration modes vary and most models are battery powered.

Intuitively, POC glucose testing may appear simple, easy and foolproof, but this is not the case and there are many problems, pitfalls and limitations that working health professionals need to be aware of. As Olansky and Kennedy (2010) state: 'common experience tells us that the majority of patients using meters for SMBG (self-monitoring of blood glucose) are unaware of the magnitude of the potential inaccuracy of results, and we suspect that many health-care providers also tend to ascribe greater accuracy than is warranted to portable glucose meter results.'

## Issues and limitations with POCT blood glucose meters

Factors that can affect blood glucose measurement are summarised in Table 9.3.

### Sample issues

At a normal haematocrit of 43%, the glucose concentration in whole blood is ~11% less than the glucose concentration in plasma; that is, whole blood glucose × 1.11 = plasma glucose. This is because whole blood comprises red cells and plasma, and red cells have lower water content (71%) compared with plasma (93%) (Wahl 2009).

There is the possibility that pseudo-hyperglycaemia can occur if a blood glucose test is performed on a patient's finger that has been in contact with glucose-rich foodstuffs and therefore, in this instance, hands should be washed before sample collection (Hirose *et al.* 2011). As a general rule, fingers should be warm and clean before lancing for measuring blood glucose.

### Device set-up issues

There are two units of measurement for glucose: mg/dL (which are used in the USA and several other countries); and mmol/L (the SI unit, which is used throughout the rest of the world). There is an 18-fold difference in units

**Table 9.2.** Comparison of selected specifications for some POCT glucose meters used in recent years in Australia

| POCT device | Image | Method principle; detection | Sample volume (μL) | Time for result (s) | Measuring range (mmol/L) | Weight (g) | Power source | Calibration |
|---|---|---|---|---|---|---|---|---|
| Roche Accu-Check® Performa | | GDH/PQQ; electrochemistry | 0.6 | 5 | 0.6–33.0 | 62 | Battery | Code chip |
| Abbott Freestyle Optium | | GDH/NAD; electrochemisty | 0.6 | 5 | 1.1–22.8 | 42 | Battery | Strip |
| HemoCue® 201 glucose | | GDH/NAD; electrochemistry | 4.0 | <40 | 0–22.2 | 350 | Battery or AC | Factory |
| Nova StatStrip® Xpress | | Modified GO; electrochemistry | 1.2 | 6 | 0.5–33.3 | 75 | Battery | Strip |

GDH = glucose dehydrogenase; GO = glucose oxidase; NAD = nicotinamide adenine dinucleotide; PQQ = pyrroloquinolinequinone

with conversion formulae being: mg/dL × 0.0555 = mmol/L; mmol/L × 18.0182 = mg/dL.

These different units can cause significant issues for the unsuspecting patient if his/her device is inadvertently set in the wrong units for their country, especially if POC glucose results are being used for insulin dosing (Lunt *et al.* 2010).

### Patient issues

There are several potential pitfalls with POC blood glucose measurement, which predominantly affect measurement in patients with certain other co-morbidities.

Patients with anaemia who have a low haematocrit (where there is increased plasma water) may have erroneously high POC blood glucose results, while patients with polycythaemia who have a high haematocrit (low plasma water) may have lower glucose results. Patients with high levels of bilirubin (greater than 300 μmol/L) may also have erroneously low glucose meter results.

In critically ill patients with poor blood flow to peripheral tissues due to shock, hypotension, peripheral vascular disease, oedema or severe dehydration (as a result of vomiting or diabetic ketoacidosis), blood glucose meter results may be lower than the glucose concentration in the central circulation.

Some biological or pharmacological products that a patient may be prescribed can also cause errors with blood glucose meter measurements, for example:

- With glucose meters that use glucose oxidase for enzymatic digestion, altered oxygen saturation states can have an effect on glucose. Critically ill patients on oxygen therapy or with impaired oxygen transport may have falsely low glucose readings at high $pO_2$ levels and falsely high glucose readings at low $pO_2$ levels, respectively.
- For glucose meters that use glucose dehydrogenase digestion coupled with PQQ, related sugars such as maltose, galactose and xylose can react like glucose, leading to false hyperglycaemia and importantly masking hypoglycaemia. Some dialysis solutions that are used for patients on peritoneal dialysis contain a compound called icodextrin, which is a large molecular weight glucose polymer. During dialysis, icodextrin is hydrolysed to maltose, maltotriose and maltotetraose, which react with the GDH/PQQ system and cause significantly overestimated glucose results.

  There have been multiple reports of icodextrin interference with blood glucose meters using the GDH/PQQ measurement system (Flore and Delanghe 2009; Movalia and Ogino *et al.* 2006; Oyibo *et al.* 2002). This problem has led to serious clinical issues and even fatalities, which in turn has resulted in many calls from professional and expert groups recommending that GDH/PQQ methods must not be used to monitor glucose in patients receiving any form of maltose.
- At therapeutic levels, most drugs do not interfere with POC glucose measurement but, at high doses, some medications including acetoaminophen (paracetamol), salicylate, dopamine, mannitol and ascorbic acid can give erroneously low or high glucose results, depending on the method used.

#### Environmental issues

Extremes of temperature, humidity and altitude can cause deterioration of glucose test strips and affect the accuracy of POC glucose measurements.

The range of limitations described above highlight two key messages. Firstly, sound training, continuing education and quality surveillance for all operators of glucose meters is the key to ensuring that these devices are used appropriately as part of a sustainable POC glucose monitoring program. In relation to quality testing, QC should ideally be performed when:

- a strip lot number is changed
- a new container of strips is opened

**Table 9.3.** Factors that can affect the accuracy of POC blood glucose measurement

| Category | Example | Effect on blood glucose measurement |
|---|---|---|
| Pre-analytical | Sample type | Glucose concentration in whole blood is 11% less than glucose concentration in plasma |
| | Sample collection | Contamination of test finger surface with glucose-rich foodstuffs may cause pseudo-hyperglycaemia |
| | Meter set-up | Meters inadvertently set to wrong reporting units (mmol/L *v.* mg/dL) may cause gross errors in interpretation of results |
| Patient's pathophysiological status/presence of interfering substances | Haematocrit (HcT) | Patients with low HcT may have falsely high blood glucose results<br>Patients with high HcT may have falsely low blood glucose results |
| | Oxygen saturation | Patients on oxygen therapy or with impaired oxygen transport may have erroneously low blood glucose results at high $pO_2$ or falsely high blood glucose at low $PO_2$ levels, if glucose is measured on a meter using glucose oxidase |
| | Peritoneal dialysis | Patients having peritoneal dialysis containing icodextrin may have factitiously high blood glucose levels, if glucose is measured by a meter using glucose dehydrogenase/PQQ |
| | Medications | Patients taking high doses of paracetamol may have falsely elevated blood glucose results (CLSI 2015) |
| Environmental | Temperature and humidity | Test strip deterioration may occur if strips are exposed to extremes of temperature or humidity |

**Table 9.4.** Evolution of analytical goals for total error (accuracy) for glucose measurement proposed by the Clinical and Laboratory Standards Institute (CLSI) and the International Standards Organization (ISO)

| Source of goal (year) | Width of goal | For glucose less than: | Width of goal | For glucose greater than or equal to: | For what percentage of samples tested |
|---|---|---|---|---|---|
| NCCLS (now CLSI) (1994) | ± 0.83 mmol/L (15 mg/dL) | 5.5 mmol/L (100 mg/dL) | ± 20% | 5.5 mmol/L (100 mg/dL) | 95% |
| ISO 15197 (2003) | ± 0.83 mmol/L (15 mg/dL) | 4.2 mmol/L (75 mg/dL) | ± 20% | 4.2 mmol/L (75 mg/dL) | 95% |
| CLSI (2013)[a] | ± 0.67 mmol/L (12 mg/dL) | 5.55 mmol/L (100 mg/dL) | ± 12.5% | 5.55 mmol/L (100 mg/dL) | 95% |
| ISO 15197 (2013)[b] | ± 0.83 mmol/L (15 mg/dL) | 5.55 mmol/L (75 mg/dL) | ± 15% | 5.55 mmol/L (75 mg/dL) | 95% |

[a]The CLSI 2013 guideline (page 12) also states, in addition to the above goal: the sum of the number of individual results with (i) errors that exceed 20% at glucose concentrations ≥4.2 mmol/L (75 mg/dL) and (ii) errors that exceed >0.83 mmol/L (15 mg/dL) at concentrations <4.2 mmol/L should not exceed 2% of all results. This aligns with the 2003 ISO goal except the goal requires 98% rather than 95% of values to meet the goal.
[b]The ISO 2013 guideline (page 20) also states that for design verification studies performed by trained operators: the sum of individual glucose measured values shall fall within zones A and B of the Consensus Error Grid (CEG) for type 1 diabetes (ISO 2013; Parkes *et al.* 2000). The ISO 2013 guidelines also provide, for the first time, acceptance criteria for glucose meters used in accuracy verification studies by patients (reflecting the importance of accurate self-monitoring measurements), as well as criteria for the assessment of interferents (including haematocrit).

- batteries need replacing
- verifying performance to investigate possible test strip deterioration
- questionable results are obtained and before resuming routine patient testing (CLSI 2015).

Secondly, the challenge for the diagnostic pathology industry is to develop better or improved methods that minimise these interferences (Karon *et al.* 2008; Kost *et al.* 2008).

## Analytical performance

Clearly there are several pre-analytical issues and confounding factors affecting POC blood glucose measurement, but what benchmarks have been set for analytical quality and what is known about the analytical performance characteristics of these devices?

### Analytical goals for glucose

Multiple performance goals for total analytical error of POC glucose meters have been proposed over the past 30 years by different expert groups, professional associations and PT program organisers (Tables 9.4 and 9.5). Although the goals were initially couched in terms of total error, many subsequent papers represent them as goals for accuracy, with very limited mention of required goals for imprecision being available in the literature.

**Table 9.5.** Examples of analytical goals for total error for POCT glucose meter measurement proposed by bodies other than CLSI or ISO (Source: adapted in part from Fraser and Scott 2010)

| Source of goal | Year | Width of goal |
|---|---|---|
| American Diabetes Association | 1987 | Total error (pre-analytical plus analytical) <10% for glucose 1.7–22.2 mmol/L (30–400 mg/dL) 100% of the time |
| Clinical Laboratory Improvement Amendments | 1988 | Meters should be within 10% of the target value or ± 0.3 mmol/L (± 6 mg/dL), whichever is larger |
| National Academy of Clinical Biochemistry/American Diabetes Association | 2002 | Total allowable error (including bias and imprecision) of 7.9% |
| College of American Pathologists PT Program for glucose meters | 2005 | Meters should be within ± 20% or ± 0.66 mmol/L (± 12 mg/dL) of the peer group mean; for laboratory measurements the goal is within ± 10% or ± 0.33 mmol/L (± 6 mg/dL) of the peer group mean |
| Westgard website | 2015 | Imprecision ≤2.9%, bias ≤2.2% and total error ≤6.9% (based on biological variation) |

These goals vary considerably and are quite complex to interpret, making it difficult for potential users of this technology to decide which goal to use and which meter to select for their intended use (Fraser and Scott 2010; Sacks *et al.* 2011).

The most widely quoted goals for total error (accuracy) of glucose meters have been those proposed by the CLSI and the International Standards Organization (ISO); both bodies have recently released updated goals that feature stricter criteria and that align more closely with each other (Table 9.4). In basic terms, they both require 95% of the test comparisons to fall within an absolute limit below a selected glucose concentration and within a percentage limit above that concentration (Fig. 9.4). They differ in the width of the absolute limit (CLSI 0.67 mmol/L [12 mg/dL]; ISO 0.83 mmol/L [15 mg/dL]) and the width of the percentage limit (CLSI 12.5%; ISO 15%) below and above a glucose concentration of 5.55 mmol/L (100 mg/dL).

A different, more clinical approach to the question 'how good should glucose meters be?' was developed by Clarke *et al.* (1987) and later revised by Parkes *et al.* (2000); here, error grids were developed to align a specific level of clinical risk to a potential error in POCT glucose measurement. The grid plots the deviation of the POCT glucose result from the laboratory result, which may fall into one of five different zones that have been assigned a graded clinical risk from having 'no effect on clinical action' to having 'dangerous consequences' (Fig. 9.5).

In the example shown, all comparative glucose measurements fell within the 'no clinical effect zone' (zone A) and so this meter would be classed as analytically sound and fit for clinical use under this grid system. The ISO 2013 guidelines now use the error grid concept as part of its acceptance criteria for glucose meter performance stating: '99% of individual glucose measured values shall fall within zones A and B of the Consensus Error Grid (CEG) for type 1 diabetes.'

Using simulated modelling of errors in insulin dose as a different clinical approach for goal setting, Karon *et al.* (2010) found that large improvements in glycaemic control, rates of hypoglycaemia, and decreases in the rates of (two-category) insulin dosing errors in 'tight glycaemic control' protocols occurred when the total error of glucose measurement fell from 20%, through 15% to 10%. Breton and Kovatchev (2010) showed that, for a reference laboratory blood glucose concentration of 3.3 mmol/L (60 mg/dL), the probability of missing a hypoglycaemic event is 0% with an error rate in blood glucose measurement from 0 to 5%, but the probability increases to 1% at an error rate of 10%, 3.5% with an error rate of 15% and reaches 10% with an error rate of 20% (Fig. 9.6). Both Breton and Kovatchev (2010) and Karon *et al.* (2010) concluded that

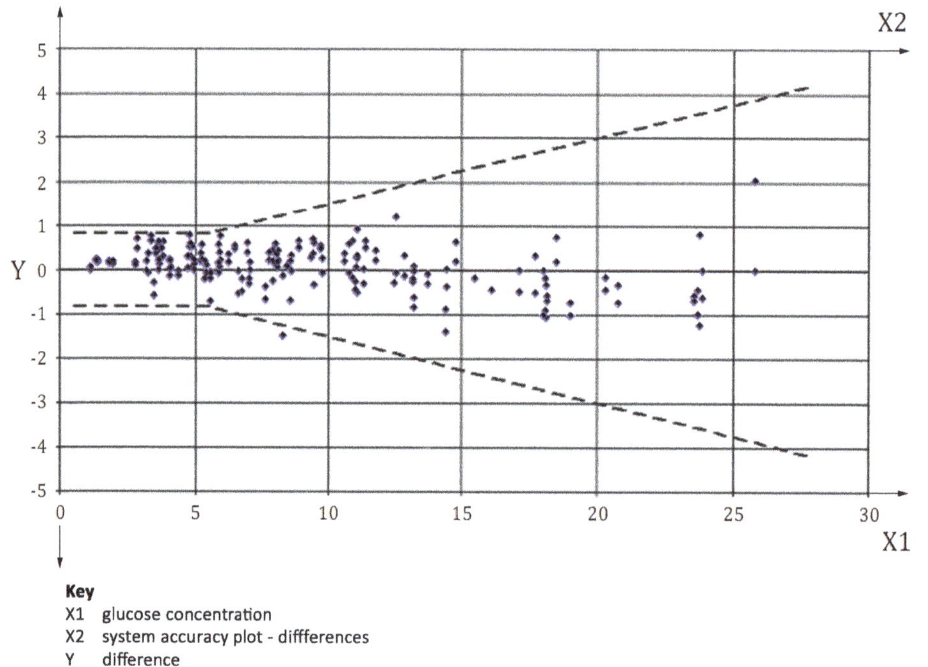


**Fig. 9.4.** Example of system accuracy plot. (Source: ISO 15197 Figure 1– reproduced with permission from SAI Global Ltd under Licence 1511-c089)

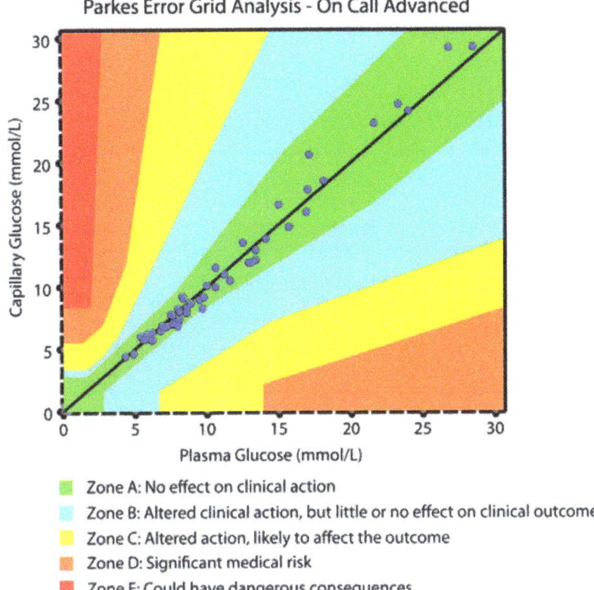


**Fig. 9.5.** Grid analysis, relating level of clinical risk to a potential error in POC blood glucose measurement. (Source: Reproduced with permission from Lunt *et al.* 2010. ©New Zealand Medical Journal)

older CLSI and ISO acceptance criteria, which allowed 20% total allowable error in glucose meters, were not optimal for patient management in tight glycaemic control where intensive insulin therapy is required.

Therefore, across the past 30 years, proposed analytical goals have turned full circle, with a total error goal of 10% proposed in 1987 by the ADA now becoming the optimal goal for POC glucose measurement for tight glycaemic control and/or for management of insulin titration for type 1 diabetes patients.

#### What is the state-of-the-art performance for current glucose meters?

There is a multitude of published evaluations on the performance of glucose meters from across the world, with the number of publications increasing every year in recent times (Thorpe 2013). Examples of recent multi-device evaluation studies include an Australian study of six meters in an antenatal diabetes clinic (Perera *et al.* 2011), a European evaluation of five glucose meters commonly available from pharmacies (Tack *et al.* 2012), a UK study of six common meters used in a diabetes outpatient clinic (Stadelmann Diaw *et al.* 2013), and two German studies involving 12 and 43 glucose meters used for patient self-testing, respectively (Freckmann *et al.* 2012, 2014).

These papers vary in their study design, the meters tested and the performance goals used, which makes comparative conclusions difficult to draw. Thorpe (2013) identified several weaknesses in recently published evaluations and, in an attempt to harmonise future studies of glucose meters, developed a useful checklist to assess analytical accuracy (as well as interferents); this checklist covered selection of a reference laboratory method, comparison of 'like with like' sample types, number of

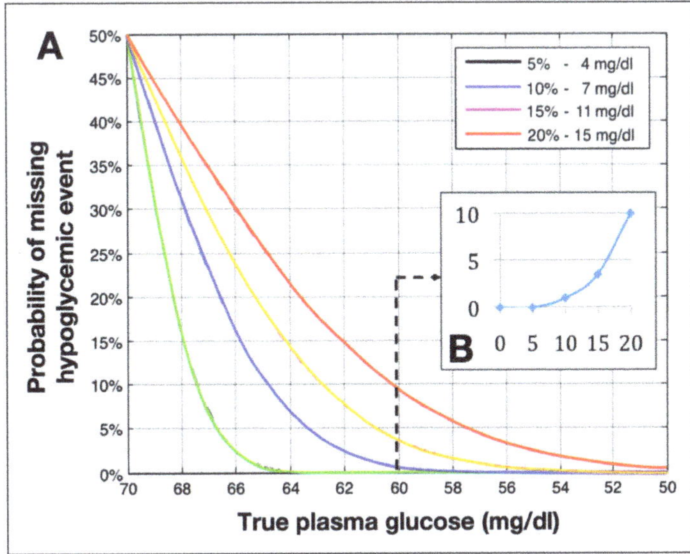


**Fig. 9.6.** Probability of blood glucose measurement missing hypoglycaemia as a function of blood glucose concentration and permitted error. (Source: Reproduced with permission from Breton and Kovatchev 2010)

**Table 9.6.** Recent consensus statements on the analytical performance of blood glucose meters

| Author | Statement |
|---|---|
| CLSI 2013 | 'The analytical uncertainty of a POCT glucose meter system [remains] greater than that of laboratory analysers' |
| CLSI 2015 | 'Most blood glucose meters are less accurate than laboratory instruments; with certain systems, significant errors in blood glucose testing results may occur if the operator does not understand the potential limitations of the system' |
| Sacks *et al.* 2011 | 'The imprecision of the results, coupled with the substantial differences among meters, precludes the use of glucose meters from the diagnosis of diabetes and limits their usefulness in screening for diabetes ... there are insufficient published data outcome to support the role for portable meters and fingerstick blood samples in the diagnosis of diabetes or for population screening' |
| Fraser and Scott 2010 | 'It is well known that glucose meters have inferior imprecision to central laboratory or blood gas analysers and can display large mean differences from laboratory methods' |

samples required, spread of glucose concentrations, accuracy criteria and strip lot numbers.

Unfortunately, despite technological advances, recent guidelines and recommendations from professional bodies and expert groups conclude that the analytical performance of blood glucose meters continues to be inferior to the laboratory measurement of this analyte (Table 9.6).

In terms of imprecision, laboratories in Australia can generally achieve an analytical imprecision (CV%) of 2.5% or less for glucose measurement, whereas the imprecision of glucose meters is in many cases approximately double that of laboratory methods. Fraser and Scott (2010) quote data from the 2009 College of American Pathologists PT program, which showed that the within-method imprecision (CV%) for 16 glucose meter methods (over 25 000 sites) ranged from 4 to 14%, while the within-method imprecision for 29 laboratory methods for glucose (across more than 5700 laboratories) was between 2.5 and 4.3%.

## Is the self-monitoring of blood glucose levels clinically effective?

The self-monitoring of blood glucose (SMBG) is a huge industry in its own right, but which patient groups benefit most from self-monitoring and what is the evidence to support the argument that self-monitoring is clinically effective?

The ADA's view is that: 'SMBG is recommended for all insulin-treated patients with diabetes' and 'SMBG [should] be carried out greater than or equal to three-times per day by patients on insulin therapy (injections or pumps)' (Sacks *et al.* 2011).

Evidence for the effectiveness of SMBG in patients with non-insulin treated type 2 diabetes patients has been the subject of considerable debate over many years. Montagnana *et al.* (2009) examined 12 studies on the subject and stated: 'For type 2 diabetic patients non-insulin-treated, a unanimous consensus on the real clinical usefulness of SMBG is still lacking.' The ADA view is that: 'In patients with type 2 diabetes treated with diet and oral agents, SMBG may help achieve better control ... [but] data are insufficient to claim an associated improvement of health outcomes' (Sacks *et al.* 2011). A recent meta-analysis also concluded: 'Evidence ... was not convincing for a clinically meaningful effect on clinical management of non-insulin treated type 2 diabetes by self-monitoring of blood glucose levels compared with management without self-monitoring ...' (Farmer *et al.* 2012).

## Continuous blood glucose monitoring – a way for the future?

Continuous blood glucose monitoring (CGM) is an example of a minimally invasive diagnostic POC technology.

With CGM, a sensor is implanted subcutaneously and glucose in the interstitial fluid is measured continuously by a detection system in the sensor, which uses enzyme, electrode or fluorescent methods (and assumes that the glucose concentration of interstitial fluid correlates with the blood glucose levels). The range of CGM devices available on the market is ever increasing (Vashist 2013). Most are compact, lightweight, portable or wearable, can transmit results electronically and feature early warning alarms for low and high glucose levels.

Some of the advantages of CGM include:

- CGM detects short episodes of hypoglycaemia that may be missed by blood glucose meters
- CGM detects sharp spikes in glucose levels during the day that may be missed by glucose meters

- Average blood glucose concentration during the night is lower than the day; therefore multiple daily blood glucose measurements tend to overestimate average glucose over the whole day
- CGM can be linked with insulin pumps.

Newer generation devices are now available/under development, which use non-invasive (rather than minimally invasive) technologies (such as Raman spectroscopy, near infrared occlusion spectroscopy, electromagnetism or heat capacity) to continuously monitor blood glucose levels (Vashist 2013); these devices are called non-invasive glucose monitoring devices (NGM).

Some of these devices now have the capability of wirelessly transmitting results to a smartphone, which can, for example, track trends and send medication alerts (Omre 2010). Key challenges for glucose monitoring devices (both CGM and NGM) are to make them cost effective, improve their precision and specificity for glucose detection, improve their signal-to-noise ratio and sensitivity, and reduce the need for calibration.

## REFERENCES


ADA (American Diabetes Association) (2012a) Diagnosis and classification of diabetes mellitus. *Diabetes Care* **35**(Supplement 1), S64–S71. doi:10.2337/dc12-s064

ADA (2012b) Standards of medical care in diabetes – 2012. *Diabetes Care* **35**(Supplement 1), S11–S63. doi:10.2337/dc12-s011

ADA (2015) Standards of medical care in diabetes – 2015. *Diabetes Care* **38**(Supplement 1), S1–S93.

Amos A, McCarty D, Zimmet P (1997) The rising global burden of diabetes and its complications: estimates and projections to the year 2010. *Diabetic Medicine* **14**, S7–S85. doi:10.1002/(SICI)1096-9136(199712)14:5+<S7::AID-DIA522>3.3.CO;2-I

Breton MD, Kovatchev BP (2010) Impact of blood glucose self-monitoring errors on glucose variability, risk for hypoglycaemia, and average glucose control in type 1 diabetes: an *In Silico* study. *Journal of Diabetes Science and Technology* **4**, 562–570. doi:10.1177/193229681000400309

Chen L, Magliano DJ, Zimmet PZ (2012) The worldwide epidemiology of type 2 diabetes mellitus – present and future perspectives. *Nature Reviews. Endocrinology* **8**, 228–236. doi:10.1038/nrendo.2011.183

Clarke WL, Cox D, Gonder-Frederick LA, Carter W, Pohl SL (1987) Evaluating clinical accuracy of systems for self-monitoring of blood glucose. *Diabetes Care* **10**, 622–628. doi:10.2337/diacare.10.5.622

CLSI (Clinical and Laboratory Standards Institute) (2013) *Point-of-Care Blood Glucose Testing in Acute and Chronic Care Facilities. CLSI Guideline POCT 12-A3.* Clinical and Laboratory Standards Institute, Wayne PA, USA.

CLSI (2015) *Glucose Monitoring in Settings Without Laboratory Support. Guideline POCT 13.* Clinical and Laboratory Standards Institute, Wayne PA, USA.

Diabetes Forecast (2013) *Blood Glucose Meters 2013*, <www.diabetesforecast.org>.

Farmer A, Perera R, Ward A, Henegan C, Oke J, Barnett AH, *et al.* (2012) Meta-analysis of individual patient data in randomised trials of self monitoring of blood glucose in people with non-insulin treated type 2 diabetes. *British Medical Journal* **344**, e486. doi:10.1136/bmj.e486

Flore K, Delanghe J (2009) Analytical interferences in point-of-care testing glucometers by icodextrin and its metabolites: an overview. *Peritoneal Dialysis International* **29**, 377–383.

Fraser CG, Scott MG (2010) Analytical performance requirements for point-of-care testing: glucose as an example. In *Point-of-Care Testing: Needs, Opportunity and Innovation.* (Eds C Price, A St John and L Kricka) pp. 145–156. AACC Press, Washington DC, USA.

Freckmann G, Schmid C, Baumstark A, Pleus S, Link M, Haug C (2012) System accuracy evaluation of 43 blood glucose monitoring systems for self-monitoring of blood glucose according to DIN EN ISO 15197. *Journal of Diabetes Science and Technology* **6**, 1060–1075. doi:10.1177/193229681200600510

Freckmann G, Baumstark A, Schmid C, Pleus S, Link M, Haug C (2014) Evaluation of 12 blood glucose monitoring systems for self-testing: system accuracy and measurement reproducibility. *Diabetes Technology & Therapeutics* **16**, 113–122. doi:10.1089/dia.2013.0208

Hirose T, Mita T, Fujitani Y, Kawamori R, Watada H (2011) Glucose monitoring after fruit peeling: pseudohyperglycemia when neglecting hand washing before fingertip blood sampling. *Diabetes Care* **34**, 596–597. doi:10.2337/dc10-1705

Huckle D (2006) Point-of-care diagnostics: will the hurdles be overcome this time? *Expert Review of Medical Devices* **3**, 421–426. doi:10.1586/17434440.3.4.421

IDF (International Diabetes Federation) (2015) *IDF Diabetes Atlas.* 7th edn. International Diabetes Federation, Brussels, Belgium, <http://www.diabetesatlas.org/resources/2015-atlas.html>.

IDF Guideline Development Group (2014) Global guideline for type 2 diabetes. *Diabetes Research and Clinical Practice* **104**, 1–52. doi:10.1016/j.diabres.2012.10.001

ISO (International Organization for Standardization) (2013) In vitro *Diagnostic Test Systems – Requirements for Blood-Glucose Monitoring Systems for Self-Testing in Managing Diabetes Mellitus. ISO 15197.* International Organization for Standardization. Geneva, Switzerland.

Karon BS, Griesmann L, Scott R, Bryant SC, Dubois JA, Shirey TL, *et al.* (2008) Evaluation of the impact of haematocrit and other interference on the accuracy of hospital-based glucose meters. *Diabetes Technology & Therapeutics* **10**, 111–120. doi:10.1089/dia.2007.0257

Karon BS, Boyd JC, Klee GG (2010) Glucose meter performance criteria for tight glycaemic control estimated by simulation modelling. *Clinical Chemistry* **56**, 1091–1097. doi:10.1373/clinchem.2010.145367

King H, Aubert D, Herman W (1998) Global burden of diabetes, 1995-2025: prevalence, numerical estimates and projections. *Diabetes Care* **21**, 1414–1431. doi:10.2337/diacare.21.9.1414

Kost GJ, Tran NK, Louie RF, Gentile NL, Abad VJ (2008) Assessing the performance of handheld glucose testing for critical care. *Diabetes Technology & Therapeutics* **10**, 445–451. doi:10.1089/dia.2008.0049

Lunt H, Florkowski C, Bignall M, Budgen C (2010) Capillary glucose meter accuracy and sources of error in the ambulatory setting. *The New Zealand Medical Journal* **123**, 123–131.

Minges KE, Zimmet P, Magliano DJ, Dunstan DW, Brown A, Shaw JE (2011) Diabetes prevalence and determinants in Indigenous Australian populations: a systematic review. *Diabetes Research and Clinical Practice* **93**, 139–149. doi:10.1016/j.diabres.2011.06.012

Montagnana M, Caputo M, Giavarina D, Lippi G (2009) Overview on self-monitoring of blood glucose. *Clinica Chimica Acta* **402**, 7–13. doi:10.1016/j.cca.2009.01.002

Movalia M, Ogino M (2006) Point of care glucose testing in neonatal hypoglycaemia. *Point of Care* **5**, 95–99. doi:10.1097/01.poc.0000232027.69785.f5

NHS (National Health Service) (2008) *Buyer's Guide Blood Glucose Systems CEP 08008*. Purchasing and Supply Agency. Centre for Evidence-based Purchasing, NHS, London, UK, <http://www.clinbiochem.info/buyersguideglucose2008.pdf>.

Olansky L, Kennedy L (2010) Finger-stick glucose monitoring – issues of accuracy and specificity. *Diabetes Care* **33**, 948–949. doi:10.2337/dc10-0077

Omre AH (2010) Bluetooth low energy: wireless connectivity for medical monitoring. *Journal of Diabetes Science and Technology* **4**, 457–463. doi:10.1177/193229681000400227

Oyibo S, Pritchard G, Mclay L, Laing I, Gokal R, Boulton A (2002) Blood glucose overestimation in diabetic patients on continuous ambulatory peritoneal dialysis for end-stage renal disease. *Diabetic Medicine* **19**, 693–696. doi:10.1046/j.1464-5491.2002.00753.x

Parkes JL, Slatin SL, Pardo S, Ginsberg BH (2000) A new consensus error grid to evaluate the clinical significance of inaccuracies in the measurement of blood glucose. *Diabetes Care* **23**, 1143–1148. doi:10.2337/diacare.23.8.1143

Perera NJ, Molyneaux L, Constantino MI, McGill M, Yue DK-S, Twigg SM (2011) Suboptimal performance of blood glucose meters in an antenatal diabetes clinic. *Diabetes Care* **34**, 335–337. doi:10.2337/dc10-1457

RACGP and DA (Royal Australian College of General Practitioners and Diabetes Australia) (2014) *General Practice Management of Type 2 Diabetes*. RACGP and DA, Melbourne.

Saaristo T, Peltonen M, Lindström J, Saarikoski L, Sundvall J, Eriksson JG, *et al.* (2005) Cross-sectional evaluation of the Finnish Diabetes Risk Score: a tool to identify undetected type 2 diabetes, abnormal glucose tolerance and metabolic syndrome. *Diabetes & Vascular Disease Research* **2**, 67–72. doi:10.3132/dvdr.2005.011

Sacks DB, Arnold M, Bakris GL, Bruns DE, Horvath AR, Kirkman MS, *et al.* (2011) Guidelines and recommendations for laboratory analysis in the diagnosis and management of diabetes mellitus. *Clinical Chemistry* **57**, e1–e47. doi:10.1373/clinchem.2010.161596

Shaw JE, Sicree RA, Zimmet PZ (2010) Global estimates of the prevalence of diabetes for 2010 and 2030. *Diabetes Research and Clinical Practice* **87**, 4–14. doi:10.1016/j.diabres.2009.10.007

Sluss P (2006) Bedside blood glucose testing systems: current technology. *Point of Care* **5**, 121–125. doi:10.1097/01.poc.0000232579.98643.2f

St John A, Price C (2014) Existing and emerging technologies for point-of-care testing. *The Clinical Biochemist Reviews* **35**, 155–167.

Stadelmann Diaw C, Piol N, Urfer J, Werner D, Roth-Kleiner M (2013) Prospective evaluation of three point of care devices for glycemia measurement in a neonatal intensive care unit. *Clinica Chimica Acta* **425**, 104–108. doi:10.1016/j.cca.2013.07.021

Tack C, Pohlmeier H, Behnke T, Schmid V, Grenningloh M, Forst T, *et al.* (2012) Accuracy evaluation of five blood glucose monitoring systems obtained from the pharmacy: a European multicentre study with 453 subjects. *Diabetes Technology & Therapeutics* **14**, 330–337. doi:10.1089/dia.2011.0170

Thorpe GH (2013) Assessing the quality of publications evaluating the accuracy of blood glucose monitoring systems. *Diabetes Technology & Therapeutics* **15**, 253–259. doi:10.1089/dia.2012.0265

Vashist SK (2013) Continuous glucose monitoring systems: a review. *Diagnostics* **3**, 385–412. doi:10.3390/diagnostics3040385

Wahl HG (2009) How accurately do we measure blood glucose levels in intensive care unit (ICU) patients? *Best Practice & Research. Clinical Anaesthesiology* **23**, 387–400. doi:10.1016/j.bpa.2009.09.003

WHO (World Health Organization) (2006) *Definition and Diagnosis of Diabetes Mellitus and Intermediate Hyperglycaemia*. WHO, Geneva, Switzerland, <http://www.who.int>.

WHO (2011) Use of glycated haemoglobin (HbA1c) in the diagnosis of diabetes mellitus. *Diabetes Research and Clinical Practice* **93**, 299–309. doi:10.1016/j.diabres.2011.03.012

Wild S, Roglic G, Green A, Sicree R, King H (2004) Global prevalence of diabetes: estimates for the year 2000 and projections for 2030. *Diabetes Care* **27**, 1047–1053. doi:10.2337/diacare.27.5.1047

Zhang P, Zhang X, Brown J, Vistisen D, Sicree R, Shaw J, *et al.* (2010) Global healthcare expenditure on diabetes for 2010 and 2013. *Diabetes Research and Clinical Practice* **87**, 293–301. doi:10.1016/j.diabres.2010.01.026

Zimmet P, Alberti KGMM, Shaw J (2001) Global and societal implications of the diabetes epidemic. *Nature* **414**, 782–787. doi:10.1038/414782a

# 10 Point-of-care testing for diabetes: haemoglobin A1c

*Mark Shephard, Jonathan Shaw and Paul Zimmet*

**Summary**

Haemoglobin A1c (HbA1c) is the universally accepted 'gold standard' pathology test for monitoring glycaemic control in patients with established diabetes. HbA1c provides a measure of glycaemic control over the preceding 3–4 months, reflecting the progressive glycation of haemoglobin during the life span of red blood cells. POC HbA1c testing is now widely used in primary care settings throughout the world and is one of the most topical, widely debated and researched subjects in the contemporary point-of-care testing (POCT) arena. Recently both the clinical use of HbA1c for the diagnosis of diabetes (as opposed to management of this condition) and the units for reporting HbA1c results (either a percentage or a new SI unit, mmol/mol) have been heavily debated in the medical/scientific literature. Both issues have implications for HbA1c measurement by POCT.

## INTRODUCTION

### What is haemoglobin A1c (HbA1c)?

In normal adults, haemoglobin (Hb) comprises mainly HbA (representing 97% of the total haemoglobin) with small amounts of HbA2 (2.5%) and HbF (0.5%).

HbA1c is formed by glucose attaching to the N-terminal valine of the β chain of haemoglobin in the red blood cells of the body (Goodall 2005; Goodall *et al.* 2007; John *et al.* 2007). HbA1c is often loosely referred to in the literature as glycated haemoglobin or glycohaemoglobin (GHb). Importantly, glycation of haemoglobin can involve the binding of other sugars and can occur at sites other than the β chain. Total glycated haemoglobin (GHb) therefore refers broadly to all glycated haemoglobins, whereas HbA1c refers to the specific molecular form described above.

HbA1c provides a measure of glycaemic control over the preceding 3–4 months, with this time period being generally reflective of the progressive glycation of haemoglobin across the lifespan of the red blood cell (~120 days). However, the HbA1c result is 'time-weighted', with 50% of the result reflecting the glycaemic control in the 30 days immediately before sample collection, with a further 25% reflecting the period from 30 to 60 days and the remaining 25% the period from 60 to 120 days before specimen collection (Barker *et al.* 2011; Goodall *et al.* 2007).

Both HbA1c and glucose provide complimentary information on a person's glycaemic status, but many patients with diabetes may not understand the differences between the HbA1c and the glucose test. Table 10.1 lists some of these differences. A significant advantage of HbA1c is that it can be measured on a random sample throughout the day, making sample collection more convenient for the person with diabetes.

**Table 10.1.** Differences between the HbA1c and glucose tests

| Parameter | HbA1c | Glucose |
|---|---|---|
| Snapshot of glycaemia | Long term | At the instant in time the sample was collected |
| Frequency of testing for management | Periodic (once every 3–4 months or as clinically required) | Multiple times per day if on insulin |
| Optimum target for management[a] | <7% (range 6.5–7.5%)<br>53 mmol/mol (range 48–58 mmol/mol) | 4–8 mmol/L (72–144 mg/dL) [fasting]<br>4–10 mmol/L (72–180 mg/dL) [post-prandial] |
| Preferred sample | Random | Fasting |
| Stability | Small degree of biological variation within an individual | Large degree of biological variation within an individual |
| Units of measurement | %; mmol/mol | mmol/L; mg/dL |

[a]Optimal management targets recommended by the RACGP and DA (2014)

Most clinical guidelines recommend an optimal HbA1c target of 7% (range 6.5–7.5%) or 53 mmol/mol (48–58 mmol/mol) for persons with diabetes (RACGP and DA 2014). Some guidelines state that a goal for HbA1c of <6.5% (48 mmol/mol) can be appropriate for selected patients, such as those with short duration of diabetes, provided this can be achieved without significant episodes of hypoglycaemia (ADA 2012). For patients with long-standing diabetes, these targets may be impossible to achieve. However, *any* reduction in HbA1c over time will provide a positive outcome for the individual with diabetes. In type 1 diabetes, the Diabetes Control and Complications Trial (DCCT) showed that each 10% reduction in HbA1c – for example, from 12 to 10.8% or 8 to 7.2% – was associated with an ~45% lower risk for the progression of diabetic retinopathy (Sacks *et al.* 2011). In type 2 diabetes, data from the CORE Diabetes Model also showed a 1 percentage point decrease in HbA1c resulted in a reduction of the cumulative incidence of retinopathy and macular oedema by 37%, peripheral vascular disease by 43%, nephropathy by 37%, neuropathy by 37% and myocardial infarction by 14% (Fig. 10.1) (Palmer *et al.* 2004).

## METHODS FOR MEASUREMENT OF HbA1c

There are more than 100 laboratory devices/assays currently available worldwide to measure HbA1c (Sacks 2012). In Australia, almost 30 different devices for HbA1c are registered with the RCPA Quality Assurance Program's Glycohaemoglobin Program for laboratories.

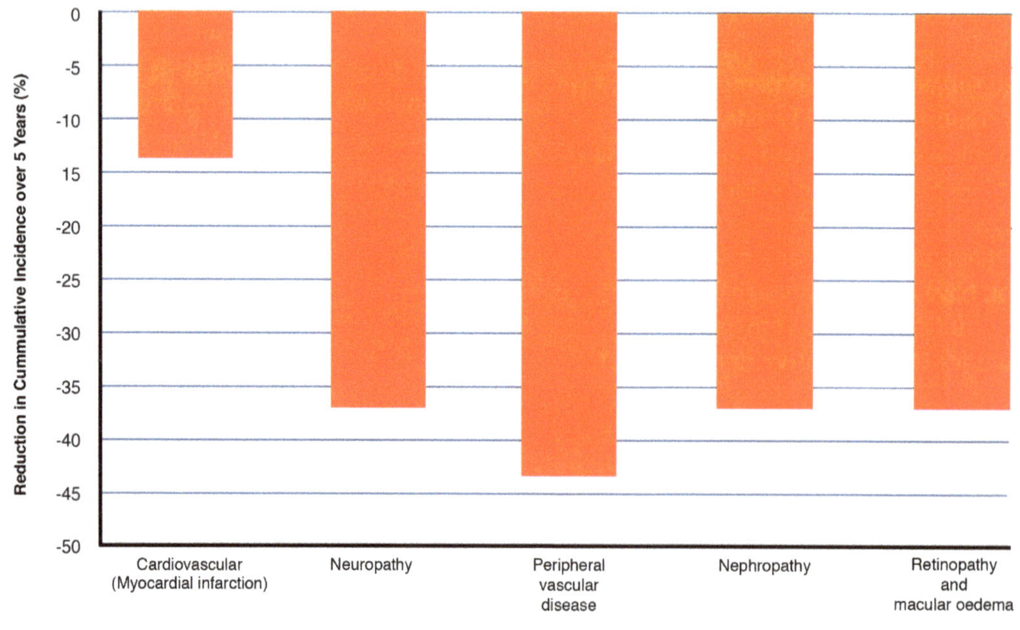


**Fig. 10.1.** The impact on diabetes complications by reducing HbA1c by 1%. (Source: adapted from Palmer *et al.* 2004)

**Table 10.2.** Some of HbA1c POCT devices on the global market over the past decade

| POCT device name | Manufacturer |
|---|---|
| DCA Vantage® | Siemens |
| Afinion™ | Alere |
| cobas® b 101 | Roche Diagnostics |
| Quo-Test™ | Quotient Diagnostics |
| HemoCue® HbA1c 501 | Radiometer |
| SD A1cCare™ | SD Biosensor |
| B-analyst | Menarini Diagnostics |
| LABGEO$^{PT10}$ | Samsung |
| i-CHROM™ | *In vitro* Technologies |
| A1CNow® | Bayer Diabetes Care |
| Nycocard™ | Axis-Shield |
| InnovaStar® | DiaSys Diagnostics |
| Clover™ | Infopia |
| D-10™ | Bio-Rad Laboratories |
| In2it® | Bio-Rad Laboratories |
| Micromat™ II | Bio-Rad Laboratories |
| PDQ | Primus |

In terms of POCT devices, there have been more than 15 devices on the global market over the past decade (Table 10.2).

The Siemens DCA test system (the Vantage® and its now obsolete predecessor the DCA 2000) has maintained a large share of the global market for HbA1c POCT since the early 1990s but there is an ever-increasing range of other HbA1c POCT devices becoming available. Just in the past 3–5 years, the cobas® b 101, SD A1cCare™, B-analyst, LABGEO$^{PT10}$ and HemoCue® HbA1c 501 have made their market debut. The Primus PDQ (now obsolete) and Bio-Rad D-10™ have been classed as POCT devices because they can be wheeled on a trolley from a laboratory to a diabetes clinic, but they are relatively large and very heavy bench-top devices (both weighing over 20 kg) and, in practice, are more suited to a satellite laboratory than a clinic setting.

Table 10.3 compares and contrasts some of the features of some of these POCT HbA1c devices.

In summary:

- Most POCT devices listed measure HbA1c either by immunoassay or boronate affinity chromatography, where HbA1c is separated and measured based on the structural differences between glycated and non-glycated products.
- Only 1–10 µL of capillary or venous whole blood is needed to perform the HbA1c test by point-of-care methods.
- Time for HbA1c result varies from 3 to 10 min.
- Most devices (except the D10 and the now obsolete PDQ) are very portable and light-weight, ranging from <1 kg to 5 kg.
- The In2it, SD A1cCare, A1CNow and Nycocard use battery as well as AC power.
- Measuring ranges are wide.
- The Clover, SD A1cCare, cobas b 101 and B-analyst reagents can be stored at room temperature, which is a significant advantage in developing countries
- Many devices measure disease markers other than HbA1c in their test profile.

A particular issue with the Afinion and B-analyst is that they only measure HbA1c on proficiency testing (PT) material of fresh whole blood origin (and not lyophilised or haemolysed material) due to the nature of their reagent test system (Lenters-Westra and Slingerland 2014). This limits the capacity to monitor and report on the analytical performance of these devices.

## Analytical goals for HbA1c POCT

HbA1c POCT devices should be able to produce test results that are both:

- *accurate* (i.e. obtain the 'true' result on a sample), because there are key clinical targets for HbA1c such as the diagnostic cut-point of 6.5% (48 mmol/mol) and the goal for optimum glycaemic control of 7% (53 mmol/mol), and
- *precise* (i.e. obtain reproducible results), because HbA1c is measured serially on patients over time and the test needs to distinguish clinically significant changes in an individual's glycaemic control, rather than have them masked by 'analytical noise' due to imprecise measurements). Table 10.4 illustrates the effect of increasing imprecision on the width of the (95%) confidence interval around the observed HbA1c result and on the ability to distinguish whether a clinically significant change between two serial results has occurred (Goodall *et al.* 2007; Shephard 2006).

## How accurate and precise then should HbA1c testing be?

The American National Glycohemoglobin Standardization Program (NGSP) currently sets a window of ±6% for

**Table 10.3.** Comparison of selected specifications for some HbA1c POCT devices

| POCT device | Photo | Method principle | Sample volume (µL) | Time for result (mins) | Measuring range (%; mmol/mol) | Weight (kg) | Power source | Long-term reagent storage | Other tests measured |
|---|---|---|---|---|---|---|---|---|---|
| DCA Vantage® | 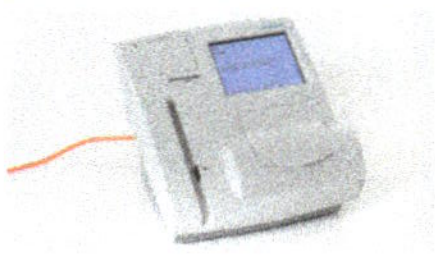 | Immunoassay | 1 | 6 | 2.5–14; 4–130 | 3.9 | AC | 2–8°C | Urine ACR |
| Afinion™ | 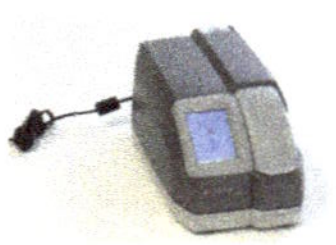 | Boronate affinity chromatography | 1.5 | 3 | 4–15; 20–140 | 5 | AC | 2–8°C | Urine ACR, lipids, CRP |
| cobas® b 101 | 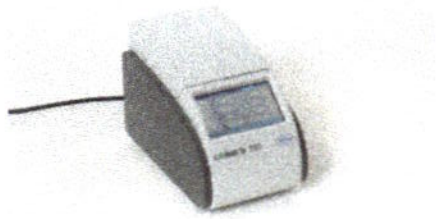 | Immunoassay | 2 | 6 | 4–14; 20–130 | 2 | AC | Room Temperature | Lipids |
| Quo-Test™ | 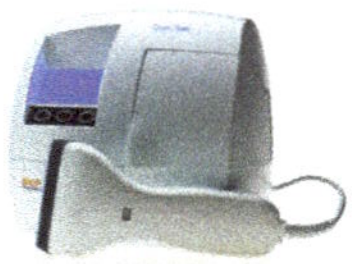 | Boronate affinity chromatography | 4 | 5 | 4–15; 20–162 | 1.3 | AC | 2–8°C | None |
| HbA1c 501 | 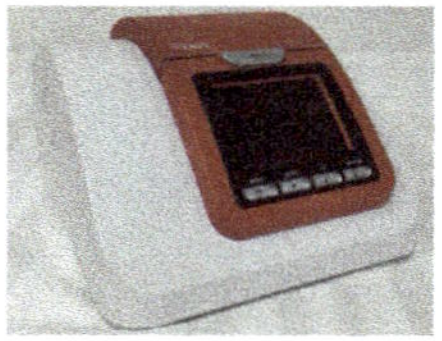 | Boronate affinity chromatography | 4 | 5 | 4–14, 20–140 | 1.6 | AC | 2–32°C | None |
| SD A1cCare™ | 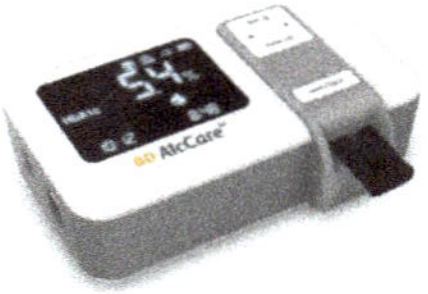 | Immunoassay | 5 | 3 | 4–15; 20–140 | 0.45 | AC and Battery | Room temperature | None |
| A1CNow® | 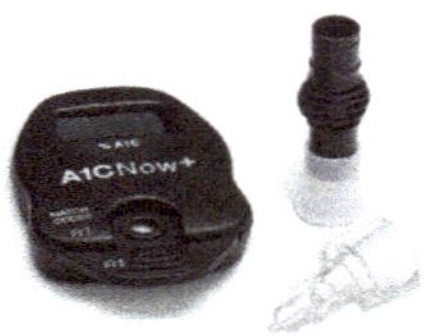 | Immunoassay | 5 | 5 | 4–13; 20–119 | <0.1 | Battery | 2–8°C | None |

| POCT device | Photo | Method principle | Sample volume (μL) | Time for result (mins) | Measuring range (%; mmol/mol) | Weight (kg) | Power source | Long-term reagent storage | Other tests measured |
|---|---|---|---|---|---|---|---|---|---|
| LABGEO$^{PT10}$ | | Immunoassay | 1 | 7 | 4–12; 20–108 | 2 | AC | 2–8°C | Hepatic and renal markers, lipids, electrolytes |
| Nycocard™ | | Boronate affinity chromatography | 5 | 3 | 4–15; 20–140 | 0.54 | Battery | 2–8°C | Urine albumin, D-dimer, CRP |
| InnovaStar® | | Immunoassay | 10 | 6.5 | 3–14; 9–130 | 4 | AC | 2–8°C | Glucose, CRP |
| Clover™ | | Boronate affinity chromatography | 4 | 4 | 4–14; 20–130 | 1.4 | AC | Room temperature | None |
| D-10™ | | Ion-exchange HPLC | 5 | 6.5 | 3.8–18.5; 18–179 | 35 | AC | Primer: 2–8°C Buffer: Room temperature | β-Thalassaemia |

**Table 10.4.** Effects of increasing imprecision on the 95% confidence interval of an HbA1c result and a note on the ability to distinguish when a clinically significant change has occurred in a patient's glycaemic status

| Imprecision | HbA1c value | Standard deviation (s.d.) | Result has 95% probability of lying within range (±2 s.d.) | Width of mean ±s.d. range |
|---|---|---|---|---|
| CV 4% | 6.5% | 0.26 | 5.98–7.02% | 1.04 |
| | 7% | 0.28 | 6.44–7.56% | 1.12 |
| | 8% | 0.32 | 7.36–8.64% | 1.28 |
| | 10% | 0.4 | 9.2–10.8% | 1.6 |
| CV 3% | 6.5% | 0.195 | 6.11–6.89% | 0.78 |
| | 7% | 0.21 | 6.58–7.42% | 0.84 |
| | 8% | 0.24 | 7.52–8.48% | 0.96 |
| | 10% | 0.3 | 9.4–10.6% | 1.2 |
| CV 2% | 6.5% | 0.13 | 6.24–6.76% | 0.52 |
| | 7% | 0.14 | 6.72–7.28% | 0.56 |
| | 8% | 0.16 | 7.68–8.32% | 0.64 |
| | 10% | 0.2 | 9.6–10.4% | 0.8 |

Note: Two serial measurements must differ by >2.77 s.d. for there to be at least a 95% probability that they are analytically different (Fraser 2001). Therefore, for an HbA1c result of 7.0% measured with a CV% of 4%, 3% and 2%, the two serial HbA1c results would need to differ by more than 0.8% (0.28 × 2.77), 0.6% (0.21 × 2.77) and 0.4% (0.14 × 2.77), respectively, for the physician to be confident that a clinically significant change in glycaemic status has occurred in that patient.

allowable bias (accuracy) relative to a standard reference laboratory mean (with 95% of the set of samples tested needing to be within this limit) in order to gain level II laboratory or manufacturer method certification for HbA1c (NGSP 2015).

There is a large body of literature on the topic of analytical goals for imprecision for HbA1c, particularly for HbA1c measured in NGSP units (Goodall *et al.* 2007; Sacks *et al.* 2011; Shephard 2006). Around the year 2000, a between-method coefficient of variation (CV) of 5% was considered acceptable imprecision. However, with continued improvements in the standardisation of HbA1c methods, tighter imprecision goals are now recommended. In 2011, the American Association of Clinical Chemistry and the American Diabetes Association (ADA) concluded the desired imprecision goal for HbA1c should be <3.5% (inter-site) and <2% (intra-site); for a single method, the goal should be <3% (inter-site) (Sacks *et al.* 2011). Lenters-Westra and Slingerland (2014) state the intra-laboratory goal for imprecision should be <2% in NGSP units and <3% in SI units.

Within Australia, there is general consensus that a CV of ≤2% is the optimal analytical goal for HbA1c, with ≤3% being the desired goal and ≤4% being the minimum goal for HbA1c devices (no matter whether the device is used in the laboratory or at the point of care) (Shephard 2006). As detailed earlier in the book, an optimal goal describes the standard of analytical performance that the very best methods for a particular test can achieve; the desirable goal is the performance generally achievable by most methods for a test; and the minimum goal is a measure of the widest allowable standard of analytical performance that methods for a test should be able to achieve. These levels of imprecision (2%, 3% and 4%) are generally consistent with the current analytical performance achieved by the top 20%, 50% and 75% of Australian laboratories, respectively. These goals are also currently used in the national QAAMS POCT program for diabetes management in Indigenous medical services in Australia (Shephard *et al.* 2015).

In terms of total allowable error (the sum of bias and imprecision), the Royal College of Pathologists of Australasia Quality Assurance Programs have recently set goals of ±0.4 up to 6.7% and 6% at >6.7% (NGSP units) and ±4 up to 45 mmol/mol and 8% at >45 mmol/mol (SI units) (RCPA QAP 2015).

### Which POCT devices can meet these analytical goals?

There are many POCT device evaluations for HbA1c in the published literature, including several well-researched multi-device evaluations over the past decade.

The well-designed study of St John *et al.* (2006) obtained data on accuracy, precision and user-friendliness of the DCA 2000, A1CNow, Nycocard and Cholestech GDX using both laboratory technicians and nurses as POCT operators. The authors concluded that only the DCA system could be recommended for HbA1c testing outside the laboratory, with this device being the only one capable of achieving a between-batch imprecision of <5%. The analytical performance achieved by nursing staff was similar to laboratory technicians for all devices, except the Nycocard where performance was poorer. The DCA system was rated by nurses as the most user-friendly device.

Morandi *et al.* (2011) retrospectively analysed over 55 000 HbA1c proficiency testing results obtained from 1999 to 2008 by laboratories participating in PT schemes from Switzerland and France. They concluded 'the best global precision performances were obtained by professional laboratories and medical offices using DCA 2000 devices', with a general improvement of (weighted) yearly imprecision being observed (from 4.3% in 2000 to 2.8% in 2008 in the Swiss program).

The National Health Service Purchasing and Supply Agency (NHS 2008) evaluated the DCA Vantage, Afinion, in2it, A1CNow and Nycocard. They concluded the devices exhibiting the best analytical performance were the DCA Vantage, Afinion and in2it. The Afinion displayed the best imprecision (total CV of 1.1% at HbA1c levels of 5.6% and 10%), followed by the DCA Vantage and in2it (CVs <2.8 and 3.3% for the different HbA1c levels tested). In terms of accuracy, the in2it gave best agreement with laboratory results (average bias 0.08%), with the DCA Vantage and Afinion showing a rise in bias at higher HbA1c levels (above 9% and 10%, respectively).

In 2010, Lenters-Westra and Slingerland published a landmark paper in which they evaluated the performance of 8 HbA1c POCT devices using CLSI protocols for precision and accuracy, with the latter assessed using the mean of three certified secondary reference measurement procedures. Two reagent lot numbers were used across the evaluation. They determined which devices met NGSP certification criteria for a level II laboratory (precision: total CV <3%; accuracy: the 95% confidence interval of the difference between each POCT method and the laboratory within ±0.85% HbA1c [as indicated previously, this has now been revised to 6% since the beginning of 2014]). The devices evaluated were the DCA Vantage, Afinion, in2it, Nycocard, Clover, InnovaStar, A1CNow and Quo-test. They concluded that only two of the eight devices (the DCA Vantage and Afinion) met the acceptable NGSP precision criteria of having a total CV <3% within the clinical range. In terms of accuracy, all devices showed variability in bias between the two lot numbers of reagents tested. (Lenters-Westra and Slingerland 2010).

Lenters-Westra and Slingerland repeated their study in 2014, because several new devices had entered the POCT market since their initial study. Using the same protocols, which included three certified International Federation of Clinical Chemistry (IFCC) as well as NGSP reference materials, seven devices were evaluated: DCA Vantage, Afinion, InnovaStar, cobas b 101, B-analyst, Quo-Test and a variant of the latter called the Quo-Laboratory (Lenters-Westra and Slingerland 2014). In this evaluation, they concluded that four of the devices (DCA Vantage, Afinion, cobas b 101 and B-analyst) met performance criteria for accuracy and precision. The InnovaStar, Quo-Test and Quo-Laboratory devices displayed a negative bias compared with the reference measures.

In the Australian QAAMS program for HbA1c POC testing in Aboriginal and Torres Strait Islander medical services, imprecision for the DCA Vantage (and its predecessor DCA 2000) has been tracked constantly for the past 16 years using both quality control (QC) and PT testing. For PT, the quality of analytical performance observed in the QAAMS Program has continued to improve over the past decade and continues to meet analytical goals. The performance of QAAMS participants can be directly compared with Australian laboratories for HbA1c testing because QAAMS and the laboratory-based RCPA QAP Glycohaemoglobin Program use identical material (Fig. 10.2). For the past 8 years, there has been no statistically significant difference between the imprecision achieved by QAAMS sites and Australian laboratories, with the median imprecision for HbA1c PT testing on the DCA Vantage averaging 2.47% ±0.15 for QAAMS sites and 2.45% ±0.26 for Australian laboratories (all methods) ($P = 0.08$).

## THE CLINICAL, OPERATIONAL AND COST-EFFECTIVENESS OF POCT FOR HbA1c

The ADA's Standards of Medical Care in Diabetes 2015 states: the 'use of point-of-care testing for A1c provides opportunities for more timely treatment.' (ADA 2015). This is certainly the case, but does access to POCT assist in improving clinical outcomes for patients?

In 2011, a systematic review and meta-analysis on the clinical effectiveness of HbA1c POCT for diabetes

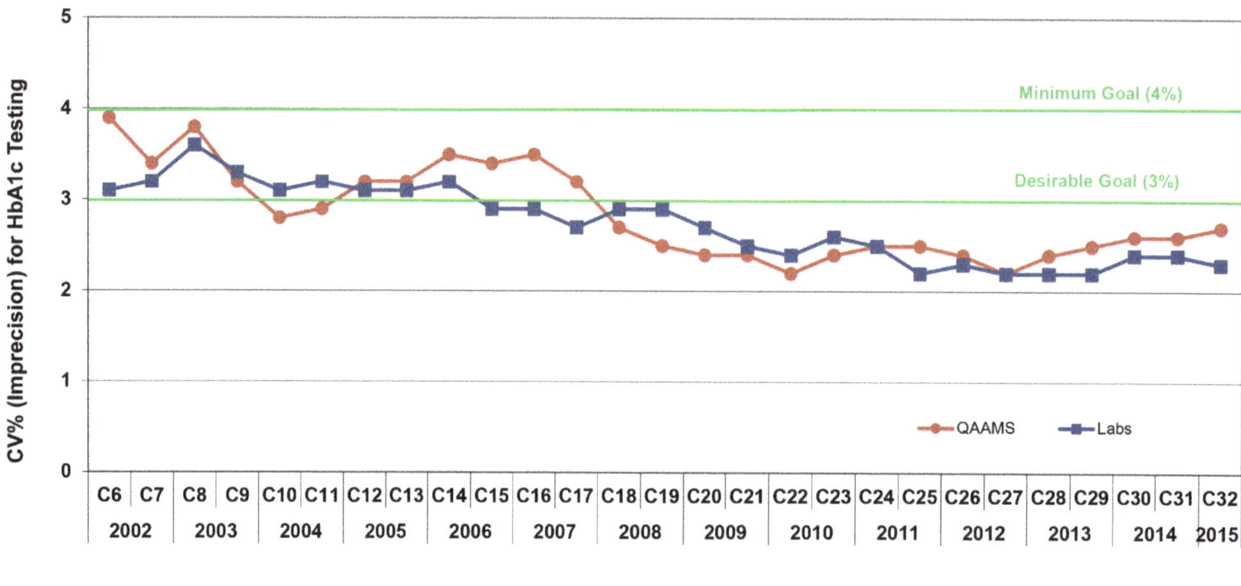


**Fig. 10.2.** Comparative imprecision (median CV%) observed for HbA1c quality assurance testing in QAAMS (by POCT) and in Australian laboratories (all methods) from 2002 to 2015.

management was published (Al-Ansary *et al.* 2011). The research team identified seven randomised controlled trials for inclusion in their study. Two were conducted in primary care settings, and five in ambulatory clinics in secondary care settings. The DCA 2000 was used in five of the seven trials, with two involving the A1CNow. Three DCA studies reported the change in mean HbA1c over the study duration (Agus *et al.* 2010; Bubner *et al.* 2009; Cagliero *et al.* 1999). Agus *et al.* (2010) conducted a 12-month prospective randomised single centre trial of POCT in which 215 children with type 1 diabetes attending an urban paediatric medical centre initially participated. In the POCT group, HbA1c decreased significantly from baseline at 3 months (by –0.2%), but returned to baseline at 6, 9 and 12 months. In the control group, HbA1c levels were unchanged at 3, 6 and 9 months but increased significantly (by +0.27%) at 12 months. Bubner *et al.* (2009) undertook a multi-centre cluster randomised controlled trial of POCT in 53 Australian general practices involving 4968 patients with different chronic disease including 1967 with type 1 or 2 diabetes. This trial reported the POCT group had a 9.3% higher proportion of patients with an HbA1c within the target range of ≤7% compared with the control group (65.5% compared with 56.2%; $P$ <0.001) at the end of the 18-month trial. Cagliero *et al.* (1999) conducted a randomised controlled trial in 201 type 1 and insulin-treated type 2 diabetes patients attending an academic diabetes centre. HbA1c levels decreased significantly at 6 and 12 months in the POCT group (by –0.57% and –0.40%, respectively) but did not change in the control group. Overall, the results of the meta-analysis of these three studies (Al-Ansary *et al.* 2011) showed a (non-significant) reduction of 0.09% (95% CI – 0.21 to 0.02) in HbA1c in the POCT group compared with the group receiving standard treatment. Although data were also collected on the change in proportion of patients reaching a target HbA1c of <7% in these three studies, treatment intensification and heterogeneity in the populations studied and how measures were reported precluded pooling of data and meta-analysis (Al-Ansary *et al.* 2011).

In another systematic review of POCT in general practice, Gialamas *et al.* (2010) identified a further two randomised controlled trials on the clinical effectiveness of POCT for diabetes management (Khunti *et al.* 2006; Miller *et al.* 2003). Miller *et al.* (2003) conducted a prospective controlled trial in 597 type 2 diabetes patients attending a rural primary care clinic. They reported that there was greater intensification of insulin therapy in the patient group having access to POCT at the time of consultation compared with the patient group who did not have POCT at this time (51% versus 32%). The HbA1c fell modestly but significantly from 8.4 to 8.1% ($P$ = 0.04) in the POCT group at their 4–6 month follow-up visit, but there was no change in HbA1c in the control group. Khunti *et al.* (2006) conducted a randomised controlled trial involving 681 type 2 diabetes patients attending eight general practices in Leicestershire, UK, with patients receiving their results by POCT at the time of consultation or from the central laboratory. This group found there was no significant difference in the proportion of patients within the therapeutic range (HbA1c <7%) between these groups (37% intervention *v.* 38% control) at 12 months follow-up.

In terms of operational effectiveness, several studies and reviews have reported positive levels of both operator and patient satisfaction with HbA1c POCT across different health sectors (e.g. Indigenous and non-Indigenous, hospital and primary care settings) and different geographic locations (urban, rural and remote) (Grieve *et al.* 1999; Laurence *et al.* 2010a; Shephard 2006b; Shephard *et al.* 2005, 2015a,b). A small number of studies report no difference in patient satisfaction.

There is limited published information on the cost effectiveness of HbA1c POCT from randomised controlled studies (Al-Ansary *et al.* 2011). In the first major study in this area, Grieve *et al.* (1999) found that the cost of HbA1c measurement with POCT was higher than by standard laboratory methods (£23 versus £14), but importantly they also found POCT reduced the number of clinic visits from 2.28 to 1.81, which resulted in an equivalent final cost for POCT and usual care. Khunti *et al.* (2006) found the mean annual cost per patient for the POCT group was slightly less than for standard care (£371 versus £390) but not statistically significantly different. Laurence *et al.* (2010b) found the overall cost per patient for the POCT group was almost identical to the usual care group (A$3676 versus A$3672).

## ISSUES AND LIMITATIONS WITH HbA1c TESTING

### Units of measurement for HbA1c

Over the past 30 or more years, HbA1c has been reported in percentage terms (i.e. HbA1c as a percentage of total haemoglobin). However, across the mid-1980s and early 1990s in particular, there was considerable variability between HbA1c methods globally, and different calibration systems were used across methods. This led to several countries developing their own national standardisation programs.

In 1996, the USA introduced the NGSP, in which the single laboratory method used in the DCCT Trial (the BioRex 70 HPLC system) was chosen as the reference method (Sacks 2012). The NGSP program was adopted widely in the USA and many other countries of the world, including Australia. However, the NGSP reference method measured several other haemoglobin-sugar complexes as well as HbA1c and therefore overestimated the true HbA1c by a factor of between 10% and 40%, depending on the HbA1c concentration (Jones *et al.* 2011). Also, at around the same time in the mid-1990s, Japan and Sweden developed separate national systems using different reference methods.

To tackle this lack of standardisation between countries, the IFCC (through its Working Group on HbA1c Standardisation) spent more than a decade developing a new international reference system for HbA1c with the aim of achieving global harmonisation of HbA1c methods (both laboratory and POCT). The new IFCC reference system included two equivalent reference methods (Goodall 2005; John *et al.* 2007), as well as a new SI (Systeme International) unit of measurement, known as mmol/mol (i.e. mmol of HbA1c per mol of haemoglobin, expressed as a whole number). The IFCC reference system provided a much more scientifically valid and accurate measure of HbA1c.

In 2007, a global consensus statement was published by four leading diabetes organisations and professional bodies endorsing the IFCC measurement system and the new units (Consensus Committee 2007). A further consensus statement supporting global standardisation and endorsing the new SI unit of measurement was released in 2010 (Hanas and John 2010). The conversion between the two measurement units is described by the following two equations (Jones *et al.* 2011; Sacks 2012):

$$\text{HbA1c SI unit (mmol/mol)} = 10.93 \times \text{HbA1c NGSP unit (\%)} - 23.50$$

$$\text{HbA1c NGSP unit (\%)} = 0.915 \times \text{HbA1c SI unit (mmol/mol)} + 2.15$$

There is also a simple rule, called the 'minus two minus two rule', which enables health professionals to quickly calculate the mmol/mol equivalent from the % term (Barker *et al.* 2011). For example, for an HbA1c of 7% in the old units, minus two from 7 equals 5 and minus two from 5 equals 3, giving a result of 53 mmol/mol in the new units. This rule works for HbA1c in whole percentage numbers from 4 to 13% inclusive. To further aid health professionals, several societies and program networks have included conversion calculators on their websites (including the QAAMS Program: http://www.qaams.org.au/resources/hba1c_converter).

What is the status of the global uptake of the new units? Several countries 'led the charge' early and are now reporting HbA1c in the new SI units only; these include New Zealand, the United Kingdom, Germany, Italy, The Netherlands, and Sweden (Sacks 2012). Some countries, including the USA, Canada and Japan have chosen not to adopt the new SI unit and continue to report NGSP (%) units only. Other countries such as Australia transitioned to the reporting of dual units in July 2011, with the intent of reporting only the new SI units after July 2013; however, at the time of writing, the switch to the single new SI units has not occurred (Jones *et al.* 2011; Sacks 2012). It is important to emphasise that, regardless of the units used, the standard of analytical performance of HbA1c testing has improved markedly in the past decade and is independent of the unit of measurement.

## The use of POCT HbA1c results for diagnosis

In 2009, an International Expert Committee published a paper that recommended that consideration be given to use of the HbA1c assay for the diagnosis of diabetes, using an HbA1c level of ≥6.5% (48 mmol/mol) as a cut-off point for diagnosing diabetes (International Expert Committee 2009). The rationale behind the use of the 6.5% cut-off was that, above this level, the prevalence of moderate retinopathy begins to increase exponentially (Colagiuri *et al.* 2011). This is the same rationale for the choice of cut-off points for glucose, and indeed HbA1c performs just as well as glucose in identifying those who are at risk of retinopathy.

The use of HbA1c as a diagnostic tool has been the subject of considerable debate ever since but the World Health Organization, the International Diabetes Federation, the American Diabetes Association and several countries, including the USA, UK, Australia and New Zealand endorsed the use of HbA1c for this purpose (ADA 2015; d'Emden *et al.* 2012; IDF Guideline Development Group 2014; John *et al.* 2012; New Zealand Society for the Study of Diabetes 2012; WHO 2011).

HbA1c has advantages over glucose in terms of its use as a diagnostic test. These are summarised in Table 10.5 (Bonora and Tuomilehto 2011; International Expert Committee 2009).

There are also some limitations with its use. HbA1c is more expensive than the glucose test (but less expensive than an OGTT). There are several clinical conditions that can cause falsely low or high HbA1c results (regardless of whether the test is used for diagnosis or management) (ADA 2015; d'Emden *et al.* 2012, 2015; John *et al.* 2012). Conditions that affect red blood cell turnover/survival and congenital haemoglobin variants (haemoglobinopathies) may cause false levels of HbA1c to be reported. Haemolytic anaemia, acute blood loss, malaria, chronic renal failure and severe liver disease reduce red cell survival and may cause lower HbA1c values, while iron deficiency can lead to an increase in HbA1c. A reduction in average red blood cell lifespan, resulting from erythropoietin therapy, splenomegaly, rheumatoid arthritis and antiretroviral drugs, can result in a lower HbA1c concentration, whereas splenectomy increases erythrocyte lifespan and hence HbA1c. Ageing can increase HbA1c values, while ethnic differences in HbA1c have also been reported (John *et al.* 2012).

Congenital variants of haemoglobin can also cause false HbA1c results to be reported. Lenters-Westra and Slingerland (2014) studied the effect of HbA1c variants on selected POCT devices. They found the DCA Vantage, cobas b 101, Quo-Test and InnovaStar were not affected by Hb AS, Hb AC, Hb AD, Hb AE or increased A2, except for the cobas b 101, which showed a 17% increase in HbA1c levels with the Hb AE variant, and the DCA Vantage, which showed a 6.9% increase with Hb AC. All

**Table 10.5.** Advantages of using HbA1c as a diagnostic test, compared with glucose

| Advantages of HbA1c over glucose |
|---|
| Better index of overall glycaemic exposure (and risk for long-term complications) |
| Can be performed on a random sample (no need for fasting or timed samples) |
| Greater pre-analytical stability (glucose decreases by 5–7%, around 0.5 mmol/L, per h in whole blood in the absence of the correct preservative [Bonora and Tuomilehto 2011]) |
| Less biological day-to-day variability |
| Less affected by acute perturbations in glucose levels (that can occur with stress or illness) |
| Past issues with method standardisation are no longer a problem |

devices reported between 10 and 20% lower values with the Hb F variant. Despite the long list of conditions that can interfere with HbA1c assays, they are uncommon in most populations, and thus for most individuals, HbA1c is a reliable diagnostic test.

**Are POCT methods good enough to be used for diagnosis?**

For HbA1c to be used as a diagnostic test, the device/method used needs to be both accurate and precise. For imprecision, Shaw *et al.* (2011) state: '… it would be reasonable to think that a laboratory can be relied on, in the context of using HbA1c as a diagnostic tool, if the routine coefficient of variation is ≤3% (the 2010 accreditation target used by the NGSP) … and the external quality assurance results are consistently within … allowable limits of performance.'

The following statements have appeared in the recent literature in relation to the use of HbA1c POCT devices for the diagnosis of diabetes:

- 'Point-of-care instruments have not yet been shown to be sufficiently accurate or precise for diagnosing diabetes.' (International Expert Committee 2009)
- 'The ADA cautions that point-of-care devices for measuring HbA1c should not be used for diagnosis.' (Sacks *et al.* 2011)
- 'Point-of-care assays are not sufficiently accurate at this time to use for diagnostic purposes.' (American Diabetes Association 2010).

These statements blanketing all POCT devices under the same umbrella are unjustified and it is more scientifically valid to look at each POCT device individually and to objectively assess the evidence base for their accuracy and precision. If an individual POCT device meets the analytical criteria for being suitable to use for diagnosis, then it should not be excluded from use for this purpose. For example, Lenters-Westra and Slingerland (2014) evaluated the analytical performance of POCT devices with a sample at an HbA1c of 6.5% (48 mmol/mol) relative to the mean of three certified IFCC and NGSP secondary reference measurement procedures (SRMP) and with two reagent lot numbers. There was no statistically significant difference between the mean of the SRMPs and the cobas b 101, B-analyst and Afinion for either lot number; for the DCA Vantage there was a difference of 1.1 mmol/mol (46.9 versus 48 mmol/mol) for the first lot number. As reported earlier, each of these devices exhibited acceptable imprecision with both SI and NGSP units.

Given the significant advantages of POCT being undertaken close to the patient, the consistent analytical performance of selected POCT devices already on the market and the continuing improvements in technology, POCT is likely to play a greater role in the diagnosis of patients with diabetes into the future.

## REFERENCES


ADA (American Diabetes Association) (2010) Standards of medical care in diabetes – 2010. *Diabetes Care* **33**(Supplement 1), S11–S61. doi:10.2337/dc10-S011

ADA (2012) Standards of medical care in diabetes – 2012. *Diabetes Care* **35**(Supplement 1), S11–S63. doi:10.2337/dc12-s011

ADA (2015) Standards of medical care in diabetes – 2015. *Diabetes Care* **38**(Supplement 1), S1–S93.

Agus MS, Alexander JL, Wolfsdorf JI (2010) Utility of immediate haemoglobin A1c in children with type I diabetes mellitus. *Pediatric Diabetes* **11**, 450–454. doi:10.1111/j.1399-5448. 2009.00635.x

Al-Ansary L, Farmer A, Hirst J, Roberts N, Glasziou P, Perera R, *et al.* (2011) Point-of-care testing for HbA1c in the management of diabetes: a systematic review and meta-analysis. *Clinical Chemistry* **57**, 568–576. doi:10.1373/clinchem.2010.157586

Barker G, Shephard MDS, Goodall I, Oberstellar E, Jones G (2011) Measuring change. *Australian Doctor* **Nov**, 33–36.

Bonora E, Tuomilehto J (2011) The pros and cons of diagnosing diabetes with A1c. *Diabetes Care* **34**(Supplement 2), S184–S190. doi:10.2337/dc11-s216

Bubner TK, Laurence CO, Gialamas A, Yelland LN, Ryan P, Willson KJ, *et al.* (2009) Effectiveness of point-of-care testing for therapeutic control of chronic conditions: results from the PoCT in General Practice Trial. *The Medical Journal of Australia* **190**, 624–626.

Cagliero E, Levina EV, Nathan DM (1999) Immediate feedback of HbA1c levels improves glycemic control in type 1 and insulin-treated type 2 diabetic patients. *Diabetes Care* **22**, 1785–1789. doi:10.2337/diacare.22.11.1785

Colagiuri S, Lee C, Wong T, Balkau B, Shaw J, Borch-Johnsen K (2011) Glycemic thresholds for diabetes-specific retinopathy: implications for diagnostic criteria for diabetes. *Diabetes Care* **34**, 145–150. doi:10.2337/dc10-1206

Consensus Committee (2007) Consensus Statement on the worldwide standardization of the haemoglobin A1c measurement. *Diabetes Care* **30**, 2399–2400.

d'Emden M, Shaw J, Colman P, Colagiuri S, Twigg S, Jones G, *et al.* (2012) The role of HbA1c in the diagnosis of diabetes mellitus in Australia. *The Medical Journal of Australia* **197**, 1–3.

d'Emden MC, Shaw JE, Jones GJ, Cheung NW (2015) Guidance concerning the use of glycated haemoglobin (HbA1c) for the diagnosis of diabetes mellitus. *The Medical Journal of Australia* **203**, 89–90. doi:10.5694/mja15.00041

Fraser CG (2001) *Biological Variation: From Principles to Practice*. AACC Press, Washington, DC, USA.

Gialamas A, St John A, Laurence CO, Bubner TK, members of the PoCT Management Committee (2010) Point-of-care testing for patients with diabetes, hyperlipidaemia or coagulation disorders in the general practice setting: a systematic review. *Family Practice* **27**, 17–24. doi:10.1093/fampra/cmp084

Goodall I (2005) HbA1c standardisation. Destination-global IFCC standardisation. How, why, where and when. A tortuous pathway from kit manufacturers, via inter-laboratory lyophilized and whole blood comparisons to designated national comparison schemes. *The Clinical Biochemist Reviews* **26**, 5–19.

Goodall I, Colman P, Schneider H, McLean M, Barker G (2007) Desirable performance standards for HbA1c analysis – precision, accuracy and standardisation. *Clinical Chemistry and Laboratory Medicine* **45**, 1083–1097.

Grieve R, Beech R, Vincent J, Mazurkiewicz J (1999) Near patient testing in diabetes clinics: appraising the costs and outcomes. *Health Technology Assessment* **3**, 1–74.

Hanas R, John G, the International HbA1c Consensus Committee (2010) Consensus statement on the worldwide standardization of the hemoglobin A1c measurement. *Clinical Chemistry* **56**, 1362–1364. doi:10.1373/clinchem.2010.150540

IDF Guideline Development Group (2014) Global guideline for type 2 diabetes. *Diabetes Research and Clinical Practice* **104**, 1–52. doi:10.1016/j.diabres.2012.10.001

International Expert Committee (2009) International expert committee report on the role of the A1C assay in the diagnosis of diabetes. *Diabetes Care* **32**, 1327–1334. doi:10.2337/dc09-9033

John W, UK Department of Health Advisory Committee on Diabetes (2012) Expert position statement: use of HbA1c in the diagnosis of diabetes mellitus in the UK. The implementation of World Health Organization guidance 2011. *Diabetic Medicine* **29**, 1350–1357. doi:10.1111/j.1464-5491.2012.03762.x

John W, Mosca A, Weykamp C, Goodall I (2007) HbA1c Standardisation: history, science and politics. *The Clinical Biochemist Reviews* **28**, 163–168.

Jones G, Barker G, Goodall I, Schneider H-G, Shephard M, Twigg S (2011) Change of HbA1c reporting to the new SI units. *The Medical Journal of Australia* **195**, 45–46.

Khunti K, Stone M, Burden A, Turner D, Raymond N, Burden M, *et al.* (2006) Randomised controlled trial of near-patient testing for glycated haemoglobin in people with type 2 diabetes mellitus. *British Journal of Best Practice* **56**, 511–517.

Laurence CO, Gialamas A, Bubner T, Yelland L, Willson K, Ryan P, *et al.* (2010a) Patient satisfaction with point-of-care testing in general practice. *The British Journal of General Practice* **60**, e98–e104. doi:10.3399/bjgp10X483508

Laurence CO, Moss JR, Briggs NE, Beilby JJ for the Point of Care Testing Trial Management Group (2010b) The cost-effectiveness of point of care testing in a general practice setting: results from a randomised controlled trial. *BMC Health Services Research* **10**, 165. doi:10.1186/1472-6963-10-165

Lenters-Westra E, Slingerland RJ (2010) Six of eight haemoglobin A1c point-of-care instruments do not meet the general accepted analytical performance criteria. *Clinical Chemistry* **56**, 44–52. doi:10.1373/clinchem.2009.130641

Lenters-Westra E, Slingerland RJ (2014) Three of 7 hemoglobin A1c point-of-care instruments do not meet generally accepted analytical performance criteria. *Clinical Chemistry* **60**, 1062–1072. doi:10.1373/clinchem.2014.224311

Miller CD, Barnes CS, Phillips LS, Ziemer DC, Gallina DL, Cook CB, *et al.* (2003) Rapid A1c availability improves clinical decision-making in an urban primary care clinic. *Diabetes Care* **26**, 1158–1163. doi:10.2337/diacare.26.4.1158

Morandi P-A, Deom A, Kesseler D, Cohen R (2011) Retrospective analysis of 55,769 HbA1c EQA results obtained from professional laboratories and medical offices participating in surveys organized by two European EQA centres over a nine-year period. *Journal of Clinical Laboratory Analysis* **25**, 337–343. doi:10.1002/jcla.20482

National Glycohemoglobin Standardization Program (2015) *Protocol Standardisation and Certification of Methods by Manufacturers*, <http://www.ngsp.org/protcert.asp>.

New Zealand Society for the Study of Diabetes (2012) New role of HbA1c in diagnosing type 2 diabetes. *Best Practice Journal* **42**, 14–19.

NHS (National Health Service) (2009) *Point of Care Devices for the Measurement of HbA1c and Low Concentration Albumin in Urine (CEP08057)*. NHS Purchasing and Supply Agency, London, UK.

Palmer AJ, Roze S, Valentine WJ, Minshall ME, Foos V, Lurati FM, *et al.* (2004) The CORE diabetes model: projecting long-term clinical outcomes, costs and cost effectiveness of interventions in diabetes mellitus (Types 1 and 2) to support clinical and reimbursement decision-making. *Current Medical Research and Opinion* **20**(Supplement 1), S5–S26. doi:10.1185/030079904X1980

RACGP and DA (Royal Australian College of General Practitioners and Diabetes Australia) (2014) *General Practice Management of Type 2 Diabetes*. Royal Australian College of General Practitioners and Diabetes Australia. Melbourne.

RCPA QAP (2015) *2015–2016 Allowable Limits of Performance*. Royal Australasian College of Pathologists Quality Assurance Programs.

Sacks DB (2012) Measurement of haemoglobin A1c. A new twist to the path to harmony. *Diabetes Care* **35**, 2674–2680. doi:10.2337/dc12-1348

Sacks DB, Arnold M, Bakris GL, Bruns DE, Horvath AR, Kirkman MS, *et al.* (2011) Guidelines and recommendations for laboratory analysis in the diagnosis and management of diabetes mellitus. *Clinical Chemistry* **57**, e1–e47. doi:10.1373/clinchem.2010.161596

Shaw J, d'Emden M, Goodall I (2011) Is Australia ready to use glycated haemoglobin for the diagnosis of diabetes? *The Medical Journal of Australia* **195**, 7–8.

Shephard MDS (2006a) Analytical goals for point-of-care testing used for diabetes management in Australian health care settings outside the laboratory. *Point of Care* **5**, 177–185.

Shephard MD (2006b) Cultural and clinical effectiveness of the 'QAAMS' point-of-care testing model for diabetes management in Australian Aboriginal medical services. *The Clinical Biochemist Reviews* **27**, 161–170.

Shephard MD, Mazzachi BC, Shephard AK, McLaughlin KJ, Denner B, Barnes G (2005) The impact of point of care testing on diabetes services along Victoria's Mallee Track: results of a community-based diabetes risk assessment and management program. *Rural and Remote Health* **5**, 371, <http://www.rrh.org.au/articles/subviewnew.asp?ArticleID=371>.

Shephard M, Spaeth B, Motta L, Shephard A (2015a) Point-of-care testing in Australia: practical advantages and benefits of community resiliency for improving outcomes. In *Global Point-of-Care – Strategies for Disasters, Emergencies, and Public Health Resilience.* (Eds G Kost and C Curtis) pp. 527-535. AACC Press, Washington DC, USA.

Shephard M, O'Brien C, Burgoyne A, Croft J, Garlett T, Barancek K, *et al.* (2015b) Review of the cultural safety of a national Indigenous point-of-care testing program for diabetes management. *Australian Journal of Primary Health* (Online September). doi:10.1071/PY15050

St John A, Davis TME, Goodall I, Townsend MA, Price CP (2006) Nurse-based evaluation of point-of-care assays for glycated haemoglobin. *Clinica Chimica Acta* **365**, 257–263. doi:10.1016/j.cca.2005.09.003

WHO (World Health Organization) (2011) Use of glycated haemoglobin (HbA1c) in the diagnosis of diabetes mellitus. *Diabetes Research and Clinical Practice* **93**, 299–309. doi:10.1016/j.diabres.2011.03.012

# 11 Point-of-care testing for kidney disease

*Mark Shephard and Timothy Mathew*

**Summary**

Chronic kidney disease (CKD) is a global public health problem. Escalation in CKD is driven by the increasing prevalence of diabetes, hypertension, obesity and ageing. CKD identification can be performed in primary care with point-of-care testing (POCT) as part of this approach. Two POC tests for the diagnosis and management of CKD are estimated glomerular filtration rate (eGFR), calculated from the blood/serum creatinine, and urine albumin:creatinine ratio (ACR). POCT for creatinine is limited by standardisation issues, differences between whole blood and serum/plasma matrices, and poor precision at low creatinine concentrations. Issues with urine ACR POCT include standardisation, sample requirements, and reporting and interpretation of urine albumin/ACR results.

## INTRODUCTION

The last 15 years has seen a substantial change in the knowledge and understanding of kidney disease from a clinical and epidemiological sense (Levey and Coresh 2012). Prior to then, kidney disease was recognised only when symptoms developed. The concept that early signs of kidney disease might have clinical impact had not been considered.

In 1999, a formula was published to estimate eGFR using serum creatinine (Levey *et al.* 1999). In 2002, a new definition of CKD was published, along with a staging schema (based on GFR) that enhanced assessment and management of the disease (National Kidney Foundation 2002). This widely accepted staging approach was modified in 2011 to include albuminuria – allowing improved correlation of CKD staging with clinical risk of progression of CKD and of cardiovascular events (Levey *et al.* 2011).

CKD is a silent condition with a low rate of community awareness and low rate of recognition in general practice, leading to underestimation of its contribution to morbidity and mortality. Because early CKD is probably 50 times as frequent as end-stage kidney failure (ESKF), we are only just beginning to comprehend the scope of the problem attributable to CKD. Fortunately, biomarker testing for the identification of asymptomatic early CKD can most effectively be done (from the viewpoint of cost and yield) by targeting the high-risk groups opportunistically in primary practice.

## GLOBAL BURDEN OF KIDNEY DISEASE

Non-communicable diseases (NCDs) are now the most frequent worldwide cause of morbidity and premature death. In 2008, cancer, cardiovascular disease, respiratory disease and diabetes were prioritised as primary targets for a global action plan aimed at prevention and control of NCDs (WHO 2008). CKD is a significant contributor to the morbidity and mortality in these chronic conditions – particularly cardiovascular disease and diabetes.

The full contribution of CKD to the burden of disease locally and globally is still being elucidated. Available data show considerable variation in the prevalence of CKD by US State, geographical region and by country (McClellan *et al.* 2012; McCullough *et al.* 2012). There is limited evidence from developing countries. A consistent finding is an increasing rate of CKD prevalence with age and a reduced prevalence of the more severe stages of CKD.

The Global Burden of Disease Study reported an 82% increase in CKD deaths from 1990 to 2010 (Lozano *et al.* 2012). A simulation model using the lifetime risk approach concluded that over half of all adults aged 30–64 years in the US were likely to develop CKD (Hoerger *et al.* 2015). The US disability-adjusted life year ranking for all diseases show that CKD jumped from number 28 to number 18 from 1990 to 2010 (US Burden of Diseases Collaborators 2013). Reduced kidney function was one of six new risk factors added to the comparative risk assessment in the Global Burden of Disease Study in 2013 and was ranked seventh for attributable disability adjusted life years in developed countries (GBD 2013 Risk Factor Collaborators 2015).

In 2012, the Australian Health Survey found self-reported CKD was recognised in only 1 in 11 adults who had CKD by biomarker testing. Ten per cent of adults had biomarker evidence of CKD, with the prevalence rising with age (to 43% in those over 75 years) (National Health Measures Survey 2013).

The full cost of CKD to government and society has only been published recently. The cost of ESKF programs in Australia in 2007 was around A$1 billion per year and growing at 4% per year (AIHW 2013). The AusDiab study suggested the cost of CKD for the health system and society was up to A$9.6 billion in 2012 (Wyld *et al.* 2015). Individuals with CKD incurred 85% higher health-care costs and 50% higher government subsidies than individuals without CKD.

## PATHOPHYSIOLOGY, RISK FACTORS AND COMPLICATIONS OF KIDNEY DISEASE

The pathophysiology of CKD is complex and varies from having an immunological, structural, vascular, inflammatory or genetic basis or an admixture of these mechanisms. The top four causes of treated ESKF in Australia currently are diabetes (35%), glomerulonephritis (19%), hypertension (14%) and polycystic kidney disease (6%) (ANZDATA Registry 2015). The incidence rate of ESKF is age dependent, with the rate in the over 75 year cohort being almost 10 times that of those aged 20–44 years.

The fixed risk factors for CKD are family history of kidney failure, past episodes of acute kidney injury, increasing age, low birthweight and male gender. Modifiable (behavioural) risk factors include tobacco smoking, physical inactivity and poor nutrition. Biomedical factors include hypertension, diabetes, cardiovascular disease, obesity and systemic kidney inflammation. There is significant overlap in the CKD behavioural risk factors with those for diabetes, cardiovascular disease and other non-communicable diseases.

The rate of CKD is significantly increased in all CKD stages in Aboriginal and Torres Strait Islander people, in those with lower socioeconomic status and in people living remotely (AIHW 2009, 2013).

The complications of CKD are diverse and complex (Table 11.1) but rarely cause symptoms until the GFR is <30 mL/min.

**Table 11.1.** Complications of CKD (signs and symptoms)

| Stages of CKD | Signs and symptoms |
|---|---|
| Early CKD (Stages 1–3a) | Hypertension |
| | Progression reduction of GFR |
| | Cardiovascular events |
| | Albuminuria |
| Moderate CKD (Stages 3b and 4) | Anaemia |
| | Depression |
| | Hyperkalaemia |
| | Malnutrition |
| | Mineral and bone disorder |
| | Muscle cramps |
| Severe CKD (Stages late 4 and 5) | Acidosis |
| | Pruritis |
| | Restless legs |
| | Anorexia |
| | Nausea and vomiting |
| | Lethargy |
| | Confusion, twitching, convulsions and coma |

**Table 11.2.** Approximate equivalents between urine ACR and other measures of protein excretion

| Term | Urine ACR (mg/mmol)[a] | 24 h urine albumin (mg/day) | Urine PCR (mg/mmol) | 24 h urine protein (mg/day) |
|---|---|---|---|---|
| Microalbuminuria | Male: 2.5–25<br>Female: 3.5–35 | 30–300 | Male: 4–40<br>Female: 6–60 | 50–500 |
| Macroalbuminuria | Male: >25<br>Female: >35 | >300 | Male: >40<br>Female: >60 | >500 |

[a]To convert urinary ACR values in mg/mmol to mg/g multiply by 8.85

## THE DETECTION AND MONITORING OF CKD

CKD embraces many underlying causes of kidney damage and kidney dysfunction. The tendency to regard CKD as a single entity, and an end diagnosis in itself, should be avoided and the actual cause of CKD always determined and managed. The clinical course of CKD varies with each underlying diagnosis and, within a specific condition (e.g. IgA nephropathy), there is great variation in the clinical expression of kidney disease, its rate of progression and its complications.

The diagnosis of CKD and its clinical monitoring are wholly dependent on two biomarkers:

- eGFR, which is calculated from the blood/serum creatinine, and
- a urine test for albumin (or protein). Current global consensus is that albuminuria is most reliably measured by a urine albumin:creatinine ratio (ACR) on a first morning sample (Johnson 2011; Johnson *et al.* 2012b; Miller *et al.* 2009; Sacks *et al.* 2011).

It is necessary to perform *both tests* as part of a kidney health check (along with a blood pressure measurement).

Serum creatinine measurements are influenced by age, gender, race, body size, muscle mass, consumption of cooked meat, interference with creatinine excretion (trimethoprim, fenofibrate) and biological variation. Calculation of eGFR from creatinine has used formulae such as the Modification of Diet in Renal Disease (MDRD) study equation (Levey *et al.* 1999) or the Chronic Kidney Disease Epidemiology Collaboration (CKD-EPI) equation, with the latter now preferred (Florkowski and Chew-Harris 2011; Johnson *et al.* 2012a; Jones 2015; KDIGO 2013). Current eGFR formulae are adjusted for improvements to the standardisation of serum creatinine methods (with traceability to an international standard, isotope dilution mass spectrometry [IDMS], reducing instrument-to-instrument variation and improving precision) (Mathew *et al.* 2007; Peake and Whiting 2006). One consequence of standardisation is a downward adjustment of creatinine concentration by ~20% compared with a decade ago, leading to older formulae, such as the Cockcroft-Gault equation, consistently underestimating GFR.

The presence of albuminuria adds substantially to the morbidity risk at all stages of CKD. The terms normo-, micro- and macro-albuminuria have been widely used (Table 11.2) but are now considered of limited clinical value, given the continuous spectrum of albuminuria and the arbitrariness of cut-off points (Jones 2015; Watts *et al.* 2015); they are likely to be replaced with the single term 'albuminuria'.

Monitoring established CKD is still performed by quantifying proteinuria (using a urine protein:creatinine ratio or timed collection) rather than albuminuria.

Testing for CKD is recommended (on cost-effective grounds) only for those groups at high risk for CKD (Table 11.3) (Mathew and Corso 2009; RACGP 2012). An algorithm summarising the initial detection of CKD in general practice and the risks associated with each stage of CKD has been published by Kidney Health Australia (2015) (Fig. 11.1).

## POINT-OF-CARE TESTING FOR CREATININE

### Devices currently available

Numerous types of POCT devices for measuring creatinine in whole blood, serum or plasma are available globally (a representative example being provided in Table 11.4). Devices can be divided into those that are primarily blood gas analysers (offering creatinine as a metabolite they measure) and 'non blood gas' analysers.

Table 11.5 summarises the non-analytical specifications of selected devices currently in Australasia (Shephard 2011). Method principles are based on a cascade of enzymatic reactions, followed by either photometric or electrochemical detection. There has been recent international attention to align all methods for creatinine (including point-of-care) to isotope dilution mass spectrometry (IDMS) equivalent standards (Myers *et al.* 2006). The ABL Flex is IDMS-

## Algorithm for initial detection of CKD

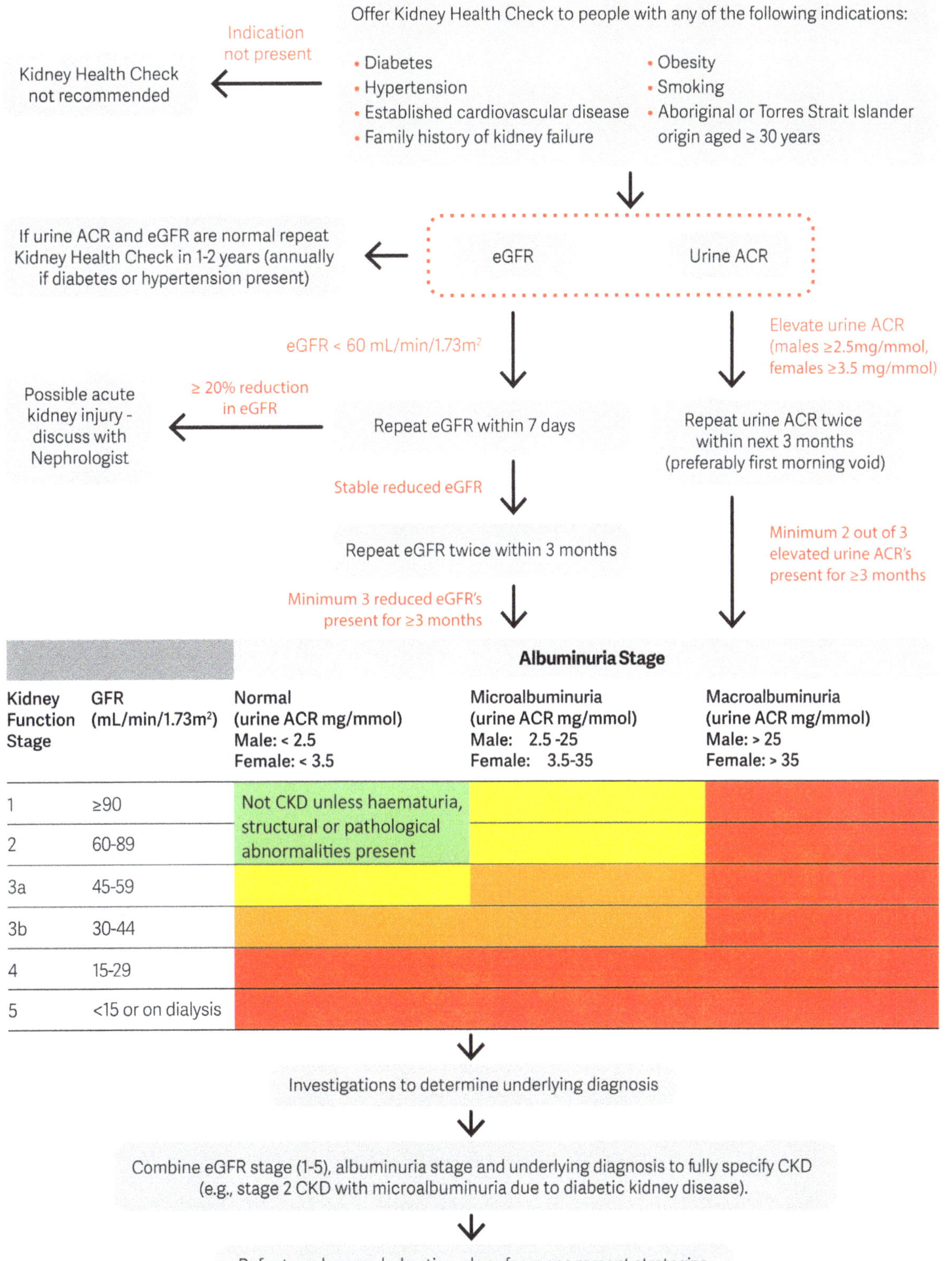


| Kidney Function Stage | GFR (mL/min/1.73m²) | Normal (urine ACR mg/mmol) Male: < 2.5 Female: < 3.5 | Microalbuminuria (urine ACR mg/mmol) Male: 2.5 -25 Female: 3.5-35 | Macroalbuminuria (urine ACR mg/mmol) Male: > 25 Female: > 35 |
|---|---|---|---|---|
| 1 | ≥90 | Not CKD unless haematuria, structural or pathological abnormalities present | | |
| 2 | 60-89 | | | |
| 3a | 45-59 | | | |
| 3b | 30-44 | | | |
| 4 | 15-29 | | | |
| 5 | <15 or on dialysis | | | |

**Fig. 11.1.** Algorithm for initial detection of CKD. (Source: Reproduced with permission from Kidney Health Australia 2015)

**Table 11.3.** Early detection of CKD using the kidney health check (Sources: Mathew and Corso 2009; RACGP 2012)

| Indications for assessment | Recommended assessments | Frequency |
|---|---|---|
| Diabetes | Urine ACR, eGFR, blood pressure | Every 1–2 years |
| Hypertension | | |
| Established cardiovascular disease | If urine ACR positive repeat twice over 3 months (preferably first morning void) | |
| Family history of kidney failure | | |
| Obesity (BMI ≥30 kg/m$^2$) | | |
| Smoker | If eGFR <60 mL/min/1.73 m$^2$ repeat within 7 days | |
| Aboriginal or Torres Strait Islander origin aged ≥30 years | | |

aligned, while most other devices are traceable to IDMS through Standard Reference Materials (SRM) from the National Institute of Standards and Technology (NIST). Equivalence between whole blood and plasma creatinine assumes 'healthy mean values' for haematocrit and both red blood cell and plasma water mass. In many disease states, these parameters may cause disparity between reported whole blood and plasma creatinine concentrations (Straseski *et al.* 2011). Devices such as the ABL, epoc, StatSensor and Reflotron can provide an automatic calculation of eGFR. The epoc, i-STAT and NovaStat are handheld devices with capacity for battery operation. Apart from the StatSensor, all other devices can test for other analytes.

## Analytical goals for POCT creatinine

Analytical goals for creatinine from biological variation allow for a minimum total error of 11.4% (comprising an imprecision goal of 3.2% and a goal for bias of 5.1%), desirable total error of 7.6% (2.2% for imprecision and 3.4% for bias) and optimal total error of 3.8% (1.1% for imprecision and 1.7% for bias) (Myers *et al.* 2006). Westgard (2015) has recently updated the desirable goals for serum creatinine to 8.9% for total error, 3.0% for imprecision and 4.8% for bias.

The Laboratory Working Group of the National Kidney Disease Education Program (NKDEP) stated that the combination of systematic bias and random error should not give rise to an error in eGFR calculation of >10%. This goal is a trade-off between imprecision and bias, with the lower the method bias, the wider the allowable imprecision. The NKDEP also stated that, after recalibration to IDMS, imprecision should be <8% and bias relative to IDMS should be <5% at a serum creatinine concentration of 88.4 μmol/L (1 mg/dL) (Myers *et*

**Table 11.4.** Examples of POCT devices for creatinine available globally

| Type | Device | Manufacturer | In Australia and/or New Zealand |
|---|---|---|---|
| Blood gas | i-STAT® | Abbott POC | Yes |
| | ABL 700/800 Flex | Radiometer Medical ApS | Yes |
| | IRMA TRUpoint® | International Technidyne Corporation (ITC) | No |
| | Stat Profile® Critical Care Xpress | Nova Biomedical | No |
| | GEM® Premier™ 4000 | Instrumentation Laboratory | Yes |
| | epoc® | Alere | Yes |
| Non blood gas | Stat Sensor® | Nova Biomedical | Yes |
| | Piccolo xpress® | Abaxis | Yes |
| | Reflotron® Plus | Roche | Yes |
| | Fuji Dri-Chem NX500 | FujiFilm, Japan | Yes |
| | LABGEO$^{PT10}$ Blood Analyzer | Samsung | Yes |
| | Pentra C200 | Horiba, France | No |

**Table 11.5.** Non-analytical specifications of selected POCT devices for creatinine available in Australia and New Zealand

| Device | i-STAT | ABL 800 Flex | Reflotron | Dri-Chem NX500 IE/E | StatSensor-I | Piccolo | epoc | LABGEO$^{PT10}$ |
|---|---|---|---|---|---|---|---|---|
| Photo | | | | | | | | |
| Manufacturer | Abbott POC | Radiometer | Roche | Fuji Film | Nova Biomedical | Abaxis | Alere | Samsung |
| Consumable | Cartridge | Sensor Cassette | Dry strip | Dry slide | Dry strip | Rotor | Smart Cartridge | Cartridge |
| Sample type | Whole blood (A,V,C) | Whole blood (A,V,C), serum, plasma | Whole blood (V,C), serum, plasma | Whole blood, serum, plasma | Whole blood (A,V,C) | Whole blood, serum, plasma | Whole blood (A,V,C) | Whole blood, serum, plasma |
| Sample volume (μL) | 65 | 125 (C)/250 (syr) | 30 | 10 | 1 | 9 | 92 | 70 |
| Time for result (min) | 2 | 1 | 2 | 5 | 0.5 | 12 | 0.5 min from sample introduction | 7 |
| Measuring range (μM) | 18–1768[a] | 10–2000 | 45–884 | 18–2122 | 27–1056 | 18–1768 | 27–1326 | 8.84–1768 |
| eGFR calculation | No | Yes | Yes | No | Yes | No | Yes | No |
| Size | Handheld | Bench-top | Bench-top | Bench-top | Handheld | Bench-top | Handheld | Bench-top |
| Weight (kg) | 0.7 | 33 | 5 | 24 | 0.4 | 5 | 0.7 | 2 |
| Power | AC or battery | AC | AC | AC | AC or battery | AC | AC or battery | AC |
| Examples of other analytes | Elu, BGas, metabs, Hb, coag, cardiac | Elu, BGas, metabs | Elu, Hb, metabs, lipids, enzymes | Elu, metabs, lipids, enzymes | nil | Elu, metabs, lipids, liver function | Elu, metabs (glucose, lactate), Bgas | Elu, lipids, liver function, HbA1c |

Note: A = arterial, V = venous, C = capillary; syr = syringe; AC = mains power; Elu = electrolytes, BGas = blood gas, metabs = metabolites, Hb = haemoglobin

[a]To convert creatinine from μmol/L to mg/dL, multiply by 0.0113

Source: Adapted from Shephard (2011) with permission from the Australasian Association of Clinical Biochemists

*al.* 2006). (The <8% imprecision goal includes inter-laboratory variation.)

The allowable limit of performance (a total error goal) for blood creatinine in the RCPA Quality Assurance Program's General Chemistry Program in Australasia has been ±8 μmol/L up to 100 μmol/L and 8% for concentrations ≥100 μmol/L since 2010.

## Current analytical performance and clinical utility of POCT devices for creatinine

### Large-scale, multi-device evaluations

In 2010, the National Health Service (NHS) Purchasing and Supply Agency (UK) published an in-house analytical evaluation on seven POC creatinine devices – the i-STAT, Piccolo Xpress, Dri-Chem 4000 (now superseded by NX500), Pentra C200, ABL 800 Flex, Reflotron Plus and IRMA TRUpoint (NHS 2010).

Most devices in this evaluation showed a positive bias of 10–15% relative to the IDMS method. For devices using whole blood as their preferred sample type, the Piccolo and i-STAT displayed best agreement with IDMS. For those using serum or plasma, the Piccolo and Dri-Chem devices showed closest agreement.

Using the 5-day CLSI EP15-A protocol for imprecision, none of the seven devices met the minimum goal from biological variation (at the time, 3.2%) at the lowest creatinine concentration tested (70 μmol/L). The best imprecision at this concentration was observed with the Pentra (3.6%), followed by the i-STAT (4.1%).

The NHS study also looked at the effect of the accuracy of each POCT device (relative to the IDMS method) on eGFR results for a 60-year-old white male at six different creatinine concentrations. At IDMS creatinine concentrations of 30, 60 and 300 μmol/L, differing accuracy bases between the POCT devices did not change CKD staging. At concentrations of 90, 120 and 150 μmol/L, the i-STAT, ABL (both sample types) and Piccolo (whole blood) recorded the same CKD staging as IDMS results at all concentrations. The i-STAT and the ABL were the only devices that were interference-free for bilirubin, glucose, haemoglobin and lipids.

Lomakin and Tobar (2014) reviewed the analytical quality of multiple POC creatinine devices when used for detecting patients at risk of contrast-induced nephropathy (CIN). CIN refers to acute kidney injury that can occur after the administration of iodinated contrast media (e.g. in computed tomography [CT] or magnetic resonance imaging [MRI] studies) in hospital patients. CIN is the third leading cause of hospital-acquired renal failure (Dimeski *et al.* 2013) and is characterised by a transient rise in creatinine of more than 44 μmol/L (0.5 mg/dL) or a 25% increase in creatinine above baseline level 48 h after administration of contrast media (Lomakin and Tobar 2014). Patients with pre-existing kidney impairment are at greatest risk, with up to 70% of patients with severe chronic kidney disease being at risk of developing CIN (Haneder *et al.* 2012). A rapid, accurate measure of POC creatinine immediately before contrast agents would therefore be a clinically efficient application of this test (Lee-Lewandrowski *et al.* 2012; You *et al.* 2013).

Lomakin and Tobar identified 13 studies from 1279 papers (across acute and non-acute care settings) that met the authors' inclusion and exclusion criteria related to diagnostic accuracy and clinical outcomes. These studies used the ABL Flex, StatProfile CCX, Nova 16, i-STAT, Reflotron Plus and StatSensor devices; the last device being evaluated in five of the 13 studies. Overall concordance between POCT and laboratory results was 'moderate'; overall mean differences were generally low but 95% limits of agreement were often ±35 μmol/L. Concordance decreased with increasing creatinine. Sensitivities and specificities of >80% for detecting patients at risk of CIN were reported for the StatProfile CCX, StatSensor (at one of two centres), ABL Flex and i-STAT devices.

### Smaller scale or single evaluations

The StatSensor (Nova Biomedical) device can measure whole blood creatinine on a capillary (finger-prick) sample with results, including a calculated eGFR, available in 30 s. However, multiple evaluations have found this device exhibits poor between-day imprecision (from 8 to 15% or 1.5 to 6-fold greater than laboratory methods), poor between-device agreement, and a significant concentration-dependent negative bias with whole blood samples (Dimeski *et al.* 2013; Korpi-Steiner *et al.* 2009; Schnabl *et al.* 2010; Shephard *et al.* 2010; Straseski *et al.* 2011). IDMS alignment failed to rectify the ability to accurately identify patients with an eGFR of <60 mL/min/1.73 m$^2$, with many falsely low eGFR results requiring laboratory confirmation (Shephard *et al.* 2010).

Straseski *et al.* (2011) similarly found that almost a quarter of all creatinine results measured (27 of 119) in their evaluation of the StatSensor versus a laboratory IDMS method differed by >44 μmol/L (0.50 mg/dL) and, among the discordant group, 86% had eGRF values <30 mL/min/1.73 m$^2$. They concluded that haematocrit, plasma water and red cell water all contributed to the negative interference observed (and explained 91% of the variance seen) with whole blood creatinine measurement on the StatSensor.

van Lint *et al.* (2015) reported the StatSensor had potential for monitoring serial creatinine levels in recently transplanted patients. The StatSensor correctly identified a percentage change in creatinine concentration of >10% (true positives) in 70% of recently transplanted patients monitored for ~10 days post-transplant.

In Australia, the i-STAT device is used for monitoring whole blood creatinine levels (as well as other metabolic parameters) in several large-scale POCT networks in the Northern Territory, Queensland and New South Wales (Shephard *et al.* 2015). It has proven robust and reliable in the challenging rural and remote environments where these networks are based. The i-STAT was also used in the Kidney Evaluation for You (KEY) Study: a partnership between Kidney Health Australia and the Flinders University International Centre for Point-of-Care Testing (Mathew *et al.* 2010). KEY was a targeted community-based screening program for CKD risk involving 402 patients from urban, rural, and remote communities. The i-STAT measured whole blood creatinine, from which the eGFR and CKD staging were calculated 'on the spot' and fed back to patients. Prior to field use, the i-STAT underwent an IDMS alignment, after which bias averaged 0.2%. Imprecision was 5.5% (from 100 duplicate patient analyses) and 4.5% from QC testing ($n$ = 16) (Shephard *et al.* 2011b). Dimeski *et al.* (2013) evaluated the i-STAT and StatSensor in 40 hospital patients using different sample types. For the i-STAT, a small positive bias of 6–9% was observed, while between-day imprecision was 4.9–5.6%. Dopamine (at concentrations between 40 and 200 mg/L) caused a significant concentration-dependent positive interference. Korpi-Steiner *et al.* (2009) evaluated the i-STAT, ABL 800 Flex and StatSensor devices in 266 patients before CT scans. The ABL 800 displayed better concordance with the laboratory than the i-STAT, but the i-STAT had highest sensitivity (97%) for an eGFR cut-off of 60 mL/min/1.73 m$^2$.

Tirimacco *et al.* (2015) evaluated the new creatinine cartridge on the epoc and reported equivalent performance to the i-STAT.

The ABL 700/800 Flex devices are well represented in the Blood Gases and Co-oximetry Program run by the RCPA Quality Assurance Programs Pty Ltd (87 participants). In a recent QAP testing cycle (55, 2015), the median imprecision for creatinine on the ABL 700/800 devices was 5.2%. Insufficient data was available to comment on other POC creatinine devices.

### Limitations and challenges with POC creatinine measurement

Globally, most devices exhibit varying degrees of inaccuracy and poor precision at low creatinine concentrations (<120 μmol/L), concentrations which may (depending on age and sex) often correspond closely to an eGFR cut off of 60 mL/min/1.73 m$^2$ and Stage 3 CKD. Creatinine measurement in whole blood is challenging due to the complexity of its matrix and influences arising from different disease states.

With the global prevalence of CKD increasing, analytically sound POCT methods for identifying CKD risk are needed. POCT creatinine measurement also has a role in identifying patients at risk of CIN. A POCT device fit-for-purpose in these settings requires capillary sampling, fast result turnaround, automatic eGFR calculation, and sound analytical performance to correctly categorise risk of CKD and CIN. Currently no device fulfils these requirements. Opportunities remain to use POC creatinine testing in other clinical settings, such as pharmacies and disaster management.

Given these limitations, other biomarkers have been proposed to detect kidney injury/dysfunction. These include cystatin-C, liver fatty acid binding protein, urinary neutrophil gelatinase-associated lipocalin (NGAL), urinary kidney injury molecule-1 (KIM-1), urinary tissue inhibitor of metalloproteinase-2 (TIMP-2) and insulin-like growth factor binding protein 7 (IGFBP7) (Coca *et al.* 2008; Lomakin and Tobar 2014). Point-of-care options for some of these tests are now available or under development, including the Eurolyser SMART and CUBE devices for cystatin C, the Alere Triage® NGAL Test, the RenaStick test for urinary KIM-1 (Parikh 2009; Vaidya *et al.* 2009) and new POC assays for TIMP-2 and IGFBP7 (Endre and Pickering 2014).

## POINT-OF-CARE TESTING FOR ALBUMINURIA

Albumin is the main protein filtered through the kidneys and passed in the urine; it represents more than 80% of the total protein of normal urine. There are a multitude of pathology tests for the measurement of urine albumin or

**Table 11.6.** List of tests for the measurement of urine albumin or protein

| Test | Units of measurement |
|---|---|
| 24-h urine collection for albumin or protein[a] | mg/day |
| Urine albumin excretion rate | μg/min |
| Urine albumin | mg/L |
| Urine albumin:creatinine ratio (ACR) | mg/mol |
| Urine protein:creatinine ratio (PCR) | mg/mmol |
| Urine dipsticks | Qualitative or semiquantitative measurement of albumin, protein, ACR or PCR |

[a]The 24-h collection (for albumin or protein) has traditionally been the gold standard collection for routine laboratory practice, but it is subject to inaccuracies due to incomplete collection of all urine voided, inaccurate timing, and appreciable intra-individual biological variation due to varying activity, hydration and diet (Miller *et al.* 2009)

protein (Table 11.6) and a range of POCT devices to measure these tests. As mentioned, urine albumin:creatinine ratio (ACR), calculated by dividing the urine albumin concentration by the urine creatinine concentration, is the current preferred measurement to detect kidney damage in most countries. Urine creatinine is co-measured with urine albumin because it corrects or adjusts for variations in urine concentration. The first morning void is the specimen of choice because it has the lowest biological variability and is often the most concentrated sample for the day.

## Devices currently available to measure albumin and protein in urine

### Qualitative and semi-quantitative methods

Urine dipsticks contain a series of dry reagent pads impregnated with chemicals attached to a plastic test strip. Each pad measures a specific and separate test including protein, as well as glucose, ketones, blood, nitrites and leucocytes, bilirubin, urobilinogen, pH and specific gravity. Siemens Multistix® and Roche Combur-Test® are examples of dipsticks measuring profiles of these urinary constituents. Their main limitations are:

- Pads are visually read and most require a timed reaction, with both factors contributing to considerable operator variability.
- Urine protein provides only a crude estimate of the albumin (or protein) in urine and lacks analytical sensitivity for detecting low levels of albuminuria (Sacks *et al.* 2011).

Immunoassay methods for urine albumin resulted in a second wave of dipsticks that provide a semiquantitative measure of urine microalbumin and/or urine ACR. Examples include the Siemens Microalbustix™ and Microalbumin strips, Roche Chemstrip® Micral strip and Genzyme Diagnostics Immunodip®.

Nagrebetsky *et al.* (2013) evaluated the Micral test and the Microalbustix visual-read dipsticks among 98 type 2 diabetes patients from four general practices. Although dipstick testing decreased costs, both dipsticks displayed suboptimal performance (Microalbustix: sensitivity 33%; Micral: specificity 44%).

Devices that automate the reading of dipsticks have been developed, including the Siemens Clinitek series, with the latest model being the Clinitek Status® Plus. Using Clinitek Microalbumin strips, this device provides a graded result (UACR normal, abnormal [microabuminuria] or high abnormal [macroalbuminuria] in 60–90 s).

McTaggart *et al.* (2012) studied 600 patients mainly with diabetes ($n$ = 274) and hypertension ($n$ = 262) in a primary care setting and showed the semiquantitative ACR test (using Microalbumin reagent strips on the Clinitek Status) was a good rule-out test for albuminuria (negative predictive value 95%, negative likelihood ratio 0.21), but its ability to rule in albuminuria was less exact (positive predictive value 51%, positive likelihood ratio 4.2). Guy *et al.* (2009) studied 86 patients with CKD attending a hospital renal outpatient clinic and confirmed McTaggart's findings. However, Graziani *et al.* (2009) reported an improved positive likelihood ratio of >10 in both diabetic ($n$ = 259) and general populations ($n$ = 201) for the Microalbumin/Clinitek system, indicating improved ability as a rule-in test. McTaggart's group evaluated the test in primary care, while the Guy and Graziani studies assessed the test in the laboratory.

McTaggart *et al.* (2014) conducted a systematic review and meta-analysis of both semiquantitative and quantitative POC tests for albuminuria, which included 16 studies and results from 3356 patients (mainly with diabetes or hypertension and from primary or secondary ambulatory care settings). Semiquantitative ACR testing (using the Siemens Clinitek and Aution [Arkray, Kyoto, Japan] devices) did not have the required diagnostic accuracy for screening patients at risk of kidney disease. The performance of the quantitative ACR test (using the Siemens DCA) was equivalent to the laboratory (pooled sensitivity 96%, specificity 98% and negative likelihood ratio 0.04). This sensitivity estimate met the ADA and NHS targets of 95% (NHS 2009; Sacks *et al.* 2011).

#### Quantitative methods

Table 11.7 summarises examples of POCT devices that provide quantitative measurement of urine ACR and/or urine albumin. All devices measure urine albumin by immunoassay. For urine creatinine, the DCA Vantage uses a colourimetric assay involving 3,5-dinitrobenzoic acid, while the Afinion uses a modified peroxidase-coupled kinetic enzymatic method with colourimetric detection. Measuring ranges for urine albumin at the low end of their detection range (5 mg/L) are 60-times more sensitive than urine dipsticks (with a 1+ protein result equivalent to 300 mg/L). Upper level of measurement varies between 150 and 300 mg/L.

### Analytical Goals for Albuminuria

The NHS (2009) and Sacks *et al.* (2011) state the analytical imprecision (CV%) of quantitative methods for measuring low levels of albuminuria should be <15%. This goal is based on biological variation data and the premise that the analytical CV should be less than half the biological CV.

In Australia, the following analytical goals for imprecision (CV%) have been used in the QAAMS POCT Program and the Point-of-Care Testing in General Practice Trial: <10% for urine albumin; <6% for urine creatinine and <12% for urine ACR (Shephard 2006; Shephard and Gill 2005; Shephard *et al.* 2009).

Lambers-Heerspink *et al.* (2008) quote US Food and Drug Administration criteria that state the imprecision goal for urine albumin is a CV% of ≤10% for 10 consecutive measurements, while, for accuracy, 95% of urine albumin values should be within 30% (or 10 mg/L) of the laboratory-determined values.

### A review of the current analytical performance of POCT devices for the quantitative measurement of albuminuria

In 2009, the NHS (National Health Service) Purchasing and Supply Agency in the UK conducted an evaluation of the DCA Vantage, Afinion, HemoCue and Nycocard (NHS 2009). For urine albumin, the DCA Vantage showed best agreement with the laboratory method but had a positive bias at 250 mg/L. Bias was close to zero for all devices except the HemoCue, which underestimated urine albumin (mean bias –4.4 mg/L). For urine ACR, the DCA Vantage and Afinion agreed well with the laboratory but showed greater scatter at higher ACR values.

The median imprecision (CV%) from proficiency testing for urine ACR (and urine albumin and urine creatinine) on the DCA 2000/Vantage devices in the QAAMS Program over the past 10 years is shown in Fig. 11.2.

**Table 11.7.** Selected specifications for POCT devices for the quantitative measurement of albuminuria

| Device | DCA Vantage®[a] | Afinion™ | HemoCue® | Nycocard™ | Eurolyser Smart |
|---|---|---|---|---|---|
| Method principle | A: Immunoassay<br>C: Colourimetric | A: Immunoassay<br>C: Colourimetric | A: Immunoassay | A: Immunoassay | A: Immunoassay |
| Reporting range | A: 5–300 mg/L<br>C: 1–44 mmol/mol | A: 5–200 mg/L<br>C: 2–30 mmol/mol | A: 5–150 mg/L | A: 5–200 mg/L | A: 5–400 mg/L |
| Reagent | Cartridge | Cartridge | Cuvette | Test disc | Cuvette |
| Sample volume (µL) | 40 | 3.5 | 18 | 50 | 20 |
| Time for result (min) | 7 | 5 | 1.5 | 3 | 6 |
| Size (cm) | 29 × 28 × 25 | 17 × 32 × 12 | 17 × 12 × 7 | 20 × 17 × 7 | 26 × 14.5 × 14 |
| Weight (kg) | 4 | 5 | 0.35 | 0.54 | 3.4 |
| Power | AC | AC | AC | AC or DC | AC |

Note: A = urine albumin; C = urine creatinine
[a]DCA Vantage superseded the DCA 2000 in 2008

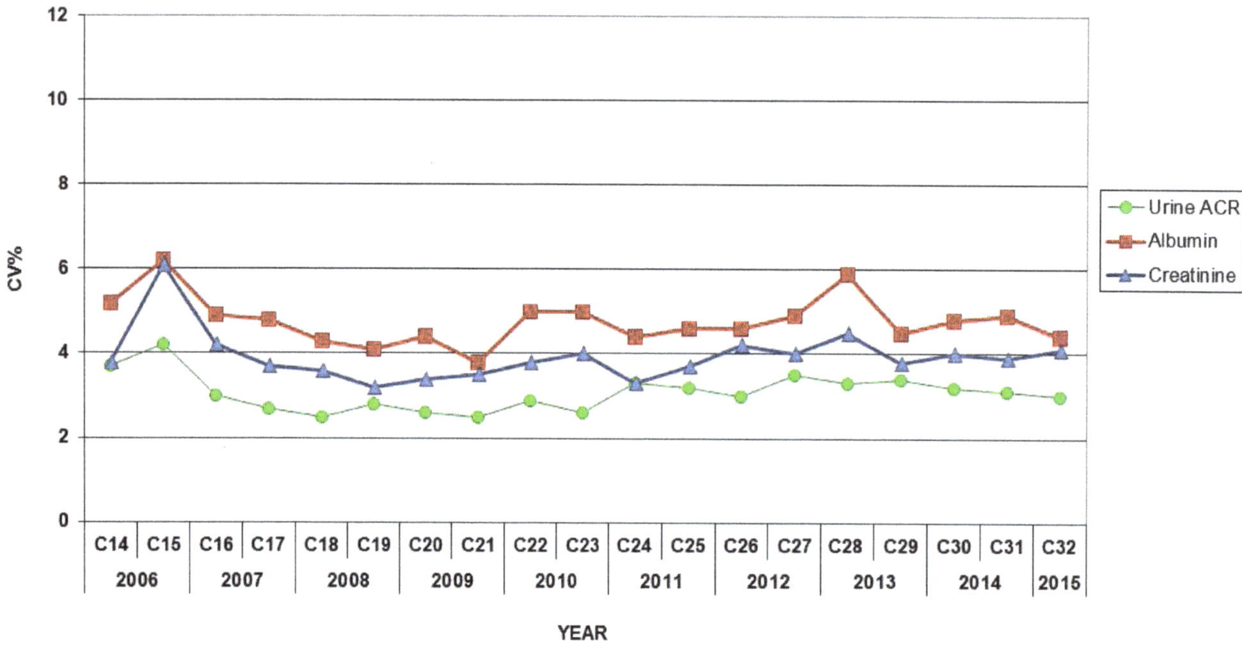


**Fig. 11.2.** Imprecision for albuminuria POCT in the QAAMS program: 2006–2015.

These samples have concentrations ranging from 1 to 25 mg/mmol for urine ACR, 20 to 250 mg/L for urine albumin and 9 to 26 mmol/L for urine creatinine. The imprecision for all analytes has consistently met the goals (of 12%, 6% and 10%) for these tests, averaging CVs of 3.1% (s.d. 0.44), 4.8% (0.57) and 3.9% (0.62), respectively, across the past decade.

Omoruyi *et al.* (2012) evaluated the Afinion and DCA Vantage. They reported that between-day and total imprecision using bi-level QC material ($n$ = 28) was <8% for all three tests (albumin, creatinine and ACR) on the Afinion and <9% on the DCA Vantage. A negative concentration dependent bias was observed with the Afinion at ACR values >5 mg/mmol ($n$ = 88 spot urines).

Several other papers have evaluated the HemoCue urine albumin analyser. Sarafidis *et al.* (2008) compared the HemoCue, Clinitek Microalbumin and the ChemStrip Micral tests with the laboratory using 165 spot urines; good correlation between the HemoCue and laboratory urine albumin results ($r^2$ = 0.90) was observed but data on mean bias and confidence intervals was not provided. They also reported 92% sensitivity, 98% specificity, 92% positive predictive value and 98% negative predictive value with the HemoCue for detection of microalbuminuria.

Lambers Heerspink *et al.* (2008) measured urine albumin in 259 patients using the HemoCue device and a laboratory nephelometer. The HemoCue showed a negative bias with urine albumin concentrations above 20 mg/L and 94% of samples had urine albumin concentrations within 30% or 10 mg/L of those determined by the laboratory. Within-run imprecision for urine albumin ranged from 4.9 to 8%.

## Limitations and challenges with POC measurement of albuminuria

### Physiological and pathophysiological factors

Urine albumin excretion exhibits high levels of biological variation. Sacks *et al.* (2011) report within-person variation (CV) in albumin excretion was 36% for urine albumin and 31% for urine ACR among health volunteers (and even higher in diabetes patients).

Transient increases in urine albumin excretion (leading to false positive measurements) have been reported following exercise, urinary tract infections, acute febrile illnesses and postural changes (Martin 2011; Miller *et al.* 2009), as well as short-term hyperglycaemia, marked hypertension, heart failure and hyperlipidaemia (Sacks *et al.* 2011).

### Lack of global standardisation of urine albumin methods

Global harmonisation of urine albumin methods is urgently needed. A joint Working Party of the National Kidney Education Program (NKDEP) and the International Federation of Clinical Chemistry (IFCC) was formed to develop a reference system for urine albumin (Martin 2011). Currently most methods (including POCT) are traceable to a diluted certified reference material CRM470 (now called 'ERM-DA 470'; Institute for Reference Materials and Measurements, Belgium, a serum protein reference material with an albumin concentration of 39.7 g/L) (Miller *et al.* 2009).

#### Collection and stability of urine albumin

For routine testing, fresh, midstream urine is the specimen of choice, with urine albumin being stable for 7 days when stored refrigerated or at room temperature. Urine albumin shows no decreases when stored long term (over 160 days) at −80°C, but decreases by 0.27% per day at −20°C (Miller *et al.* 2009; Sacks *et al.* 2011). Therefore, if urine needs to be frozen, it should be at around −70°C.

If the urine sample for testing is cloudy due to precipitate or cellular components, it should be centrifuged before storage and analysis. Refrigerated urine should be warmed to room temperature before measurement to dissolve precipitates that may have adsorbed albumin. Often a clear urine sample can turn cloudy upon overnight refrigeration due to the precipitation of urate.

#### Lack of global consensus on preferred specimen for albuminuria

A single specimen of choice needs to be adopted globally for both detection and monitoring of albuminuria (Johnson 2011). Miller *et al.* (2009) assessed several guidelines, recommendations and position statements; eight recommended early or first morning urine collections, but seven recommended random or 'spot' urine collections. There is more chance of a false positive sample with a random urine (due to larger biological variation and the effects of exercise and posture). A random sample that is positive for albuminuria should ideally be repeated on a first morning sample. The Australasian Proteinuria Consensus Working Group recommend a first void spot urine sample for urine ACR measurement, but where a first void sample is not possible or practical, a random spot urine specimen is acceptable (Johnson *et al.* 2012b).

#### Lack of global consensus on units of reporting for urine ACR

Most countries (including Australia and the UK) report urine ACR in units of mg albumin/mmol creatinine; however, several professional bodies (e.g. the National Kidney Foundation and American Diabetes Association) still quote ACR in mg/g or µg/mg units. The conversion factor is 1 mg/g or 1 µg/mg = 0.113 mg/mmol.

#### Lack of global consensus regarding confirmation of diagnosis of albuminuria

The timeframe for confirmation of the diagnosis of (micro) albuminuria following a single raised urine ACR is variable. The American Diabetes Association (ADA) allows 3–6 months for repeat testing and verification of microalbuminuria (Sacks *et al.* 2011). The International Diabetes Federation state that, if the ACR is raised above the microalbuminuria range, ACR should be repeated twice over the following 4 months (IDF Guideline Development Group 2014). The Australasian Proteinuria Consensus Working Group recommend repeat urine ACR testing should be conducted twice within a 3-month period, with two of three ACR results being abnormal to establish persistent albuminuria (Johnson *et al.* 2012b).

#### Lack of global consensus for cut-offs for stages of albuminuria

Urine ACR levels varies with age, sex and ethnicity. Johnson *et al.* (2012b) note that urine creatinine excretion is influenced by muscle mass, with excretion in males 40–50% higher than in women. Most countries and professional organisations specify gender-specific cut-offs for urine ACR, with some minor differences (Johnson 2011). In Australia, the recommended ACR cut-off for microalbuminuria and macroalbuminuria in males is 2.5–25 mg/mol and >25 mg/mmol, respectively; while for women it is 3.5–35 mg/mmol and >35 mg/mol (Johnson *et al.* 2012b). The ADA has retained a single cut-off criteria with no gender difference, e.g. <30 µg/mg [3.4 mg/mmol] for normal, 30–300 µg/mg [3.4 to 34 mg/mmol] for microalbuminuria ('high albuminuria') and >300 µg/min [>34 mg/mmol] for macroalbuminuria ('very high' albuminuria) (Sacks *et al.* 2011).

These differences in global reporting units, preferred specimens, confirmation protocols and interpretative cut-offs 'reflects national or regional preferences and are not likely to be resolved in the short-term' (Miller *et al.* 2009).

#### Antigen excess and the 'Hook effect'

Some physiological and clinical conditions can result in a transient (false positive) elevation of urine ACR. It is less well known that a false negative urine albumin (and hence ACR) result can occur when a patient has gross proteinuria (>1000 mg/L), due to the flooding of available antibody in the reagent system by an abundance of albumin (known as 'antigen excess' or 'the Hook effect'). For this reason, a dipstick test for urine protein should ideally be performed before a urine ACR test to ensure that the patient does not already have well-established kidney disease (protein ≥2+) and that the sample would therefore not be suitable for POC urine ACR analysis.

## ACKNOWLEDGEMENT

Some sections of text from the creatinine section of this chapter were reproduced/modified with permission of the Australasian Association of Clinical Biochemists (Source: Shephard 2011).

## REFERENCES

AIHW (Australian Institute of Health and Welfare) (2009) 'An overview of chronic kidney disease in Australia'. AIHW, Canberra.

AIHW (2013) 'Chronic kidney disease: regional variation in Australia'. AIHW, Canberra.

ANZDATA Registry (2015) *37th Report, Chapter 1: Incidence of End Stage Kidney Disease.* Australia and New Zealand Dialysis and Transplant Registry, Adelaide, <http://www.anzdata.org.au>.

Coca SG, Yalavarthy R, Concato J, Parikh CR (2008) Biomarkers for the diagnosis and risk stratification of acute kidney injury. *Kidney International* **73**, 1008–1016. doi:10.1038/sj.ki.5002729

Dimeski G, Tilley V, Jones B, Brown N (2013) Which point-of-care creatinine analyser for radiology: direct comparison of the i-Stat and StatStrip creatinine methods with different sample types. *Annals of Clinical Biochemistry* **50**, 47–52. doi:10.1258/acb.2012.012081

Endre ZH, Pickering JW (2014) Cell cycle arrest biomarkers win race for AKI injury. *Nature Reviews. Nephrology* **10**, 683–685. doi:10.1038/nrneph.2014.198

Florkowski CM, Chew-Harris JSC (2011) Methods of estimating GFR – different equations including CKD-EPI. *The Clinical Biochemist Reviews* **32**, 75–79.

GBD (Global Burden of Disease) 2013 Risk Factor Collaborators (2015) Global, regional and national comparative risk assessment of 79 behavioural, environmental and occupational, and metabolic risks or clusters of risks in 188 countries, 1990–2013: a systematic analysis for the Global Burden of Disease Study 2013. *The Lancet* **386**, 2287–2323.

Graziani MS, Gambaro G, Mantovani L, Sorio A, Yabarek T, Abaterusso C, *et al.* (2009) Diagnostic accuracy of a reagent strip for assessing urinary albumin excretion in the general population. *Nephrology, Dialysis, Transplantation* **24**, 1490–1494. doi:10.1093/ndt/gfn639

Guy M, Newall R, Borzomato J, Kalra P, Price C (2009) Diagnostic accuracy of the urinary albumin: creatinine ratio determined by the CLINITEK Microalbumin and DCA 2000+ for the rule-out of albuminuria in chronic kidney disease. *Clinica Chimica Acta* **399**, 54–58. doi:10.1016/j.cca.2008.09.006

Haneder S, Gutfleisch A, Meier C, Brade J, Hannak D, Schoenberg SO, *et al.* (2012) Evaluation of a handheld creatinine measurement device for real-time determination of serum creatinine in radiology departments. *World Journal of Radiology* **4**, 328–334. doi:10.4329/wjr.v4.i7.328

Hoerger TJ, Simpson SA, Yarnoff BO, Pavkov ME, Burrows NR, Saydah SH, *et al.* (2015) The future burden of CKD in the United States: a simulation model for the CDC CKD initiative. *American Journal of Kidney Diseases* **65**, 403–411. doi:10.1053/j.ajkd.2014.09.023

IDF Guideline Development Group (2014) Global guideline for type 2 diabetes. *Diabetes Research and Clinical Practice* **104**, 1–52. doi:10.1016/j.diabres.2012.10.001

Johnson D (2011) Global proteinuria guidelines: are we nearly there yet? *The Clinical Biochemist Reviews* **32**, 89–95.

Johnson DW, Jones GR, Mathew TH, Ludlow M, Doogue MP, Jose MD *et al.* (2012a) Chronic kidney disease and the automatic reporting of estimated glomerular filtration rate: new developments and revised recommendations. *The Medical Journal of Australia* **197**, 222–223.

Johnson DW, Jones GR, Mathew TH, Ludlow MJ, Chadban SJ, Usherwood T, *et al.* (2012b) Chronic kidney disease and measurement of albuminuria or proteinuria: a position statement. *The Medical Journal of Australia* **197**, 224–225. doi:10.5694/mja11.11468

Jones GRD (2015) Adventures with creatinine and eGFR – a national, international and personal story. *The Clinical Biochemist Reviews* **36**, 75–82.

KDIGO (2013) Clinical practice guideline for the evaluation and management of chronic kidney disease. *Kidney International. Supplement* **3**, 1–150.

Kidney Health Australia (2015) *Chronic Kidney Disease (CKD) Management in General Practice.* 3rd edn. Melbourne, <http://www.kidney.org.au/HealthProfessionals/CKDManagementinGeneralPractice/tabid/789/Default.aspx>.

Korpi-Steiner NL, Williamson EE, Karon BS (2009) Comparison of three whole blood creatinine methods for estimation of glomerular filtration rate before radiographic contrast media administration. *American Journal of Clinical Pathology* **132**, 920–926. doi:10.1309/AJCPTE5FEY0VCGOZ

Lambers Heerspink H, Witte E, Bakker S, de Jong P, de Zeeuw D, Gansevoort R (2008) Screening and monitoring for albuminuria: the performance of the HemoCue point-of-care system. *Kidney International* **74**, 377–383. doi:10.1038/ki.2008.186

Lee-Lewandrowski E, Chang C, Gregory K, Lewandrowski K (2012) Evaluation of rapid point-of-care creatinine testing in the radiology service of a large academic medical center; impact on clinical operations and patient disposition. *Clinica Chimica Acta* **413**, 88–92. doi:10.1016/j.cca.2011.05.006

Levey AS, Coresh J (2012) Chronic kidney disease. *Lancet* **379**, 165–180. doi:10.1016/S0140-6736(11)60178-5

Levey AS, Bosch JP, Lewis JB, Greene T, Rogers N, Roth D (1999) A more accurate method to estimated glomerular filtration rate from serum creatinine: a new prediction equation. *Annals of Internal Medicine* **130**, 461–470. doi:10.7326/0003-4819-130-6-199903160-00002

Levey AS, De Jong PE, Coresh J, El Nahas M, Astor BC, Matushita K, *et al.* (2011) The definition, classification and prognosis of chronic kidney disease: a KDIGO controversies report. *Kidney International* **80**, 17–28. doi:10.1038/ki.2010.483

Lomakin FM, Tobar C (2014) Accuracy of point-of-care serum creatinine devices for detecting patients at risk of contrast-induced nephropathy: a critical overview. *Critical Reviews in Clinical Laboratory Sciences* **51**, 332–343. doi:10.3109/10408363.2014.937794

Lozano R, Naghavi M, Lim S, Shibuya K, Aboyans V, Abraham J, *et al.* (2012) Global and regional mortality from 235 causes of death for 20 age groups in 1990 and 2010: a systematic analysis for the Global Burden of Disease Study 2010. *Lancet* **380**, 2095–2128. doi:10.1016/S0140-6736(12)61728-0

Martin H (2011) Laboratory measurement of urine albumin and urine total protein in screening for proteinuria in chronic kidney disease. *The Clinical Biochemist Reviews* **32**, 97–102.

Mathew T, Corso O (2009) Early detection of chronic kidney disease in Australia: which way to go? *Nephrology* **14**, 367–373. doi:10.1111/j.1440-1797.2009.01113.x

Mathew T, Johnson DW, Jones GRD (2007) Chronic kidney disease and automatic reporting of estimated glomerular filtration rate: revised recommendation. *The Medical Journal of Australia* **87**, 459–463.

Mathew T, Corso O, Ludlow M, Boyle A, Cass A, Chadban S, *et al.* (2010) Screening for chronic kidney disease in Australia: a pilot study in the community and workplace. *Kidney International* **77**(Supplement 116), S9–S16. doi:10.1038/ki.2009.538

McClellan AC, Plantinga L, McClellan WM (2012) Epidemiology, geography, and chronic kidney disease. *Current Opinion in Nephrology and Hypertension* **21**, 323–328. doi:10.1097/MNH.0b013e3283521dae

McCullough K, Sharma P, Ali T, Khan I, Smith WC, McCleod A, *et al.* (2012) Measuring the population burden of chronic kidney disease: a systematic literature review of the estimated prevalence of impaired kidney function. *Nephrology, Dialysis, Transplantation* **27**, 1812–1821. doi:10.1093/ndt/gfr547

McTaggart M, Price C, Pinnock R, Stevens P, Newall R, Lamb E (2012) The diagnostic accuracy of a urine albumin-creatinine ratio point-of-care test for detection of albuminuria in primary care. *American Journal of Kidney Diseases* **60**, 787–794. doi:10.1053/j.ajkd.2012.05.009

McTaggart MP, Newall RG, Hirst JA, Bankhead CR, Lamb EJ, Roberts NW, *et al.* (2014) Diagnostic accuracy of point-of-care tests for detecting albuminuria. A systematic review and meta-analysis. *Annals of Internal Medicine* **160**, 550–557. doi:10.7326/M13-2331

Miller W, Bruns D, Hortin G, Sandberg S, Aakre K, McQueen M, *et al.* (2009) Current issues in measurement and reporting of urinary albumin excretion. *Clinical Chemistry* **55**, 34–38.

Myers GL, Miller WG, Coresh J, Fleming J, Greenberg N, Greene T, *et al.* (2006) Recommendations for improving serum creatinine measurement: a report from the Laboratory Working Group of the National Kidney Disease Education Program. *Clinical Chemistry* **52**, 5–18. doi:10.1373/clinchem.2005.0525144

Nagrebetsky A, Jin J, Stevens R, James T, Adler A, Park P, *et al.* (2013) Diagnostic accuracy of urine dipstick testing in screening for microalbuminuria in type 2 diabetes: a cohort study in primary care. *Family Practice* **30**, 142–152. doi:10.1093/fampra/cms057

National Health Measures Survey (2013) *Australian Health Survey: Biomedical Results for Chronic Diseases, 2011–2012.* Canberra.

National Kidney Foundation (2002) K/DOQI clinical practice guidelines for chronic kidney disease: evaluation, classification and stratification. *American Journal of Kidney Diseases* **39**(Supplement 1), S1–S266.

NHS (National Health Service) (2009) *Point of Care Devices for the Measurement of HbA1c and Low Concentration Albumin in Urine (CEP08057).* NHS Purchasing and Supply Agency, London, UK.

NHS (2010) *Point of Care Tests for the Measurement of Blood Creatinine (CEP10042).* NHS Purchasing and Supply Agency, London, UK.

Omoruyi F, Mustafa G, Okorodudu A, Petersen J (2012) Evaluation of the performance of urine albumin, creatinine and albumin-creatinine ratio assay on two POCT analyzers relative to a central laboratory method. *Clinica Chimica Acta* **413**, 625–629. doi:10.1016/j.cca.2011.12.013

Parikh C (2009) A point-of care device for acute kidney injury: a fantastic, futuristic, or frivolous 'measure'? *Kidney International* **76**, 8–10. doi:10.1038/ki.2009.125

Peake M, Whiting M (2006) Measurement of serum creatinine – current status and future goals. *The Clinical Biochemist Reviews* **27**, 173–184, <http://www.aacb.asn.au/documents/item/1202>.

RACGP (Royal Australian College of General Practitioners) (2012) *Guidelines for Preventive Activities in General Practice.* 8th edn. The Royal Australian College of General Practitioners, South Melbourne, Australia.

Sacks D, Arnold M, Bakris G, Bruns D, Horvath A, Kirkman M, *et al.* (2011) Guidelines and recommendations for laboratory analysis in the diagnosis and management of diabetes mellitus. *Clinical Chemistry* **57**, e1–e47. doi:10.1373/clinchem.2010.161596

Sarafidis P, Riehle J, Bogojevic Z, Basta E, Chugh A, Bakris G (2008) A comparative evaluation of various methods for microalbuminuria screening. *American Journal of Nephrology* **28**, 324–329. doi:10.1159/000111825

Schnabl K, Bagherpoor S, Diker P, Cursio C, DuBois J, Yip P (2010) Evaluation of the analytical performance of the Nova StatSensor creatinine meter and reagent strip technology for whole blood testing. *Clinical Biochemistry* **43**, 1026–1029. doi:10.1016/j.clinbiochem.2010.04.055

Shephard M (2006) Analytical goals for point-of-care testing used for diabetes management in Australian health care settings outside the laboratory. *Point of Care* **5**, 177–185.

Shephard M (2011) Point-of-care testing and creatinine measurement. *The Clinical Biochemist Reviews* **32**, 109–114.

Shephard MDS, Gill JP (2005) An innovative Australian point-of-care model for urine albumin:creatinine ratio testing that supports diabetes management in indigenous medical services and has international application. *Annals of Clinical Biochemistry* **42**, 208–215. doi:10.1258/0004563053857806

Shephard M, Shephard A, Watkinson L, Mazzachi B, Worley P (2009) Design, implementation and results of the quality control program for the Australian government's point of care testing in general practice trial. *Annals of Clinical Biochemistry* **46**, 413–419. doi:10.1258/acb.2009.009045

Shephard M, Peake M, Corso O, Shephard A, Mazzachi B, Spaeth B, *et al.* (2010) Assessment of the Nova StatSensor whole blood point-of-care creatinine analyzer for the measurement of kidney function in screening for chronic kidney disease. *Clinical Chemistry and Laboratory Medicine* **48**, 1113–1119. doi:10.1515/CCLM.2010.238

Shephard A, Shephard M, Halls H, Corso O, Mathew T (2011) Innovative use of point-of-care testing for chronic kidney disease screening. *Point of Care* **10**, 98–101. doi:10.1097/POC.0b013e31821c6bd0

Shephard MDS, Spaeth B, Motta LA, Shephard A (2015) Point-of-care testing in Australia: practical advantages and benefits of community resiliency for improving outcomes. In *Global Point of Care. Strategies for Disasters, Emergencies and Public Health Resilience.* (Eds GJ Kost and CM Curtis) pp. 527-535. AACC Press, Washington DC, USA.

Straseski J, Lyon M, Clarke W, DuBois J, Phelan L, Lyon A (2011) Investigating interferences of a whole-blood point-of-care creatinine analyser: comparison to plasma enzymatic and definitive creatinine methods in an acute-care setting. *Clinical Chemistry* **57**, 1566–1573. doi:10.1373/clinchem.2011.165480

Tirimacco R, Simpson PA, Siew L, Cowley P, Velleman N, Tidemann PA (2015) Evaluation of creatinine and chloride on the epoc blood gas and electrolyte point of care analyser. *The Clinical Biochemist Reviews* **36**, S30.

US Burden of Disease Collaborators (2013) The State of US Health, 1990–2010. Burden of diseases, injuries and risk factors. *Journal of the American Medical Association* **310**, 591–608.

Vaidya VS, Ford GM, Waikar SS, Wang Y, Clement M, Ramirez V, *et al.* (2009) A rapid urine test for early detection of kidney injury. *Kidney International* **76**, 108–114. doi:10.1038/ki.2009.96

van Lint C, van der Boog P, Romijn F, Schenk P, van Dijk S, Rövekamp T, *et al.* (2015) Application of a point of care creatinine device for trend monitoring in kidney transplant patients: fit for purpose? *Clinical Chemistry and Laboratory Medicine* **53**, 1547–1556. doi:10.1515/cclm-2014-0932

Watts AK, Dwyer KM, Ekinci EI, Jerums G, MacIsaac RJ (2015) The shifting paradigm in albuminuria in diabetic kidney disease. *Medicine Today* **16**, 34–38.

Westgard J (2015) *Desirable Specifications for Total Error, Imprecision, and Bias, Derived from Intra- and Inter-Individual Biologic Variation*, <http://www.westgard.com/biodatabase1.htm>.

WHO (World Health Organization) (2008) *2008–2013 Action Plan for the Global Strategy for the Prevention and Control of Non-Communicable Diseases: Prevent and Control Cardiovascular Diseases, Cancers, Chronic Respiratory Disease and Diabetes.* WHO, Geneva, Switzerland.

Wyld ML, Lee CM, Zhuo X, White S, Shaw JE, Morton RL, *et al.* (2015) Cost to government and society of chronic kidney disease stage 1-5: a national cohort study. *Internal Medicine Journal* **45**, 741–747. doi:10.1111/imj.12797

You JE, Chung YE, Park JW, Lee W, Lee HJ, Chung TN, *et al.* (2013) The usefulness of rapid point-of-care creatinine testing for the prevention of contrast-induced nephropathy in the emergency department. *Emergency Medicine Journal* **30**, 555–558. doi:10.1136/emermed-2012-201285

# 12 Point-of-care testing for cardiovascular disease

*Heather Halls, Anne Shephard and Ken Sikaris*

**Summary**

Cardiovascular disease is a burgeoning global health issue, with common risk factors being obesity, hypertension, dysglycaemia and dyslipidaemia. Total cholesterol and HDL cholesterol are now considered the most relevant clinical markers of lipid dysfunction. POCT for lipids on capillary blood samples is widely available for assessment of cardiovascular risk and for management of patients with lipid disorders. Most POCT devices are portable and have connectivity capability, making them suitable for use in a range of community settings. Although most devices measure total cholesterol and triglyceride well, the analytical performance for HDL cholesterol is of major concern. There is some evidence for the clinical effectiveness of lipid POCT but cost effectiveness studies are lacking.

## INTRODUCTION

Cardiovascular disease (CVD), which includes coronary heart disease, stroke and heart failure, is the leading cause of death worldwide, being responsible for 31% (~17.5 million) of all deaths in 2012 (WHO 2015). Of these deaths, an estimated 42% were due to coronary heart disease and 38% were due to stroke. More than 75% of all deaths due to CVD occur in low or middle income countries. In Australia, CVD causes ~30% of deaths, with coronary heart disease the leading cause of mortality (AIHW 2014). Improvements in CVD management have resulted in fewer deaths but an increase in hospitalisations.

The risk factors for CVD are best summarised as 'the deadly quartet' and include obesity, hypertension, dysglycaemia and dyslipidaemia. Obesity and hypertension are easily assessed at the point of care. Point-of-care testing (POCT) for blood glucose has been available for decades and more recently POCT devices for lipids are widely available.

At present, 63% of Australians are overweight (BMI 25–30 kg/m$^2$) or obese (BMI ≥30 kg/m$^2$) according to government surveys (ABS 2015). It is therefore surprising that 'obesity' is not in the top 30 reasons for consulting a general practitioner (GP) (BEACH 2014). Furthermore, obesity is not even in the top 20 pathology generating problems experienced by primary care physicians, with being 'overweight' scraping in at number 20 (AAPP 2008).

The apparent neglect of obesity as a clinical issue, this most common component of the deadly quartet, is made up for by the investigations surrounding hypertension, high cholesterol and diabetes, which affects 1:9, 1:14 and 1:20 Australians, respectively (ABS 2015), and also represent at least three of the top five reasons for pathology test growth (AAPP 2008).

Dysglycaemia, typically caused by insulin resistance and progressing to type 2 diabetes, is both difficult to define and assess. The difficulty in defining dysglycaemia is best illustrated by the different definitions of prediabetic 'impaired fasting glycaemia' (IFG), which the World Health Organization (and Australia) classifies as a fasting glucose level of 6.1–6.9 mmol/L (WHO 1999), whereas in the USA it is delineated at 5.6–6.9 mmol/L (ADA 2005). Blood glucose levels are variable, with 95% confidence intervals for daily variation being ± 15% for fasting glucose and ± 30% for random blood glucose levels. This variability is recognised clinically as a general rule to never diagnose dysglycaemia or diabetes on the basis of a single glucose value.

The difficulties with blood glucose assessment have been reduced with a more stable marker reflecting long-term glucose levels, namely HbA1c (see Chapter 10). The relationship of HbA1c, dysglycaemia and cardiovascular disease is very important because it has clearly been shown that a HbA1c between 5.5 and 6.4% (NGSP)/37–46 mmol/mol (IFCC) is a zone in which macrovascular risk rises exponentially (Selvin *et al.* 2010).

The 'lipid hypothesis' asserted high concentrations of cholesterol in the blood cause heart disease but has undergone major modification because not all forms of cholesterol in the blood are harmful, hence the distinction between 'good' and 'bad' cholesterol (Yang 2005). High density lipoprotein cholesterol (HDL-C) is considered good, while high levels of low density lipoprotein cholesterol (LDL-C) are considered bad. The 'diet-heart hypothesis' asserted that saturated fats elevate blood cholesterol and, given that elevated blood cholesterol is linked to heart disease, saturated fats are a major cause of heart disease (Steinberg 2004). Numerous studies have demonstrated that medications that lower LDL-C reduce CVD risk. Despite the importance of cholesterol or LDL-C in atherosclerosis theories, the dyslipidaemia associated with prediabetes and obesity only includes high triglycerides and low HDL-C in the metabolic syndrome definitions of the WHO (WHO 1999), National Cholesterol Education Panel (NCEP 2001) and International Diabetes Federation (IDF 2006).

HDL-C is also an integral part of all the most highly predictive lipid formulae; LDL-C/HDL-C, non-HDL-C (TC minus HDL-C) and TC/HDL-C, while high triglycerides has been found to have little predictive power independently of low HDL-C (Yarnell *et al.* 2001).

Most modern theories of atherogenesis recognise that not all LDL-C is bad and the normal large buoyant LDL is not harmful, while the small dense forms of LDL-C are truly atherogenic (St-Pierre *et al.* 2005). The cause of small dense LDL-C is linked to the high triglyceride (TG) levels seen in prediabetes and the interaction between the triglyceride containing very low density lipoprotein (VLDL) and the normal large buoyant LDL-C particle, which is facilitated by the enzyme cholesterol ester transfer protein (CETP). High triglycerides not only result in the generation of small dense LDL-C but also lead to the fall in HDL-C (Vergès 2009). It seems that the measurement of low HDL-C is a better indicator of high triglycerides than measuring triglycerides themselves. This is probably because triglycerides have much more day-to-day variability and also that the triglyceride distribution is skewed and not conducive to parametric statistics. Triglycerides vary with meals, hence the need for overnight fasting; however, total cholesterol (TC) and HDL-C vary negligibly during the typical day (Miida *et al.* 2002).

In terms of CVD risk assessment, the most modern approach is to avoid the highly variable triglyceride levels, preclude fasting, and just measure TC and HDL-C. The ratio (TC/HDL-C) or difference (TC minus HDL-C) is then calculated as the risk predictor.

In terms of cardiovascular risk assessment of the deadly quartet, the clinician certainly has available immediately (i) the patient's overweight/obesity status and (ii) the patient's blood pressure. POCT can provide (iii) a reliable measure of dysglycaemia (HbA1c) and (iv) the most relevant measures of dyslipidaemia using TC and HDL-C – and both these blood tests can be performed on finger-prick samples taken in the clinic on non-fasting patients.

## POINT-OF-CARE TESTING FOR LIPIDS

### Devices currently available

There are several POCT devices for lipid profiling currently available on the market (Table 12.1). These devices may be used for screening and risk assessment as well as long-term monitoring of patients already on treatment.

Lipid POCT devices use solid phase technology to separate blood cells from plasma and then measure TC, HDL-C and TG on the plasma fraction using enzymatic methods with colourimetric detection. No POCT methods measure LDL-C directly but instead use the Friedewald formula (LDL-C [mmol/L] = TC – HDL-C – TG/2.2) (Friedewald *et al.* 1972). This formula, however, is only valid if the sample has a TG concentration below 4.5 mmol/L. An LDL-C result will not be available above this TG concentration.

**Table 12.1.** Some examples of POCT devices for lipids available globally

| Device | Manufacturer | In Australia and/or New Zealand |
|---|---|---|
| Cholestech LDX® | Alere | Yes |
| CardioChek® PA | PTS Diagnostics | Yes |
| Piccolo Xpress® | Abaxis | Yes |
| cobas b101 | Roche | Yes |
| Afinion™ | Alere | Yes |
| LABGEO$^{PT10}$ | Samsung | Yes |
| SD *LipidoCare*® | SD Biosensor | Yes |
| multiCare in | Biochemical Systems International | No |
| Accutrend® Plus | Roche | Yes |

Table 12.2 summarises the specifications of selected devices currently in Australasia.

Most POCT lipid devices now offer a full lipid panel of TC, HDL-C, TG and LDL-C, with the sample applied to a cartridge, cassette, disc or strip. Some manufacturers also offer less expensive cassettes or strips that measure some, but not all, lipid panels in varying combinations.

## Analytical goals for POCT lipids

Accurate and precise measurement of lipids is necessary to ensure patients receive appropriate classification of cardiovascular risk and/or suitable treatment strategies. The National Cholesterol Education Program (NCEP) was convened in the mid-1980s to develop guidelines and educate the public and medical professionals about the relationship between elevated cholesterol and coronary heart disease. In 1988, an NCEP expert laboratory panel published recommendations that set targets for allowable bias, imprecision and total analytical error for cholesterol measurement. These were followed in 1995 with guidelines for measuring LDL-C, HDL-C and TG (Warnick *et al.* 2002).

Analytical performance targets for measuring lipids are listed in Table 12.3. The total error goals set by NCEP are generally consistent with allowable limits of performance (ALP) set by the Royal College of Pathologists of Australasia Quality Assurance Programs General Chemistry Program (RCPA QAP 2015). The Westgard QC website lists optimal, desirable and minimal specifications for lipid measurement, calculated from biological variation (Westgard 2015).

A recommendation for analytical goals specifically for lipid POCT performed outside the laboratory was published by Shephard (2006). Biological variation, NCEP analytical goals and the state-of-the art performance of laboratories participating in the RCPA Quality Assurance Programs Special Lipid Program were considered when setting recommended optimal, desirable and minimum goals. Desirable imprecision goals of 3% for TC, 5% for TG, 4% for HDL-C and 4% for LDL-C were proposed. These goals were used when assessing analytical performance for lipids in the Australian Point-of-Care Testing in General Practice Trial (Shephard *et al.* 2009).

Manufacturers are able to validate the calibration of their lipid devices against the Cholesterol Reference Method Laboratory Network (CRMLN) that is maintained by the Centers for Disease Control and Prevention (USA). The CRMLN compares (POCT) lipid devices with reference methods and certifies those that meet the NCEP guidelines for acceptable analytical performance for the measurement of TC, HDL-C and TG. A list of devices and reagents certified between 2013 and 2015 is available on the CDC website (CDC 2015).

## A review of the current analytical performance and clinical utility of POCT devices for lipid testing

There are limited recent evaluations of the performance of POCT devices for lipid testing. Most studies are small scale (2–3) or single device studies that evaluate the device from a strictly analytical perspective (iCCnet CHSA 2013; Gialamas *et al.* 2010; Jain *et al.* 2014; Joergensen and Sais Zidek 2014; Matteucci *et al.* 2014; Méndez-González *et al.* 2009; Motta *et al.* 2015; Rapi *et al.* 2009; Simpson *et al.* 2010; Whitehead *et al.* 2014a).

The analytical performance of the Cholestech LDX has been evaluated in several studies (Gialamas *et al.* 2010; Motta *et al.* 2015; Whitehead *et al.* 2014a).

**Table 12.2.** Non-analytical specifications of selected POCT devices for lipids available in Australia and New Zealand

| Device | Cholestech LDX | CardioChek PA | Piccolo Xpress | cobas b 101 | Afinion | LABGEO$^{PT10}$ | SD *LipidoCare* |
|---|---|---|---|---|---|---|---|
| Manufacturer | Alere | PTS Diagnostics | Abaxis | Roche | Alere | Samsung | SD Biosensor |
| Method principle | Enzymatic colourimetric | Enzymatic colourimetric | Enzymatic colourimetric | Enzymatic colourimetric | Enzymatic colourimetric | Enzymatic colourimetric | Enzymatic colourimetric |
| CRMLN traceable | Yes | Yes | Yes | Yes | Yes | No | No |
| Consumable | Cassette | Strip | Disc | Disc | Cartridge | Cartridge | Strip |
| Sample type | Whole blood (V,C) | Whole Blood (V,C) | Whole blood (V,C) or serum, plasma | Whole blood (V,C), plasma | Whole blood (A,V,C), serum, plasma | Whole blood (V,C), serum, plasma | Whole blood, serum, plasma |
| Sample volume (µL) | 40 | 15 | 100 | 19 | 15 | 70 | Single – 10<br>Multi – 35 |
| Time for result (min) | 5 | 1 | 12–13 | 6 | 8 | 7 | 3 |
| Measuring range (mmol/L) | TC 2.59–12.9<br>HDL-C 0.39–2.59<br>TG 0.51–7.34 | TC 2.59–10.36<br>HDL-C 0.65–2.20<br>TG 0.56–5.65 | TC 0.52–13.5<br>HDL-C 0.39–2.59<br>TG 0.23–5.65 | TC 1.28–12.95<br>HDL-C 0.38–2.60<br>TG 0.50–7.35 | TC 2.59–12.95<br>HDL-C 0.39–2.59<br>TG 0.51–7.34 | TC 1.84–11.68<br>HDL-C 0.51–3.60<br>TG 0.71–7.20 | TC 2.59–11.64<br>HDL-C 0.65–2.46<br>TG 0.51–7.34 |
| Size | Bench-top | Handheld | Bench-top | Bench-top | Bench-top | Bench-top | Handheld |
| Weight (kg) | 1.0 | 0.16 | 5 | 2 | 5 | 2 | 0.7 |
| Power | AC | Battery | AC | AC | AC | AC | Battery |
| Connectivity | Yes | Yes | Yes | Yes | Yes | Yes | Yes |
| Other analytes | Glucose | Glucose, ketones, creatinine | ELU, liver function, metabs | HbA1c | HbA1c, urine ACR, CRP | HbA1c, ELU, liver function, kidney, function | Glucose |

Note: A = arterial, V = venous, C = capillary; AC = mains power; ELU = electrolytes, metabs = metabolites, CRP = C-reactive protein

**Table 12.3.** Analytical goals for lipid measurement

| Analyte | Imprecision (CV %) | | Bias (%) | | Total error (%) | | |
|---|---|---|---|---|---|---|---|
| | NCEP | Westgard (desirable) | NCEP | Westgard (desirable) | NCEP | Westgard (desirable) | RCPA QAP ALP |
| Total cholesterol | 3.0 | 2.98 | 3.0 | 4.1 | 9.0 | 9.01 | 6.0 |
| HDL cholesterol | 4.0 | 3.65 | 5.0 | 5.61 | 13.0 | 11.63 | 12.0 |
| LDL cholesterol | 4.0 | 3.9 | 4.0 | 5.46 | 12.0 | 11.9 | na[a] |
| Triglyceride | 5.0 | 9.95 | 5.0 | 9.57 | 15.0 | 25.99 | 12.0 |

[a]na = not available

Whitehead *et al.* (2014a) evaluated the Cholestech LDX in a laboratory and field study using the TC/HDL-C cassette. Inter-batch imprecision for both analytes was slightly above NCEP guidelines but consistent with the minimum imprecision goals recommended by Shephard (2006). The Cholestech showed good agreement with the Roche laboratory method for TC (bias –1.8%) but there was a mean negative bias of –11.6% for HDL-C, with greatest bias observed at HDL-C concentrations <1.1 mmol/L. There was no interference from haematocrit, with the LDX displaying an error message if the haematocrit was higher than its operating range of 30–49%. Ascorbic acid (at plasma concentrations reflective of those expected in individuals taking supplements) had a negative effect on TC and HDL-C measurements.

Gialamas *et al.* (2010) examined results from the POCT in General Practice Trial conducted in 2005–2007. Both laboratory and Cholestech LDX POCT results were available on ~800 samples. On average, the LDX underestimated TC and HDL-C but overestimated TG compared with laboratory results, but a limitation of this study was the variability in laboratory methods used because it was not feasible to have one reference laboratory due to the geographic spread of practices in the Trial. Motta *et al.* (2015) also found lower TC and HDL-C and higher TG results compared with the laboratory. The Cholestech LDX met the desirable analytical goals for imprecision for TG only and was not able to meet even the minimal goal for HDL-C.

Whitehead *et al.* (2014a) also evaluated the analytical performance of the CardioChek analyser. The CardioChek did not perform as well as the Cholestech and was unable to meet NCEP imprecision criteria for TC or HDL-C; however, the device did meet the minimum imprecision goals recommended by Shephard (2006) for POCT lipid analysis. The CardioChek showed significant negative bias for TC (mean difference –17.6%) and HDL-C (mean difference –12.7%). Haematocrit and ascorbic acid interfered negatively with both TC and HDL-C results. The CardioChek did not suppress results when haematocrit was outside its operating range and in fact reported erroneous TC and HDL-C results. In an earlier study by Méndez-González *et al.* (2009), the CardioChek demonstrated poor analytical performance and was generally unable to meet NCEP guidelines.

Importantly, ease of use of the two POCT devices was also evaluated in the Whitehead *et al.* study (2014a). Operators at health clinics reported the LDX was easier to use than the CardioChek, where the menu system was found to be difficult to navigate and more complex. The CardioChek's capillary specimen collection devices were considered difficult to use and often many attempts were required to provide a suitable specimen for analysis. The authors identified the following limitations with both devices: inability to restrict user access, no prompts to perform QC testing, lack of full connectivity, difficulty in collecting adequate capillary sample and the potential for the reporting units to be changed by the operator.

Matteucci *et al.* (2014) published a study on the CardioChek PA and their efforts to work with the manufacturer to improve the performance of this analyser. Initial assessment of the analyser in 2011 showed that TC and HDL-C results were significantly different to the laboratory results and imprecision did not meet NCEP guidelines with within-run CVs >6% for all analytes. There was also significant variation in results between different analysers and strip lot numbers. Following this evaluation, improvements were made to both strips and the device by the manufacturer. In March 2013, after these improvements, there was no significant difference between the CardioChek PA and the laboratory result for TC, HDL-C and TG, with consistent results across devices and strip lot numbers. Collaboration with the manufacturer resulted in significant improvements to the device such that it met NCEP guidelines for total error for TC and HDL-C (Matteucci *et al.* 2014).

While the Cholestech LDX and CardioChek PA have been available for many years, the Piccolo Xpress, Afinion and cobas b 101 are more recent additions to the POCT lipid analyser market. A limited number of evaluations of their analytical performance is available. Motta *et al.* (2015) found the Piccolo met the optimal imprecision goal and NCEP total error guidelines for all four lipids (TC, HDL-C, TG and LDL-C). The device showed good agreement with the laboratory for TC, HDL-C and TG. LDL-C showed a negative bias (mean bias ≥7%). An evaluation of the device by Simpson *et al.* (2010) demonstrated the device met NCEP guidelines for imprecision for TC and TG. The Piccolo did not meet NCEP guidelines for HDL-C (CV 5.4%) but was consistent with the minimum POCT goals of Shephard (2006). This study showed good agreement between the device and the laboratory for all lipid analytes.

The Afinion AS100 analyser has been evaluated in a clinical setting to assess CVD risk (Jain *et al.* 2014). The device showed a concentration dependent negative bias compared with the laboratory for TC at concentrations <3.6 mmol/L with similar results seen for TG. HDL-C showed a negative bias compared with the laboratory method at concentrations <1.0 mmol/L. However, the device was able to give good agreement with the laboratory when calculating cardiac risk using the QRISK algorithm used in the National Health Service in Britain.

A Korean study of the performance of the Samsung LABGEO$^{PT10}$ (Jeong *et al.* 2013) found both within run and total CVs of <10% for TC, TG and HDL-C with correlation coefficients of ≥0.98 for comparisons of these three fractions with other methods. Values were also consistent between whole blood, plasma and serum for TC and TG, but HDL-C concentrations in whole blood were 0.2 mmol/L and 0.15 mmol/L higher than for plasma and serum respectively.

The most recently available POCT lipid analyser is the cobas b 101. A 2013 evaluation showed good correlation with laboratory results for TC, HDL-C and TG (iCCNet CHSA 2013). A negative bias was observed for TC (–5.7%) and HDL-C (–1.4%) and a positive bias for TG (3.5%). Total error for all analytes met NCEP guidelines. Joergensen and Sais Zidek (2014) also reported similar results in their evaluation of the b 101.

Rapi *et al.* (2009) evaluated the small, low cost multiCare in POCT device that measures TC and TG on separate strips. Mean imprecision (CV) was 4.5% for TC and 3.3% for TG. Compared with the laboratory method, the device showed a positive bias for TC (mean bias 3.5%) and a negative bias for TG (mean bias –2.4%). Testing was also performed by patients who were able to produce comparable results to professional POCT operators. The authors suggest the device may be suitable for screening in low resource settings because the device is small, very portable and battery operated; both the device and strips are inexpensive compared with other instruments available, and test strips do not require refrigeration. However, a recent evaluation (Conti *et al.* 2015a) of the Accutrend and the multiCare in with the Roche Cobas 6000 laboratory analyser found a much better correlation with the laboratory analyser for TC with the Accutrend Plus ($r^2$ = 0.83) compared with the multiCare in ($r^2$ = 0.34). The findings of this small study agreed with Finderle *et al.* (2009) who found the Accutrend gave results that correlated well with the laboratory method for both TC and TG, whereas the results with the multiCare in were poor for TC ($r$ = 0.57 for serum and $r$ = 0.60 for plasma).

## Summary of limitations and challenges with POC lipid measurement

The ability to develop a POCT device that is able to measure all lipid fractions (TC, HDL-C, TG and LDL-C) to the highest analytical standards has proved challenging. Historically, the older devices such as the Cholestech LDX and CardioChek have struggled to meet NCEP guidelines for analytical quality. Newer devices such as the Piccolo Xpress and cobas b 101 appear to have better analytical quality, but there is still limited published information available on the performance of these devices. At the time of writing, no independent evaluations of the newest device the SD *LipidoCare* were available so its analytical performance remains unknown.

The volume of sample required for lipid analysis can also be problematic. Ideally a capillary specimen is the easiest and preferred specimen to collect for POCT lipid testing. Most devices require a sample volume over 35 µL to perform lipid analysis. Capillary specimens of 30–40 µL can be difficult to collect without 'milking' the finger resulting in dilution of the specimen with tissue fluid. Sample volumes over 50 µL require a venous specimen, and therefore the Piccolo Xpress (100 µL sample volume) cannot analyse finger-prick samples.

All POCT methods are limited by the fact they do not measure LDL-C directly but use the Friedewald formula to calculate LDL-C, which is only applicable if the TG concentration is <4.5 mmol/L.

## THE APPLICATION AND EFFECTIVENESS OF POC LIPID TESTING

### Screening for lipid abnormalities and assessment of cardiovascular risk in high-risk groups

In 2005, the Flinders University International Centre for Point-of-Care Testing partnered with Mallee Track Health and Community Service in rural Victoria, Australia, to establish and manage a POCT service to improve diabetes management in communities in the region (Shephard *et al.* 2005). In the first phase of the 'Diabetes Management along the Mallee Track' program, a community-based risk assessment was undertaken, which included the measurement of a lipid profile on the Cholestech LDX. Of the 320 community members who had a random TC POCT performed, 38% (116) had elevated TC (>5.5 mmol/L) and were referred to the health service for follow up.

As part of the NHS Health Checks pilot program, Jain *et al.* (2011) measured lipids on the Cholestech LDX in residents of South Asian origin living in Northern London. Samples from all subjects ($n$ = 406) were tested by POCT and the laboratory, and JBS2, Framingham, ETHRISK and QRISK2 CVD risk scores were calculated using the results of both methods. Risk scores calculated using POCT results agreed with those using laboratory results in between 89 and 95% of cases. Further analysis revealed that discrepancies in HDL-C were responsible for most of the observed difference. The authors concluded POCT was suitable for CVD risk screening in the NHS program.

Whitehead *et al.* (2014b) extended the use of POCT as part of NHS Health Checks by using both the Cholestech LDX and the Cardiochek to measure TC and HDL-C in a series of voluntary community health check clinics in Wolverhampton, England. Dependent on the risk assessment used, the Cholestech misclassified some subjects as having high risk while the Cardiochek misclassified some clients as having low risk.

Jones *et al.* (2013) conducted POCT for lipid measurement in an ethnic population (South Asian Canadians) at high risk for CVD in Alberta, Canada. Ethnic community volunteers were trained to conduct a CVD risk assessment and test for TC and HDL-C on the Cholestech LDX. 58% of those tested ($n$ = 288) were found to have elevated TC/HDL-C ratios. Assessments were faxed to the patient's GP and, where appropriate, patients were referred to a local CVD assessment clinic or chronic disease management program. After 9 months, 100 of the initial participants were re-tested. The average TC/HDL-C ratio fell significantly from 5.80 to 4.76. Most participants reported that they had visited their family doctor to discuss their assessment, with 22% receiving a change to their medication.

As part of the evaluation of the multiCare in device reported earlier, Rapi *et al.* (2009) determined the sensitivity and specificity of this device for detecting hypercholesterolemia (95.7% and 61.9%) and hypertriglyceridaemia (98% and 93.5%); they concluded that this low-cost device was suitable for epidemiological studies examining various aspects of cardiovascular risk. In 2013, this group incorporated measurement of TC and TG by the multiCare in device into a large cross sectional survey of three regions in Yemen to determine the prevalence of hypercholesterolaemia (11.7% in men, 15.5% in women) and hypertriglyceridaemia (39.6% in men, 36.4% in women) in 10 242 subjects aged between 15 and 69 years (Modesti *et al.* 2012). Vetrano *et al.* (2013) screened 1100 consecutive volunteers for TC using the multiCare in at shopping centres in 7 Italian cities and found a high incidence of elevated cholesterol, with only 34% of volunteers (who were not taking cholesterol-lowering medications) recording a level <5.0 mmol/L.

A recent large-scale study by Zang *et al.* (2015) measured lipids on the CardioChek to determine the prevalence of dyslipidaemia in an outpatient setting in Guangzhou, China. Of 4012 patients, 1993 (49.7%) were found to have dyslipidaemia, although only 101 (5.1%) were taking lipid lowering medication. The authors suggest that expansion of POCT testing for lipids is practical and clinically useful in a large country such as China.

POCT for lipids has also been incorporated into programs to screen for (and manage) chronic kidney disease. The KEY (Kidney Evaluation for You) study was the first comprehensive primary health care screening program in Australia to use POCT for the early detection of chronic kidney disease (CKD), and included on-site exit interviews to discuss the patient's CKD risk score, and follow-up with their GPs (Mathew *et al.* 2010; Shephard *et al.* 2011). POC tests performed included HbA1c, urine ACR, creatinine (and eGFR), glucose, haemoglobin and total cholesterol (measured using the Cholestech LDX). Of 402 high-risk patients screened across three testing sites in remote South Australia, rural Queensland and urban Western Australia, 34% ($n$ = 103) had elevated cholesterol.

## Clinical effectiveness of POCT for lipids for chronic disease management

The Australian Government's Point-of-Care Testing in General Practice Trial was a multicentre cluster randomised control trial carried out in urban, rural and remote Australian general practices (Bubner *et al.* 2009; Laurence *et al.* 2008). This trial is described in detail in Chapter 27. As part of the trial, 1463 patients on lipid-lowering medication had lipid testing performed by the laboratory, while 2356 patients on similar medication had lipid testing performed on the Cholestech LDX by a trained practice nurse.

The main clinical effectiveness outcome measures were the proportion of patients and tests with results in the target range and the percentage of patients who demonstrated an improvement in lipid levels from baseline over the 18 month trial (Bubner *et al.* 2009). For all three measures of clinical effectiveness, POCT for TC and TG was shown to be non-inferior (i.e. the same or better) than laboratory testing. However, HDL-C was inferior to laboratory testing with each measure. For example, for TC 21.6% of patients had tests in the target range following 18 months of laboratory testing whereas 38.7% were in the target range after POCT (difference = 17%; 95% CI: 13.0–21.1%; $P$ <0.001). Three-quarters (74.2%) of patients accessing POCT had a lower TC at the conclusion of the trial, whereas this percentage was only 57.4% in patients tested by the laboratory. Failure to demonstrate any benefit of POCT for HDL-C may have been partly due to the poor analytical performance of the Cholestech LDX for this analyte during the trial.

The Diabetes Management along the Mallee Track program, mentioned previously, comprises not only a community risk assessment arm but also a management arm for patients with established diabetes; these patients have regular POCT for HbA1c, urine ACR and lipids as part of their management (Motta *et al.* 2015; Shephard *et al.* 2005). POCT is performed by a trained community nurse and the patient visits their GP after POCT has been performed to discuss the results (which are now uploaded directly to the GP's patient management system). Ten months after introducing this service, total cholesterol levels in the patient group ($n$ = 52 at the time) decreased from 4.64 (± 1.0) mmol/L to 4.28 (± 0.9) mmol/L (p = 0.01). This program has been supporting the community for more than a decade now; following a review of the service in 2010, lipids are now being performed on the Piccolo device (Motta *et al.* 2015). Assessments of stakeholder satisfaction a decade apart showed that greater than 95% of patients were satisfied with the availability of immediate results, more than 90% had confidence in the accuracy of their POCT result and 94% (2005 study) indicated that POCT improved their self-motivation to look after their diabetes (Motta *et al.* 2015; Shephard *et al.* 2005).

## POCT for lipids in pharmacy settings

The benefits of POCT in community pharmacies, including for lipids, has been widely reviewed (Kirkbride 2010; Lippi *et al.* 2010; St John 2010) and is discussed in detail in Chapter 34.

Donyai and Van den Berg (2009) found that 35% of around 8000 individuals who had a POC TC test as part of a screening program run by a large pharmacy chain were at high or moderate risk of CVD. They concluded that patients unlikely to undergo a risk assessment at a traditional health clinic could potentially be reached by pharmacy screening.

Several studies have been reported where POCT for lipids in pharmacies has been incorporated into a pharmacist-led program to increase general health and wellbeing of the community serviced by the pharmacy or to manage chronic disease (Cranor 2003; Peterson *et al.* 2004; Tsuyuki *et al.* 2002; Yamada *et al.* 2005; Oyetayo *et al.* 2011). These studies have each demonstrated a statistically significant improvement in at least one lipid fraction. For example, in the Peterson study, 94 patients discharged from hospital with CVD were randomised into a control group who received standard care and an intervention group who received home visits from a pharmacist who conducted POCT for TC using the Roche Accutrend. The pharmacist also educated patients on healthy lifestyle and monitored medication compliance and effectiveness. At the end of the 6-month study, 44% of patients in the intervention group had TC values below 4.0 mmol/L compared with 24% in the control group ($P$ = 0.06). A satisfaction survey indicated that patients and doctors were positive about the program benefits, with 97% of patients responding that the quality of the service was 'excellent'.

In an effort to enhance wellbeing of university employees, Fanous *et al.* (2014) instigated a pharmacist-directed walking program. Prior to the commencement of the walking program, each of the 144 participant's lipid levels were measured by POCT to enable the pharmacist to provide immediate feedback and education on desirable goals, risks of high lipids and strategies to bring the levels into the target range. Forty-nine had low HDL-C values and 36 had elevated TG values. At the completion of the 12-week program, although there was no change in the proportion of patients who had elevated TG, the percentage of participants with low HDL-C levels fell significantly from 51 to 28%.

Kirkbride (2010) concluded that more carefully planned, longer, ideally randomised studies with larger numbers of participants are needed to demonstrate the clinical and cost effectiveness of the use of POC lipid testing in pharmacies. In most, if not all cases, studies have not been able to investigate the benefit to outcomes of introducing POCT for lipids as a single factor rather than as part of a more comprehensive pharmacist-led program.

### Economic benefits of POCT for lipids

Detailed studies on the economic effectiveness of POCT for lipids, regardless of the community setting involved, are very limited.

In the Point-of-Care Testing in General Practice Trial, Laurence *et al.* (2010) concluded that the cost per patient of performing lipids (and HbA1c and INR) by POCT for patient management was more than by laboratory testing, although these differences were not significant. They also suggested that POC lipid testing resulted in higher medication costs, presumably due to enhanced treatment, with a component contributed by improved medication compliance.

Conti *et al.* (2015b) carried out a small pharmacy-based study using the Accutrend Plus or the multiCare in in 33 pharmacies in Malta. Via a survey, they determined how much patients were willing to pay for POC lipid testing, the average price charged and the cost of performing the test. They concluded the Accutrend would recoup costs within the first year of use while the multiCare in would not recoup costs within 10 years (the expected lifetime of the device). In addition, the average cost of the tests charged was ~30% more than the patients were willing to pay.

## REFERENCES


AAPP (Australian Association of Pathology Practices) (2008) *An analysis of Pathology Test Use in Australia*. University of Sydney, Sydney.

ABS (Australian Bureau of Statistics) (2015) *National Health Survey, First Results*. ABS Catalogue 4364.0.55.001. Commonwealth Australian Bureau of Statistics, Commonwealth of Australia, Canberra.

ADA (American Diabetes Association) (2005) Diagnosis and classification of diabetes mellitus. *Diabetes Care* **28**(Supplement 1), S37–S42. doi:10.2337/diacare.28.suppl_1.S37

AIHW (Australian Institute of Health and Welfare) (2014) *Cardiovascular disease, diabetes and chronic kidney disease – Australian facts: Morbidity–Hospital care*. Australian Institute of Health and Welfare. Cardiovascular, diabetes and chronic kidney disease series no. 3. Cat. no. CDK 3. Canberra.

BEACH (2014) *General Practice Activity in Australia 2013–2014*. General Practice Series Number 36. Bettering the Evaluation of Care and Health, Sydney University Press, <http://ses.library.usyd.edu.au/bitstream/2123/11882/4/9781743324226_ONLINE.pdf>.

Bubner TK, Laurence CO, Gialamas A, Yelland LN, Ryan P, Willson KJ, *et al.* (2009) Effectiveness of point-of-care testing for therapeutic control of chronic conditions: results from the PoCT in General Practice Trial. *The Medical Journal of Australia* **190**, 624–626.

CDC (Centers for Disease Control and Prevention) (2015) *Cholesterol Reference Method Laboratory Network Clinical Laboratory Certification Program*, CDC, <http://www.cdc.gov/labstandards/crmln.html>.

Conti R, Azzopardi LM, Serracino-Inglott A (2015a) The correlation of Accutrend Plus® and Multicare-In® for the total cholesterol parameter with standard lab results. *International Journal of Clinical Pharmacy* **37**, 212.

Conti R, Azzopardi LM, Serracino-Inglott A (2015b) An economic and feasibility testing for point-of-care testing for total cholesterol using Accutrend Plus® and Multicare-In®. *International Journal of Clinical Pharmacy* **37**, 270–271.

Cranor CW (2003) The Ashville Project: long-term clinical and economic outcomes of a community pharmacy diabetes care program. *Journal of the American Pharmaceutical Association* **43**, 173–184. doi:10.1331/108658003321480713

Donyai P, Van den Berg M (2009) Coronary heart disease risk screening: the community pharmacy Healthy Heart Assessment Service. *Pharmacy World & Science* **31**, 643–647. doi:10.1007/s11096-009-9338-4

Fanous A, Kier K, Rush M, Terrell S (2014) Impact of a 12-week, pharmacist-directed walking program in an established employee preventive care clinic. *American Journal of Health-System Pharmacy* **71**, 1219–1225. doi:10.2146/ajhp130484

Finderle P, Prah M, Prezelj M (2009) Measurement of cholesterol and triglycerides by two POCT instruments: Accutrend GCT and Multicare. *Clinical Chemistry and Laboratory Medicine* **47**(Supplement), S325.

Friedewald WT, Levy RI, Fredrickson DS (1972) Estimation of the concentration of low-density lipoprotein cholesterol in plasma, without the use of preparative ultracentrifuge. *Clinical Chemistry* **18**, 499–502.

Gialamas A, Laurence CO, Yelland LN, Tideman P, Worley P, Shephard MD, *et al.* (2010) Assessing agreement between point of care and laboratory results for lipid testing from a clinical perspective. *Clinical Biochemistry* **43**, 515–518. doi:10.1016/j.clinbiochem.2009.11.014

iCCnet (Integrated Cardiovascular Clinical Network) CHSA (2013) *Roche cobas b101 HbA1c and Lipids Evaluation*, iCCnet, <http://www.appn.net.au/Data/Sites/1/appn/05instrumentevaluations/02evaluationreports/aacbb101report.pdf>.

IDF (International Diabetes Federation) (2006) *The IDF Consensus Worldwide Definition of the Metabolic Syndrome*, IDF, <https://www.idf.org/webdata/docs/IDF_Meta_def_final.pdf>.

Jain A, Persaud JW, Rao N, Harvey D, Robertson L, Nirmal L, *et al.* (2011) Point of care testing is appropriate for National Health Service health check. *Annals of Clinical Biochemistry* **48**, 159–165. doi:10.1258/acb.2010.010195

Jain A, Rao N, Sharifi M, Bhatt N, Patel P, Persaud JW, *et al.* (2014) Evaluation of the Afinion™ AS100 analyser in a community setting. *Atherosclerosis* **236**, e306–e307.

Jeong T-D, Kang HJ, Kim MS, Kim SY, Lee W, Chun S, *et al.* (2013) Evaluation of the performance of LABGEO PT hepatic test 9. *Laboratory Medicine Online* **3**, 138–144. doi:10.3343/lmo.2013.3.3.138

Joergensen B, Sais Zidek A (2014) A new point-of-care analyser for rapid and precise determination of lipid profile and HbA1c. *Atherosclerosis* **235**, e288. doi:10.1016/j.atherosclerosis.2014.05.867

Jones C, Nanji A, Mawani S, Davachi S, Ross L, Vollman A, *et al.* (2013) Feasibility of community-based screening for cardiovascular risk in an ethnic community: the South East Asian Cardiovascular Health Assessment and Management Program (SA-CHAMP). *BMC Public Health* **13**, 160. doi:10.1186/1471-2458-13-160

Kirkbride R (2010) Point-of-care testing in the community pharmacy. In *Point-of-Care Testing*. 3rd edn. (Eds C Price, A St John and L Kricka) pp. 323–334. AACC Press, Washington DC, USA.

Laurence C, Gialamas A, Yelland L, Bubner T, Ryan P, Wilson K, *et al.* (2008) A pragmatic cluster, randomised trial to evaluate the safety, clinical effectiveness, cost effectiveness and satisfaction with point of care testing in a general practice setting – rationale, design and baseline characteristics. *Trials* **9**, 50. doi:10.1186/1745-6215-9-50

Laurence CO, Moss JR, Briggs NE, Beilby JJ (2010) The cost-effectiveness of point of care testing in a general practice setting: results from a randomised controlled trial. *BMC Health Services Research* **10**, 165. doi:10.1186/1472-6963-10-165

Lippi G, Plebani M, Favaloro E, Trenti T (2010) Laboratory testing in pharmacies. *Clinical Chemistry and Laboratory Medicine* **48**, 943–953. doi:10.1515/CCLM.2010.184

Mathew T, Corso O, Ludlow M, Boyle A, Cass A, Chadban S, *et al.* (2010) Screening for chronic kidney disease in Australia: a pilot study in the community and workplace. *Kidney International* **77**(Supplement 116), S9–S16. doi:10.1038/ki.2009.538

Matteucci E, della Bartola L, Rossi L, Pellegrini G, Giampietro O (2014) Improving CardioChek PA analytical performance: three year study. *Clinical Chemistry and Laboratory Medicine* **52**, 1291–1296. doi:10.1515/cclm-2013-1084

Méndez-González MD, Bonet-Marqués R, Ordoñez-Llanos J (2009) Lipid profile in ambulatory patients using 3 point-of-care devices and comparison with reference methods. *Point of Care* **8**, 110–116. doi:10.1097/POC.0b013e3181b31692

Miida T, Nakamura Y, Mezaki T, Hanyu O, Maruyama S, Horikawa Y, *et al.* (2002) LDL-cholesterol and HDL-cholesterol concentrations decrease during the day. *Annals of Clinical Biochemistry* **39**, 241–249. doi:10.1258/0004563021901946

Modesti P, Rapi S, Bamoshmoosh M, Baldereschi M, Massetti L, Padeletti L, *et al.* (2012) Impact of one or two visits strategy on hypertension burden estimation in HYDY, a population-based cross-sectional study: implications for healthcare resource allocation decision making. *BMJ Open* **2**, e001062. doi:10.1136/bmjopen-2012-001062

Motta LA, Shephard MDS, Halls HJ, Barnes G, Senior J (2015) Optimizing point-of-care for diabetes management in a rural Australian general practice. *Point of Care* **14**, 25–31. doi:10.1097/POC.0000000000000047

NCEP (National Cholesterol Education Program) (2001) *Third Report of the National Cholesterol Education Program Expert Panel on Detection, Evaluation, and Treatment of High Blood Cholesterol in Adults (Adult Treatment Panel III) Executive Summary*. National Institutes of Health, National Heart, Lung and Blood Institute, Bethesda MD, USA.

Oyetayo O, James C, Martinez A, Roberson K, Talbert R (2011) The Hispanic Diabetes Management Program: impact of community pharmacists in clinical outcomes. *Journal of the American Pharmacists Association* **51**, 623–626. doi:10.1331/JAPhA.2011.09229

Peterson GM, Fitzmaurice KD, Naunton M, Vial JH, Stewart K, Krum H (2004) Impact of pharmacist-conducted home visits on the outcomes of lipid-lowering drug therapy. *Journal of Clinical Pharmacy and Therapeutics* **29**, 23–30. doi:10.1046/j.1365-2710.2003.00532.x

Rapi S, Bazzini C, Tozzetti C, Sbolci V, Amedeo Modesti P (2009) Point-of-care testing of cholesterol and triglycerides for epidemiologic studies: evaluation of the multicare-in system. *Translational Research; the Journal of Laboratory and Clinical Medicine* **153**, 71–76. doi:10.1016/j.trsl.2008.11.010

RCPA QAP (Royal College of Pathologists of Australasia Quality Assurance Programs) (2015) *General Chemistry 2015–2016 Allowable Limits of Performance*, RCPA QAP.

Selvin E, Steffes MW, Zhu H, Matsushita K, Wagenknecht L, Pankow J, *et al.* (2010) Glycated hemoglobin, diabetes, and cardiovascular risk in nondiabetic adults. *The New England Journal of Medicine* **362**, 800–811. doi:10.1056/NEJMoa0908359

Shephard M (2006) Analytical goals for point-of-care testing used for diabetes management in Australian health care settings outside the laboratory. *Point of Care* **5**, 177–185.

Shephard MD, Mazzachi BC, Shephard AK, McLaughlin KJ, Denner B, Barnes G (2005) The impact of point of care testing on diabetes services along Victoria's Mallee Track:

results of a community-based diabetes risk assessment and management program. *Rural and Remote Health* **5**, 371. <http://www.rrh.org.au/articles/subviewnew.asp?ArticleID=371>

Shephard M, Shephard A, Watkinson L, Mazzachi B, Worley P (2009) Design, implementation and results of the quality control program for the Australian government's point of care testing in general practice trial. *Annals of Clinical Biochemistry* **46**, 413–419. doi:10.1258/acb.2009.009045

Shephard A, Shephard M, Halls H, Corso O, Mathew T (2011) Innovative use of point-of-care testing for chronic kidney disease screening. *Point of Care* **10**, 98–101. doi:10.1097/POC.0b013e31821c6bd0

Simpson P, Jolly L, Tirimacco R, Gill J, Tideman P (2010) Evaluation of the lipid panel on the Abaxis Piccolo Xpress to determine its potential as a point-of-care instrument in a nonlaboratory setting. *Point of Care* **14**, 25–31.

St John A (2010) The evidence to support point-of-care testing. *The Clinical Biochemist Reviews* **31**, 111–119.

St-Pierre AC, Cantin B, Dagenais GR, Mauriège P, Bernard PM, Després JP, *et al.* (2005) Low-density lipoprotein subfractions and the long-term risk of ischemic heart disease in men: 13-year follow-up data from the Québec Cardiovascular Study. *Arteriosclerosis, Thrombosis, and Vascular Biology* **25**, 553–559. doi:10.1161/01.ATV.0000154144.73236.f4

Steinberg D (2004) Thematic review series: the pathogenesis of atherosclerosis. An interpretive history of the cholesterol controversy: part I. *Journal of Lipid Research* **45**, 1583–1593. doi:10.1194/jlr.R400003-JLR200

Tsuyuki RT, Johnson JA, Teo KK, Simpson SH, Ackman ML, Biggs RS, *et al.* (2002) A randomized trial of the effect of community pharmacist intervention on cholesterol risk management: the Study of Cardiovascular Risk Intervention by Pharmacists (SCRIP). *Archives of Internal Medicine* **162**, 1149–1155. doi:10.1001/archinte.162.10.1149

Vergès B (2009) Lipid modification in type 2 diabetes: the role of LDL and HDL. *Fundamental & Clinical Pharmacology* **23**, 681–685. doi:10.1111/j.1472-8206.2009.00739.x

Vetrano D, Martone A, Mastropaolo S, Tosato M, Colloca G, Marzetti E, *et al.* (2013) Prevalence of the seven cardiovascular health metrics in a Mediterranean country: results from a cross-sectional study. *European Journal of Public Health* **23**, 858–862. doi:10.1093/eurpub/ckt130

Warnick GR, Myers GL, Cooper GR, Rifai N (2002) Impact of the third cholesterol report from the Adult Treatment Panel of the National Cholesterol Education Program on the clinical laboratory. *Clinical Chemistry* **48**, 11–17.

Westgard J (2015) *Desirable Specifications for Total Error, Imprecision, and Bias, Derived from Intra- and Inter-Individual Biologic Variation*, <http://www.westgard.com/biodatabase1.htm>.

Whitehead SJ, Ford C, Gama R (2014a) A combined laboratory and field evaluation of the Cholestech LDX and CardioChek PA point-of-care testing lipid and glucose analysers. *Annals of Clinical Biochemistry* **51**, 54–67. doi:10.1177/0004563213482890

Whitehead S, Ford C, Gama R (2014b) The impact of different point-of-care testing lipid analysers on cardiovascular disease risk assessment. *Journal of Clinical Pathology* **67**, 535–539. doi:10.1136/jclinpath-2013-202123

WHO (World Health Organization) (1999) *Definition, Diagnosis and Classification of Diabetes Mellitus and its Complications.* WHO, Geneva, Switzerland, <http://apps.who.int/iris/bitstream/10665/66040/1/WHO_NCD_NCS_99.2.pdf>.

WHO (2015) *Cardiovascular Diseases (CVDs) Fact Sheet No 317.* WHO, Geneva, Switzerland, <http://www.who.int/mediacentre/factsheets/fs317/en/>.

Yamada C, Johnson J, Robertson P, Pearson G, Tsuyuki R (2005) Long term impact of a community pharmacist intervention on cholesterol levels in patients at high risk. *Pharmacotherapy* **25**, 110–115. doi:10.1592/phco.25.1.110.55619

Yang B (2005) A change of heart: how the people of Framingham, Massachusetts, helped unravel the mysteries of cardiovascular disease. *Discovery Medicine* **5**, 104–111.

Yarnell JW, Patterson CC, Sweetnam PM, Thomas HF, Bainton D, Elwood PC, *et al.* (2001) Do total and high density lipoprotein cholesterol and triglycerides act independently in the prediction of ischemic heart disease? Ten-year follow-up of Caerphilly and Speedwell Cohorts. *Arteriosclerosis, Thrombosis, and Vascular Biology* **21**, 1340–1345. doi:10.1161/hq0801.093505

Zhang P, He L, Guo Y, Liu P, Li G, Wang L, Liu Y (2015) Blood lipid profiles and factors associated with dyslipidemia assessed by a point-of-care testing device in an outpatient setting: a large-scale cross-sectional study in Southern China. *Clinical Biochemistry* **48**, 586–589. doi:10.1016/j.clinbiochem.2015.03.008

# 13 Point-of-care testing for the management of oral anticoagulants

*Paul Harper and Bronwyn Sheppard*

**Summary**

Warfarin is the most commonly used oral anticoagulant worldwide, with approximately 1% of the population in developed countries taking this medication. Warfarin has a narrow treatment range, where too much can cause life-threatening bleeding and not enough can increase the risk of thrombosis that can lead to major disability or even death. Patients on warfarin require a regular blood test, international normalised ratio (INR), to maintain safe control. Point-of-care testing (POCT) for INR is now used in several models of care including patient self-testing, pharmacy-based services and mobile services in remote regions. In this chapter, we review the data from clinical trials, meta-analyses and a Cochrane review that demonstrate the clinical and economic benefits of POCT for warfarin management. We also describe examples of successful models to illustrate the improved safety and clinical benefit as well as the greater convenience for patients.

## INDICATIONS FOR WARFARIN

Warfarin is the best known and most widely used oral anticoagulant of the class of vitamin K antagonists; however, other preparations including acenocoumarol (sinthrome) and phenprocoumon are extensively used in Europe. These drugs function by inhibiting vitamin K thus slowing normal blood coagulation. Warfarin is prescribed for the treatment of acute venous thrombosis and pulmonary embolus and to prevent blood clots associated with mechanical heart valves. The use of warfarin increased dramatically ~20 years ago when it was shown that warfarin can significantly reduce the risk of stroke in patients with an irregular heart rate due to atrial fibrillation (Albers *et al.* 2001). The incidence of atrial fibrillation in the USA is 4.7% in people aged over 65 years, rising to 10% in men over 75 years resulting in an increasing number of elderly patients on long-term warfarin. Data from British studies showed that ~250 000 people took warfarin in the UK in 1994 and this had risen to 950 000 by 2005. Indications for the use of warfarin therapy in patients managed in community pharmacies in New Zealand are summarised in Table 13.1.

## THE IMPORTANCE OF GOOD WARFARIN CONTROL

Warfarin has a narrow therapeutic window, and maintaining stable treatment can be difficult due to many factors that influence anticoagulant control. Warfarin treatment is monitored using a simple blood test called the international normalised ratio or INR. This is a ratio

Table 13.1. Indications for long-term warfarin based on 5000 patients managed in community pharmacies (Harper *et al.* 2015)

| Indications for warfarin therapy | Mean age (years) | Proportion of patients (%) |
|---|---|---|
| Atrial fibrillation | 72 | 63 |
| Deep vein thrombosis | 60 | 10 |
| Mechanical heart valves | 59 | 12 |
| Pulmonary embolus | 62 | 7.5 |
| Others | 63 | 7.5 |

of how long the patient's blood takes to clot compared with a normal control (pooled samples from patients not taking warfarin). Different laboratory reagents produce different results, so the result is adjusted (or normalised) depending on the reagent used; a person not taking warfarin should have an INR of 1.0. For most conditions requiring anticoagulants, the aim is to maintain the INR between 2.0 and 3.0, but changes in diet, medication, exercise and lifestyle can influence control, giving results outside this range and increasing the risk of complications. Bleeding is the most serious complication, with the risk directly related to the INR value. There is a consistent increase in major bleeding (including intracranial bleeding) when the INR exceeds 4.0 (BSH-BCHS-HTTF 1990; SPORTIF III 2003) and is up to 5-fold higher when the INR exceeds 7.0 (Palareti *et al.* 1996).

The main reason for prescribing warfarin is to prevent blood clots or thromboses without causing bleeding, so the ideal way to monitor the efficacy and safety of warfarin treatment is to measure the number of bleeds and thromboses that occur. This data is difficult to collect because it involves extensive review of medical records. An easier way to monitor control is to measure the amount of time the INR is within the therapeutic range (the TTR). This is a surrogate measure but has been shown to correlate with complications. Two large clinical trials (Akins *et al.* 2007; SPORTIF III 2003) showed that patients on warfarin with good control (INR within range 75% of the time) had an annual mortality of 1.69% and major bleeding events of 1.58%, whereas the poorly controlled patients (INR within the therapeutic range <60% of the time) had an annual mortality of 4.2% and major bleeding of 3.85%. More recent studies have confirmed these findings. Overall, these studies estimate that patients with a TTR of 70% have a complication rate (bleeding or thrombosis) of ~1 per 100 patient years, which increases ~5 fold when the TTR drops to below 40%.

## REGULAR LABORATORY TESTS ARE INCONVENIENT

Conventional anticoagulant monitoring is carried out through an anticoagulant clinic, or by the patient's family doctor or a specialist physician. The patient attends a laboratory or clinic for blood sample collection. The sample is sent to the laboratory for INR testing, which may take several hours. Later, the patient is contacted and given advice about the warfarin dose and the date of the next test. The process is inconvenient and time consuming and likely to have an impact on compliance. In a conventional anticoagulant clinic, most stable patients would have a test approximately once a month, but in some clinics the interval is extended to 6 weeks between tests.

## ADVANTAGES OF POINT-OF-CARE TESTING

It is now possible to measure the INR using a POCT device. Several different devices are available: larger devices designed for use in hospitals, doctor's surgeries or pharmacies and smaller handheld devices for patients to use at home. These alleviate some of the problems seen with the present process of warfarin management (Table 13.2). Specific additional advantages are discussed in the various models of care described below.

## POINT-OF-CARE TESTING DEVICES FOR INR

POCT devices to measure INR are available for both professional use and patient self-testing (Table 13.3). Professional use devices are recommended for healthcare professionals operating Anticoagulation Management Services (AMS) and for use in hospitals. They enable the service to comply with POC regulatory requirements (e.g. ISO 22870:2006) and to achieve quality testing and good patient care.

**Table 13.2.** Comparison between warfarin management by the laboratory and by POCT

| **Problems with laboratory-based warfarin management** | |
|---|---|
| Time consuming | Patient has to travel to a laboratory and wait for a blood sample. |
| Venous blood sample | Older patients and those requiring regular blood tests often have poor venous access, making blood collection difficult. |
| Disjointed service | Venous sample collected, sent to a laboratory for processing, result relayed to doctor, patient contacted with advice. In some services the patient has to take the lead and contact the practice for advice. Many points of potential delay and error. |
| Less frequent testing | Impractical for patients to test more frequently than once every 2 to 3 weeks |
| Less patient involvement | The patient remains remote from the process. |
| **Advantages of point-of-care testing** | |
| Rapid process | The test result is available within a few minutes. |
| Finger-prick blood sample | Many patients prefer a finger-prick blood test and useful for testing children. |
| More coordinated service | As the blood test only takes a few seconds the patient can receive immediate treatment advice. |
| More frequent testing | It is practical for patients to measure the INR every week especially if they perform self-monitoring at home (see discussion below). |
| More patient involvement | The patient can see a graphical display of results on computer screen. |
| Better anticoagulant control | The studies discussed below show that POCT improves anticoagulant control and reduces the incidence of complications. |

**Table 13.3.** Comparison of patient self-testing devices and professional use devices

| **Patient self-testing device** | **Professional use device** |
|---|---|
| Intended for use by patients for self-testing and self-management | Intended for use by health-care professionals either in primary care or in hospitals. |
| Capillary whole blood sample (1 drop) | Capillary whole blood sample (1 drop) |
| Short turnaround to get INR result | About 1 min to get INR result |
| Small, light and portable device | Larger (may include touch screen), light and portable device |
| Designed for single patient use | Designed for multiple patient use |
| Few user dependent steps. Easy user interface (e.g. one button operation). | More user dependent steps. May include touch screen with icon-based LCD display. |
| No patient ID possible (assumption is that the device will be used for a single patient) | Patient ID input possible (manual entry or barcode scanner) |
| No operator ID possible | Operator ID input possible (manual entry or barcode scanner) |
| Disposable battery | Rechargeable battery |
| Built-in quality control on every strip | Built-in quality control on every strip |
| No or limited connectivity | Connectivity (data transfer to Patient Management System/Laboratory Information System) |
| Limited on-board data storage | Larger on-board data storage including QC and calibration data |
| | Optional liquid QC (to meet regulatory requirements, such as ISO 22870) |
| | Optional operator and QC lock-outs |
| | Higher price *v.* patient self-testing device |
| Examples: CoaguChek XS, INRatio, MicroINR, QLabs Micropoint. | Examples: CoaguChek XS Plus, CoaguChek XS Pro, iSTAT, Protime InRhythm. |

The range of POCT INR devices on the global market is ever increasing (Curtis *et al.* 2012). Selected examples of commonly used INR devices include:

- the CoaguChek® range of devices including the XS, XS Plus and XS Pro, marketed by Roche Diagnostics
- the i-STAT® (Abbott Point of Care Inc.)
- the Coagu-Sense™ PT/INR Monitoring System (Coagu-Sense Inc.)
- INRatio®/INRatio®2 PT/INR Monitoring System (Alere)
- ProTime® InRhythm™ (Accriva Diagnostics).

All these devices are dedicated coagulation meters except the i-STAT, which can measure a range of other different POC tests apart from INR.

With all devices, a capillary blood sample (containing the necessary clotting factors) mixes with (usually a recombinant human) tissue thromboplastin (embedded in the reagent) to activate thrombin, which initiates clot formation. Different devices use different thrombin substrates to detect clot formation. For example, with the CoaguChek XS, thrombin cleaves the peptide substrate Electrocyme TH into a residual (inert) peptide and the electro-active phenylenediamine, which generates an electrochemical signal. The i-STAT also uses electrochemical detection but a different thrombin substrate H-D-phenylalanyl-pipecolyl-arginine-p-amino-p-methoxydiphenylamine. Thrombin cleaves this substrate to produce a chemically inert tripeptide and an electro-active compound ($NH_3^+$-$C_6H_4$-NH-$C_6H_4$-$OCH_3$). The INRatio uses electrochemical detection of changes in impedance in the sample following the cleavage of fibrinogen to fibrin by thrombin. The Coagu-Sense employs a direct micromechanical clot detection system.

A comparison of some features of the CoaguChek XS, i-STAT and INRatio systems is provided in Table 13.4.

When purchasing a POC anticoagulation monitoring device, the following considerations are recommended (Anticoagulation Europe). The device should have:

- been evaluated by a credible, independent agency such as the NHS Purchase and Supply Agency Centre for Evidence-Based Purchasing (CEP), UK or Scandinavian Evaluation of Laboratory Equipment for Primary Health Care (SKUP) and found to be safe and accurate for use in clinic or at home
- an International Sensitivity Index (ISI) of close to 1.0, in line with WHO recommendations, which specify that ISIs should be between 0.9 and 1.7 but that ISIs towards the lower end of the scale are preferable (WHO 1999)
- a means for providing both internal quality control (QC) and external proficiency testing (PT)/quality assessment (EQA)
- appropriate precision and accuracy for the clinical need; low coefficients of variation of 4–5% that closely match laboratory analysers are preferable
- data management capabilities that match your requirements (e.g. results transferred electronically to patient records)
- value-added support services provided by the manufacturer and/or distributor (e.g. training and/or training materials and helpline)

Specific considerations for patient self-testers should also include:

**Table 13.4.** Comparison of selected specifications of common INR devices

| Parameter | CoaguChek XS | iSTAT | INRatio |
|---|---|---|---|
| Method principle | | | |
| Substrate | Electrocyme TH | PPAAM[a] | Fibrinogen |
| Detection | Electrochemical | Electrochemical | Impedance |
| Reagent | Strip | Cartridge | Strip |
| Sample volume (μL) | 10 | 20 | 14 |
| Size (cm) | 14 × 8 × 3 | 21 × 6 × 5 | 15 × 7 × 5 |
| Weight (g) | 175 | 520 | 260 |
| Calibration traceable to | WHO rTF/95 | WHO rTF/95 | WHO rTF/95 |
| ISI | 1.0 | 1.05 | 1.0 |

[a]H-D-phenylalanyl-pipecolyl-arginine-p-amino-p-methoxydiphenylamine

- your physician's or anticoagulation clinic personnel's recommendation, based on their experience and knowledge of the instruments
- other patients' experience and satisfaction with their home monitoring device, and the educational and support services provided to them by the manufacturer and/or distributor.

## POINT-OF-CARE TESTING IN CLINICAL PRACTICE

### In hospital use

The main focus of this chapter is on the use of POCT in the community, but it is important to recognise that POCT is also used for INR measurement in hospitals where a rapid result may assist clinical management, for example, in the emergency department, the intensive care unit or theatre.

### Community-based services

#### Community pharmacy anticoagulant management

With the introduction of mobile POCT devices, it has become possible to move anticoagulant monitoring into community pharmacies. The Community Pharmacy Anticoagulant Management Service (CPAMS) in New Zealand is an example of how POCT and decision support software can be integrated via the internet to provide a national service with data accessible to all health-care professionals involved in the service.

#### Community Pharmacy Anticoagulant Management Service

CPAMS was introduced in New Zealand in 2010 to improve anticoagulant control and relieve the workload of general practitioners. A pilot was carried out in 25 pharmacies and achieved a high level of anticoagulant control with a TTR >75%, which was significantly higher than achieved by the standard service provided by family doctors (Harrison *et al.* 2015). The pilot was expanded over the next 3 years and is now available in 150 pharmacies providing management for over 5000 patients.

*Outline of the service*

The patients attend a local community pharmacy at their convenience. They are interviewed by a trained pharmacist who asks if they have had any bleeding, changes in medication or hospital visits since their last test. The pharmacist carries out the INR test on a POC device (Roche CoaguChek XS Plus) using a finger-prick blood sample. The results are automatically transferred to a decision support software (DSS) program that provides immediate treatment advice. The patient receives a printed dosing calendar to take away and is advised when to come for the next test. They also receive an email reminder when the next test is due. The results are automatically sent to the family doctor's patient management system.

*Advantages of the Community Pharmacy Anticoagulant Service*

Prior to the introduction of CPAMS, the majority of patients in New Zealand had their anticoagulant care supervised by general practitioners (GPs). An audit of anticoagulant management in Auckland showed that GPs achieved a TTR of around 50% (Young *et al.* 2004). CPAMS has led to an improvement in anticoagulant control with a TTR consistently around 75% and this has been maintained over 2 years as the service has expanded (Harper *et al.* 2015).

Factors that potentially contribute to the improved control include:

- developed in collaboration with the New Zealand Pharmaceutical Society, the POC device provider (Roche Diagnostics), the DSS provider (INR Online Ltd), health-care professionals and district health boards
- appropriate training for pharmacists with an assessment process
- pharmacists working in partnership with doctors under a Standing Order, which is an agreement delegating the pharmacists authority to manage warfarin within certain parameters
- a computerised system enabling accurate data collection and record keeping
- validated DSS providing automated dosing (Harper *et al.* 2014)
- a recall process that lists all patients due for testing each day and highlights those who are overdue
- automatic email reminders.

A survey of the pilot study (Shaw *et al.* 2014) showed that pharmacists derived satisfaction from the expansion of their role. Many felt that their clinical skills and knowledge were previously underused and they welcomed the challenge of developing a new model of care that made better use of these. The pharmacists also enjoyed the opportunity to develop a closer relationship with their patients.

The survey also showed that the majority of GPs and practice nurses who responded thought that CPAMS had saved them time and some doctors were pleased to have the responsibility for day-to-day management of warfarin patients taken on by the pharmacist.

Feedback from patients was also positive; many preferred to have a finger-prick blood test and liked the convenience of being able to drop-in for a blood test without an appointment. Patients also felt more involved with their care and had a greater understanding of their condition by getting immediate advice and being able to discuss their management with the pharmacists at the time of the test.

#### Nurse-led service in a remote Indigenous community

In the CPAMS model, the patient came to the pharmacy for testing, but in remote regions it may be more appropriate to take the device to the patient. This is particularly important in areas where there is poor access to laboratory services and there may be delays in giving treatment advice. This type of service has been introduced on the East Cape in New Zealand (Fig. 13.1); this is a remote region with a large Maori population with difficult access to health care.

Prior to the introduction of the nurse-led service, warfarin management was complex: a blood sample was collected at a remote site and taken by road to the nearest laboratory, which could take up to 6 h. The sample was processed the next day and the result was relayed back to the patient's doctor. The practice nurse would then contact the patient, which was often difficult because many patients are from a low socioeconomic group and some do not have access to a phone.

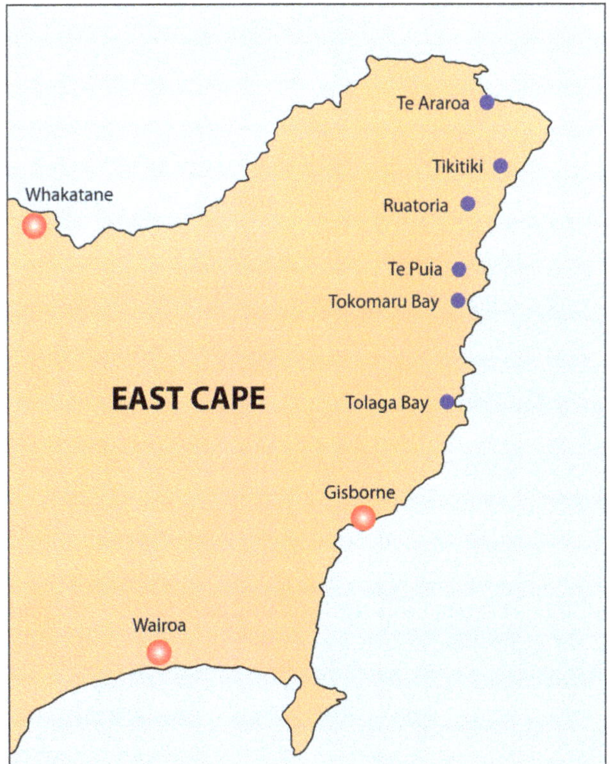


**Fig. 13.1.** East Cape of New Zealand. Dots represent remote clinics using POCT. Gisborne has the nearest hospital laboratory.

The new POCT service has been developed as a collaboration between the local Maori health-care provider, Ngati Porou Hauora, Roche New Zealand, INR Online Ltd and the Flinders University International Centre for Point-of-Care Testing. A nurse travels to six sites on the East Cape, carries out POCT, enters the results into the DSS via a laptop linked to the internet and receives immediate treatment advice for the patient. The whole process takes only a few minutes.

The service has several benefits:

- *Improved anticoagulant control* – overall the TTR improved from 60 to 69%, but the patients with poor control before the new service benefited most. Fig. 13.2 shows that patients with good control before the POC service continued to have good control (Fig. 13.2A), but those with poor control showed a significant improvement (Fig. 13.2B) with 10 patients achieving a TTR of greater than 60% (Fig. 13.2C).
- *More efficient service* – results are available within minutes and the patient can be given advice immediately.
- *More patient involvement and a more culturally acceptable process* – the introduction of this service emphasised the importance of close collaboration with the patients involved. Discussion with Māori health-care leaders revealed that Māori were more comfortable with a finger-prick blood test rather than a venous sample, as they could see at all times how their blood was handled. They also liked the immediacy of the testing and advice, and felt they could take more ownership of the process. Previously, the participants had felt more disconnected from the service because the testing was carried out remotely, but with local testing participants gained a much better understanding of the whole process and why testing was necessary.

## Self-monitoring and self-management

As POCT devices have developed and become smaller and more portable, it has become possible for patients to use these devices at home for either 'self-monitoring', where they perform their own INR test and contact a medical professional for treatment advice, or

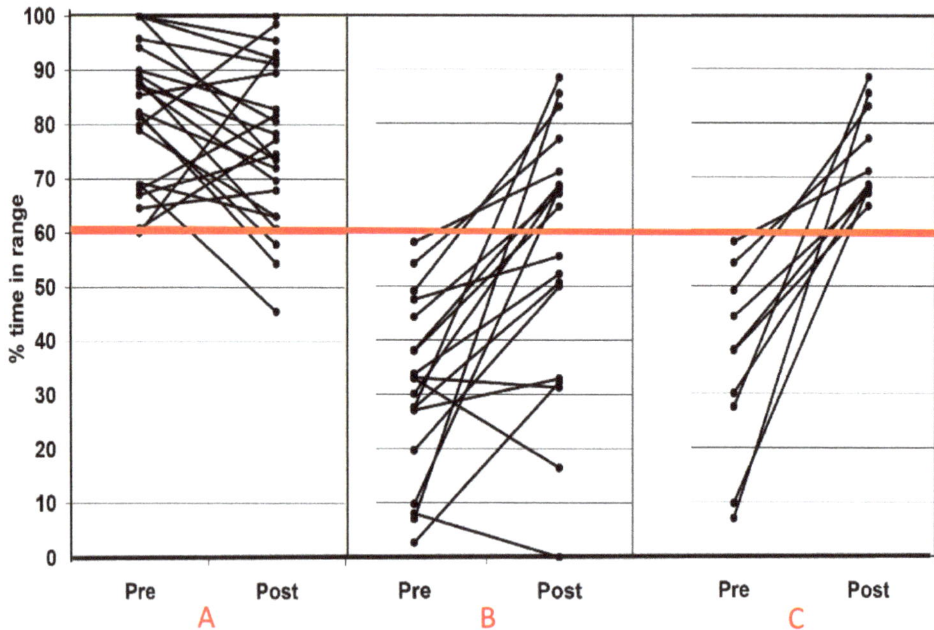


**Fig. 13.2.** Time in therapeutic range before and after the introduction of POCT with decision support software (A) Patients with TTR >60% prior (*n* = 20); (B) patients with TTR <60% prior (*n* = 19); (C) patients with TTR <60% prior and >60% post the change (*n* = 10).

'self-management', where they take complete control of their treatment performing the INR test and adjusting the warfarin dose as required.

### Self-monitoring

Evidence that more patient involvement improved outcomes has come from several studies. One of the earliest studies using POCT was reported in 1989, which showed that patients on home monitoring supervised by a clinician achieved a significantly better time in range than in a clinic based service (90% compared with 66%). Other small studies have shown a similar trend, but one criticism of these is that there is a high degree of patient selection; patients were only included if they were willing and able to use a POC device. The problem of selection bias was partly rectified in the study by Beyth *et al.* (2000) where patients were selected on an intention to treat basis with only a limited number of exclusion criteria. Patients were randomised to either supervised treatment with POCT (163 patients) or standard warfarin care (162 patients). All patients were included in the outcome analysis, but, of the 163 patients in the intervention group, only 96 (60%) used POCT; in spite of this, the outcomes showed a significantly better time in range (56% versus 32%) and significantly less bleeding in this group.

### Self-management

The concept of self-management, where the patient manages their own treatment was introduced in the 1990s. A study in Germany (Sawicki 1999) showed that a wide range of patients could be taught to make their own dose adjustments. In this study, 179 patients were randomised to either self-management or usual care. Patients in the self-management group achieved better control than the standard care group, but this did not reach statistical significance; however, the study demonstrated the concept was manageable and a patient survey of quality of life showed a significant improvement in the self-management patients. Similar studies in the Netherlands (Cromheecke *et al.* 2000) and UK (Fitzmaurice *et al.* 2002) also confirmed the feasibility of the concept, with a trend towards better control in the self-managing patients. A much larger study reported in 2001 (Körtke and Korfer 2001) involving over 600 patients with valve replacements confirmed a statistically significant improvement in anticoagulant control. Patients using self-management achieved a time in range (INR 2.5–4.5) of 79% compared with only 62% in those using standard care. This study also showed a significant reduction in major thrombosis and bleeding in the patients on self-management, which was particularly pronounced during the first few months of anticoagulant treatment.

#### Meta-analyses

Further support for the benefits of self-testing came from a meta-analysis published in 2006 (Heneghan *et al.* 2006). This reviewed the data from 14 randomised controlled trials and looked at the TTR and the rate of complications in various groups. Eleven trials reported the time in the therapeutic range and all 11 showed improvement in the self-monitoring group, with six reaching statistical significance. In addition, more than half of the trials reported that the incidence of thrombosis was significantly lower in the patients performing self-monitoring and self-management, with the rate of thrombosis less than half of the control group in those self-monitoring. The reduction in the incidence of major bleeding was reduced by one-third in those self-monitoring, but did not reach statistical significance in those using self-management.

The data of the above analysis was updated in 2010 in a Cochrane review (Garcia-Alamino *et al.* 2010) examining a further four randomised trials to include 18 trials involving over 4700 patients. This confirmed that both self-monitoring and self-management halved thrombo-embolic events (RR 0.50, 95% CI 0.36–0.69, *P* <0.0001) and was able to show this benefit in specific subgroups including patients with mechanical heart valves (RR 0.53, 95% CI 0.30–0.91, *P* <0.02). The review also included sufficient data on mortality (4305 participants, 137 events) to calculate a benefit. Despite only one trial showing a significant reduction in mortality, the pooled estimate indicated that self-monitoring and self-management were associated with an overall reduction in mortality from all causes when compared with standard therapy (RR 0.64, 95% CI 0.46–0.89, *P* <0.007).

One criticism of these reviews is that the analysis is based on data from randomised trials and therefore only includes a selected population, which does not reflect the outcomes that might be expected in a 'real-world' population. This has been resolved in a cohort study from Switzerland (Jenner *et al.* 2015) reviewing data from over 1100 patients using self-management with median follow-up of over 4 years. The study included all patients trained to perform self-management in one centre between 1998 and 2009 with no specific exclusions and therefore represents a real-life cohort. These patients achieved a TTR of 80% and the complication rate was similar to the rate reported in randomised studies.

#### Who should be considered for self-testing?

Most studies using self-testing show that not all patients are able to use the POC device and some have difficulty making dose adjustments. The experience from Germany, where over 60 000 patients use self-testing, was that ~50% of patients on long-term anticoagulation were suitable for home testing. To some extent, this is related to the patient's motivation because one study (Voller *et al.* 2001) showed that 70% of patients with heart valves were willing to try self-testing but only 40–50% with atrial fibrillation were. Table 13.5 lists criteria that have been suggested for selecting appropriate patients for self-testing (Douketis and Singh 2006).

#### What training is required?

Most clinical trials comparing self-management with standard care have based training on the model introduced in Germany where patients attend two or three training courses run by health-care professionals and all patients undergo some form of assessment to ensure they are able to use the POC device and understand dose adjustments. Interestingly a study by Khan *et al.* (2004) showed that education alone improved TTR. In their study, 85 patients attended a 2-h training session; half were randomised to self-management and the others continued with usual care. Both groups showed a significant improvement in TTR (education alone TTR improved from 61 to 70%, education and self-management TTR improved from 57 to 71%) showing that patient's involvement and understanding is a key part of good warfarin management.

**Table 13.5.** Patients who may benefit most from self-management

| Patients who could be considered for warfarin self-management |
|---|
| Require long-term (more than 6 months) or life-long warfarin therapy for a mechanical prosthetic heart valve, valvular heart disease, chronic atrial fibrillation, or recurrent venous thromboembolism |
| No visual impairment that precludes a finger-prick method of blood sampling and use of the portable coagulometer |
| The cognitive ability to receive training about anticoagulation self-monitoring |
| Willingness to take an active role in their health-care management |
| Self-monitoring of anticoagulation may be especially useful in people who live in remote areas or travel frequently |

**Table 13.6.** Theoretical and practical components of patient training

| **Theoretical aspects of training** |
|---|
| Theoretical aspects of anticoagulation management |
| How to monitor, and the frequency of coagulation monitoring |
| Problems with monitoring |
| Interaction between anticoagulants and other medications |
| Influences of nutrition, alcohol, intercurrent illness and travel |
| Recognising and treating complications |
| The target INR for their condition and the importance of maintaining the INR within 0.5 of the target |
| **Practical aspects of training** |
| Operating the coagulation monitor |
| Practising a coagulation test |
| Practising a quality control test |
| Performing finger-stick procedure |

Tables 13.6 lists the training recommended in the British Committee for Standards in Haematology guidelines.

### How do patients adjust their dose?

The key difference between self-monitoring and self-management is that patients using self-management adjust their own warfarin dose and decide when to do their next INR test. Several algorithms have been suggested to aid the patient to make the correct decision. Table 13.7 is an example of a simple algorithm to help patients make a dose adjustment when the INR is between 1.5 and 4.0. Other authors have used more complex algorithms such as a two-stage process with a dose management card and dose adjustment card (Jenner *et al.* 2015).

**Table 13.7.** Protocol used by patients to adjust dose of warfarin (Source: adapted from Sidhu and O'Kane 2001)

| INR value | Action taken by patient |
|---|---|
| <1.5 | Contact doctor for advice |
| 1.5–1.9 | Increase dose of warfarin by 1 mg daily |
| 2.0–2.5 | Same dose of warfarin |
| 2.6–4.0 | Decrease dose of warfarin by 1 mg daily |
| >4.0 | Contact doctor for advice |

Note: If the patient fluctuated between ranges very often, the dose increment was changed to 0.5 mg daily rather than 1 mg

### Anticoagulant decision support software

Several computerised anticoagulant management programs have been developed. The benefit of computerised dosing was most convincingly shown in a large multicentre trial of 13 000 patients that demonstrated that clinical events occurred less frequently with computer-assisted dosing and the TTR was significantly improved by computer assistance ($P < 0.001$) (Poller *et al.* 2008).

Computer systems have largely been used in anticoagulant clinics, but a recent study in 2010 linked patients directly to DSS via the internet (Harper and Pollock 2011). Forty-one patients were trained how to perform an INR test on a CoaguChek device and then enter their INR result into the decision support software via a webpage (INR Online Ltd) from home. The computer software immediately provided the patient with dosing advice and when to perform the next test. If the results were outside a specified range, the supervising doctor was automatically informed to review the results and provide the patient with updated advice via email. Patients using this model achieved a TTR of 82%. The service also received positive feedback from the patients because they knew their treatment was supervised and they were not making treatment decisions entirely alone. The system also ensured that their records were complete and available to other health-care professionals.

The American College of Chest Physicians Guidelines (Gyatt *et al.* 2012) recommends a dosing algorithm for warfarin management with the following statement:

> '*For dosing decisions during maintenance VKA (Vitamin K antagonists) therapy, we suggest using validated decision support tools (paper nomograms or computerized dosing programs) rather than no decision support (Grade 2C).*'

## GUIDELINES

Clinical guidelines for POCT have largely focussed on patient self-monitoring or self-management. Although self-testing has been available for several years, international guidelines have only recently been developed. The American College of Chest Physician Guidelines (2012), which are widely used by clinicians, discuss the benefits of self-testing and include the following recommendation:

> *'For patients treated with VKAs who are motivated and can demonstrate competency in self-management strategies, including the self-testing equipment, we suggest patient self-management rather than usual outpatient INR monitoring (Grade 2B). For all other patients, we suggest monitoring that includes the safeguards in our best practice statement. (Gyatt et al. 2012).'*

In September 2014, The National Institute for Healthcare and Excellence (NICE) in the UK published guidelines for self-monitoring for patients with atrial fibrillation or mechanical heart valves (NICE 2014). These recommended self-monitoring with POCT for patients on long-term anticoagulants who preferred to use self-monitoring and were both physically and cognitively able to do so. They recommend that patients should be trained and that their testing equipment is regularly checked against a health-care professional's coagulometer, which is checked using an external quality assurance scheme. They also advise that patient's records are kept and shared appropriately.

The British Committee for Standards in Haematology also published guidelines in 2014 (Jennings *et al.* 2014); these make similar recommendations but have a more extensive discussion of the place of quality assurance.

## COST-EFFECTIVENESS

POCT clearly has clinical benefits but it is only likely to be widely used if the treatment is cost-effective. Cost–benefit analysis of anticoagulant therapy is complex. Basically patient self-management (PSM) has an upfront cost for the equipment and patient training, which is above the cost of the existing service, but PSM uses less laboratory services and patients have fewer hospital visits potentially saving money. However, the main potential saving from patient self-management is the reduction in medical complications. Wan *et al.* (2008) in a review of 34 000 patients showed a clear correlation between TTR and the incidence of both thrombosis and major bleeding.

Fig. 13.3 is adapted from this study and illustrates the approximate incidence of complications at various TTRs. Clearly if a patient achieves a TTR of 80% the incidence of complications is low and the health cost reduced and the cost of one Quality Adjusted Life Year (QALY) gained is low. In fact, the current costs of suboptimal oral anticoagulation should not be underestimated and are substantial. A US economic model reported that if 50% of those currently receiving warfarin had optimal anticoagulation, 9852 emboli would be prevented at a saving of US$13 billion (Caro 2004).

Several cost–benefit analyses have been carried out over the last few years but they show surprisingly different outcomes. A UK study in 2006 (Jowett *et al.* 2006) reported that PSM was more expensive (£417 pa) than current routine care (£122 pa) and estimated that patient self-monitoring would cost the NHS £8–14 million per year; they concluded that PSM is unlikely to be cost-effective. However, a German study of PSM following heart valve replacement (Müller and Bergemann 2001) concluded that the incidence of lethal strokes may be reduced by PSM at an acceptable cost-effectiveness ratio and other studies have also shown a cost benefit (Lafata *et al.* 2000; Regier *et al.* 2006).

Most models do not take into account the increased convenience and the potential for lower personal costs for individual patients, particularly if the individuals live remotely. The Canadian Agency for Drugs and Technologies in Health (CADTH) found that patient self-testing/monitoring (PST) compared with traditional laboratory

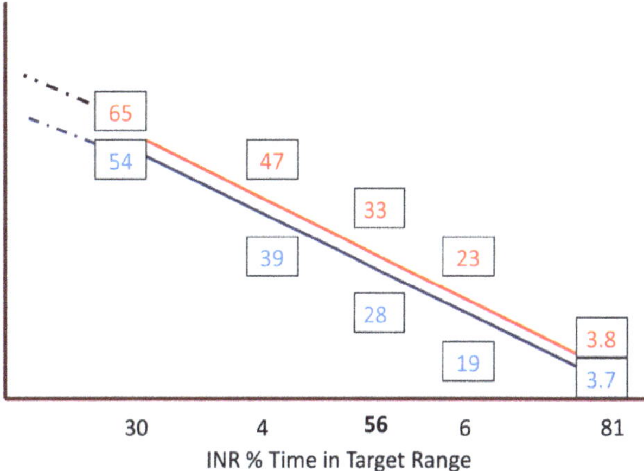


**Fig. 13.3.** Rates of major bleeding (red) and thrombosis (blue) per 1000 patient years against the time in therapeutic range (TTR) based on data from 38 atrial fibrillation trials.

tests was deemed not to be cost effective based on QALY gained. However, when a societal perspective was adopted and patient travel and time costs (as well as those of their caregivers) were included, PST was determined to be cost-saving. Overall, most models support PSM as a cost-effective management option.

## CONTROVERSIES

POCT for warfarin management has evolved relatively quickly and as a result there are some areas of practice that cause controversy. Some issues that have not been completely resolved and need to be considered when establishing a new POC service are briefly highlighted below.

### Who maintains and provides oversight of the POC device and service?

In the past, all blood tests were performed within a laboratory and were supervised by laboratory scientists. The same was true for POCT when it was first introduced because it was only available within the hospital. However, with the development of POCT in the community, it has become less clear who should provide maintenance and ensure appropriate quality control. In some regions, the laboratory still maintains some oversight but in others the responsibility falls on the user.

### What is the role of quality testing for POC monitoring of the INR?

In laboratories, it is standard practice to perform regular quality control testing on INR analysers and it is expected that laboratories will participate in external PT/QA programs to ensure that their results are within specified limits and are reliable. The place of these quality testing procedures in newer POC INR devices is less clear because there is less that the user can do to adjust measurement and most of the technology to measure the INR is in the test strip, which is disposed of each time a test is performed.

The current British recommendations for patient self-testing/self-management are that, if liquid QC samples are available, they should be run at least when testing with a new batch of test strips or if an unexpectedly high or low result occurs, and at least once every 6 months (Jennings *et al.* 2014).

An alternative view is that, while quality control remains important for POC devices, most of it is in-built in the device or test-strip itself. If a quality control sample gives a result outside the required range, the user only has one option: to not use the device. Therefore it is difficult to see the value of quality control testing for individual users.

For health-care professionals, accredited PT programs are available and established for several POCT devices, such as the UK National External Quality Assessment Scheme (UK NEQAS) or Royal College of Pathologists of Australasia (RCPA QAP). However, PT schemes for patients are not currently available.

When POCT was first introduced, clinicians and laboratory scientists were naturally concerned that the results may not be comparable with standard laboratory tests. This led to the practice of parallel testing where a patient would have a test performed on the POC device and also have a blood sample taken at the same time for a laboratory INR test to ensure comparable results. The British Guidelines recommend this type of testing approximately every 6 months for patients using self-management, but the interpretation of results can be difficult. It is well recognised that different methodologies will give different results and there is no global consensus on what degree of difference between POCT and laboratory results is acceptable and what should be done if the difference is outside a specified range. This type of testing can be confusing for patients because they may be told two different INR results on the same day and don't know which to accept for their own dose adjustment. It is strongly recommended that patients conduct serial INR measurements using a single POCT device and do not swap or alternate INR testing between POC and laboratory methods.

Current British Guidelines (Jennings *et al.* 2014) state that:

- when comparing capillary POCT results on a patient's own device and a device used in an anticoagulation clinic (whether it be in a primary care or hospital setting), results should be within 0.5 INR of each other (provided the patient and clinic use the same device); the clinic device should also be externally assessed through an accredited PT program, and,
- when testing a capillary sample and at the same time collecting a venous sample for testing in a hospital laboratory, again results should be within 0.5 INR of each other.

### Taking action on a high INR result

If a patient INR of between 4.5 and 8.0 is obtained with a POCT device, the test should be repeated to ensure that the prolonged result is not a consequence of poor sample quality. The second result should be within 0.5 INR of the first. If an INR result of greater than 8.0 is confirmed with repeat testing, patients should seek medical advice promptly, and a venous sample should be sent to the laboratory, because clinical decisions may be affected by the degree of INR prolongation.

### Who owns the data?

In the past, the process for reviewing and interpreting laboratory results was the responsibility of the requesting physician. In most modern laboratories the results are automatically transmitted to the doctor's patient management system and are accessible to all health-care workers involved in a patient's care. With POCT, particularly self-management, the patient is responsible for handling the results and they may not all be available to the supervising clinician, which can potentially impact on their medical care.

## CONCLUSIONS

POCT for warfarin management is now well established and has several advantages over laboratory or general practice-based services. The main benefit is the improved clinical outcome with better anticoagulant control, fewer complications and a lower mortality. This has been confirmed by numerous clinical trials and two large meta-analyses. In spite of this, few health services fully fund POCT. From our experience, POCT for warfarin should be part of a coordinated service and does require collaboration from all parties involved. There is a need for adequate training, good data collection, close medical supervision and regular audit to ensure that the service delivers safe effective care.

## REFERENCES


Akins PT, Feldman HA, Zoble RG, Newman D, Spitzer SG, Diener HC, *et al.* (2007) Secondary stroke prevention with ximelagatran versus warfarin in patients with atrial fibrillation: pooled analysis of SPORTIF III and V clinical trials. *Stroke* **38**, 874–880. doi:10.1161/01.STR.0000258004.64840.0b

Albers GW, Amerenco P, Easton JD, Sacco RL, Teal P (2001) Antithrombotic and thrombolytic therapy for ischemic stroke. *Chest* **119**(1, Supplement), 300S–320S. doi:10.1378/chest.119.1_suppl.300S

Beyth RJ, Quinn L, Landfeld S (2000) A multicomponent intervention to prevent major bleeding complications in older patients receiving warfarin. *Annals of Internal Medicine* **133**, 687–695. doi:10.7326/0003-4819-133-9-200011070-00010

BSH-BCSH-HTTF (British Society for Haematology-British Committee for Standards in Haematology-Haemostasis and Thrombosis Task Force) (1990) Guidelines on oral anticoagulation. 2nd edn. *Journal of Clinical Pathology* **43**, 177–183.

Caro JJ (2004) An economic model of stroke in atrial fibrillation: the cost of suboptimal oral anticoagulation. *The American Journal of Managed Care* **10**, S451–S461.

Cromheecke ME, Levi M, Colly LP, de Moi BJ, Prins MH, Hutten BA, *et al.* (2000) Oral anticoagulation self-management and management by a specialist anticoagulation clinic: a randomised cross-over comparison. *Lancet* **356**, 97–102. doi:10.1016/S0140-6736(00)02470-3

Curtis CM, Kost GJ, Louie RF, Sonu RJ, Ammirati EB, Sumner S (2012) Point-of-care hematology and coagulation testing in primary, rural, emergency and disaster care scenarios. *Point of Care* **11**, 140–145. doi:10.1097/POC.0b013e31825a9d3a

Douketis JD, Singh D (2006) Self-monitoring and self-dosing of oral anticoagulation improves survival. *Evidence-Based Cardiovascular Medicine* **10**, 124–126. doi:10.1016/j.ebcm.2006.04.021

Fitzmaurice DA, Murray ET, Gee KM, Allan TF, Hobbs FD (2002) A randomised controlled trial of patient self management of oral anticoagulation treatment compared with primary care management. *Journal of Clinical Pathology* **55**, 845–849. doi:10.1136/jcp.55.11.845

Garcia-Alamino JM, Ward AM, Alonso-Coello P, Perera P, Bankhead C, Fitzmaurice D, *et al.* (2010) Self-monitoring and self-management of oral anticoagulation (Review). *San Paolo Medical Journal* **128**, 246. doi:10.1590/S1516-31802010000400015

Gyatt GH, Aki EA, Crowther M, Gutterman DD, Schuunemann HJ (2012) Executive summary: antithrombotic therapy and prevention of thrombosis, 9th ed: American College of Chest Physicians evidence-based clinical practice guidelines. *Chest* **141**(Supplement 2), 7S–47S. doi:10.1378/chest.1412S3

Harper P, Pollock D (2011) Improved anticoagulant control in patients using home international normalized ratio testing and decision support provided through the Internet. *Internal Medicine Journal* **41**, 332–337. doi:10.1111/j.1445-5994.2010.02282.x

Harper P, Harper J, Hill C (2014) An audit of anticoagulant management to assess anticoagulant control using decision support software. *BMJ Open* **4**, e005864. doi:10.1136/bmjopen-2014-005864

Harper P, McMichael I, Griffiths D, Harper J, Hill C (2015) The community pharmacy-based anticoagulation management service achieves a consistently high standard of anticoagulant care. *The New Zealand Medical Journal* **128**, 35–44.

Harrison J, Shaw JP, Harrison JE (2015) Anticoagulation management by community pharmacists in New Zealand: an evaluation of a collaborative model in primary care.

*International Journal of Pharmacy Practice* **23**, 173–181. doi:10.1111/ijpp.12148

Heneghan C, Allonso-Coello P, Garcia-Alamino JM, Perera R, Meats E, Glasziou P (2006) Self-Monitoring of oral anticoagulation: a systematic review and meta-analysis. *Lancet* **367**, 404–411. doi:10.1016/S0140-6736(06)68139-7

Jenner KM, Simmons BJ, Delate T, Clark NP, Kurtz D, Witt DM (2015) An education program for patient self-management of warfarin. *The Permanente Journal* **19**, 33–38.

Jennings I, Kitchen D, Keeling D, Fitzmaurice D, Heneghan C (2014) Patient self-testing and self-management of oral anticoagulation with vitamin K antagonists: guidance from the British Committee for Standards in Haematology. *British Journal of Haematology* **167**, 600–607. doi:10.1111/bjh.13070

Jowett S, Bryan S, Murray E, McCahon E, Rafferty J, Hobbs FD, Fitzmaurice D (2006) Patient self-management of anticoagulation therapy: a trial-based cost-effectiveness analysis. *British Journal of Haematology* **134**, 632–639. doi:10.1111/j.1365-2141.2006.06243.x

Khan TI, Kamali F, Kesteven P, Avery P, Wynne H (2004) The value of education and self-monitoring in the management of warfarin therapy in older patients with unstable control of anticoagulation. *British Journal of Haematology* **126**, 557–564. doi:10.1111/j.1365-2141.2004.05074.x

Körtke H, Korfer R (2001) International normalized ratio self-management after mechanical heart valve replacement: is an early start advantageous? *The Annals of Thoracic Surgery* **72**, 44–48. doi:10.1016/S0003-4975(01)02656-X

Lafata JE, Martin SA, Kaatz S, Ward RE (2000) Anticoagulation clinics and patients self-testing for patients on chronic warfarin therapy: cost effectiveness analysis. *Journal of Thrombosis and Thrombolysis* **9**, S13–S19. doi:10.1023/A:1018704318655

Müller E, Bergemann R (2001) Economic analysis of bleeding and thromboembolic sequelae after heartvalve replacement. *European Heart Journal* **3**(Supplement 17), Q65–Q69. doi:10.1016/S1520-765X(01)90046-X

NICE (National Institute for Health and Care Excellence) (2014) *Atrial Fibrillation and Heart Valve Disease: Self-Monitoring Coagulation Status Using Point-of-Care Coagulometers (the CoaguChek XS system and the INRatio2 PT/INR monitor).* NICE, London, UK, <https://www.nice.org.uk/guidance/dg14/resources>.

Palareti G, Leali N, Coccheri S, Poggi M, Manotti C, D'Angelo A, *et al.* (1996) Bleeding complications of oral anticoagulant treatment: an inception-cohort, prospective collaborative study (ISCOAT). *Lancet* **348**, 423–428. doi:10.1016/S0140-6736(96)01109-9

Poller L, Keown M, Ibrahim S, Lowe G, Moia M, Turpie AG, *et al.* (2008) An international multicenter randomized study of computer-assisted oral anticoagulant dosage vs. medical staff dosage. *Journal of Thrombosis and Haemostasis* **6**, 935–943. doi:10.1111/j.1538-7836.2008.02959.x

Regier DA, Sunderji R, Lynd LD, Gin K, Marra CA (2006) Cost effectiveness of self-managed versus physician managed oral anticoagulation therapy. *Canadian Medical Association Journal* **174**, 1847–1852. doi:10.1503/cmaj.051104

Sawicki PT (1999) A structured teaching and self-management program for patients receiving oral anticoagulation. A randomized controlled trial. *Journal of the American Medical Association* **281**, 145–150. doi:10.1001/jama.281.2.145

Shaw J, Harrison J, Harrison J (2014) A community pharmacist-led anticoagulation management service: attitudes towards a new collaborative model of care in New Zealand. *International Journal of Pharmacy Practice* **22**, 397–406. doi:10.1111/ijpp.12097

Sidhu P, O'Kane HO (2001) Self-managed anticoagulation: results from a two-year prospective randomized trial with heart valve patients. *The Annals of Thoracic Surgery* **72**, 1523–1527. doi:10.1016/S0003-4975(01)03049-1

SPORTIF III (Executive Steering Committee on behalf of the SPORTIF III Investigators) (2003) Stroke prevention with the oral direct thrombin inhibitor ximelagatran compared with warfarin in patients with non-valvular atrial fibrillation (SPORTIF III): randomised controlled trial. *Lancet* **362**, 1691–1698. doi:10.1016/S0140-6736(03)14841-6

Voller H, Dovifat C, Glatz J (2001) Home management of anticoagulation. *European Heart Journal Supplements* **3** (Supplement Q), Q44–Q49. doi:10.1016/S1520-765X(01)90042-2

Wan Y, Heneghan C, Perera R, Roberts N, Hollowell J, Glasziou P, *et al.* (2008) Anticoagulation control and prediction of adverse events. *Circulation: Cardiovascular Quality and Outcomes* **1**, 84–91. doi:10.1161/CIRCOUTCOMES.108.796185

WHO (World Health Organization) (1999) *Annex 3. Guidelines for Thromboplastins and Plasma Used to Control Anticoagulant Therapy.* WHO Technical Report Series. No. 889. WHO, Geneva, Switzerland.

Young L, Ockelford P, Harper P (2004) Audit of community-based anticoagulant monitoring in patients with thromboembolic disease: is frequent testing necessary? *Internal Medicine Journal* **34**, 639–641. doi:10.1111/j.1445-5994.2004.00690.x

# 14 Point-of-care testing for markers of haematology disorders

*Michelle Williamson*

**Summary**

The uptake of point-of-care testing (POCT) for haematology markers has continued to grow throughout the world due to the increasing demand to reduce turnaround times to improve patient care. Recent advances in technology have resulted in the development of numerous haematology devices designed to be used in a number of different clinical settings within hospitals and primary care facilities. This chapter will explore the clinical use and POCT devices available for measuring full blood count, platelet count, haemoglobin, white blood cells, coagulation markers (excluding INR) and D-dimer.

## FULL BLOOD COUNT

The full blood count (FBC) is one of the most commonly performed pathology tests, providing useful information on the general health of the patient. The FBC includes the measurement of the haemoglobin (Hb), white blood cell count (WBC) including three or five part white blood cell differential, platelet count, red cell count (RBC) and red cell indices. The parameters used most by clinicians include the Hb, WBC and platelet count.

The FBC is important in the diagnosis and monitoring of several different clinical conditions, some of which include:

- anaemia
- infection
- leukaemia
- drug and radiation therapy
- abnormal bleeding or clotting.

### Which POCT devices are currently on the global market?

There are several different point-of-care (POC) FBC analysers available on the market to suit different working environments such as sites inside and outside the hospital (Table 14.1) (Briggs *et al.* 2008).

FBC analysers available on the market for POCT are generally bench-top analysers weighing 15 kg or more that include all the main parameters (Hb, WBC and platelet count) for an FBC and provide either a 3- or 5-part white blood cell differential (Table 14.2). These analysers are mostly too large and heavy to be used at the patient's bedside but are found in accident and emergency departments (ED), intensive care units (ICU), outpatient departments and medical clinics (Briggs *et al.* 2012).

FBC analysers with a 5-part WBC differential provide an absolute count for all of the peripheral blood's

Table 14.1. Sites for FBC POCT

| Sites for hospital POCT | Sites for outside hospital POCT |
|---|---|
| Intensive care units | Ambulances |
| Accident and emergency departments | General practitioners and health centres |
| Operating theatres and post-operative care units | Workplaces |
| Renal dialysis units | Health-care screening clinics |
| Neonatal units | Pharmacies |
| Outpatient departments | |
| Research laboratories | |

five white cells: neutrophils, lymphocytes, monocytes, eosinophils and basophils. FBC analysers with a 3-part WBC differential generally report granulocytes (neutrophils, eosinophils and basophils), lymphocytes and monocytes (Table 14.3). One of the main advantages of the pocH-100i and XP series (Sysmex Corporation, Kobe, Japan) is that they offer an absolute count for neutrophils with their 3-part differential measurement. This is important, because the neutrophil count is one of the most important parameters most clinicians require in an after-hours scenario, along with Hb and platelets (Williams 2011).

There are also FBC analysers that include other analytes, such as the Microsemi CRP (HORIBA, Kyoto, Japan). This analyser can simultaneously measure a FBC including a 3-part white blood cell differential and C-reactive protein (CRP), a marker used to assist in the diagnosis of infection. An instrument such as this is likely to be found in emergency departments and neonatal intensive care units.

The most common sample type required for FBC analysis is venous whole blood. Several analysers are able to perform a FBC using capillary blood; however, this often requires removing the lid manually from the capillary sample tube in order to analyse the sample or making up a dilution depending on the minimum volume requirements of the analyser. Capillary blood collection has been shown to be reliable when compared with venous blood for the FBC parameters (Ponampalam *et al.* 2012). Capillary blood collection is relatively simple compared with venous blood collection because it does not require the same level of phlebotomy expertise.

In Australia, POCT for FBC is limited outside of a laboratory; however, in other countries, FBC testing at the POC is more common. In the United Kingdom (UK), there are FBC analysers in mental health units for monitoring the WBC and neutrophil counts for patients prescribed the drug Clozapine (Briggs *et al.* 2012). Another example in the UK includes the Frimley Park Hospital NHS Foundation Trust, which has eight remote bidirectional FBC analysers located in the emergency department, oncology clinics, health-care centres and satellite community hospital that is overseen by a POC team and fully complies with their accreditation body, the Clinical Pathology Accreditation (CPA) (http://www.horiba.com/fileadmin/uploads/Medical-Diagnostics/Documents/Feedback/case_study_frimley_park_hospital.pdf).

## Overview of the performance of the POCT FBC devices and current limitations/issues

Several of the POC FBC analysers listed above are used within a small laboratory or in locations overseen by laboratory staff and the performance characteristics are comparable to other haematology analysers.

It is important that the operator of any FBC analyser, including those at the POC, are given appropriate training and undergo regular competency assessment to ensure that they are able to interpret spurious or unexpected FBC results. Some manufacturers and suppliers have recognised the need for this and as a result have developed training programs, e-learning programs and online competency testing (Briggs *et al.* 2012).

Table 14.2. Bench top FBC analysers

| FBC and 5-part WBC differential | Weight (kg) | FBC and 3-part WBC differential | Weight (kg) |
|---|---|---|---|
| Sysmex XS-1000i | 24 | Sysmex pocH-100i | 14 |
| ABX Pentra 60 | 35 | Sysmex XP-300 | 28 |
| ABX Pentra 60 C+ | 35 | Sysmex XP-100 | 28 |
| Pentra ES 60 | 35 | ABX Micros ES 60 | 16 |
| Yumizen H500 | 23 | Microsemi CRP | 19 |
| | | Norma Icon | 10 |

**Table 14.3.** Three part differential analysers

| 3-part differential analysers | WBC differential |
|---|---|
| Sysmex pocH-100i | Neutrophils, lymphocytes, mixed (monocytes, eosinophils and basophils) |
| Sysmex XP-300 | Neutrophils, lymphocytes, mixed (monocytes, eosinophils and basophils) |
| Sysmex XP-100 | Neutrophils, lymphocytes, mixed (monocytes, eosinophils and basophils) |
| ABX Micros 60 | Lymphocytes, monocytes and granulocytes (neutrophils, eosinophils and basophils) |
| Norma Icon | Lymphocytes, MID cells (mid-sized cells) and granulocytes (neutrophils, eosinophils and basophils) |

### Future directions, new or emerging technologies and global trends

The FBC continues to be one of the most useful haematology markers for clinicians to use for the treatment of their patients. A growing need for affordable FBC testing at the POC has been recognised by manufacturers. Research and development continues to investigate different technologies to provide a POC FBC analyser suitable to be used by non-laboratory staff in regions where laboratory testing is unavailable or too far away to provide an effective diagnosis and treatment.

The ultimate FBC analyser for use at the POC would include the following features:

- FBC including a 5-part differential
- portable
- easy to use
- maintenance free
- robust
- small sample volume – includes capillary collection
- fast
- cost effective
- performance characteristics of a laboratory analyser
- data management system – includes operator and patient identification and connectivity.

A POC FBC analyser not yet commercially available with several of the features listed above is the HemoScreen (Pixcell Medical Technologies, Israel) (Fig. 14.1). This analyser includes a 5-part white blood cell differential performed on a finger stick blood collection using a single-use cartridge. It is currently undergoing clinical validation studies and the first model has been approved by the European regulatory authority in June 2013. It is expected to be commercially available by the end of 2016.

In the USA, a team of engineers has demonstrated that a mobile phone attached to a portable imaging cytometry platform can measure red and white blood cells and Hb (Zhu *et al.* 2013). A minimum sample of 10 µL is required for the test, which can be collected via a venous or finger-stick sample. Fluorescent and bright-field images of blood samples are captured using separate optical attachments to the mobile phone. The images are rapidly processed through a custom-developed smart application running on the phone to perform the analysis. Results obtained for the red and white blood cells and Hb were comparable to a standard bench-top haematology analyser.

The mobile phone is an ideal platform to develop diagnostic tests, especially at the POC, due to the rapid advancement in mobile phone technology, widespread connectivity of the existing wireless telecommunication infrastructure and the massive volume of mobile phone users (Zhu *et al.* 2013). It is likely that mobile phone technology will continue to advance to a level where it will be routinely used for supporting diagnostic tests in developing countries due to its cost effectiveness and ease of use.

## PLATELET COUNT

Platelets, also called thrombocytes, are blood cell fragments that are required to form part of a clot to prevent bleeding if a blood vessel is damaged. The platelet count is a diagnostic test that determines the number of platelets in a patient's blood, with the normal range for platelets in adults being 150–400 × $10^9$/L. The platelet count is an important marker in both the diagnosis and monitoring of several disease states that may affect the process of blood clotting. A decrease in platelet numbers is called thrombocytopenia and is often associated with bleeding disorders. An increase in platelets is called thrombocytosis and can indicate disorders of the bone marrow. There are several causes of an abnormal platelet count (Table 14.4).

In developing countries where viral infections such as dengue fever, malaria and HIV are common, it can be difficult to obtain a platelet count due to the expense of a FBC analyser. In these regions, the platelet count is

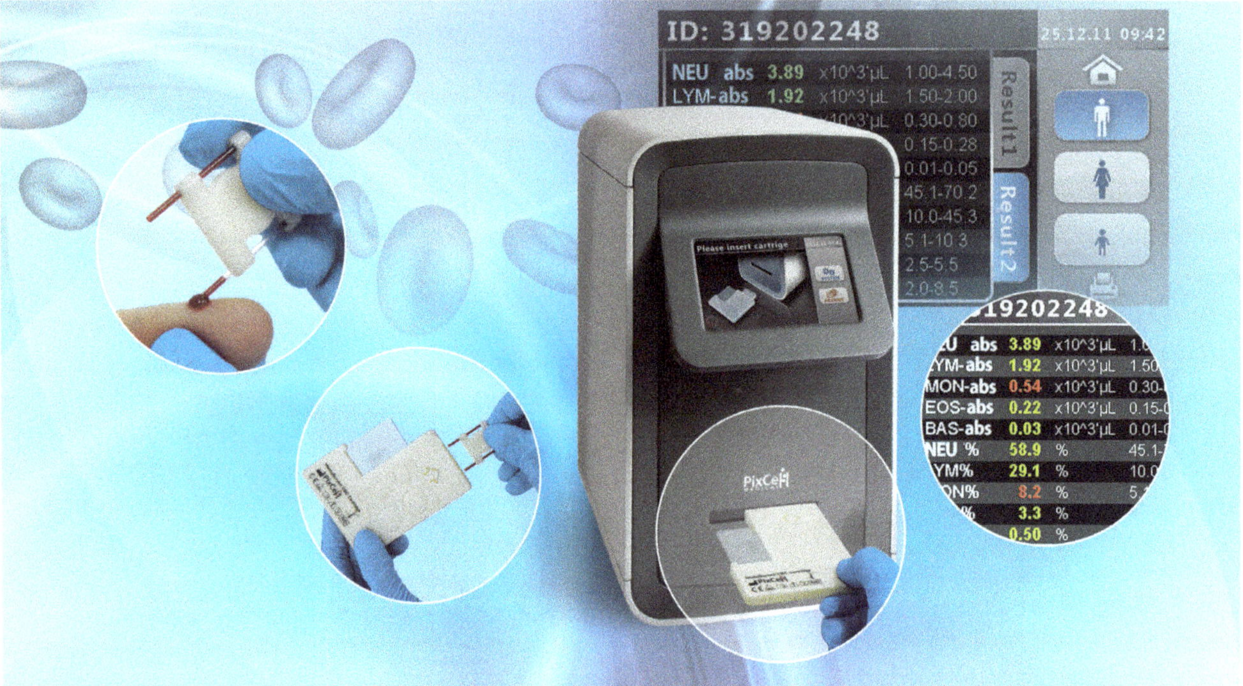


Fig. 14.1. HemoScreen FBC analyser.

typically performed manually, which is labour intensive and requires an experienced laboratory technician.

## Which POCT devices are currently on the global market?

There are four main method principles used in obtaining a platelet count: manual phase contrast microscopy, impedance, optical light scatter/fluorescence and flow cytometry (Briggs *et al.* 2007).

The manual methods include the direct platelet count using a counting chamber (haemocytometer) and the indirect method where the platelet count is determined by using a blood film. The manual methods are time-consuming and there is in an increased risk of obtaining an inaccurate result due to several variables including incorrect dilution of sample and platelet clumping (Briggs *et al.* 2007). The FBC analysers currently on the market employ one or two of the other principles to determine the platelet count.

Currently there is no standalone POC device available commercially that measures the platelet count only. An analyser available that measures and monitors platelet function that also includes a platelet count is the ICHOR®II Analyzer (Helena Laboratories) used with Plateletworks reagents. This analyser provides the basic haematology parameters including RBC, WBC, Hb,

Table 14.4. Causes of an abnormal platelet count

| Thrombocytopenia | Thrombocytosis |
|---|---|
| Viral infection | Iron deficiency anaemia |
| Bone marrow disorders | Haemolytic anaemia |
| Drugs | Absence of a spleen |
| Autoimmune disorders | Cancer |
| Liver disease | Inflammatory or infectious diseases |
| Sepsis | Acute bleeding and blood loss |
| Platelet consumption – disseminated intravascular coagulation, thrombotic thrombocytopenia purpura (TTP) and haemolytic uraemic syndrome (HUS) | Myeloproliferative neoplasms |

mean cell volume (MCV), mean cell haemoglobin (MCH), mean cell haemoglobin concentration (MCHC) and platelet count. Platelet function devices will be discussed in more detail in the coagulation section of the chapter.

### Overview of the performance of POCT devices for platelet count and current limitations/issues

There are limitations to the measurement of the platelet count regardless of whether it is automated or manual. Several factors can influence the accuracy of the platelet count. A falsely low platelet count can be caused by poor or difficult venepuncture and overfilling of the sample tube. One of the primary causes for a falsely high platelet count is due to the presence of fragmented red cells or severe microcytosis (small RBCs) and it can also occur when there is bacterial overgrowth in the blood. Most analysers will generate a flag or a warning indicating an erroneous result. Samples with unexpected counts in relation to the clinical setting or those that generate specific flags require additional investigation.

### Future directions, new or emerging technologies and global trends

Due to the expense and difficulty in obtaining an accurate platelet count in developing countries, potential solutions are being developed to tackle this problem. A team in Indonesia is currently developing an automated platelet counter for resource poor settings to replace the manual platelet count. Software is being developed to analyse images of the blood to obtain an accurate platelet count. The technology is based on a conventional microscope equipped with a digital camera linked to a personal computer, which can capture and analyse microscope images of blood samples (Lazuardi *et al.* 2013).

## HAEMOGLOBIN

Haemoglobin (Hb) is responsible for transporting oxygen from the lungs to the rest of the body and is an important clinical parameter for assessing anaemia in both chronic and acute conditions. Anaemia can be defined as a low blood concentration of Hb. The World Health Organization publication: *Haemoglobin Concentrations for the Diagnosis of Anaemia and Assessment of Severity* (WHO 2011) provides the definition of mild to severe anaemia (Table 14.5).

In 2008, the WHO published the *Worldwide Prevalence of Anaemia 1993–2005*, estimating that anaemia affects 1.62 billion people (95% CI: 1.50–1.74 billion) (WHO 2008). In 2015, the WHO published *The Global Prevalence of Anaemia in 2011*, which describes the prevalence of anaemia for the year 2011 in preschool-age children (6–59 months) and women of reproductive age (15–49 years). This document estimates anaemia affects around 29% (496 million) of non-pregnant women and 38% (32.4 million) of pregnant women globally. The prevalence of anaemia was highest in south Asia and central and west Africa. The most common cause of anaemia is iron deficiency due to poor nutrition (Table 14.6).

Anaemia is a widespread public health issue that affects low, middle and high income earners and has significant adverse health consequences, as well as adverse impacts on social and economic development (WHO 2015). In 2012, the World Health Assembly set a target of a 50% reduction of anaemia in women of reproductive age by 2025 (WHO 2014). The WHO *Global Nutrition Targets 2025: Anaemia Policy Brief* provides a framework for action. Globally, the prevalence of anaemia fell by 12% between 1995 and 2011; from 33 to 29% in non-pregnant women and from 43 to 38% in pregnant women,

**Table 14.5.** Haemoglobin levels (g/L) to diagnose anaemia at sea level

| | | Anaemia | | |
|---|---|---|---|---|
| **Population** | **Non-anaemia** | **Mild** | **Moderate** | **Severe** |
| Children aged 6–59 months | 110 or higher | 100–109 | 70–99 | lower than 70 |
| Children aged 5–11 years | 115 or higher | 110–114 | 80–109 | lower than 80 |
| Children aged 12–14 years | 120 or higher | 110–119 | 80–109 | lower than 80 |
| Non-pregnant women (aged 15 years and above) | 120 or higher | 110–119 | 80–109 | lower than 80 |
| Pregnant women | 110 or higher | 100–109 | 70–90 | lower than 70 |
| Men (aged 15 years and above) | 130 or higher | 110–129 | 80–109 | lower than 80 |

**Table 14.6.** Common causes of anaemia

| Common causes of anaemia |
|---|
| Nutritional deficiencies (iron, folate, riboflavin, vitamin A and B12) |
| Loss of blood (traumatic injury, surgery, bleeding, colon cancer) |
| Acute and chronic infections (malaria, tuberculosis, dengue fever, HIV) |
| Bone marrow problems (replacement of bone marrow by cancer) |
| Suppression by chemotherapy drugs |
| Kidney failure |
| Parasitic infections (hookworm, ascaris and schistosomiasis) |
| Abnormal haemoglobin (sickle cell anaemia) |

indicating that it is possible to reduce prevalence. However, urgent action is required to reach the 2025 target. Guidelines for the prevention, control and treatment of anaemia in women of reproductive age have been developed by the WHO to assist countries reaching the target (*WHO Guidelines on Nutrition*; http://www.who.int/publications/guidelines/nutrition/en/).

## Which POCT devices are currently on the global market?

Hb is the most common haematology marker used to diagnose and monitor anaemia at the POC (Briggs *et al.* 2012). Hb POC devices, also commonly referred to as haemoglobinometers, are used in several different settings as described in Table 14.1. They are also commonly used in blood collection sites to screen potential blood donors.

In 1995, the development of the haemoglobin colour scale (HbCS) began in response to the recognised need for a simple, rapid and cheap method for estimating Hb that could be used on a fingerstick collection and in situations where there was no laboratory and where the diagnosis of anaemia relied on clinical symptoms. The HbCS became commercially available in 2001 and is commonly used in the developing world (WHO 2004). The method is based on comparing the colour of a drop of blood absorbed onto special filter paper against a standardised colour scale provided on a laminated card in increments of 2 g/dL. Due to the nature of this method, the results can be quite subjective.

In 2008, the International Council for Standardization in Haematology (ICSH) in conjunction with Eurotrol, B.V. (https://eurotrol.com/) released a new lot of the haemiglobincyanide (HiCN) standard. This standard is used for the standardisation and calibration of both laboratory based FBC analysers and POC instruments (Davis and Jungerius 2010).

There are several POC devices for measuring Hb that are affordable, portable and easy to use with some factory calibrated using the ICSH HiCN standard (Table 14.7).

The most commonly used and extensively studied POC Hb device is the HemoCue® (Radiometer), a small handheld device used in many different clinical settings (Sireci 2015). There are three different models of the HemoCue available: the older versions, HemoCue Hb201$^{+}$ and HemoCue Hb201 DM, are based on an azidemethaemoglobin reaction similar to the ICSH reference method and the newer version, HemoCue Hb301, which has been calibrated against the ICSH HiCN standard.

The DiaSpect Tm (DiaSpect Medical GmbH, Sailauf, Germany) POC device provides a Hb result in under 2 s and is factory calibrated against the ICSH HiCN standard. One of the main advantages of this Hb device is that the microcuvettes are unaffected by moisture or temperature and can be used until expiration date after opening the reagent bag. Also, the microcuvettes have a long shelf life of 2.5 years from the date of production. This device is used widely in humid countries such as Indonesia, India and Malaysia.

Other devices used at the POC to obtain an Hb include bench-top and handheld blood gas machines commonly located in ICUs, EDs and operating theatres, with the method of measurement based on either conductivity or spectrophotometry. Examples of devices that employ conductivity as the method for determining the Hb include the Abbott i-STAT® (Abbott Laboratories, Abbott Park, Illinois PA, USA) and the Alere epoc® Blood Analysis System (Alere, Waltham MA, USA). These devices do not measure Hb directly but rather calculate it from the haematocrit.

Non-invasive methods are now available to measure the Hb; these include the NBM 200 and NBM 200MP monitors (OrSense, Nes Ziona, Israel), which take optical measurements after temporary blood flow occlusion using a pneumatic finger cuff. The devices are approved for use in both the European and US market, but they are not yet commercially available in Australia. The advantages of this method include cost reduction, speed, eliminating the risk of infection and improved patient comfort. The NBM 200MP continuously measures multiple blood parameters,

Table 14.7. Examples of haemoglobinometers

| Device | Measuring range (g/L) | Test time (s) | Method principle |
|---|---|---|---|
| HemoCue Hb201+ | 0–256 | <60 | Photometric |
| HemoCue Hb301 | 0–256 | <10 | Photometric |
| DiaSpect Tm | 30–255 | <2 | Photometric |
| DiaSpect Haemoglobin T Low | 0.3–30 | <2 | Photometric |
| HemoControl | 0–256 | 25 | Photometric |
| BeneCheck | 70–260 | 10 | Electrochemistry |
| CERA-CHECK Hb Plus | 20–260 | <5 | Electrochemistry |
| Hemochroma PLUS | 0–270 | 3 | Absorptiometry |
| URIT-12 | 40–240 | <10 | Optical Reflectance |

including Hb levels, oxygen saturation of Hb ($SpO_2$), low perfusion oximetry, pulse rate and plethysmogram.

### Overview of the performance of POCT Hb devices and current limitations/issues

There have been several publications about haemoglobinometers, particularly the HemoCue. Overall, studies comparing the HemoCue systems with laboratory systems have shown acceptable agreement with laboratory-based haemoglobin measurements in a variety of clinical settings; however, some studies have shown significant bias with standard laboratory analysers (Sireci 2015).

The conductivity methods do provide an accurate haematocrit (Hct) result in normal subjects; however, results can be erroneously high or low during haemodilution or the alteration of plasma proteins, electrolytes or triglycerides (Briggs *et al.* 2012). Hb results from instruments such as these should be interpreted with caution, particularly those based in operating theatres and intensive care units where physiological changes in the patients are more likely.

Devices such as the non-invasive NMB 200 product range are commonly used in blood collection centres to screen potential blood donors. Although the non-invasive method has significant advantages over other haemoglobinometers, it does have disadvantages as well, particularly accuracy and precision when compared with other haemoglobinometers. Abhay Singh *et al.* completed a study in 2015 evaluating various methods of POC testing in blood donors and compared the NBM 200, DiaSpect and HemoControl (EKF diagnostic GmbH) to the laboratory analyser KX-21 (Sysmex, Kobe, Japan). The NBM 200 was found to be unsuitable when compared with the other haemoglobinometers due to its lack of desired sensitivity (71.7%) (Singh *et al.* 2015). However, in another study the non-invasive method was determined to be a reasonable first line approach for pre-donation Hb screening but a second method should be available to re-test those with Hb levels below the acceptable donor cut-off level of 125 g/L for females and 135 g/L for males (Sümnig *et al.* 2015).

Hb results performed on haemoglobinometers should be reviewed with caution, particularly when the results determine the decision to transfuse blood. The results should be considered in association with the patient's clinical presentation. If it is not consistent with the patient symptoms, then an Hb should be performed in a laboratory to confirm the POC result.

### Future directions, new or emerging technologies and global trends

The relatively new non-invasive method for measuring Hb is promising. These devices have been used across the world for several years and offer a simple, non-invasive, portable and an easily operable system that does not require the services of experienced or skilled staff (Kumar and Ranganathan 2013). Non-invasive devices are likely to become a more popular choice, particularly in blood donor screening areas and developing countries where cost is a major factor.

## WHITE BLOOD CELL COUNT

The WBC count is a diagnostic test that determines the number of white blood cells in a patient's blood. The normal range for the WBC in adults is 4.00–11.00 × $10^9$/L. There are five different types of WBCs in the peripheral blood: neutrophils, lymphocytes, monocytes, eosinophils and basophils (Table 14.8).

**Table 14.8.** White blood cell reference ranges

| White blood cell | Reference range (×10$^9$/L) | High count | Low count |
|---|---|---|---|
| Neutrophil | 2.0–7.0 | Neutrophilia | Neutropenia |
| Lymphocyte | 1.5–4.0 | Lymphocytosis | Lymphopenia |
| Monocyte | 0.2–0.8 | Monocytosis | Monocytopenia |
| Eosinophil | 0–0.45 | Eosinophilia | |
| Basophil | 0–0.2 | Basophilia | |

WBCs, also known as leucocytes, are cells of the immune system that fight foreign bodies and infection. A low WBC count is termed leucopenia and is often associated with bone marrow deficiency, certain viral infections and severe bacterial infection. An elevated WBC count, also referred to as leucocytosis, is usually caused by bacterial infections, tissue damage and inflammatory diseases (Zhang *et al.* 2015). The WBC count and differential is an important test in the diagnosis, treatment and monitoring of the disease states listed in Table 14.9.

## Which POCT devices are currently on the global market?

In poorly resourced regions where FBC analysers are unavailable, WBC counts and differentials are performed using a manual method. The WBC count is performed by dispensing a measured amount of diluted blood into a counting chamber (haemocytometer) where the WBCs are counted using the gridlines of the haemocytometer as a guide. The WBC differential is performed on a stained blood film under a microscope and the sub-types calculated. This technique is time consuming, labour intensive and requires a high level of training (Majors *et al.* 2014).

**Table 14.9.** Causes of leucopenia and leucocytosis

| Leucopenia | Leucocytosis |
|---|---|
| Viral infections | Infection |
| Chemotherapy | Inflammation: burns, tissue necrosis |
| Leukaemia | Stress |
| Malnutrition | Drugs |
| Parasitic diseases | Trauma: splenectomy |
| Medications | Haemolytic anaemia |
| AIDS | Acute leukaemia |
| Aplastic anaemia | Chronic leukaemia |
| Myelodysplastic syndromes | Myeloproliferative disorders |

The development of POC devices that measure the WBC count has been quite slow when compared with other POC devices such as the haemoglobinometers (Briggs *et al.* 2012). In 2008, the HemoCue® WBC (Radiometer) was introduced onto the market. This was closely followed by the HemoCue® WBC Diff (Radiometer) (Fig. 14.2). The HemoCue WBC provides an absolute WBC count as opposed to the HemoCue WBC Diff, which provides both an absolute WBC count and a 5-part differential.

The HemoCue system employs imaging analysis to count the white blood cells and perform the 5-part differential (HemoCue WBC DIFF system). The system requires ~10 µL of capillary or venous EDTA blood and provides a result in 3 min for the HemoCue WBC and within 5 min for the HemoCue WBC DIFF. The measuring range for WBC for both systems are 0.3–30.0 × 10$^9$/L and results lower than 0.3 (LLL) or greater than 30.0 (HHH) are flagged.

## Overview of the performance of POCT devices for WBC count and current limitations/issues

The HemoCue WBC provides a simple method to obtain reliable measurements with an accuracy that is comparable to that of a standardised reference analyser. It is a suitable alternative to a FBC analyser in a clinical setting where an analyser is not available, such as medical clinics in remote or rural locations and developing countries. Inaccurate WBC readings may result in the presence of significant numbers of reticulocytes or normoblasts (immature red blood cells) where they will be counted as white blood cells, resulting in an erroneously high WBC count (Osei-Bimpong *et al.* 2009).

The analytical performance characteristics and usefulness of the HemoCue WBC DIFF was evaluated in a remote Aboriginal medical service, where access to pathology services is difficult due to the location (Spaeth *et al.* 2015). A venous sample was collected and sent to a laboratory for analysis on the Sysmex XE-2100. A fingerstick sample was also collected at the same time and tested on the HemoCue WBC DIFF. The study established that the HemoCue WBC DIFF was user-friendly and demonstrated sound analytical performance characteristics for total WBC and differential (except for monocytes), making it a useful device for POCT in regions with limited access to a laboratory service.

### Future directions, new or emerging technologies and global trends

There is a recognised need for an affordable WBC count, particularly in developing countries. As a result, several new technologies are under development. A group in Singapore is developing a disposable device that semi-quantifies WBCs via a paper-based vertical flow platform (Zhang *et al.* 2015). They were able to differentiate an abnormal WBC count from a normal WBC count in 15 μL of blood by visualising the intensity of the test spot. According to the authors, the proposed platform shows great promise and with several improvements it has the potential to provide a quick, simple and cheap alternative for poorly resourced regions.

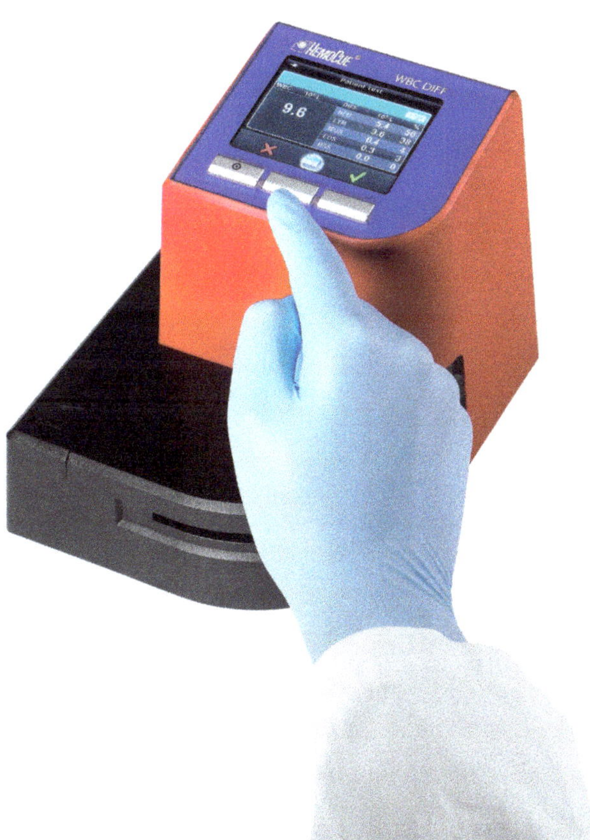


**Fig. 14.2.** The HemoCue WBC DIFF point-of-care device.

Another new technology in development is a disposable cartridge and image analysis algorithm that can be used with a single drop of blood and returns a WBC count and a 3-part differential in under 5 min (Majors *et al.* 2014). The cartridge is composed of a glass slide, a layer of transfer tape and a glass coverslip and incorporates acridine orange for cell staining and cell differentiation. A portable microscope has been designed and is currently in the prototype phase. This method would be suitable for low-resource regions that do not have access to trained technicians or expensive FBC analysers and will allow clinicians to perform a WBC count and differential at the POC.

There are other methods being developed, as described in the FBC section, where the mobile phone is being used to count blood cells and determining haemoglobin intensity. Considerable investment is being made by several research and development groups to create a device that will provide a cost-effective solution for developing countries with little or no access to a laboratory service.

## COAGULATION

Haemostasis is the process by which loss of blood is stopped after an injury. Abnormalities in haemostasis can result in bleeding or blood clots. Coagulation testing is important in monitoring the haemostatic status of the patient.

A standard coagulation profile, generally performed in the laboratory, includes the prothrombin time (PT) and internationalised normal ratio (INR), activated partial thromboplastin time (APTT), platelets and fibrinogen; however, this does not cover all causes of bleeding tendencies.

There are several different clinical settings where coagulation at the POC occurs including operating theatres, catheterisation laboratories and cardiac theatres, ICUs, EDs, renal clinics and extracorporeal membrane oxygenation (ECMO) sites. The tests available on POC instruments are listed in Table 14.10.

The PT/INR test is the subject of a separate chapter in this book (Chapter 13).

The APTT is a test used as part of a screen to assess the overall haemostasis of a patient and to monitor heparin therapy. It is one of the most commonly requested coagulation tests along with the PT/INR. The APTT is widely used in general wards perioperatively in patients at high risk of thromboembolism who are on prophylactic heparin. The ACT is more commonly performed at the POC

**Table 14.10.** Coagulation tests available at the point of care

| POC tests available |
|---|
| Prothrombin time (PT) |
| Internationalised normalised ratio (INR) |
| Activated partial thromboplastin time (APTT) |
| Activated clotting time (ACT) |
| Platelet function |
| D-dimer |
| Viscoelastic methods:<br>– Thromboelastography (TEG®)<br>– Rotational Thromboelastometry (ROTEM®) |

than in the laboratory and is used to guide high-dose anticoagulation with heparin in patients during cardiopulmonary bypass (CPB), ECMO and haemodialysis.

Platelet function is commonly determined at the POC, with a variety of devices available. These devices are used to detect platelet dysfunction or inhibition and to evaluate the effect of antiplatelet medications. Globally, the PFA-100 is the most common primary haemostasis screening instrument and has recently upgraded to the INNOVANCE® PFA-200 system (Siemens Healthcare, Marburg, Germany) (Favaloro and Bonar 2014).

Viscoelastic tests provide rapid information about global clotting in whole blood with a graphical display of clot development, stabilisation and dissolution that reflects *in vivo* haemostasis. They are widely used in the setting of liver transplants, cardiac surgery, trauma and obstetrics. The two devices most commonly used are thromboelastography (TEG®; Hemonetics Corporation, Braintree AM, USA) and rotational thromboelastometry (ROTEM®; TEM International GmbH, Munich, Germany). The use of viscoelastic tests has been shown to reduce overall transfusion requirements because it allows for specific treatment based on individual needs, resulting in minimal haemostatic intervention (Mallett and Armstrong 2015).

## Which POCT devices are currently on the global market?

Some POC devices that perform APTT, ACT or platelet function tests are listed in Tables 14.11 and 14.12.

## Overview of the performance of POCT coagulation devices and current limitations/issues

There are several publications on coagulation tests at the POC. One of the common issues identified was comparing results from POC devices with laboratory instruments largely due to the different sample types and methodology. POC coagulation tests are generally performed with whole blood, as opposed to citrate plasma used on laboratory testing platforms.

Quality control of POC coagulation devices is often difficult due to the lack of QC material (e.g. PFA-100) or it is overlooked/neglected by the end user. It is important that there is a quality management system in place that incorporates sample collection, the analytical process and the interpretation of the data presented.

## Future directions, new or emerging technologies and global trends

Evidence is growing that POC coagulation tests result in fewer transfusions, improved patient outcomes and reduced hospital costs (Mallett and Armstrong 2015). Several sites are incorporating POC coagulation testing into their patient blood management (PBM) protocols.

A recent study completed at The Prince Charles Hospital, Brisbane, Australia focussed on the POC coagulation testing component of a bleeding management treatment protocol in detecting, managing and monitoring critical bleeding in cardiac surgery patients (Pearse *et al.* 2015). A ROTEM and Multiplate analyser were placed in a laboratory adjacent to the cardiac OT and ICU with results streamed live to the appropriate OT or ICU. The 12-month study demonstrated POCT improved patient

**Table 14.11.** POC devices for APTT and ACT

| APTT and ACT POC devices | POC tests measured | Manufacturer |
|---|---|---|
| GEM PCL | PT, APTT, ACT-LR, ACT and Citrate PT | Instrumentation Laboratory |
| Hemochron® Signature Elite | ACT+, ACT-LR, PT, Citrate PT, APTT, and Citrate APTT | Accriva Diagnostics |
| Hemochron® Response | ACT | Accriva Diagnostics |
| i-STAT | ACT | Abbott Point of Care |
| ACT Plus® System | ACT | Medtronic |
| Actalyke® XL | ACT | Helena Laboratories |

Table 14.12. POC devices for platelet function

| Platelet function POC devices | Manufacturer |
|---|---|
| ICHOR Haematology Analyzer with Plateletworks reagents | Helena Laboratories, Beaumont TX, USA |
| PFA-100® System | Siemens Healthcare Diagnostics, Deerfield IL, USA |
| INNOVANCE® PFA-200 System | Siemens Healthcare Diagnostics, Deerfield IL, USA |
| Multiplate® Analyzer | Roche Diagnostics, Indianapolis IN, USA |
| VerifyNow | Accumetrics, San Diego CA, USA |

outcomes through the significant reduction in blood transfusion, cost savings, increased awareness of the need for a PBM program, adoption of bleeding management supported by POC coagulation testing into orthopaedic surgery, general surgery and general ICU and the implementation of anaemia management for all patients.

Coagulation at the POC can improve haemostatic management and reduce overall transfusion rates when compared with standard management (Mallett and Armstrong 2015). It is likely that more sites will continue to adopt POC coagulation testing and incorporate it into their PBM protocol, particularly due to the need to reduce unnecessary blood and blood product transfusions, reduce costs and improve patient outcomes.

## D-DIMER

D-dimer is a small protein fragment produced by the breakdown of a blood clot (fibrinolysis) in the body. D-dimers are present in small quantities in the blood in most healthy individuals; increased levels in the blood indicate increased clotting activity in the blood (Table 14.13). The D-dimer test is most commonly used in EDs to rule out the possibility of a deep vein thrombosis (DVT) or pulmonary embolism (PE). D-dimer is used in conjunction with various other clinical diagnostic algorithms including the widely used Wells Score. The Wells Score is calculated by completing an assessment of the patient's clinical features for PE and DVT. There are two Wells Score clinical prediction rules – one for DVT and one for PE – with the final score predicting the probability of PE and DVT. A negative D-dimer test when applying the Wells score always demonstrates the absence of thrombosis and PE (Fries and Streif 2015).

The D-dimer is also used to diagnose and monitor treatment for patients with disseminated intravascular coagulation (DIC), a serious or even life threatening condition caused by abnormal activation of blood clotting mechanisms. In ICUs, patients tend to have very high D-dimer levels due to the nature of their clinical situation, such as surgical trauma, infection, sepsis or other history or underlying conditions (Fries and Streif 2015). Decreasing levels of D-dimer in patients with DIC indicate that treatment is effective while an increasing level may indicate that treatment is not working.

### Which POCT devices are currently on the global market?

Quantitative and qualitative D-dimer assays are available for use at the POC. There are several testing platforms available to measure the D-dimer, which include small bench-top analysers, portable meters and rapid test strips (Table 14.14). The small bench-top analysers and portable meters also perform several other assays considered

Table 14.13. Causes for elevated D-dimer level

| Causes for elevated D-dimer levels | |
|---|---|
| Deep vein thrombosis | Surgery |
| Pulmonary embolism | Infection |
| Disseminated intravascular coagulation | Pregnancy |
| Acute myocardial infarction | Inflammation |
| Atherosclerosis | Age |
| Trauma | Cancer |
| Hepatic disease | Thrombolytic therapy |
| Sepsis | |

urgent in the emergency care setting such as cardiac markers. Cardiac markers are often included to assist in the differential diagnosis of patients with a suspected DVT or PE.

### Overview of the performance of POCT D-dimer devices and current limitations/issues

Several studies have been undertaken to compare the accuracy and precision of POC D-dimer devices. One study comparing five POC D-dimer devices used for the exclusion of a clinically suspected DVT showed negative predictive values higher than 98% for all devices, demonstrating that they have good performance characteristics to aid in safe and cost-effective exclusion of DVTs (Geersing *et al.* 2010).

The introduction of the D-dimer test at the POC requires careful consideration. Poor standardisation among D-dimer assays necessitates clinical validation before implementation (Oude Elferink *et al.* 2015). It is essential that cut-off values for the exclusion of DVT have been established for the specific method selected in a comprehensive evaluation (Perry *et al.* 2010). The values on a POC D-dimer device may not align perfectly with the laboratory D-dimer, which could potentially create confusion in the interpretation of the result. It is essential that appropriate training is provided in both the operation of the device and the interpretation of the results.

### Future directions, new or emerging technologies and global trends

Overcrowding in EDs is a common problem, resulting in new strategies being developed to minimise the patient's length of stay. As new POC tests become available, there is an increasing opportunity to implement rapid testing to improve turnaround time in EDs. A US-based study evaluated the impact of implementing a rapid whole blood quantitative D-dimer test in an ED and found there was significant decrease in the mean and median ED length of stay (Lee-Lewandrowski *et al.* 2009).

Considering most patients present to their treating medical practitioner before going to hospital, primary care is becoming an ideal setting to introduce a D-dimer test at the POC. Excluding a DVT at the primary care setting would in many cases eliminate the need for referrals to central laboratories or diagnostic services (Geersing *et al.* 2010).

## EXAMPLE OF A WORKING MODEL FOR POC TESTING FOR HAEMOGLOBIN

*POCT for haemoglobin: an effective approach to develop social responsibility and address iron deficiency anaemia in women and children of rural Pakistan. Synopsis prepared by Professor Mark Shephard (Flinders University) and Dr Rukhsana Ayub (Associate Professor and Head of Department, Health Professions Education, Al Nafees College and Hospital, Islamabad, Pakistan).*

Anaemia is a major public health problem with a particularly high prevalence in developing countries. Estimates of the prevalence of anaemia in Pakistan vary somewhat. Through a global collaboration between the Al Nafees Medical College in Pakistan, the Flinders University International Centre for Point-of-Care Testing in Australia and the Begum Mehmooda Welfare Trust of Pakistan, a study was undertaken in 2014 to identify the rates of anaemia in a small mountain community of Haripur in rural Pakistan. The study incorporated POCT

**Table 14.14.** D-dimer POCT devices

| D-dimer POCT devices | Testing platform | Assay |
|---|---|---|
| PATHFAST™ | Small bench-top analyser | Quantitative |
| VIDAS® | Small bench-top analyser | Quantitative |
| AQT90 FLEX | Small bench-top analyser | Quantitative |
| Stratus®CS 200 Acute Cardiac™ Care | Small bench-top analyser | Quantitative |
| Alere Triage®MeterPro | Portable meter | Quantitative |
| Roche Cardiac Reader | Portable meter | Quantitative |
| Roche Cobas®h 232 POC System | Portable meter | Quantitative |
| Alere Nycocard™ Reader II | Portable meter | Quantitative |
| Clearview Simplify® | Rapid test | Qualitative |

for haemoglobin to detect anaemia, health education and promotion, and was also interwoven with a service-learning program designed to promote social responsibility in undergraduate medical students.

Undergraduate medical students and community workers were trained and certified to conduct POCT for haemoglobin on the HemoCue Hb301 device. Women and children from the community had their haemoglobin levels tested and those who were diagnosed with anaemia were given immediate treatment with either dietary iron supplementation and/or deworming medication (mebendazole). An education campaign was also delivered to the participants of the study. Haemoglobin levels were tested again at 8 weeks post-intervention.

Initial POCT screening for haemoglobin found that 52.9% of women and 46.9% of children tested were classified as anaemic (Hb <120 g/L). The average haemoglobin concentration increased significantly post-intervention both in women (by an average of 12 g/L) and in children (by an average of 10 g/L) (paired $t$-test: $t = 7.9$ and 5.6, $P$ <0.001 and <0.001, respectively).

The program significantly increased the number of haemoglobin tests conducted in the community. Rates of anaemia were found to be higher (in women) and lower (in children) than the current WHO estimates for rural Pakistan. POCT enabled immediate treatment of anaemia and the undergraduate medical students experienced involvement in community health interventions, which contributed to their learning.

## REFERENCES


Briggs C, Harrison P, Machin A (2007) Continuing developments with the automated platelet count. *International Journal of Laboratory Hematology* **29**, 77–91. doi:10.1111/j.1751-553X.2007.00909.x

Briggs C, Carter J, Lee S-H, Sandhaus R, Simon-Lopez R, Corrons V (2008) ICSH Guideline for worldwide point-of-care testing in haematology with special reference to the complete blood count. *International Journal of Laboratory Hematology* **30**, 105–116. doi:10.1111/j.1751-553X.2008.01050.x

Briggs C, Kimber S, Green I (2012) Where are we at with point-of-care testing in haematology? *British Journal of Haematology* **158**, 679–690. doi:10.1111/j.1365-2141.2012.09207.x

Davis B, Jungerius B (2010) International Council for Standardization in Haematology technical report 1-2009: new reference material for haemiglobincyanide for use in standardization of blood haemoglobin measurements. *International Journal of Laboratory Hematology* **32**, 139–141. doi:10.1111/j.1751-553X.2009.01196.x

Fries D, Streif W (2015) Point-of-care testing in critically ill patients. *Seminars in Thrombosis and Hemostasis* **41**, 75–83. doi:10.1055/s-0035-1544184

Favaloro E, Bonar R (2014) External quality assessment/proficiency testing and internal quality control for the PFA-100 and PFA-200: an update. *Seminars in Thrombosis and Hemostasis* **40**, 239–253. doi:10.1055/s-0034-1365844

Geersing G, Toll D, Hanssen K, Oudega R, Blikman M, Wijland R, *et al.* (2010) Diagnostic accuracy and user-friendliness of 5 point-of-care D-dimer tests for the exclusion of deep vein thrombosis. *Clinical Chemistry* **56**, 1758–1766. doi:10.1373/clinchem.2010.147892

Kumar R, Ranganathan H (2013) Noninvasive sensor technology for total hemoglobin measurement in blood. *Journal of Industrial and Intelligent Information* **1**, 243–246. doi:10.12720/jiii.1.4.243-246

Lazuardi L, Sanjaya G, Candradewi I, Holmner A (2013) Automatic platelets counter for supporting dengue case detection in primary health care in Indonesia. *Studies in Health Technology and Informatics* **192**, 585–588.

Lee-Lewandrowski W, Nichols J, Van Cott E, Grisson R, Louissaint A, Benzer T, *et al.* (2009) Implementation of a rapid whole blood D-dimer test in the emergency department of an urban academic medical centre. *American Journal of Clinical Pathology* **132**, 326–331. doi:10.1309/AJCP6US3ILGEAREE

Majors C, Pawlowski M, Tkaczyk T, Richards-Kortum R (2014) Low-cost disposable cartridge for performing a white blood cell count and partial differential at the point-of-care. In *Health Innovations and Point of Care Technologies Conference.* 8–10 October, Seattle WA, USA. p. 10–13. Institute of Electrical and Electronics Engineers: Engineering in Medicine and Biology Society, Piscataway NJ, USA.

Mallett S, Armstrong M (2015) Point-of-care monitoring of haemostasis. *Anaesthesia* **70**(Supplement 1), 73–77. doi:10.1111/anae.12909

Osei-Bimpong A, Jury C, McLean R, Lewis S (2009) Point-of-care method for total white cell count: an evaluation of the HemoCue WBC device. *International Journal of Laboratory Hematology* **31**, 657–664. doi:10.1111/j.1751-553X.2008.01093.x

Oude Elferink RF, Loot AE, Van De Klashorst CG, Hulsebos-Huygen M, Piersma-Wichers M, Oudega R (2015) Clinical evaluation of eight different D-dimer tests for the exclusion of deep vein thrombosis in primary care patients. *Scandinavian Journal of Clinical and Laboratory Investigation* **75**, 230–238. doi:10.3109/00365513.2014.993697

Pearse BL, Smith I, Faulke D, Wall D, Fraser JF, Ryan EG, *et al.* (2015) Protocol guided bleeding management improves cardiac surgery patient outcomes. *Vox Sanguinis* **109**, 267–279. doi:10.1111/vox.12279

Perry D, Fitzmaurice D, Kitchen S, Mackie I, Mallett S (2010) Point-of-care testing in haemostasis. *British Journal of Haematology* **150**, 501–514. doi:10.1111/j.1365-2141.2010.08223.x

Ponampalam R, Chong S, Tan S (2012) Comparison of full blood count parameters using capillary and venous samples in patients presenting to the emergency department. *International Scholarly Research Network (ISRN) Emergency Medicine* **2012**, Article ID 508649. doi:10.5402/2012/508649

Singh A, Dubey A, Sonker A, Chaudhary R (2015) Evaluation of various methods of point-of-care testing of haemoglobin concentration in blood donors. *Blood Transfusion* **13**, 233–239.

Sireci A (2015) Hematology testing in urgent care and resource-poor settings. *Clinics in Laboratory Medicine* **35**, 197–207. doi:10.1016/j.cll.2014.10.009

Sümnig A, Hron G, Westphal A, Petersmann A, Kohlmann T, Greinacher A, *et al.* (2015) The impact of non-invasive, capillary, and venous haemoglobin screening on donor referrals and the hemoglobin content of red blood cells concentrates: a prospective study. *Transfusion* **55**, 2847–2854. doi:10.1111/trf.13241

Spaeth B, Shephard M, McCormack B, Sinclair G (2015) Evaluation of HemoCue white blood cell differential counter at a remote health centre in Australia's Northern Territory. *Pathology* **47**, 91–95.

WHO (World Health Organization) (2004) *Haemoglobin Colour Scale – Operational Research Agenda and Study Design.* Department of Essential Health Technologies, WHO, Geneva, Switzerland.

WHO (2008) *Worldwide Prevalence of Anaemia 1993–2005.* WHO, Geneva, Switzerland.

WHO (2011) *Haemoglobin Concentrations for the Diagnosis of Anaemia and Assessment of Severity.* Vitamin and Mineral Nutrition Information System, WHO, Geneva, Switzerland.

WHO (2014) *Global Nutrition Targets 2025: Anaemia Policy Brief.* WHO, Geneva, Switzerland.

WHO (2015) *The Global Prevalence of Anaemia in 2011.* WHO, Geneva, Switzerland.

Williams C (2011) Evaluation of the Sysmex pocH-100i analyser for use in remote laboratory settings. *Australian Journal of Medical Science* **32**, 11–15.

Zhang Y, Bai J, Wu H, Ying J (2015) Trapping cells in paper for white blood cell count. *Biosensors & Bioelectronics* **69**, 121–127. doi:10.1016/j.bios.2015.02.019

Zhu H, Sencan I, Wong J, Dimitroc S, Tseng D, Nagashima K, *et al.* (2013) Cost-effective and rapid blood analysis on a cell-phone. *Lab on a Chip* **13**, 1282–1288. doi:10.1039/c3lc41408f

# 15 Point-of-care testing for electrolytes and acid-base imbalances

*Cameron Martin*

**Summary**

Routine blood gas and electrolyte analysis is a sophisticated and important part of both laboratory and point-of-care testing (POCT) in the 21st century. As the science of emergency medicine has advanced, so has gas and electrolyte analysis to where it is now a routine part of patient management in acute and intensive care situations. Scientific instrument manufacturers have risen to the challenge by designing and producing a range of reliable point-of-care analysers that fit applications from the smallest remote health clinic, to the largest emergency or intensive care unit. The laboratory, and laboratory scientists, have an important role to play in the education of clinicians who use and base patient management on results from these analysers.

## INTRODUCTION

Unless one includes the early days of Greek medicine, when the visual examination of bodily fluids, notably urine, was of particular importance, the measurement of gas partial pressure and electrolytes in blood has the honour of being one of the first examples of true modern POCT in use, dating back to the 1950s.

The American anaesthetist Severinghaus and his technician Bradley are credited with inventing the first serviceable blood gas analyser in 1958 (Severinghaus and Freeman 1958). The Danish company Radiometer, along with Beckman Instruments, Instrumentation Laboratory, and others, began manufacturing commercial blood gas analysers shortly after. Today, most major medical device manufacturers build, or supply, a blood gas analyser of some type.

The design, refinement and, above all, reliability of bench-top blood gas analysers progressed steadily through the 1960s and 70s and by the early 1980s had reached sufficient sophistication to be moved from the laboratory, once again back to the point of care (POC), as long as there was a supervising laboratory not too far away! These instruments, of course, are still extensively used in medical laboratories.

In modern blood gas analysers, gas partial pressures and electrolytes are still measured using electrodes. Although the design and reliability may have improved, the basic principle remains the same as Severinghaus's original analyser from 1958.

Later modifications to the basic electrode design have meant that solid state, or printed electrodes on silicon, ceramic or plastic substrates could be used to make highly stable, compact and reliable, disposable cartridge-based analysers (Lauks 2005; Lauks *et al.* 1992). These have formed the basis for both smaller analysers with single-use cartridges, and larger bench-top analysers where the cartridge contains all the elements needed for repeated calibration, quality control and cleaning. These cartridges are used for multiple test cycles and then, when exhausted, simply removed from the analyser and replaced with a new one.

Single-use cartridge based gas analysers, such as the i-STAT® (Abbott Point of Care) and the epoc® (Alere) designed specifically for POC use and users, has pushed the ready availability of gases and electrolytes further afield into rural and remote areas, and military and civilian first response units.

Finally, several manufacturers offer small, portable, cartridge-based POCT general chemistry analysers, capable of performing a limited range of common chemistry tests including basic electrolytes.

## WHY MEASURE BLOOD GASES AND ELECTROLYTE BALANCES?

The advances of critical care medicine over the last 50 years have helped drive a similar demand for advances in blood gas and electrolyte analysis, because the two are inexorably linked. Ironically many of the terms and concepts used are actually much older, having been carried across from earlier research in physical chemistry.

To sustain life, humans (and other mammals) must maintain blood gas, pH, and electrolyte balances within closely defined limits. The accurate measurement of blood gases and electrolytes, and calculation of acid base balance, is essential to the management of patients who, for various reasons, may be unable to maintain this balance without clinical intervention.

## BASICS

In 1909, Soren Sorenson introduced the concept of *pH*, which is the negative log of the hydrogen (hydronium) ion activity in water (Alberty and Silbey 1996). It must be remembered that pH was originally devised for use in physical chemistry. In translation to use in medicine, the seemingly narrow reference range of 7.34 to 7.44 commonly used, in fact, represents a surprisingly wide latitude for bodily response. Likewise, due to the negative log, somewhat confusingly, an *increase* in hydronium ion corresponds to a *decrease* in pH and vice versa.

Approximately 50 years later, Astrup *et al.* introduced the concept of *base excess* (BE) as a measure of the bodily acid base balance (Astrup *et al.* 1960). BE can be estimated from the bicarbonate ion concentration and the pH using the equation:

$$BE = 0.93 \times [HCO_3^-] + 13.77 \times pH - 124.58$$

In practice, this estimates the amount of acid to return *in vitro* blood to normal pH (7.40) under standard conditions (at 37°C at a $PCO_2$ of 40 mmHg). A negative BE is essentially an excess of acid; likewise, a positive BE indicates reduced acid, or excess base (alkali). The reference range is commonly quoted as: BE = (–2) – (+2) mmol/L (Painter *et al.* 1994).

*Standard base excess* uses the above base equation, but incorporates a correction factor for the buffering effect of haemoglobin (Hb) at a standardised anaemic Hb concentration of 50 g/L. This estimates the amount of acid or alkali to return the whole body, including the extra cellular fluid (ECF) component, to normal pH (7.40) under standard conditions (Grogono 2015).

The *anion gap* (AG) is the difference in the measured cations (+) and measured anions (–) in body fluids such as plasma, serum or (less commonly) urine. The commonly used equation is:

$$\text{Anion gap} = (\text{Sodium } [Na^+] + \text{Potassium } [K^+]) - (\text{Chloride } [Cl^-] + \text{Bicarbonate } [HCO_3^-])$$

In practice, the potassium $[K^+]$ component is not included in some versions of this equation due to the normally minimal contribution by potassium.

The anion gap is widely used when trying to identify the cause of metabolic acidosis.

The reference range classically quoted in acid base literature is 8–16 mmol/L; however, 4–12 mmol/L is commonly recommended now that electrolytes are usually measured by ion selective electrodes (ISE) rather than flame photometry (Cadogan and Nickson 2015).

*Blood gases* are measured as *partial pressure of gases dissolved in blood*; this means that, in a mixture of gases, the gas under analysis is presumed to fill the same volume as if the space contained that gas alone.

Blood gas partial pressures are still commonly reported in mmHg, a convention harking back to the days when mercury manometers were used to measure gas partial pressure. They are, however, more correctly expressed in the SI unit, kilopascals (KPa).

Blood gases are normally reported as 'P' for partial pressure, the source (arterial or venous), and the particular gas under analysis, in the form: $PaCO_2$ = XX mmHg for an arterial gas, for example.

The reference range for adult arterial gases is:

$PaO_2$ at sea level (765 mmHg) 75-100 mmHg

$PaCO_2$ at sea level (765 mmHg) 35–45 mmHg (Painter *et al.* 1994).

The corresponding venous gas values are:

$PvO_2$ at sea level 30–40 mmHg
$PvCO_2$ at sea level 41–51 mmHg (Painter *et al.* 1994).

Another gas not uncommonly measured in emergency medicine is carbon monoxide (CO). As there are no specific electrodes designed to measure CO, this is measured by co-oximetry in blood gas analysers. *In vivo* CO becomes irreversibly bound to haemoglobin (Hb) forming carboxyhaemoglobin (COHb), which can be measured by its spectral shift from normal oxy and de-oxy Hb in blood gas analysers capable of performing co-oximetry (Nikkanen and Skolnick 2011; Pathway Medicine 2015).

Another parameter often reported is *oxygen saturation* ($SO_2$). In large bench-top analysers, this is measured by spectral shift using the analyser's co-oximetry module, much like CO. Each haemoglobin molecule can bind up to four oxygen atoms. Once all four sites are occupied, the molecule is said to be 'saturated'. This is accompanied by a progressive change in the colour of the molecule. The $PaO_2$ ratio of Oxy Hb to total Hb is reported as percentage saturation.

Analysers that do not have a co-oximetry module must approximate the '% Sats' by calculation using the $PO_2$, the $PCO_2$ and pH. For example, the i-STAT analyser uses the equation:

$$SO_2 = 100\ (X^3 + 150X)\ /\ X^3 + 150X + 23400$$

where X is a constant calculated from the $PO_2$, pH and $HCO_3$.

These types of equations assume several things, such as normal affinity of $O_2$ for Hb, and no interference from abnormal haemoglobins; they also do not take into account the 2,3 diphosphoglycerate (DPG) concentrations, which affect the oxygen dissociation curve. Thus they should be used more as a guide rather than exact measurements. A commonly quoted reference range for $SO_2$ (normal respiration – room air) is 95–98%.

In the blood gas context (and in large biochemistry analysers) electrolytes in whole blood, plasma, or serum, are measured using ion selective electrodes (ISEs). In most of the world, the SI unit mmol/L is used; however, in the USA the term meq/L or mEQ/L is still often used. These terms are not necessarily interchangeable because the mEQ/L unit is a measurement of both mass and charge. They are only interchangeable in the case of monovalent ions.

## EXAMPLES OF COMMON BLOOD GAS AND ELECTROLYTE ANOMALIES

Although seemingly complex at first glance, acid/base balance theory can be explained using several fairly straight forward generalisations.

### Respiratory acidosis

*Respiratory acidosis* occurs when respiratory carbon dioxide ($CO_2$) accumulates in the body. The extra $CO_2$ dissolves in the plasma where it combines with water molecules to form the weak acid, carbonic acid ($H_2CO_3$). The increased acid level lowers the pH of the plasma.

Most bodily acid comes from aerobic cellular respiration and the resulting $CO_2$ is exhaled through the lungs resulting in a normally relatively stable pH and $PCO_2$. If this process is impaired in any way, for example by acute or chronic airways obstruction, bronchiospasm or respiratory depression, 'respiratory' acidosis can result. To correct this, more $CO_2$ must be removed from the body, this being commonly done medically in the hospital by increasing the respiration by mechanical means.

### Metabolic acidosis

*Metabolic acidosis* occurs when, for various reasons, the mechanism for normal aerobic respiration is impaired. Because this acid is not respiratory in origin, then it is said to be 'metabolic'.

Normally metabolic acid is a much smaller plasma acid component than respiratory acid, and is usually regulated through the kidneys and, to a lesser extent, the liver. However, when blood supply is compromised, or normal metabolic processes are disturbed, such as in vessel obstruction with tissue ischaemia, diabetic keto-acidosis, or poisoning by various agents, metabolic acid production can increase considerably, to the point where the normal regulatory process cannot cope, resulting in a metabolic acidosis. The treatment is also 'metabolic' and may be achieved medically by the administration of bicarbonate ($HCO_3^-$) to buffer the acid and raise the pH, if the case is sufficiently serious (Brandis 2015; Grogono 2015).

### Alkalosis

Alkalosis normally results when excess acid has been removed from the bodily system, or excess bicarbonate has been introduced.

## Compensation

The diagnosis of both respiratory and metabolic acidosis, as well as alkalosis, can be complicated by the body's normal tendency to compensate. The body has several buffering systems available to counteract sudden pH changes and help drive shifts back towards equilibrium.

Normally a respiratory acidosis can at least be partially compensated by an increased respiration rate. A severe metabolic acidosis that is not fully correctable by the kidney and liver can be also partially compensated for in this manner. Chronic respiratory acidosis will also incorporate some compensation from the bicarbonate buffering system.

Likewise, a respiratory alkalosis can be compensated by a reduction in respiration rate or volume, or increased $PCO_2$ in the inspired air fraction and a metabolic acidosis by changing bicarbonate excretion by the kidney.

Clinicians need to be wary when interpreting blood gas and electrolyte results, because in some long standing chronic disturbances, the compensation may be so extreme as to almost mask the underlying condition.

## Base excess

The BE assists in the determination of the cause of an acid/base disturbance. Causes can be respiratory, metabolic or mixed. As stated above $CO_2$ comprises the respiratory component of the acid base balance, and base excess defines the metabolic component. Bicarbonate contributes the majority of the base in the BE calculation, so any disturbance of the blood bicarbonate will immediately reflect in corresponding changes in the BE value.

A high BE (>+2.0 mmol/L) indicates metabolic alkalosis and a low BE (<–2.0 mmol/L) suggests metabolic acidosis. However, compensation by the body can mask these changes, making interpretation more difficult because multiple metabolic contributions may be present at the same time.

## Anion gap

As discussed above, the AG is the difference between measured cations and anions in the body. The measured components must be as accurate as possible for the AG to be useful. Significant levels of unmeasured anions such as lactate, phosphate or β-hydroxybutyrate in ketoacidosis will increase the 'gap' and point towards a metabolic acidosis.

A summary of blood gas anomalies and their clinical causes is provided in Tables 15.1–15.5.

## Electrolytes

An electrolyte is a substance that dissociates into ions in solution and acquires the capacity to conduct electricity. Sodium, potassium, chloride, bicarbonate, calcium,

**Table 15.1.** Nomenclature associated with acidosis with varying $PaCO_2$ and base excess values (Source: adapted from Duh and Cook 2005; Painter *et al.* 1994)

| **pH <7.35** | | | **Acidosis** | | |
|---|---|---|---|---|---|
| $PaCO_2$ (mmHg) | Normal (35–45) | Low (<35) | High (>45) | High (>45) | High (>45) |
| BE (mmol/L) | Negative(<–2) | Negative(<–2) | Negative (<–2) | Normal (–2 to +2) | Positive (>+2) |
| Presumption | Primary metabolic acidosis | Primary metabolic acidosis with respiratory compensation | Mixed respiratory and metabolic acidosis | Primary respiratory acidosis | Primary respiratory acidosis with renal compensation |

**Table 15.2.** Nomenclature associated with alkalosis with varying $PaCO_2$ and base excess values (Source: adapted from Brandis 2015; Cadogan and Nickson 2015; Grogono 2015)

| **pH >7.45** | | | **Alkalosis** | | |
|---|---|---|---|---|---|
| $PaCO_2$ (mmHg) | Low | Low | Low | Normal | High |
| BE (mmol/L) | Negative | Normal | Positive | Positive | Positive |
| Presumption | Primary respiratory alkalosis with renal compensation | Primary respiratory alkalosis | Mixed respiratory and metabolic alkalosis | Primary metabolic alkalosis | Primary metabolic alkalosis with respiratory compensation |

**Table 15.3.** Causes of respiratory acidosis and alkalosis (Source: adapted from Brandis 2015; Cadogan and Nickson 2015; Grogono 2015)

| Respiratory acidosis (acute) | Respiratory acidosis (chronic) | Respiratory alkalosis (acute) | Respiratory alkalosis (chronic) |
|---|---|---|---|
| Respiratory centre depression by drugs or disease (e.g. opiates) | COPD | Hyperventilation (psychiatric, e.g. panic) | Pregnancy |
| Neuromuscular disease e.g. (Guillain-Barre Syndrome, Myasthenia gravis) | Obesity hypoventilation syndrome (Pickwickian Syndrome) | High altitude (increased respiration rate) | Pneumonia, (increased hypoxic drive) |
| | | Excessively high mechanical ventilation (Iatrogenic) | |
| | | Cerebral effects, (stroke, subarachnoid haemorrhage, meningitis) | |

**Table 15.4.** Causes of metabolic acidosis (Source: adapted from Brandis 2015; Cadogan and Nickson 2015; Grogono 2015)

| Normal anion gap (8–16 mmol/L) (drop in HCO3) | Elevated anion gap (>16) (metabolic acidosis) | Low anion gap (<8) |
|---|---|---|
| Chronic diarrhoea | Lactic acidosis | Hypoalbuminaemia (retention of chloride and bicarbonate) |
| Pancreatic fistula | Ketoacidosis | Paraproteinaemia |
| Renal failure | Chronic renal failure | Nephrotic syndrome (loss of albumin) |
| Drug intoxication TPN | Poisoning (e.g. methanol, ethanol, ethylene glycol, formaldehyde, phenformin) | Liver cirrhosis (loss of albumin) |
| Ammonium chloride and acetazolamide ingestion | Chronic alcoholism | |
| Addison's disease | | |

**Table 15.5.** Causes of metabolic alkalosis (Source: adapted from Brandis 2015; Cadogan and Nickson 2015; Grogono 2015)

| | Primary/acute | Chronic | Comment |
|---|---|---|---|
| Chloride responsive | Loss of acid (vomiting, nasogastric tubes) | Chronic vomiting (bulimia) | Acute conditions may become chronic |
| | Loss of water/excessive diuretics (contraction alkalosis) | Decreased renal perfusion (cardiac failure, cirrhosis, chronic dehydration) | |
| | Posthypercapnia ('rebound' after renal compensation for respiratory acidosis) | Long-term use of loop diuretics | Acute can follow rebound after medical administration of bicarbonate |
| Chloride resistant | Hypokalemia | Barter Syndrome<br>Giteman Syndrome | |
| | Excessive bicarbonate administration or retention | Hyperaldersteronism | |
| | Aminoglycoside toxicity | Impaired chloride ion reabsorption | |

**Table 15.6.** Nomenclature relating to abnormalities of selected electrolytes

| Analyte | Reference range (mmol/L) | Term for low/high analyte levels |
|---|---|---|
| Sodium | 135–145 | Hypo/hyper natraemia |
| Potassium | 3.5–5.0 | Hypo/hyper kalaemia |
| Chloride | 95–105 | Hypo/hyper chloraemia |
| Calcium | 1.03–1.23 (ionised) 2.00–2.60 (total) | Hypo/hyper calcaemia |

magnesium and phosphate are examples of electrolytes in bodily fluids. Electrolyte imbalances in the blood are somewhat easier to understand than blood gases – they are normal, elevated or low for various physical reasons, and disease states (Tables 15.6 and 15.7). However, electrolyte levels are also interwoven with acid–base balance, particularly the commonly measured electrolytes at the POC.

## AVAILABLE DEVICES FOR POINT-OF-CARE BLOOD GAS AND ELECTROLYTE MEASUREMENTS

A large variety of devices are used to measure blood gases and electrolytes at the POC, ranging from traditional laboratory-type 'bench-top' blood gas analysers, to smaller portable blood gas and electrolyte devices, and even smaller, dedicated POCT chemistry analysers.

In Australia, the use of large laboratory-type blood gas analysers at the POC is generally associated with a nearby laboratory. The high maintenance demand of these analysers tends to restrict their use to locations where scientific expertise and advice is readily available. These instruments are best typified by the Radiometer 800 series analysers and the Siemens RAPIDLab 1200 series.

The increasing popularity and use of large multi-use cartridge-based analysers has somewhat decreased the maintenance burden for laboratory staff; however, even with these, the testing economy of scale still tends to mean that these larger cartridge analysers are used in larger facilities, which also usually tend to have on-site laboratories.

Popular choices for the larger cartridge based analysers include the Instrumentation Laboratory GEM 3000 and 4000 series, the Radiometer 90 Flex analysers and the Siemens RapidPoint 500 series.

Once a new test cartridge is installed and calibrated, these analysers are able to self-monitor, calibrate and quality control themselves reliably, producing results for up to 28–30 days, or until the cartridge test cycle is exhausted – whichever occurs first. This is achieved by either having multiple compartments within the cartridge assembly containing calibrators, or a separate cartridge block containing both calibrator and QC material. In the case of the GEM analysers, once a new

**Table 15.7.** A brief list of common causes of selected electrolyte disturbances

| Electrolyte | Low | High |
|---|---|---|
| Sodium | Liver disease, congestive heart failure, nephrotic syndrome, prolonged vomiting, glucocorticoid deficiency, water intoxication | Dehydration, inadequate water intake, watery diarrhoea, polyuria, sea water drowning, excess hypertonic fluid administration |
| Potassium | Inadequate intake, excessive loss, loop diuretics, high aldosterone, urinary loss, diabetic ketoacidosis, pancreatic fistula, low magnesium, alkalosis | Excessive intake of ACE inhibitors, NSAIDs, aldosterone deficiency, excessive release from cells, massive haemolysis, burns, rhabdomyolysis, tumour lysis, acidosis, Box Jellyfish sting |
| Chloride | Hypoventilation, respiratory acidosis, metabolic alkalosis (vomiting) | Large saline infusions, diarrhoea, some kidney diseases (renal tubular acidosis), some diuretics |
| Calcium | Hypoparathyroidism, chelation therapy, osteoporosis treatments, acute renal failure, chronic renal failure, vitamin D deficiency, malabsorption, pancreatitis, alkalosis | Hyperparathyroidism, various tumours, including parathyroid, squamous cell carcinoma, phaeochromocytoma, haematological malignancies such as multiple myeloma, vitamin D intoxication, aluminium intoxication |

cartridge has been installed and manually initialised by the operator with an external calibrator, the inbuilt calibrator functions as both a calibrator and QC material for the remainder of the cartridge life. At programmed time intervals, and after a set number of samples, the analyser will auto rinse, calibrate and then QC itself. The analyser has a sophisticated internal statistical analysis package to monitor and report or alert operators of any malfunction or sensor drift (St John and Ritter 2010). Radiometer and Siemens cartridge analysers use a separate calibrator and QC pack, and tend to function more like a 'traditional' gas analyser but in a more convenient form where, once the cartridge pack is loaded, the operator simply has to push a button to initiate the process. Cartridges are available in several test cycle sizes to facilitate environments with different workload requirements.

It must be remembered that, in the case of all the large bench-top analysers, including the large cartridge-based versions, the analyser 'runs' 24 h a day whether actually performing tests or not. These analysers are continually auto-performing calibration, quality control and rinse cycles, in order to be in an 'always ready' state for patient testing. The large analysers also require annual maintenance regardless of degree of use. This has an important bearing on their cost-effectiveness in low or intermittent use situations, because they have a fairly high 'fixed' running cost component. However, they are a cost-effective option in heavy use situations such as busy emergency, operating theatre or intensive care units.

However, it is the smaller single-use cartridge based analysers such as the Abbott i-STAT and the Alere epoc that have truly made blood gas and electrolyte analysis widely available. The single-use cartridges contain all the needed test components within the cartridge, have months of shelf life and auto-calibrate before use. When coupled with a small, compact, portable, 'analyser' this testing system has enabled blood gas and electrolyte analysis to be pushed out to the very front line of medicine. These analysers are often seen in smaller emergency departments, air and road ambulances, and military medical units. Because their 'down-time' costs and maintenance requirements are virtually nil, they are also often used as backup instruments by mainstream laboratories.

A very important niche use for small cartridge-based instruments is rural and remote medicine where they provide an essential primary care service in countries such as Australia, which has a relatively small population spread across a large area, with many small remote hospitals and medical centres, without on-site, or nearby, laboratories.

The emergence of large, coordinated POCT networks has further enhanced the use of small cartridge-based blood gas and electrolyte analysers in these rural and remote areas. In these networks, laboratory professionals or specialist POCT providers can support clinicians by standardising items such as analyser and test selection, and promoting common operator training, and quality standards.

In Australia, POCT networks using these small cartridge-based blood gas and electrolyte analysers are now supported by the state health authorities in Queensland, New South Wales, South Australia, Western Australia and the Northern Territory (Francis and Martin 2010; Martin 2010; Shephard *et al.* 2012, 2014).

All of these instruments measure electrolytes using a process known as direct ion selective electrode (DISE); this means that the test sample (usually whole blood) is not pre-diluted before testing. This is an important distinction from where electrolytes are measured on mainstream laboratory biochemistry analysers using an indirect ISE process, where the sample (usually serum or plasma) is pre-diluted before testing. In samples with extremely high levels of suspended fats, or plasma proteins, these indirect ISE analysers can underestimate the true electrolyte values due to a phenomenon known as the volume of distribution of water. Because the electrolytes are only dissolved in the plasma water, any other non-aqueous material filling the space of a fixed volume of sample will proportionally decrease the electrolyte readings in any method relying on a fixed sample aliquot, such as indirect ISE methods. Conversely, in situations where the plasma protein level is significantly lower than normal, the reverse can also occur for the same reasons.

Therefore POCT blood gas analysers, both bench-top and cartridge based, are valuable for checking and correcting electrolyte levels measured on indirect ISE laboratory instruments under these circumstances (Dimeski *et al.* 2012).

## OTHER DEVICES TO MEASURE ELECTROLYTES AT THE POINT OF CARE

Electrolytes can also be measured at the POC by small clinical chemistry analysers such as the Abaxis Piccolo® or Samsung LABGEO$^{PT10}$. These small compact analysers can measure a variety of common biochemical

**Table 15.8.** Commonly used blood gas analysers and applications in Australia

| Manufacturer | Model | Application | Cost per test |
|---|---|---|---|
| Radiometer<br>Siemens | ABL 800 Series[a]<br>Siemens 1200 Series[a] | Large emergency departments (ED), intensive care units, operating theatres (OT), laboratories | Lowest if correctly specified for the application |
| Radiometer<br>Siemens<br>Instrumentation Laboratory | ABL 90 Flex[b]<br>Siemens 500 Series[b]<br>GEM 3000, 4000 Series[b] | Medium-sized ED, ICU; OT; Smaller laboratory; Secondary unit for above applications | Higher than above, but still cost effective in correct application |
| Abbott<br>Alere | i-STAT[c]<br>epoc[c] | Small ED, High-dependency units, OT, rural and remote, emergency, first response units, field hospital/military, disaster relief, veterinary applications, laboratory backup unit | Highest cost per test, but must be viewed in light of total cost of applications and clinical need. Cost-effective in intermittent or low use requirement scenario |

[a]Full size bench-top blood gas analysers
[b]Multi-use cartridge-based analysers
[c]Single-use cartridge analysers

parameters such as protein, liver enzymes and metabolites, in addition to basic electrolytes.

The Abaxis Piccolo is a miniature colourimetric centrifugal analyser, and thus measures electrolytes optically rather than by ISE; as a result, electrolytes measured by this instrument may be subject to chemical interferences or may vary slightly from those of other POCT analysers using ISE technologies.

Likewise, the Samsung LABGEO[PT10] measures chemistry profiles and electrolytes optically and may also suffer from chemical interferences, which do not affect ISE-type electrolyte measurements.

These analysers are of immense use in areas such as field hospitals, remote medical practices and in veterinarian practice. Although, due to the cartridge cost, the relative cost per test is comparatively high compared with mainstream pathology, the testing numbers usually are low. Thus, because the analysers themselves are modestly priced, they can be quite cost-effective (Dimeski *et al.* 2010). Table 15.8 lists examples of common POC blood gas analysers available in Australia, the clinical settings where they have greatest application, and an estimate of their relative costs.

## THE IMPORTANCE OF OPERATOR TRAINING, ANALYSER MAINTENANCE AND CONTROL

As modern blood gas and electrolyte analysers become increasingly more reliable and automated in terms of their calibration, quality control and sample handling requirements, misconceptions tend to arise about them. 'Easy to use' does not equate to 'no user training needed' nor does 'low maintenance' equate to 'no maintenance'. It is easy for clinical users to fall into this trap, and one of the reasons that laboratory professionals should be involved in the management of POCT.

As in all other areas of POCT, correct testing procedure is essential to achieving reliable, good quality results that positively contribute to patient care. In blood gas and electrolyte analysis, the pre-analytical testing phase is particularly important. Use of an incorrect anticoagulant, poor collection technique or poor pre-treatment of samples before testing can significantly affect test results, even if the analyser used is perfectly calibrated and controlled.

Additional testing error can insidiously occur from incorrect analyser operation or calibration and maintenance issues with a particular analyser, which of course will all add to the total error in a POC test result. The exact same issues can affect a laboratory result as well, but in a laboratory a considerable amount of scientist time and effort is expended to contain and minimise these errors.

What this means is that, similar to normal laboratory practice, staff performing POCT must be properly trained in the collection of samples, and the correct use of all analysers used at the POC. POCT analysers must wherever possible be calibrated, controlled and maintained exactly as if they were located in the laboratory. If this is not done, all the advantages of having POCT results readily available are lost, if operators don't trust these results.

Suitable reference material for blood gas and electrolyte training programs, and correct analyser maintenance, can be sourced from the manufacturer's analyser manual, their website or the POCT resources listed below; there are also many other good resources on the web dealing with the pre-analytical testing phase (Gill and Shephard 2010; Gill and Watkinson 2010; Martin 2008; Shephard *et al.* 2013; Tirimacco *et al.* 2011; www.appn.net.au/training.aspx; www.aacb.asn.au/resources/poct).

## CASE STUDIES

*Please note that the following case histories are fictitious examples compiled from multiple cases drawn from both the author's experience, and those reported in the literature.*

### Case study 1

A young male is admitted to hospital suffering from symptoms of intoxication and an altered level of consciousness. His condition deteriorates, and he requires ventilation and renal dialysis. POC tests performed on admission included a blood gas with electrolytes and a full blood count. The results are shown in the table below.

**What are the abnormalities in this patient's POC test results and what are their likely causes?**

- The pH is markedly reduced, suggesting an acidosis.
- The $PCO_2$ is reduced, suggesting an attempt at respiratory compensation.
- The bicarbonate is also reduced, suggesting an attempt by the body to buffer the excess acid.
- The creatinine is raised, suggesting renal impairment.
- The lactate is raised, suggesting a possible cause for the acidosis.
- The anion gap is elevated, suggesting a metabolic acidosis.

**Diagnosis**

- The patient in fact has ethylene glycol (antifreeze) poisoning.
- The metabolic acidosis is real; however, it is probably not caused primarily by lactate.
- The lack of a leucocytosis in the blood count tends not to support lactic acidosis associated with tissue ischemia or infection.
- Ethylene glycol is metabolised by alcohol dehydrogenase to glycoaldehyde, glycolate, glyoxylate, then oxalate.
- Glycolate in the form of glycolic acid, and glycoxylate are very similar to lactate structurally, and can 'fool' the recombinant enzyme lactate sensors used in many blood gas analysers (L-lactate oxidase) resulting in a falsely elevated lactate.
- Running the sample on a laboratory analyser will usually give a correct lactate estimate.

**Case study 1**

| Test | Result | Reference range | Unit | Comment |
|---|---|---|---|---|
| pH (arterial) | 7.19* | 7.34–7.45 | | Acidosis |
| $PaCO_2$ | 20* | 32–43 | mmHg | Reduced (?compensation) |
| $PaO_2$ | 131* | 70–100 | mmHg | |
| Bicarbonate | 9.0* | 20–26 | mmol/L | Reduced (?buffering) |
| Sodium | 141 | 136–146 | mmol/L | |
| Potassium | 3.9 | 3.8–5.0 | mmol/L | |
| Calcium | 2.12 | 2.20–2.60 | mmol/L | |
| Chloride | 109 | 99–108 | mmol/L | |
| Creatinine | 201* | 58–103 | µmol/L | Raised (?renal failure) |
| Urea | 5.2 | 3.0–7.5 | mmol/L | |
| Glucose | 6.8 | 3.6–5.6 | mmol/L | |
| Lactate | 26* | 0.0–2.2 | mmol/L | Raised (?metabolic acidosis) |
| Anion gap | 26* | 5–11 | mmol/L | Raised (?metabolic acidosis) |
| White cell count | 5.0 | 4–11 | $\times 10^9$/L | |
| Haemoglobin | 12.5 | 12.3–15.3 | g/L | |
| Platelets | 245 | 150–450 | $\times 10^9$/L | |

Note: The significantly out-of-range test results have been marked with an asterisk

- The oxalate is deposited in the kidney and other tissues as calcium oxalate crystals, adding to the renal impairment already caused by glycolate.

Treatment consists of administering ethanol, which is preferentially metabolised by alcohol dehydrogenase, and supporting failing renal function with haemodialysis until the ethylene glycol and metabolites are removed by the dialysis and the recovering kidneys. Antidiuretic hormone (ADH) blocking drugs can and are also used in some applications (Head 2012; Latus *et al.* 2012; Oostvogels *et al.* 2013).

## Case study 2

An elderly man with severe chronic obstructive pulmonary disease (COPD) is admitted to hospital from the emergency department where his history is known to staff. He is a long-term smoker, and suffers from chronic bronchitis with regular exacerbations. Recently his bronchitis has again become worse with increased dyspnoea, and thick mucus production over the last couple of days. The results in the table below are from his POC blood gas at presentation.

**Case study 2**

| Test | Result | Reference range | Unit | Comment |
|---|---|---|---|---|
| pH (arterial) | 7.24* | 7.34–7.45 | | Acidosis |
| $PaCO_2$ | 70* | 32–43 | mmHg | Raised (respiratory acidosis) |
| $PaO_2$ | 51* | 70–100 | mmHg | Reduced (poor alveolar ventilation) |
| Bicarbonate | 30* | 20–26 | mmol/L | Raised (buffer) |
| $O_2$ saturation | 80 | >94 | % | Reduced (poor ventilation) |

Note: The significantly out-of-range test results have been marked with an asterisk

**What are some of the abnormalities in this patient's POC test results and what are their likely causes?**

- The pH is markedly reduced, suggesting an acidosis.
- The $PCO_2$ is increased, suggesting the acidosis is of respiratory origin.
- The bicarbonate is increased, suggesting a metabolic alkalosis in response to a chronically elevated $PCO_2$.

### Diagnosis

The patient has a primary respiratory acidosis with metabolic compensation because of his COPD. Because his condition has recently become worse, the compensation is not complete.

Unfortunately for this patient, although the exacerbations can be treated with antibiotics, steroids and bronchodilators, his episodes will probably tend to worsen as his lung function continues to decline with increasing age, and cumulative past damage.

## Case study 3

A 48 year old woman is transported by ambulance, and admitted to hospital after becoming disoriented and collapsing in the latter stages of a full marathon event run in fairly hot conditions. During the ambulance trip, suspecting dehydration/heatstroke, the woman was administered IV normal saline by paramedics, but she did not improve; indeed she seemed to deteriorate further.

Her significant results from a POCT blood gas analyser at admission are summarised in the table below.

**Case study 3**

| Analyte | Result | Reference range (mmol/L) |
|---|---|---|
| Sodium | 114* | 135–145 |
| Potassium | 3.2 | 3.2–4.5 |
| Chloride | 106 | 100–110 |
| Bicarbonate | 26 | 22–29 |
| Anon gap | 7 | 4–13 |
| Glucose | 4.1 | 3.0–7.8 |
| Urea | 8.0 | 3.0–8.0 |

Note: The significantly out-of-range test results have been marked with an asterisk

**What is the main abnormality in her POC test results?**

- The patient's sodium is markedly depressed.
- The emergency physician at the hospital, luckily for the patient, an endurance athlete himself, immediately diagnosed exercise-induced hyponatraemia, also commonly known as 'water intoxication'.

In this case, the treatment is hypertonic saline to correct the sodium rapidly with minimal extra fluid volume. This may be combined with fluid restriction, because volumes of hypotonic fluid can still remain in the gut.

When questioned after recovery, the patient admitted to drinking much more fluid than she would do normally at each water station, to ward off dehydration. She did this because of the hot day, and repeated warnings by the race promoters, but began to feel worse the further she went. This extra fluid accumulated in the body and, combined with excess sodium lost in sweat, caused the condition. Vasopressin released due to the stress of the run can complicate matters even more, by encouraging the kidneys to retain still more water. As excess water moves into the cells, due to the changed osmotic gradient, tissue oedema begins, including the brain, which can cause the neurological symptoms (Noakes and Speedy 2006; Pattison *et al.* 2011; Rosner and Kirven 2007).

## REFERENCES


Alberty R, Silbey R (1996) *Physical Chemistry.* John Wiley & Sons Inc, New York, USA.

Astrup P, Jorgenson K, Anderson OS, Engel K (1960) The acid-base metabolism: a new approach. *Lancet* **275**, 1035–1039. doi:10.1016/S0140-6736(60)90930-2

Brandis K (2015) *Acid-Base Physiology*, <http://www.anaesthesiaMCQ.com>.

Cadogan M, Nickson C (2015) *Acid Base Disorders*, <http://lifeinthefastlane.com/investigations/acid-base/>.

Dimeski G, Badrick T, St John A (2010) Ion Selective Electrodes (ISEs) and interferences – a review. *Clinica Chimica Acta* **411**, 309–317. doi:10.1016/j.cca.2009.12.005

Dimeski G, Morgan T, Presneil J, Balasubramanian V (2012) Disagreement between ion selective electrode direct and indirect sodium measurements: estimation of the problem in a tertiary referral hospital. *Journal of Critical Care* **27**, 326.e9–326.e16. doi:10.1016/j.jcrc.2011.11.003

Duh S-H, Cook JD (2005) *Laboratory Reference Range Values.* New York, USA, <http://www.stedmansonline.com/webFiles/Dict-Stedmans28/APP17.pdf>.

Francis AJ, Martin CL (2010) A practical example of PoCT working in the community. *The Clinical Biochemist Reviews* **31**, 93–97.

Gill JP, Shephard M (2010) The conduct of quality control and quality assurance testing for PoCT outside the laboratory. *The Clinical Biochemist Reviews* **31**, 85–88.

Gill J, Watkinson L (2010) Quality control and quality assurance in point of care testing. In *Point of Care Testing.* 3rd edn. (Eds CP Price, A St John and LL Kricka) pp. 225–236. AACC Press, Washington DC, USA.

Grogono AW (2015) *Acid-base Tutorial.* New Orleans, Los Angeles, <http://www.acid-base.com/terminology.php#BE2>.

Head JM (2012) *Ethylene Glycol Ingestion Masked by Concomitant Ethanol Intoxication.* British Medical Journal Case Reports, London, UK, <http://casereports.bmj.com/content/2012/bcr.12.2011.5326.abstract>.

Latus J, Kimmel M, Alscher MD, Braun N (2012) Ethylene glycol poisoning: a rare but life threatening cause of metabolic acidosis – a single centre experience. *Clinical Kidney Journal* **5**, 120–123. doi:10.1093/ckj/sfs009

Lauks IR (inventor) (2005) *Point-of-Care In-Vitro Blood Analysis System.* US Patent 6,845,327.

Lauks IR, Wieck HJ, Zelin MP, Blyskal P (inventors) (1992) *Disposable Sensing Device for Real Time Fluid Analysis.* US Patent 5,096,669.

Martin CL (2008) Quality control issues in point of care testing. *The Clinical Biochemist Reviews* **29**(Supplement 1), S79–S82.

Martin CL (2010) i-STAT – combining chemistry and haematology in PoCT. *The Clinical Biochemist Reviews* **31**, 81–84.

Nikkanen H, Skolnick A (2011) Diagnosis and management of carbon monoxide poisoning in the emergency department. *Emergency Medicine Practice* **13**, 1–14.

Noakes TD, Speedy DB (2006) Case proven: exercise associated hyponatraemia is due to over drinking. So why did it take 20 years before the original evidence was accepted? *British Journal of Sports Medicine* **40**, 567–572. doi:10.1136/bjsm.2005.020354

Oostvogels R, Kemperman H, Hubeek I, Wmt ter Braak E (2013) The importance of the osmolality gap in ethylene glycol intoxication. *British Medical Journal* **347**, f6904. doi:10.1136/bmj.f6904

Painter PC, Cope JY, Smith JL (1994) Reference ranges, Table 41-20. In *Tietz Textbook of Clinical Chemistry.* 2nd edn. (Eds CA Burtis and ER Ashwood ER) pp. 2190. WB Saunders, Philadelphia PA, USA.

Pathway Medicine (2015) *Carbon Monoxide and Oxygen Transport*, <http://pathwaymedicine.org/carbon-monoxide-and-oxygen-transport>.

Pattison DA, Walters TE, Seal E (2011) Exercise-associated hyponatraemia on the Kokoda Track. *The Medical Journal of Australia* **194**, 247–248.

Rosner MH, Kirven J (2007) Exercise-associated hyponatremia. *Clinical Journal of the American Society of Nephrology; CJASN* **2**, 151–161. doi:10.2215/CJN.02730806

Severinghaus J, Freeman B (1958) Electrodes for blood pO2 and pCO2 determination. *Journal of Applied Physiology* **13**, 515–520.

Shephard M, Spaeth B, Mazzachi B, Auld M, Schatz S, Loudon J, *et al.* (2012) Design, implementation and initial assessment of the Northern Territory Point-of-Care Testing Program. *The Australian Journal of Rural Health* **20**, 16–21. doi:10.1111/j.1440-1584.2011.01243.x

Shephard M, Halls H, McAteer B, Mazzachi M, Motta L, Spaeth B, *et al.* (2013) Management challenges for Point-of-Care Coordinators in delivering training and competency programs. *Point of Care* **12**, 84–85. doi:10.1097/POC.0b013e 318265e1c8

Shephard M, Spaeth B, Auld M, Schatz M, Lingwood A, Loudon J, *et al.* (2014) Towards sustainable point-of-care testing in remote Australia – the Northern Territory i-STAT Point-of-Care Testing Program. *Point of Care* **13**, 6–11. doi:10.1097/POC.0000000000000009

St John A, Ritter C (2010) Benchtop instruments for point of care testing. In *Point of Care Testing: Needs, Opportunity and Innovation*. 3rd edn. (Eds CP Price, A St John and LL Kricka). pp. 43–62. AACC Press, Washington DC, USA.

Tirimacco R, Glastonbury B, Laurence CO, Bubner TK, Shephard MD, Beilby JJ (2011) Development of an accreditation program for point of care testing (PoCT) in general practice. *Australian Health Review* **35**, 230–234. doi:10.1071/AH09792

# 16 Point-of-care testing of cardiac markers

*Per Venge, Bertil Lindahl and Heather Halls*

**Summary**

The management of patients presenting at the emergency department with symptoms of chest pain and/or acute dyspnoea accounts for a significant amount of emergency care resources. In the work-up of these patients, the blood measurements of cardiac troponins and brain natriuretic peptides are recommended by current guidelines. The introduction of point-of-care testing (POCT) for these biomarkers has the potential to change the work flow in the emergency department by reducing length of stay, patient suffering and costs. However, to take advantage of POCT, the brain-to-vein-to-brain time has to be adjusted with the elimination of unnecessary delays before any clinical decision and action are taken.

## INTRODUCTION

The management at the emergency department (ED) of patients presenting with symptoms of cardiac disease such as chest pain and/or acute dyspnoea accounts for a substantial proportion of emergency care resources. Patients with symptoms of cardiac disease are high-risk patients and should be effectively identified by the emergency physician in order to initiate specific clinical actions. Current recommendations identify the measurement of cardiac markers – that is, cardiac troponins (cTn) and brain natriuretic peptides (BNP) – as important parts of the diagnostic work-up, alongside other testing modalities such as ECG measurement and cardiac imaging. Occasionally, the measurement of D-dimer and blood gases may be indicated (e.g. in patients with suspected pulmonary embolism or patients suffering from cardiogenic shock). The measurement at the point-of-care (POC) is a potential strategy for the reduction in turnaround time for cardiac marker testing in the emergency setting (Storrow *et al.* 2009). In a recent survey of 2770 primary care physicians worldwide, more than 50% of general practitioners would use cTn and natriuretic peptide POCT in their practice if available. Thus, POCT cardiac markers ranked among the top four biomarkers, only surpassed by POCT assays for D-dimer and chlamydia and in the same range as POCT assays for infection and inflammation, such as C-reactive protein and white blood cell counts (Howick *et al.* 2014).

With the introduction of cTn assays with higher sensitivities and of natriuretic peptides, other important applications in addition to diagnosis have been highlighted, such as risk stratification and choice of therapy. However, these aspects are beyond the scope of this overview and we have concentrated on the use of these biomarkers in the diagnostic work-up in the hospital emergency department. This overview is a summary based on round-table discussions between experts in cardiology, emergency medicine and laboratory medicine and were reported in two recent publications (Bingisser *et al.* 2012, 2013).

## POINT-OF-CARE TESTING FOR CARDIAC TROPONIN

### What is cardiac troponin?

The troponin complex is bound to the actin filaments (myofibril complex) of striated muscle and performs a control function in muscle excitation–contraction. This complex consists of three protein subunits, troponin I (cTnI) and troponin T (cTnT), which are both specific to the heart, and troponin C (cTnC). Most of the troponin subunits (~95%) are considered to exist in the bound form with the remainder of cTnI (3–4%) and cTnT (6–8%) existing as a free pool in the cytoplasm, although this concept has been challenged recently (Starnberg *et al.* 2014). Easily releasable cTnI and cTnT are released initially following cardiac muscle damage, with further breakdown of the myofibril complex resulting in the discharge of multiple complexed forms of both cTnI and cTnT (Kemp *et al.* 2004; Korff *et al.* 2006). Manufacturers of the numerous laboratory and POCT assays for cTnI and cTnT use different antibodies to the various epitope regions on these cTn complexes, which complicates the standardisation of methods and comparison between them (Apple 2006).

### POC tests for cardiac troponin – the current state-of-the-art and future needs

The number of commercially available POCT assays with acceptable analytical sensitivity for cTn is limited; this reflects the enormous challenge in developing sensitive troponin assays for this format that are able to measure cTn concentrations at the level of a few ng/L. Thus, it is only recently that we have seen the introduction of cTn assays for the laboratory platform that qualify as so called high-sensitive (hs) assays. According to the IFCC Task Force on the Clinical Applications of Cardiac Biomarkers (Apple and Collinson 2012), an assay for cTn is considered to be an hs assay if it satisfies two criteria. Firstly, the assay should have a coefficient of variation (CV) of 10% at the 99th percentile of the reference population – but what defines a 'healthy' reference population of those without cardiac disease is a matter for debate. There is little consistency in what 'populations' device manufacturers have used to determine this 99th percentile. Secondly, the assay should be able to measure cTn values reliably, above the assay limit of detection (LoD), in at least 50% of apparently 'healthy' subjects.

Table 16.1 summarises selected currently available POC cTn assays and some of their analytical specifications, including the LoD. Traditionally, before the development of hs cTn assays, cTn concentrations were usually expressed in μg/L or even ng/mL, whereas hs cTn values are now expressed in ng/L (Chenevier-Gobeaux *et al.* 2015; Thygesen *et al.* 2012a). For comparative purposes, all assays in Table 16.1 are provided in units of ng/L.

Five of the 11 POCT devices listed weigh more than 30 kg, while the remaining devices are smaller, lightweight (<5 kg) and more portable devices.

None of the POCT assays listed in the table meet the requirements of being hs, but several actually measure cTn concentrations at the 99th percentile level with the required imprecision of <10% CV and therefore might be useful for ruling in or out patients admitted with the suspicion of acute myocardial infarction; these are the Trinity Meritas troponin I, Mitsubishi Pathfast troponin I and the Siemens Stratus CS troponin I assays. Although international cardiac societies recommend that POC devices for cTn should measure the 99th percentile values with a CV <10% and state that devices with a CV >20% should not be used, devices with an intermediate CV are not specifically precluded from use. Following the 2007 publication of the international definition of MI (Thygesen *et al.* 2007), Apple (2009) classified cTn assays into those that were guideline compliant (CV <10%) and those that were clinically usable (CV 10–19%). According to Apple and Amundson (2015), although not ideal, these assays are still 'clinically acceptable'. The i-STAT, for example, has a 99th percentile cut-off of 80 ng/L, 10% CV is achieved at 100 ng/L, with a CV of 20% reached at 70 ng/L, making the device clinically useful.

Few, if any, POCT devices are able to detect cTn at levels found in 50% of apparently disease-free individuals, unlike hs cTn assays (Thygesen *et al.* 2012c), and a recent review of POCT devices did not comment on this ability (Amundson and Apple 2015). As shown in Table 16.1, POCT assays for both cTnI and cTnT have a LoD ranging from 9.5 to 50 ng/L (and a 99th percentile upper reference limit of 10–80 ng/L). For comparison, two current hs laboratory devices, the Abbott Architect and Roche Elecsys/Modular E/cobas e, have a LoD of 1.9 and

**Table 16.1.** Some features of currently available quantitative point-of-care assay systems for measuring cardiac troponin. The table also indicates which systems have brain natriuretic peptides (BNP or NT-proBNP) on their platform.

| Brand name/company | 99th percentile upper reference limit (ng/L) | Concentrations at which 10% CV was obtained (ng/L) | Limit of detection[a] (ng/L) | Analytic TAT (min) | Device weight (g/kg) | Natriuretic peptides measured |
|---|---|---|---|---|---|---|
| i-STAT® Troponin I[H]/ Abbott | 80 | 100 | 20 | 10 | 650 g | BNP |
| Triage® troponin I[B] (old) /Alere | 50 | 400 (12% CV) | 50 | 20 | 680 g | BNP |
| Triage® troponin I[B] (contemporary)/Alere | 20 | Not stated | 10 | 20 | 680 g | BNP |
| Meritas® troponin I[B]/ Trinity | 36 | 36 | 19 | 15 | ND | BNP |
| PATHFAST® troponin I[B] /Mitsubishi | 29 | 29 (5% CV) | 19 | 17 | 33 kg | NT-proBNP |
| AQT90 Flex™troponin I[B] /Radiometer | 23 | 39 | 9.5 | 18 | 35 kg | NT-proBNP |
| AQT90 Flex™ troponin T[B] /Radiometer | 17 | 30 | 10 | 12 | 35 kg | NT-proBNP |
| RAMP® troponin I[B]/ Response Biomedical | <100 | 210 | 30 | 20 | 1.5 kg | NT-proBNP |
| Cobas h232 Cardiac T troponin T[H]/Roche | ND[b] | 100 (9%) | 50 | 14 | 650 g | NT-proBNP |
| Stratus® CS troponin I[B] /Siemens | 70 | 60 | 30 | 14 | 68 kg | NT-proBNP |
| Vidas troponin I[B]/ bioMerieux | 10 | 110 | 10 | 20 | 40 kg | NT-proBNP |

Notes: ND = not determined or not available. [B] = Bench-top instrument, [H] = Handheld instrument. Data have been obtained from assay inserts, the official home pages of the respective companies, from Amundson and Apple (2015) and Aldous *et al.* (2014).

[a]The limit of detection (LoD) is the lowest detectable analyte concentration likely to be distinguished from the limit of blank (LoB) (the concentration below which 95% of results are expected to be found when replicates of a sample containing no analyte are measured) and the limit of quantitation (LoQ) (the smallest value obtained at a predefined CV – for cTn usually 10%). LoD and LoQ define the analytical sensitivity of the assay, with assays with a low LoQ being able to detect a rise in cTn with early stage clinical signs for acute coronary syndrome (Chenevier-Gobeaux *et al.* 2015).

[b]Roche have not reported a 99th percentile for the cardiac troponin T assay, but rather have stated that a value above 100 ng/L indicates that an AMI is likely. Over the full measuring range of the assay (100–2000 ng/L), most CVs were lower than 9% (Package insert and Amundson and Apple 2015).

5 ng/L (and a 99th percentile value of 26.2 and 14 ng/L, respectively) (Aldous *et al.* 2014; Chenevier-Gobeaux *et al.* 2015).

## The clinical use of cardiac troponins in the diagnosis of the acute coronary syndrome

Increasing levels of cardiac troponins, either cTnI or cTnT, in blood signify damage to the myocardium. The detection of circulating cTn is the most sensitive and specific biochemical marker of myocardial injury that is available to the physician in clinical settings, including the ED (Saenger and Jaffe 2008).

The early identification or ruling-out of the presence of an acute coronary syndrome relies on a combination of signs and symptoms, cardiac biomarker levels and findings in the ECG. This is important, since signs and symptoms alone can be misleading, because a substantial proportion of patients present with non-specific symptoms. Cardiac biomarkers can be elevated also in conditions other than acute coronary syndromes and findings

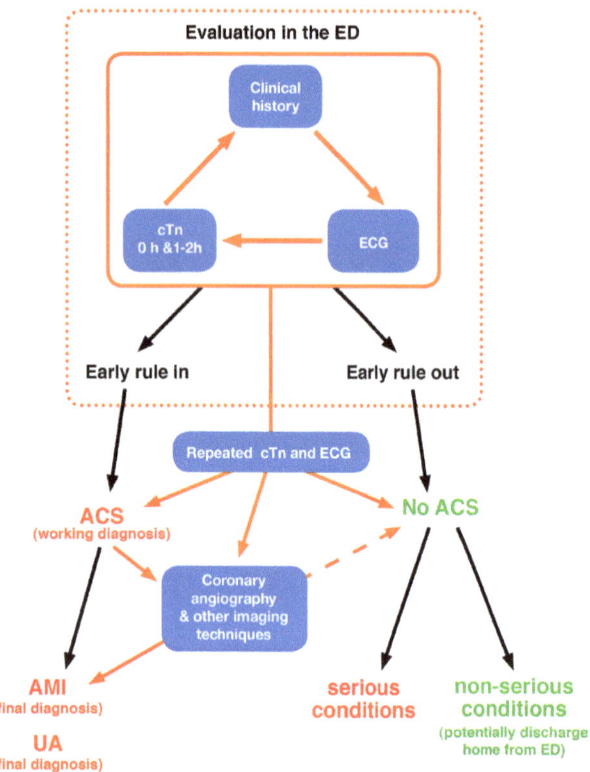


**Fig. 16.1.** Steps in the triage and management of patients presenting with suspected acute coronary syndromes.

in ECG are quite often unspecific (Body *et al.* 2010; Steurer *et al.* 2010).

Fig. 16.1 summarises key steps in the triage and management of patients presenting with suspected acute coronary syndromes (Hamm *et al.* 2011). The initial triage of a patient presenting to an ED with acute chest pain and ST segment elevation in the 12-lead ECG is usually straightforward. However, patients with suspected non-ST elevation acute coronary syndromes must be assessed using a combination of three key factors: clinical presentation, 12-lead ECG findings and measurement of cardiac biomarkers (i.e. cardiac troponins) (Fig. 16.1). The third universal definition of myocardial infarction – a collaborative consensus proposed jointly by European, American and international expert societies in 2012 (Thygesen *et al.* 2012a) – considered that a change in blood concentrations of cTn, with at least one value above the 99th percentile limit of the distribution of reference values, can be used to diagnose acute myocardial infarction when accompanied by other signs of ischaemia (symptoms or ECG changes) (Thygesen *et al.* 2007, 2010). The detection of changes in cTn levels are also included in the guidelines; that is, a rise and/or fall should be seen and detected in blood samples taken 2–3 h apart. The debate is still ongoing whether these changes should be calculated as relative changes (e.g. 50% change or as absolute changes).

Recent recommendations have noted that currently available cTn assays can contribute to rule-out protocols for myocardial infarction within 3 h of arrival at the ED (Amsterdam *et al.* 2010; Hamm *et al.* 2011). However, such protocols require the use of hs cTn assays currently only available at the clinical laboratory. Contemporary studies using sensitive cTn assays show no added value of adding other markers of myocardial damage, such as CK-MB, myoglobin or fatty-acid binding protein (Eggers *et al.* 2004, 2012). However, in the very early stage of acute myocardial infarction, the biomarker copeptin may have some value (Roffi *et al.* 2015). Copeptin is a precursor glycopeptide of arginine vasopressin (AVP), which can increase in cardiac injury at a stage before tissue necrosis (Jayasinghe *et al.* 2014). However, the introduction of the very hs cTn assays seems to make this biomarker redundant (Poldervaart *et al.* 2015).

The core principle underlying POC measurement of cTn is the reduction in turnaround time without compromising the quality of information on which clinical decisions for patients are based (Collinson 2006). A turnaround time of <1 h should be achieved, and the availability of POCT could reduce the turnaround time to <30 min. The 2011 guideline for management of non-ST elevation acute coronary syndromes noted that a rapid (2-h) rule-out protocol for acute coronary syndromes using POCT for cTn, ECG and risk scoring was found to be safe (Hamm *et al.* 2011; Than *et al.* 2011). This protocol was further modified by the guidelines in 2015 in which a safe rule-out and rule-in protocol at 0–1 h was recommended if an hs cTn test with a validated 0 h/1 h protocol is available (Roffi *et al.* 2015). Thus, the development of hs POC cTn assays is of major importance in order to reduce the time to rule-in or rule-out further. Such assays will undoubtedly be introduced to the market shortly.

POCT systems should provide quantitative, and not merely semiquantitative or qualitative, measurement of cTn to support or rule out a diagnosis of acute myocardial infarction, given the importance of detecting changes in cTn levels for a correct diagnosis (Christenson and Phillips 2011). In addition, the sensitivity of the assay system should ideally not differ from that provided by central laboratory assays. The imprecision of the measurement at the 99th percentile concentrations of cardiac troponins of healthy subjects has been highlighted as important in current management recommendations (Thygesen *et al.* 2010). Specifically, imprecision of 10% CV or less at the 99th percentile limit is desirable and, as mentioned previously, routine use of cTn assays with imprecision greater than 20% at this limit are not recommended (Jaffe *et al.* 2010).

In order to be implemented successfully, POCT for cTn should significantly reduce turnaround time without jeopardising the diagnostic performance. In particular, emergency physicians would tolerate neither a significant increase in false negative results, which might lead to discharge of patients with a persistent risk of cardiac adverse events, nor a substantial increase in false positive results with the risk of unjustified and potentially hazardous therapeutic interventions.

The safety of an accelerated 90-min protocol to exclude a diagnosis of acute myocardial infarction has been demonstrated in the ED setting using serial multi-marker POCT (cTn, CK-MB, myoglobin) (Ng *et al.* 2001). All cases of acute myocardial infarction were diagnosed within 90 min, and admissions to the coronary care unit were decreased by 40%. In addition, 90% of patients with negative cardiac biomarkers and ECG findings were discharged, with only one returning with myocardial infarction within 1 month. Another study focussed on 817 consecutive emergency department admissions for suspected acute myocardial infarction (McCord *et al.* 2001). The POCT strategy, which involved measurement of CK-MB and cTn, provided a negative predictive value of 99.6% for the diagnosis of myocardial infarction within 90 min, facilitating prompt and reliable rule-out of acute myocardial infarction. The median turnaround time for the POC tests was 24 min, compared with 71 min for the central laboratory. Recently, Aldous *et al.* (2014) compared the diagnostic ability of the new Alere Cardio3 TnI test, which runs on the Triage POCT device, with the hs Abbott Architect assay. This new test, which claims an improved sensitivity, was shown to have clinical sensitivity that was statistically comparable to the hs assay when used for an accelerated diagnostic protocol.

The Disposition Impacted by Serial Point-of-Care Markers in Acute Coronary Syndromes (DISPO-ACS) trial set out to test the hypothesis that POCT for cTnI would reduce length of stay, relative to central laboratory testing, in a large sample of 2000 patients evaluated for suspected acute coronary syndromes (Ryan *et al.* 2009). There was no overall change in length of stay. The authors concluded that reduced turnaround time of the POCT assay *per se* was insufficient to influence length of stay, and that POCT must impact on other aspects of patient management in order to translate reduced assay turnaround time to more rapid discharge. Reducing 'brain-to-brain time' (the time between a physician ordering a test and when he/she interprets its results and takes action based on predefined algorithms) was considered key to reducing overall length of stay. A previous study from the USA involved 545 patients admitted to a cardiology unit with chest pain in roughly equal proportions immediately before or after the introduction of POCT for cTnI (Apple *et al.* 2006). Charges to patients fell by 25% after the introduction of POCT, due to reduced costs associated with boarding, other departments, pharmacy, laboratories, and cardiac or non-cardiac procedures. In a study of comprehensive POCT (including cardiac biomarkers, haemoglobin, haematocrit, lactate and INR) on critically ill patients in the emergency room, the turnaround time to results was substantially reduced, as well as length of stay and the time to intravenous (IV) contrast computed tomography (CT), in particular during the night-time. Among the ED physicians who used cardiac biomarkers more widely, the ED length of stay was even shorter (Singer *et al.* 2015). Koehler *et al.* (2013) found that the satisfaction among ED health workers who performed POCT was high, while ED throughput was accelerated through the use of POCT.

The above studies were performed with current POC assays with relatively low sensitivity. With the imminent advent of hs POC cTn assays, new studies along these lines are needed to prove that results similar to current studies using hs cTn laboratory assays can be obtained (Roffi *et al.* 2015); that is, hs POC cTn assays can allow rule-in and rule-out within 0–1 h after admission with a dramatic change in turnaround time and the rapid disposition of the patient.

## POINT-OF-CARE TESTING FOR BRAIN NATRIURETIC PEPTIDES

Dyspnoea (shortness of breath) has been observed in about half of patients who received a primary diagnosis of heart failure in the ED, though it is well known to the ED physician that several other conditions present with dyspnoea, including asthma, pulmonary oedema, chronic obstructive pulmonary disease, interstitial lung disease and myocardial ischaemia. Rapid and accurate assessment of acute heart failure is therefore a priority when a patient presents with dyspnoea in an emergency setting. In recent years, the measurement of B-type natriuretic peptide (BNP) or NT-proBNP has become increasingly established for the management of patients presenting to an ED with dyspnoea or other symptoms suggestive of heart failure in order to distinguish acute heart failure from these other conditions (Thygesen *et al.* 2012b).

In response to increased myocardial stretch caused by volume and pressure overload as a result of heart failure, pre-proBNP is secreted by the ventricular myocytes and then enzymatically cleaved into BNP and the physiologically inactive NT-proBNP. Physiologically BNP acts to antagonise the effects of heart failure by reducing blood volume and pressure by several mechanisms including decreasing the release of renin and aldosterone and, at the level of the kidney, increasing the glomerular filtration rate while inhibiting renal sodium reabsorption (Kemp *et al.* 2004; Mayo *et al.* 2006).

POC measurement of cardiac biomarkers has the potential for faster turnaround times and consequent increases in the speed of diagnosis and subsequent throughput of patients within the ED. Table 16.1 highlights that all currently available POC assay systems that measure cardiac troponins also include natriuretic peptides on their test menu. The analytical challenge of establishing immunoassays for natriuretic peptides on POC platforms is far less than is the case for sensitive cTn assays. Thus, all POC tests for natriuretic peptides measure normal concentrations with acceptable performance. The decision is whether to choose assays that measure BNP or NT-proBNP. In the emergency setting with immediate testing by the POC device, the clinical performance of the two biomarkers is very similar, whereas the greater stability of NT-proBNP to storage gives this biomarker some advantages in the laboratory testing.

The use of the smaller handheld and portable POC devices for BNP and NT-proBNP has been validated in several recent studies including, for example, BNP on the Abbott i-STAT in a large regional centre in Australia (Stuckey *et al.* 2011), BNP on the i-STAT and Alere Triage in a US urban setting (Ro *et al.* 2011) and NT-proBNP on the Roche Cobas h232 (Bertsch *et al.* 2010).

Data from randomised or observational clinical studies (Lam *et al.* 2010; Meisel *et al.* 2012; Rehman *et al.* 2008) have generally demonstrated that the measurement of natriuretic peptides in the ED adds diagnostic information to other clinical measurements within a panel of biomarker and clinical measurements for the rule-in or rule-out of heart failure. Different authors and different studies have used various cut-off values for ruling in or ruling out heart failure; for example, for BNP, Maisel (2002) state that a BNP value below 100 pg/mL suggests that the patient with dyspnoea is unlikely to be suffering from heart failure, while a value above 400 pg/mL strongly suggests heart failure; however, Stuckey *et al.* (2011) uses a cut-off of 500 pg/mL or greater to rule in heart failure. With NT-proBNP, cut-off values are different again and vary significantly with age; for example, the cut-off to rule in heart failure is 450 pg/ml for patients aged <50 years, 900 pg/mL for patients 50–75 years and 1800 pg/mL for patients over 75 years (Kipper *et al.* (2015).

Importantly, the measurement of natriuretic peptides plus clinical judgment has been found to be superior to either alone. Major guidelines in the area support the measurement of natriuretic peptides most strongly where the clinical diagnosis of heart failure in patients presenting with acute dyspnoea is uncertain. A recent update of the main European guideline recommends measurement of natriuretic peptides in all patients with suspected heart failure (Thygesen *et al.* 2012b). Thus, rule-out may be possible with this measurement alone, without echocardiography, in patients with a normal ECG.

The measurement of NT-proBNP has been shown to result in significant cost savings relating to inpatient time, staff time, and usage of X-rays, echocardiography and treatments in a study of patients presenting to an ED with symptoms suggestive of heart failure (dyspnoea or peripheral oedema) (Mueller *et al.* 2006). Randomised controlled studies and prospective blinded studies have generally demonstrated reduced time to discharge following measurement versus no measurement of NT-proBNP, with a tendency to reduce costs, or reduced time in hospital at up to 1 year (Green *et al.* 2007; Moe *et al.* 2007; Siebert *et al.* 2006).

Measurement of natriuretic peptides generally results in more accurate diagnosis and improved risk stratification for patients with acute dyspnoea. Given current diagnostic performance, POCT measurement of natriuretic peptides could replace the use of central laboratories. The use of POCT systems could also be of considerable benefit in other settings, such as measurements of biomarkers made in the ambulance, should this approach be shown to provide benefits to patients. POCT biomarker measurements could also be convenient for community practice, where serial measurements of natriuretic peptides and other biomarkers could, in principle, reduce the risk of patients with heart failure presenting as an emergency, although this again requires clinical validation.

## POINT-OF-CARE TESTING FOR CARDIAC BIOMARKERS. WHY?

As outlined above, POCT for cTn and natriuretic peptides does not offer any advantages over laboratory testing regarding quality or sensitivity. Moreover, no studies have as yet specifically shown that POCT saves lives in the urban emergency setting. Why then is POCT in the emergency setting so attractive and how can we take advantage of this technology? In Fig. 16.2 the work flow of a patient coming to the ED is outlined. There are three key issues in relation to biomarker testing. *Brain 1* is the time when a decision is made to request a biomarker test, *Vein* is the time it takes to draw blood, perform the analysis and report the results and *Brain 2* the time when the results are reviewed and action taken. The time of *Brain 1* to *Vein* is considerably shorter when POCT is performed instead of laboratory testing because of transport time and other logistical issues. The *Vein* to *Brain 2* is the weak link. A common scenario is that *Brain 1* to *Vein* takes 20 min and *Vein* to *Brain 2* takes 1–2 h. Thus, in order to take full advantage of POCT, this latter time must be shortened. By shortening the time to a therapeutic decision and therapeutic manoeuvre, we reduce the suffering for our patients and can quickly refer them to settings outside the ED, relieving overcrowding. In the end, this will also reduce costs. Thus, in order to be implemented successfully, a POC test for cTn should significantly reduce turnaround time without jeopardising the diagnostic performance. To reiterate, emergency physicians would tolerate neither a significant increase in false negative results, which might lead to discharge of patients with a persistent risk of cardiac adverse events nor a substantial increase in false positives results with the risk of unjustified and potentially hazardous therapeutic interventions.

## EXAMPLES OF WORKING POINT-OF-CARE TESTING MODELS FOR CARDIAC TROPONIN IN RURAL AND REMOTE SETTINGS

POCT for cardiac markers in rural and remote medical services, paramedic or disaster situations present differing challenges to those experienced in an ED of a large urban hospital. In a rural or remote setting, the community may be serviced by a relatively small hospital or medical service, with the nearest laboratory hours or even days away. Without a POC device available, medical staff often have no option but to evacuate those presenting with symptoms of acute coronary syndrome (or acute dyspnoea) with a considerable time delay and expense.

Several studies have demonstrated the effective use of the Abbott i-STAT and the Roche Cobas h232 in rural and remote settings in Australia (Martin 2010; Shephard *et al.* 2014; Tideman *et al.* 2014). POCT for cTnT on the

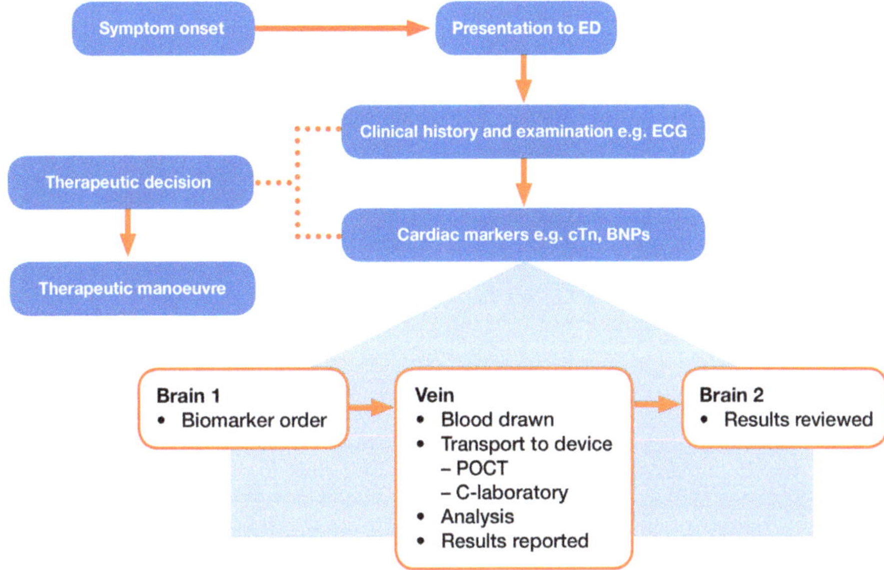


**Fig. 16.2.** Events determining turnaround time after a patient presents to the emergency department with suspected acute coronary syndrome.

Cobas h232 is one of the three key features of a cardiovascular support network that has been rolled out in regional and rural areas of South Australia since 2001 in an attempt to reduce the gap between death rates from cardiac disease between rural and metropolitan areas (Tideman *et al.* 2014). The Integrated Cardiovascular Clinical Network (iCCnet) combines quality-managed POCT with standardised risk stratification and evidence-based treatment protocols. An on-call cardiologist is available at short notice to provide consultancy to GPs and nurses, directions for on-site management and assistance with transport to a tertiary hospital if needed. By 2008, all 66 rural hospitals in South Australia were enrolled in this service. The availability of immediate assistance with cardiac patients in iCCnet was associated with a 22% relative odds reduction in 30-day mortality ($P$ = 0.007). A higher percentage of patients were transferred to hospital and the mortality was lower in those who were transferred (Tideman *et al.* 2014).

Since 2008, a partnership between the Northern Territory Government Department of Health and the Flinders University International Centre for Point-of-Care Testing has seen i-STAT devices now located in 75 remote health services for performing cTnI, along with several other tests for acute presentations (Shephard *et al.* 2014). The International Centre for Point-of-Care Testing provides staff training, manages the program's quality testing protocols, provides monthly workload statistics for the program's Management Committee and researches the evidence for the clinical and operational effectiveness of the program. Cardiac TnI POC tests were shown to comprise 22% of the tests performed on the i-STAT across the Northern Territory and there have been many cases involving cTnI POC testing that have allowed the early diagnosis of a non-ST elevation MI (non-STEMI) and/or stabilisation of patients *in situ* without the need for medical evacuation to the nearest tertiary hospital in Alice Springs or Darwin (Shephard *et al.* 2014). POCT programs such as these are applicable to developing countries where access to laboratories is very limited and costly.

## REFERENCES

Aldous S, Richards AM, George PM, Cullen L, Parsonage WA, Flaws D, *et al.* (2014) Comparison of new point-of-care troponin assay with high sensitivity troponin in diagnosing myocardial infarction. *International Journal of Cardiology* **177**, 182–186. doi:10.1016/j.ijcard.2014.09.026

Amsterdam EA, Kirk JD, Bluemke DA, Diercks D, Farkouh ME, Garvey JL, *et al.* (2010) Testing of low-risk patients presenting to the emergency department with chest pain: a scientific statement from the American Heart Association. *Circulation* **122**, 1756–1776. doi:10.1161/CIR.0b013e3181ec61df

Amundson BE, Apple FS (2015) Cardiac troponin assays: a review of quantitative point-of-care devices and their efficacy in the diagnosis of myocardial infarction. *Clinical Chemistry and Laboratory Medicine* **53**, 665–676. doi:10.1515/cclm-2014-0837

Apple F (2006) Clinical biomarkers of cardiac injury: cardiac troponins and natriuretic peptides. *Toxicologic Pathology* **34**, 91–93. doi:10.1080/01926230500431368

Apple F (2009) A new season for cardiac troponin assays: it's time to keep a scorecard. *Clinical Chemistry* **55**, 1303–1306. doi:10.1373/clinchem.2009.128363

Apple F, Collinson P (2012) Analytical characteristics of high-sensitivity cardiac troponin assays. *Clinical Chemistry* **58**, 54–61. doi:10.1373/clinchem.2011.165795

Apple FS, Chung AY, Kogut ME, Bubany S, Murakami MM (2006) Decreased patient charges following implementation of point-of-care cardiac troponin monitoring in acute coronary syndrome patients in a community hospital cardiology unit. *Clinica Chimica Acta* **370**, 191–195. doi:10.1016/j.cca.2006.02.011

Bertsch T, Chapelle J-P, Dempfle C-E, Giannitsis E, Schwab M, Zerback R (2010) Multicentre analytical evaluation of a new point-of-care system for the determination of cardiac and thromboembolic markers. *Clinical Laboratory* **56**, 37–49.

Bingisser R, Cairns C, Christ M, Hausfater P, Lindahl B, Mair J, *et al.* (2012) Cardiac troponin: a critical review of the case for point-of-care testing in the ED. *The American Journal of Emergency Medicine* **30**, 1639–1649. doi:10.1016/j.ajem.2012.03.004

Bingisser R, Cairns CB, Christ M, Collinson P, Hausfater P, Lindahl B, *et al.* (2013) Measurement of natriuretic peptides at the point of care in the emergency and ambulatory setting: current status and future perspectives. *American Heart Journal* **166**, 614–621. doi:10.1016/j.ahj.2013.06.012

Body R, Carley S, Wibberley C, McDowell G, Ferguson J, Mackway-Jones K (2010) The value of symptoms and signs in the emergent diagnosis of acute coronary syndromes. *Resuscitation* **81**, 281–286. doi:10.1016/j.resuscitation.2009.11.014

Chenevier-Gobeaux C, Bonnefoy-Cudraz E, Charpentier S, Dehoux M, Lefevre G, Meune C, *et al.* (2015) High-sensitivity cardiac troponin assays: answers to frequently asked questions. *Archives of Cardiovascular Diseases* **108**, 132–149. doi:10.1016/j.acvd.2014.11.001

Christenson RH, Phillips D (2011) Sensitive and high sensitivity next generation cardiac troponin assays: more than just a name. *Pathology* **43**, 213–219. doi:10.1097/PAT.0b013e328343762d

Collinson PO (2006) Cardiac biomarkers by point-of-care testing. In *Cardiovascular Biomarkers. Pathophysiology and Disease Management.* (Ed. DA Morrow) pp. 559–574. Humana Press, Totowa NJ, USA.

Eggers KM, Oldgren J, Nordenskjold A, Lindahl B (2004) Diagnostic value of serial measurement of cardiac markers in patients with chest pain: limited value of adding myoglobin to troponin I for exclusion of myocardial infarction. *American Heart Journal* **148**, 574–581. doi:10.1016/j.ahj.2004.04.030

Eggers KM, Venge P, Lindahl B (2012) High-sensitive cardiac troponin T outperforms novel diagnostic biomarkers in patients with acute chest pain. *Clinica Chimica Acta* **413**, 1135–1140. doi:10.1016/j.cca.2012.03.011

Green S, Redmond P, Januzzi J, Aleryani S, Lee-Lewandrowski E, Sluss P, *et al.* (2007) The impact of amino-terminal pro-brain natriuretic peptide testing on hospital length of stay and morbidity in patients with decompensated heart failure. *Archives of Pathology & Laboratory Medicine* **131**, 473–476.

Hamm CW, Bassand JP, Agewall S, Bax J, Boersma E, Bueno H, *et al.* (2011) ESC guidelines for the management of acute coronary syndromes in patients presenting without persistent ST-segment elevation: the Task Force for the management of acute coronary syndromes (ACS) in patients presenting without persistent ST-segment elevation of the European Society of Cardiology (ESC). *European Heart Journal* **32**, 2999–3054. doi:10.1093/eurheartj/ehr236

Howick J, Cals JW, Jones C, Price CP, Pluddemann A, Heneghan C, *et al.* (2014) Current and future use of point-of-care tests in primary care: an international survey in Australia, Belgium, The Netherlands, the UK and the USA. *BMJ Open* **4**, e005611. doi:10.1136/bmjopen-2014-005611

Jaffe AS, Apple FS, Morrow DA, Lindahl B, Katus HA (2010) Being rational about (im)precision: a statement from the Biochemistry Subcommittee of the Joint European Society of Cardiology/American College of Cardiology Foundation/American Heart Association/World Heart Federation Task Force for the definition of myocardial infarction. *Clinical Chemistry* **56**, 941–943. doi:10.1373/clinchem.2010.143958

Jayasinghe R, Narasimhan S, Tran T, Paskaranandadivel A (2014) Rapid rule out of myocardial infarction with the use of copeptin as a biomarker for cardiac injury. *Internal Medicine Journal* **44**, 921–924. doi:10.1111/imj.12526

Kemp M, Donovan J, Higham H, Hooper J (2004) Biochemical markers of myocardial injury. *British Journal of Anaesthesia* **93**, 63–73. doi:10.1093/bja/aeh148

Kipper B, Marston N, Maisel A (2015) Utility of B-natriuretic peptide in the diagnosis of congestive heart failure in emergency settings. In *Global Point-of-Care – Strategies for Disasters, Emergencies, and Public Health Resilience.* (Eds G Kost and C Curtis) pp. 129–134. American Association of Clinical Chemistry Press, Washington DC, USA.

Koehler J, Flarity K, Hertner G, Aker J, Stout JP, Gifford M, *et al.* (2013) Effect of troponin I point-of-care testing on emergency department throughput measures and staff satisfaction. *Advanced Emergency Nursing Journal* **35**, 270–277. doi:10.1097/TME.0b013e31829d2048

Korff S, Katus H, Giannitsis E (2006) Differential diagnosis of elevated troponins. *Heart (British Cardiac Society)* **92**, 987–993. doi:10.1136/hrt.2005.071282

Lam L, Cameron P, Schneider H, Abramson M, Muller C, Krum H (2010) Meta-analysis: effect of B-type natriuretic peptide testing on clinical outcomes in patients with acute dyspnea in the emergency setting. *Annals of Internal Medicine* **153**, 728–735. doi:10.7326/0003-4819-153-11-201012070-00006

Maisel A (2002) B-type natriuretic peptide levels: diagnostic and prognostic in congestive heart failure: What's next? *Circulation* **105**, 2328–2331. doi:10.1161/01.CIR.0000019121.91548.C2

Martin CL (2010) i-STAT – combining chemistry and haematology in PoCT. *The Clinical Biochemist Reviews* **31**, 81–84.

Mayo D, Colletti J, Kuo D (2006) Brain natriuretic peptide (BNP) testing in the emergency department. *The Journal of Emergency Medicine* **31**, 201–210. doi:10.1016/j.jemermed.2005.08.022

McCord J, Nowak RM, McCullough PA, Foreback C, Borzak S, Tokarski G, *et al.* (2001) Ninety-minute exclusion of acute myocardial infarction by use of quantitative point-of-care testing of myoglobin and troponin I. *Circulation* **104**, 1483–1488. doi:10.1161/hc3801.096336

Meisel SR, Januzzi JL, Medvedovski M, Sharist M, Shochat M, Ashkar J, *et al.* (2012) Pre-admission NT-proBNP improves diagnostic yield and risk stratification – the NT-proBNP for evaluation of dyspnoeic patients in the emergency room and hospital (BNP4EVER) study. *European Heart Journal. Acute Cardiovascular Care* **1**, 99–108. doi:10.1177/2048872612447049

Moe G, Howlett J, Januzzi J, Zowall H (2007) N-terminal pro-B-type natriuretic peptide testing improves management of patients with suspected acute heart failure. Primary results of the Canadian prospective randomized multicenter IMPROVE-CHF study. *Circulation* **115**, 3103–3110. doi:10.1161/CIRCULATIONAHA.106.666255

Mueller C, Laule-Kilian K, Schindler C, Klima T, Frana B, Rodriguez D, *et al.* (2006) Cost-effectiveness of B-type natriuretic peptide testing in patients with acute dyspnea. *Archives of Internal Medicine* **166**, 1081–1087. doi:10.1001/archinte.166.10.1081

Ng SM, Krishnaswamy P, Morissey R, Clopton P, Fitzgerald R, Maisel AS (2001) Ninety-minute accelerated critical pathway for chest pain evaluation. *The American Journal of Cardiology* **88**, 611–617. doi:10.1016/S0002-9149(01)01801-X

Poldervaart JM, Rottger E, Dekker MS, Zuithoff NP, Verheggen PW, de Vrey EA, *et al.* (2015) No added value of novel biomarkers in the diagnostic assessment of patients suspected of acute coronary syndrome. *PLoS One* **10**, e0132000. doi:10.1371/journal.pone.0132000

Rehman SU, Martinez-Rumayor A, Mueller T, Januzzi JL (2008) Independent and incremental prognostic value of multimarker testing in acute dyspnea: results from the ProBNP Investigation of Dyspnea in the Emergency Department (PRIDE) study. *Clinica Chimica Acta* **392**, 41–45. doi:10.1016/j.cca.2008.03.002

Ro R, Thode H, Taylor M, Gulla J, Tetrault E, Singer A (2011) Comparison of the diagnostic characteristics of two B-type natriuretic peptide point-of-care devices. *The Journal of*

*Emergency Medicine* **41**, 661–667. doi:10.1016/j.jemermed.2010.10.025

Roffi M, Patrono C, Collet JP, Mueller C, Valgimigli M, Andreotti F, *et al.* (2015) 2015 ESC Guidelines for the management of acute coronary syndromes in patients presenting without persistent ST-segment elevation: Task Force for the Management of Acute Coronary Syndromes in Patients Presenting without Persistent ST-Segment Elevation of the European Society of Cardiology (ESC). *European Heart Journal* (Online August), ehv320. doi.org/10.1093/eurheartj/ehv320

Ryan RJ, Lindsell CJ, Hollander JE, O'Neil B, Jackson R, Schreiber D, *et al.* (2009) A multicenter randomized controlled trial comparing central laboratory and point-of-care cardiac marker testing strategies: the Disposition Impacted by Serial Point of Care Markers in Acute Coronary Syndromes (DISPO-ACS) trial. *Annals of Emergency Medicine* **53**, 321–328. doi:10.1016/j.annemergmed.2008.06.464

Saenger AK, Jaffe AS (2008) Requiem for a heavyweight: the demise of creatine kinase-MB. *Circulation* **118**, 2200–2206. doi:10.1161/CIRCULATIONAHA.108.773218

Shephard M, Spaeth B, Mazzachi B, Auld M, Schatz S, Lingwood A, *et al.* (2014) Toward sustainable point-of-care testing in remote Australia – the Northern Territory i-STAT Point-of-Care Testing Program. *Point of Care* **13**, 6–11. doi:10.1097/POC.0000000000000009

Siebert U, Januzzi J, Beinfeld M, Cameron R, Gazelle G (2006) Cost-effectiveness of using N-terminal pro-brain natriuretic peptide to guide the diagnostic assessment and management of dyspneic patients in the emergency department. *The American Journal of Cardiology* **98**, 800–805. doi:10.1016/j.amjcard.2006.06.005

Singer AJ, Williams J, Taylor M, Le BD, Thode HC (2015) Comprehensive bedside point of care testing in critical ED patients: a before and after study. *The American Journal of Emergency Medicine* **33**, 776–780. doi:10.1016/j.ajem.2015. 03.034

Starnberg K, Jeppsson A, Lindahl B, Hammarsten O (2014) Revision of the troponin T release mechanism from damaged human myocardium. *Clinical Chemistry* **60**, 1098–1104. doi:10.1373/clinchem.2013.217943

Steurer J, Held U, Schmid D, Ruckstuhl J, Bachmann LM (2010) Clinical value of diagnostic instruments for ruling out acute coronary syndrome in patients with chest pain: a systematic review. *Emergency Medicine Journal* **27**, 896–902. doi:10.1136/emj.2010.092619

Storrow AB, Lyon JA, Porter MW, Zhou C, Han JH, Lindsell CJ (2009) A systematic review of emergency department point-of-care cardiac markers and efficiency measures. *Point of Care* **8**, 121–125. doi:10.1097/POC.0b013e3181b316b9

Stuckey L, Ward D, Negus P (2011) Correlation between point-of-care and laboratory-analyzed B-type natriuretic peptide in adult patients presenting to Nambour hospital emergency department with shortness of breath. *Point of Care* **10**, 25–27. doi:10.1097/POC.0b013e31820783ee

Than M, Cullen L, Reid CM, Lim SH, Aldous S, Ardagh MW, *et al.* (2011) A 2-h diagnostic protocol to assess patients with chest pain symptoms in the Asia-Pacific region (ASPECT): a prospective observational validation study. *Lancet* **377**, 1077–1084. doi:10.1016/S0140-6736(11)60310-3

Thygesen K, Alpert JS, White HD, Jaffe AS, Apple FS, Galvani M, *et al.* (2007) Universal definition of myocardial infarction. *Circulation* **116**, 2634–2653. doi:10.1161/CIRCULATIONAHA.107.187397

Thygesen K, Mair J, Katus H, Plebani M, Venge P, Collinson P, *et al.* (2010) Recommendations for the use of cardiac troponin measurement in acute cardiac care. *European Heart Journal* **31**, 2197–2204. doi:10.1093/eurheartj/ehq251

Thygesen K, Alpert JS, Jaffe AS, Simoons ML, Chaitman BR, White HD (2012a) Third universal definition of myocardial infarction. *European Heart Journal* **33**, 2551–2567. doi:10.1093/eurheartj/ehs184

Thygesen K, Mair J, Mueller C, Huber K, Weber M, Plebani M, *et al.* (2012b) Recommendations for the use of natriuretic peptides in acute cardiac care: A position statement from the Study Group on Biomarkers in Cardiology of the ESC Working Group on Acute Cardiac Care. *European Heart Journal* **33**, 2001–2006. doi:10.1093/eurheartj/ehq509

Thygesen K, Mair J, Giannitsis E, Muelle C, Lindahl B, Blankenburg S, *et al.* (2012c) How to use high-sensitivity cardiac troponins in acute cardiac care. *European Heart Journal* **33**, 2252–2257. doi:10.1093/eurheartj/ehs154

Tideman P, Tirimacco R, Senior D, Setchell J, Huynh L, Tavella R, *et al.* (2014) Impact of a regionalised clinical cardiac support network on mortality among rural patients with myocardial infarction. *The Medical Journal of Australia* **200**, 157–160. doi:10.5694/mja13.10645

# 17 Point-of-care testing for chlamydia, gonorrhoea and trichomoniasis

*Lisa Natoli, Louise Causer, Lara Motta, Mark Shephard and Rebecca Guy*

**Summary**

Chlamydia, gonorrhoea and trichomoniasis contribute collectively to a significant global burden of sexually transmitted infections (STIs). In low-income settings, treatment of these three curable STIs has often been based on syndromic management, which fails to detect asymptomatic cases (false negatives) and may lead to overtreatment of others (false positives). Point-of-care testing (POCT) has the potential to reduce the delays in laboratory testing and treatment of these infections but, until recently, most POCT was performed using lateral flow immunochromatographic devices with poor clinical sensitivity. The advent of new molecular-based POC test platforms with laboratory-equivalent analytical performance is revolutionising this field of STI diagnosis. A range of new molecular-based devices are likely to enter the diagnostic market in coming years.

## CLINICAL INTRODUCTION

### Global and regional burden

Chlamydia (caused by the bacterium *Chlamydia trachomatis*; CT), gonorrhoea (caused by the bacterium *Neisseria gonorrhoea*; NG) and trichomoniasis (caused by the protozoan parasite *Trichomonas vaginalis*; TV) contribute significantly to the global burden of STIs. The most recent global estimates suggest, in 2012, there were ~255 million prevalent cases of the three curable STIs among adults aged 15–49 years (Table 17.1) (Newman *et al.* 2015).

Globally, estimates of STI prevalence are generally higher among women than among men for all three infections. In women aged 15–49 years, the estimated global prevalence of chlamydia was 4.2%, gonorrhoea 0.8% and trichomoniasis 5.0%. Among men, the estimated chlamydia prevalence was 2.7%, gonorrhoea 0.6% and trichomoniasis 0.6% (Newman *et al.* 2015). Prevalence estimates for these curable STIs vary widely across the World Health Organization (WHO) regions. Based on data for 2005–2012, the estimated pooled prevalence for chlamydia were highest in the Americas and Western Pacific Region. For the other two STIs, the highest estimated prevalence rates were in the African Region (Newman *et al.* 2015).

Populations where STI prevalence is greatest include young people, men who have sex with men (MSM), female sex workers, Indigenous populations, certain racial and ethnic groups and people residing in rural areas (Kirby Institute 2015; Newman *et al.* 2015; Public Health England 2014a; Redmond *et al.* 2015; Ryder *et al.* 2012; Workowski and Bolan 2015). Trichomoniasis prevalence is higher among women than men and remains high in women above 40 years of age (Meites 2013). These STIs

Table 17.1. Global prevalence and incident estimates for 2012 (millions of cases)[a] (Source: Newman *et al.* 2015)

| Sexually transmissible infection (pathogen) | Prevalent cases | Incident cases |
|---|---|---|
| Chlamydia (Chlamydia trachomatis) | 127 | 131 |
| Gonorrhoea (Neisseria gonorrhoea) | 27 | 78 |
| Trichomoniasis (Trichomonas vaginalis) | 101 | 143 |
| All three STIs | 255 | 352 |

[a]Applying pooled estimate from 2005–2012 to the 2012 population

also impose a substantial economic burden on health systems. In the USA, for example, it was estimated that more than US$705 million was spent in 2008 to diagnose and treat the complications of chlamydia, gonorrhoea and trichomoniasis (Owusu-Edusei *et al.* 2013).

## Risk factors, pathophysiology and complications of these STIs

Risk factors commonly noted to be associated with these STIs include younger age, being female, having multiple sexual partners, inconsistent condom use, and a prior history of STIs (Holmes *et al.* 2007). In addition, broader contextual circumstances (such as poverty, involvement with crime and substance abuse) may augment sexual risk behaviours and the likelihood of exposure to infection (Buffardi *et al.* 2008).

In males, chlamydia may cause dysuria and a clear discharge (Russell *et al.* 2005) while in women, the symptoms of chlamydia can vary depending on the site of infection: infection of the urethra and lower genital tract may cause dysuria and abnormal vaginal discharge or post-coital bleeding, whereas infection of the upper genital tract can manifest as irregular uterine bleeding and abdominal or pelvic discomfort (Peipert 2003). Gonorrhoea can cause abnormal vaginal discharge, bleeding and dysuria in women, and may result in urethral discharge and dysuria in men (Bradford 2005). Trichomoniasis can result in profuse and unpleasant vaginal discharge and irritation and abdominal pain in women (Gottlieb *et al.* 2014; Kissinger 2015) and urethral discharge and dysuria in men (Petrin *et al.* 1998).

Diagnosis with these infections can have a profound psychological impact, contributing to feelings of stigma, shame and anxiety, and can negatively impact on sexual relationships and result in intimate partner violence (Gottlieb *et al.* 2014). Left untreated, these STIs can lead to consequences relating to sexual, reproductive and maternal-child health. This is especially true for women, where all three infections can lead to pelvic inflammatory disease (PID), ectopic pregnancy and tubal factor infertility (Holmes *et al.* 2007; Ljubin-Sternak and Mestrovic 2014). Several adverse pregnancy outcomes are associated with these infections including pre-term delivery, low birthweight, perinatal mortality and neonatal eye infections that can result in blindness (Gottlieb *et al.* 2014). In men, complications of these infections include prostatitis and balanoposthitis, orchitis and epididymitis, which can impact on sperm quality and male fertility (Ljubin-Sternak and Mestrovic 2014; Trojian *et al.* 2009). STIs also increase a person's susceptibility to HIV (Bernstein *et al.* 2010; Holmes *et al.* 2007).

Chlamydia, gonorrhoea and trichomoniasis infections are often asymptomatic for long periods of time. A large study of chlamydia and gonorrhoea in five countries found chlamydia to be asymptomatic in 31–98% of women and 88–100% of men; gonorrhoea was asymptomatic in 67–100% of women and 77–100% of men (Detels *et al.* 2011). Most (77%) males infected with trichomoniasis are without symptoms while the proportion of asymptomatic infections in women is between 25 and 85% (Kissinger 2015). Approximately 54% of untreated chlamydia infections will resolve within 12 months, but in a small proportion can persist for up to 4 years (Geisler 2010). Untreated gonorrhoea infections will clear within ~4 months, while trichomoniasis may persist for long periods (months to years) in women but will resolve within ~10 days in men.

All three infections are curable with widely available antibiotics, and combined with the fact that infections can be asymptomatic and persist for long periods of time, highlights the need for prompt identification and treatment of infected individuals.

## Screening guidelines for these sexually transmissible infections

Clinical guidelines in most high-income countries (Australasian Sexual Health Alliance 2015; Workowski and Bolan 2015) recommend chlamydia screening annually for young women aged <30 years (or <25 years in some jurisdictions) and also younger men in some countries, men who have sex with men (MSM), and other populations at higher risk such as Indigenous populations. Annual gonorrhoea screening is generally recommended in MSM and people from communities with a high burden of disease. Testing for chlamydia and gonorrhoea is also recommended in people with risk factors such as new or multiple sex partners, or a sex partner who has an STI, and young pregnant women. Testing for trichmoniasis is generally only conducted in women with HIV-infection and asymptomatic people in high-prevalence settings such as sexual health clinics, as well as those at high risk of infection or disease (e.g. persons with new or multiple sex partners). Screening guidelines vary by local, regional, or national epidemiology of the STIs.

In most low-income countries, detection of STIs is based on STI syndromic management guidelines using clinical criteria alone, consistent with WHO recommendations for routine care in low-income settings (WHO 2007). Syndromic management enables first-line health-care providers to commence treatment immediately, based on the most common organisms locally that cause such symptoms. Flow charts and algorithms developed by the WHO are used as a guide. A limitation of syndromic management is the potential for unnecessary treatment of patients whose symptoms are due to other causes. Unnecessary treatment carries the risk of antibiotic resistance developing and potential harm resulting from drug side effects. In addition, false positive results may result in psychosocial harm, especially if contact tracing is initiated.

## Treatment for these sexually transmissible infections

### Chlamydia

Azithromycin remains the drug of choice for uncomplicated genital chlamydia infection, although doxycycline is also used (Workowski and Bolan 2015). There has been some recent debate about whether doxycycline should replace single dose azithromycin as the first-line treatment for non-gonococcal urethritis in men, as well as for the management of rectal chlamydia (Chen and Tabrizi 2015).

### Gonorrhoea

*Neisseria gonorrhoeae* drug resistance is an increasing public health concern on a global scale. Recently there has been widespread resistance to the first- and second-line antibiotics used to treat gonorrhoea including penicillin-based regimens and fluoroquinolones (ciprofloxacin, ofloxacin or levofloxacin) (Lahra *et al.* 2012, 2015). There are also reports of increasing resistance to third generation cephalosporins, the last class of effective treatment available (Buono *et al.* 2015). Some countries have increased the recommended dose of cephalosporin, and most now advise dual therapy using an extended spectrum cephalosporin plus azithromycin (Workowski and Bolan 2015). In some remote settings (e.g. in Western and Northern Australia), antimicrobial resistance surveillance indicates continued low levels of penicillin resistance (Lahra *et al.* 2015) and penicillin-based regimens remain the treatment of choice for uncomplicated urogenital NG infection.

### Trichomoniasis

Metronidazole has been the drug of choice for *Trichomonas vaginalis* for almost 40 years. It belongs to the 5-nitroimidazole class of drugs and is efficacious in curing ~95% of cases, as are similar compounds such as tinidazole and seconidazole (Kissinger 2015).

## Uptake and timeliness of treatment in clinical practice

In low- and middle-income countries, the lack of laboratory infrastructure and affordable, easy-to-use and accurate STI tests that can be used at the point of care has meant that for the last two decades treatment of STIs has often been based on syndromic management. Considering the STI prevalence in these countries, and most infections are asymptomatic, this means syndromic management would not detect and treat most STI infections.

Despite high-quality laboratory infrastructure in most high-income countries, there can still be delays in treatment. National standards set in the UK recommend that at least 95% of chlamydia cases should be treated within 30 working days of testing (Public Health England 2014b) and in the USA national performance measures for timeliness of chlamydia treatment have been set at 14 and at 30 days (CDC 2011). Studies at sexual health clinics in several high-income countries report the median time to treatment ranges from 7 to 18 days (Geisler *et al.* 2008; Wong *et al.* 2005) while the proportion of clients treated within 7 days was reported as 45% for one study and 97% within 14 days for the other (Jones *et al.* 2011; Rukh *et al.* 2014). In high-income countries, delays have been shown to be more common in rural areas, where the distance from laboratories is great, and health centres may service populations that can be transient or mobile. Some reports have noted 20% of those diagnosed with an STI do not receive treatment and, for those treated, the average time to initiation is around 3 weeks (Guy *et al.* 2012). In Australian urban settings the corresponding figures are 3% and 3 days (Chen *et al.* 2004).

## POINT-OF-CARE TESTING DEVICE OPTIONS

### Chlamydia and gonorrhoea

There are more than 20 POC or 'rapid' immunochromatographic tests (ICTs) available globally to detect chlamydia or gonorrhoea antigen (Peeling 2012). These tests are based on lateral flow technology and most commonly employ ELISA (enzyme linked immunosorbent assay) as their method principle. They are usually available in a dipstick or card format or encased in a plastic cassette. They are simple to use (low technical complexity), require minimal training, have no (or limited) support equipment and generally produce results in <30 min.

The analytical performance of several of these rapid ICTs for chlamydia and gonorrhoea is summarised in Tables 17.2 and 17.3, respectively. In general, these rapid ICTs are plagued by poor sensitivity compared with gold standard laboratory methods. This lack of sensitivity may be explained by the following:

**Table 17.2.** Summary of analytical performance of POC tests for *Chlamydia trachomatis*

| Source | Test name (manufacturer) | POC test method | Laboratory method | Specimen type | Sensitivity (%) | Specificity (%) |
|---|---|---|---|---|---|---|
| Gaydos and Hardick 2014 | OIA (optical immunoassay) chlamydia test (Inverness, formerly BioStar) | ICT | NAAT | Cervical | 59.4–73.8 | 98.4–100 |
| Gaydos and Hardick 2014 | Clearview Chlamydia test (Alere) | ICT | PCR | Cervical | 49.7 | 97.9 |
| | | | | Vaginal | 32.8 | 99.2 |
| Gaydos and Hardick 2014 | QuickVue Chlamydia test (Quidel) | ICT | PCR | Cervical | 25–65 | 100 |
| | Chlamydia rapid test (PATH) | ICT | PCR | Vaginal | 41.4 | 89 |
| | | | | Male urine | 74.2 | 95.7 |
| Hurly *et al.* 2014 | Chlamydia rapid test (ACON Laboratories) | ICT | NAAT | Male urine | 43.8 | 98.3 |
| | | | | Vaginal | 66.7 | 91.3 |
| Sabido *et al.* 2009 | Chlamydia test card (Ultimed Products) | ICT | PCR | Cervical | 62.9 | 99.6 |
| van Dommelen *et al.* 2010 | Handilab-C (Zonda) | ICT | NAAT | Vaginal | 11.6 | 91.9 |
| van Dommelen *et al.* 2010 | Biorapid CHLAMYDIA Ag test (Biokit) | ICT | NAAT | Vaginal | 17.3 | 93.5 |
| Causer *et al.* 2015 | Diaquick CT Test (DIALAB) | ICT | NAAT | Urine (M and F) | 27.3 | 98.5 |
| Ham *et al.* 2015 | aQcare Chlamydia TRF (Medisensor Inc.) | ICT | NAAT | Urine (M and F) | 88.2 | 94.7 |
| | | | | Cervical and urethral | 93.8 | 96.8 |
| Causer *et al.* 2015 | GeneXpert CT/NG (Cepheid) | NAAT | NAAT | Urine | 100 | 99.5 |
| Gaydos and Hardick 2014 | GeneXpert CT/NG (Cepheid) | NAAT | NAAT | Cervical | 97.4 | 99.6 |
| | | | | Vaginal | 98.7 | 99.4 |
| | | | | Urine (F) | 97.6 | 99.8 |
| | | | | Urine (M) | 97.8 | 99.9 |

Note: M = male, F = female, ICT = immunochromatographic test, NAAT = nucleic acid amplification test, PCR = polymerase chain reaction

**Table 17.3.** Summary of analytical performance of POC tests for *Neisseria gonorrhoea*

| Author | Test name (manufacturer) | POC test method | Laboratory method | Specimen type | Sensitivity (%) | Specificity (%) |
|---|---|---|---|---|---|---|
| Gaydos and Hardick 2014 | GC-Check (PATH) | ICT | PCR | Cervical | 70 | 97.2 |
| | | | | Vaginal | 54.1 | 98.3 |
| Causer *et al.* 2015 | Gonorrhoea card test (Immuno-Diagnostics) | ICT | NAAT | Urine (M & F) | 66.7 | 76.9 |
| Gaydos and Hardick 2014 | NG GC OIA (Thermo BioStar) | ICT | Culture | Cervical | 60 | 89 |
| Gaydos and Hardick 2014 | Binax NOW (Inverness) | ICT | Culture | Male urine | 94 | 96 |
| Abbai *et al.* 2015 | OneStep Gonorrhea (Cortez Diagnostics Inc.) | ICT | Culture | Cervical | 0 | 98.7 |
| | | | SDA | Cervical | 7.1 | 100 |
| | | | Culture | Urethral (M) | 44.4 | 88 |
| | | | SDA | Urethral (M) | 46.4 | 91.7 |
| Gaydos and Hardick 2014 | GeneXpert CT/NG (Cepheid) | NAAT | NAAT | Cervical | 100 | 100 |
| | | | | Vaginal | 100 | 99.9 |
| | | | | Urine (M) | 98.9 | 99.9 |
| | | | | Urine (F) | 95.6 | 99.9 |
| Causer *et al.* 2015 | GeneXpert CT/NG (Cepheid) | NAAT | NAAT | Urine | 100 | 100 |

Note: SDA = strand displacement amplification, M = male, F = female, ICT = immunochromatographic test, NAAT = nucleic acid amplification test

- The lower limit of detection of most ICTs for chlamydia and gonorrhoea is between $10^4$ and $10^5$ bacteria, which is higher than that for laboratory-based detection methods. This also explains why higher sensitivities for ICTs are reported in studies involving symptomatic infections where bacterial loads are generally higher.
- The antibody–antigen reaction in the ICT format takes place over a much shorter timeframe compared with laboratory-based tests, meaning there is an inevitable trade-off between sensitivity and speed of result generation (Peeling 2012).
- ICTs are generally less sensitive for detection of antigen than antibody (Peeling 2011).

Given the overall poor performance of ICTs for chlamydia and gonorrhoea, there has been little uptake of these tests for programmatic use.

For chlamydia, nearly all studies (except one) have shown the sensitivity of rapid ICTs to be below 80%, with many reporting sensitivities below 50%, with variation according to specimen type, symptom status, background prevalence of infection and reference method (Table 17.2). Sensitivities for chlamydia can be overestimated if culture was the laboratory comparator method, since culture detects only 75–85% of infections compared with laboratory-based nucleic acid amplification (NAAT) reference techniques (Rani *et al.* 2002). Brook (2015) also conducted a literature review of chlamydia ICTs and concluded that the chlamydia rapid test was the best-performed kit available (with reported sensitivities ranging from 41 to 87% and specificities from 89 to 99.6%).

For gonorrhoea, most studies report rapid ICT sensitivities of <70% (Table 17.3) and specificities range from 77 to 100%. Brook (2015) identified the GC Check from the Program for Appropriate Technology in Health (PATH) group as the best-performed rapid IC test (with reported sensitivities ranging from 54 to 70% and specificities from 97 to 98%).

Other simple but under-used tools that might be considered to complement the POC diagnosis of chlamydia and gonorrhoea, particularly in low resource settings, include light microscopy, microscopic Gram staining and leucocyte esterase dipsticks (the latter intended to detect inflammation as a surrogate marker for urethritis due to chlamydia or gonorrhoea). Limitations of these tools include the need for invasive specimen collection, the need for technical training in microscopy and poor sensitivity and/or specificity for either or both bacterial species (Aledort *et al.* 2006; Bartelsman *et al.* 2015; Huppert *et al.* 2010). A systematic review showed that leucocyte esterase dipsticks had a much lower specificity (and positive predictive value) in women than ICT, which could be due to increased contamination of urine samples in the women by vaginal secretions and/or women being more prone to urinary tract infections when the leucocyte esterase enzyme is a marker of pyuria (Adeleke *et al.* 2009).

The recent advent of technology that combines ease of use with the high accuracy of nucleic acid amplification tests (NAATs) in a format suitable for the POC is revolutionising the field of STI diagnosis. One such device now commercially available is the GeneXpert® (Cepheid, Sunnyvale CA, USA), which can simultaneously detect chlamydia and gonorrhoea by nucleic acid amplification in a single test cartridge (the Xpert CT/NG assay) in 90 min. The self-contained, fully integrated and automated GeneXpert test system can process samples including male/female urine and provider-collected endocervical swabs or patient-collected vaginal swabs. The Xpert CT/NG assay was approved by regulatory authorities in Europe and the US Food and Drug Administration (FDA) in 2012, and was approved for diagnostic purposes in Australia by the Therapeutic Drugs Administration (TGA) in 2013. The analytical performance of the Xpert CT/NG assay for the detection of chlamydia and gonorrhoea has been confirmed by both laboratory-based and field evaluations, with these studies reporting sensitivities of greater than 97% and 96% for chlamydia and gonorrhoea, respectively, and specificities of greater than 99% for both bacteria (Causer *et al.* 2015; Gaydos and Hardick 2014; Tabrizi *et al.* 2013). Because *Neisseria gonorrhoea* is part of a family of closely related bacteria, cross reaction with other *Neisseria* species (both commensal and pathogenic) is a common problem and can lead to false positive test results (Samarawickrama *et al.* 2011). In their analytical performance study, Tabrizi *et al.* (2013) demonstrated the absence of false positive (cross-reactive) results with other *Neisseria* species or other commensal respiratory bacteria using the Xpert CT/NG assay. The use of two chromosomal targets (NG2 and NG4) for *N. gonorrhoea* by the Xpert CT/NG assay likely explains this finding.

Although the GeneXpert platform in its current format does require connection to a power source and has a relatively long turnaround time to results (90 min) compared with traditional lateral flow POC test platforms (under 30 min), it still has attributes that make it suitable for use at the POC for STI testing (Peeling 2011). These include its ease of use, high accuracy, dual infection test capability, use of easily collected specimens, minimal specimen preparation and automated result generation (Causer *et al.* 2015). As a demonstration of its suitability for use at the forefront of clinical care, the GeneXpert has recently been implemented for routine STI testing in remote Aboriginal primary care settings in Australia as part of the TTANGO (Test, Treat and Go) randomised controlled trial (Guy *et al.* 2013). This trial and selected preliminary findings are summarised in Chapter 28 as an example of a working POCT model.

In summary, the GeneXpert test system overcomes the significant performance limitations of existing ICTs for chlamydia and gonorrhoea and allows a laboratory-quality test to be available in geographically remote health services, where patients would otherwise experience treatment delays and associated sequelae of untreated infection.

## Trichomoniasis

There is limited published information about POC tests for detection of *Trichomonas vaginalis* (Table 17.4). Motile trichomonads can be seen visually by a wet microscopic examination of vaginal secretions. The most widely used ICT for trichomonas is the OSOM TV Trichomonas Rapid Test (Gaydos and Hardick 2014), which is a dipstick test that detects membrane proteins of *T. vaginalis*, has five manual steps and a turnaround time of 10 min. Reported sensitivities and specificities on vaginal swabs vary from 83 to 90% and from 98.8 to 100% (Table 17.4). Another POC test is the Affirm kit, which is a multi-analyte, nucleic acid probe-based assay system that enables the identification and differentiation of organisms associated with vaginitis (*Trichomonas vaginalis*, *Candida* sp. and *Gardnerella vaginalis*). The test requires more than 10 steps, while run time is ~45 min (Gaydos and Hardick 2014). A recent study reported poor sensitivity of 46% with this test (Cartwright *et al.* 2013).

A nucleic acid amplification (NAAT) test for *Trichomonas vaginalis* on the GeneXpert received CE-IVD marking in September 2014 and has recently been evaluated in Australia by Badman *et al.* (2015). The sensitivity and specificity observed for the 120 urine samples (60 positive and 60 negative) tested was 95% and 100%, respectively. Turnaround time is ~45 to 55 min, depending on organism

**Table 17.4.** Summary of analytical performance of POC tests for *Trichomonas vaginalis*

| Author | Test name | POC test method | Laboratory reference method | Specimen type | Sensitivity (%) | Specificity (%) |
|---|---|---|---|---|---|---|
| Gaydos and Hardick 2014 | OSOM® Trichomonas test (Sekisui Diagnostics/Genzyme Diagnostics) | ICT dipstick test | Composite of either (i) wet mount, culture, rapid test, or NAAT positive or (ii) wet mount- or culture-positive | Vaginal | 83.3–90[a] | 98.8–100[a] |
| Cartwright *et al.* 2013 | Affirm™ VPIII microbial identification test (Becton Dickinson Diagnostic Systems) | Nucleic acid probe-based assay | NAAT | Vaginal | 46.3 | 100 |
| Badman *et al.* 2015 | Xpert® TV (Cepheid) | NAAT | NAAT | Urine | 95.0 | 100 |

Note: NAAT = nucleic acid amplification test
[a]Range from three separate studies

load. Vaginal or cervical swabs can be tested along with urine samples. The capacity to perform TV plus CT/NG tests, albeit using two cartridges but on a single test platform, could significantly change the landscape for STI testing management in high burden settings with limited access to traditional based laboratory diagnosis.

The Quidel Corporation has recently launched a molecular POC test for the qualitative detection of *Trichomonas vaginalis* in vaginal samples on their AmpliVue® POC device. This test combines helicase-dependent amplification (HDA) technology with qualitative lateral flow detection. The helicase enzyme is used to separate the DNA into single strands, eliminating the need for thermocycling to promote amplification. A recent evaluation showed the device identified all of the culture and wet mount cases of *Trichomonas vaginalis* (Gaydos et *al.* 2015).

## POC tests for chlamydia, gonorrhoea and trichomoniasis in the diagnostic pipeline

There are several other promising POC tests on the horizon (Fig. 17.1), some of which will be described briefly.

The Atlas Genetics io™ test system uses a small, low-cost, simple-to-use instrument (the io™ reader) and a test-specific disposable cartridge (the io™ cartridge). Several test platforms are under development including a CT, a combination CT/NG test and a TV test. The device uses PCR technology with electrochemical detection based on differential pulse voltammetry with results available in ~30 min (Pearce *et al.* 2011).

Molbio Diagnostics has developed a portable multiplex platform for infectious disease tests called the Truelab™ real time micro PCR System and tests for CT and NG are under development. The Alere™ i-Platform uses isothermal NAAT technology for the qualitative detection of infectious disease tests including influenza A and B and *Streptococcus* A, with a CT/NG test being under development.

A low-cost POC test for chlamydia based on microwave-accelerated metal-enhanced fluorescence (MAMEF) technology has recently been described (Melendez *et al.* 2013; Zhang *et al.* 2011). This technology combines the microwave-based lysing of cells and DNA fragmentation with microwave-accelerated metal-enhanced detection of chlamydia DNA. Although the test remains under development and requires further optimisation, the low-power microwave acceleration has the potential capacity to significantly reduce the turnaround time of test results.

More recently, molecular POC technology has advanced further to include a minimally instrumented paper-based molecular diagnostic for the detection of chlamydia (Linnes *et al.* 2014). Although this is not commercially available it demonstrates proof of concept, combining molecular technology and POC technology in its truest sense. Similarly, Krõlov *et al.* (2014) recently used recombinase polymerase amplification technology to detect *C. trachomatis* in urine. This has proven feasible, sensitive and rapid, and has the potential to translate into a future POC diagnostic platform.

Other devices with CT, NG or TV tests under development include the RT-CPA (Ustar Biotechnologies), PanNAT® (Micronics) and GeneXpert® Omni (Cepheid).

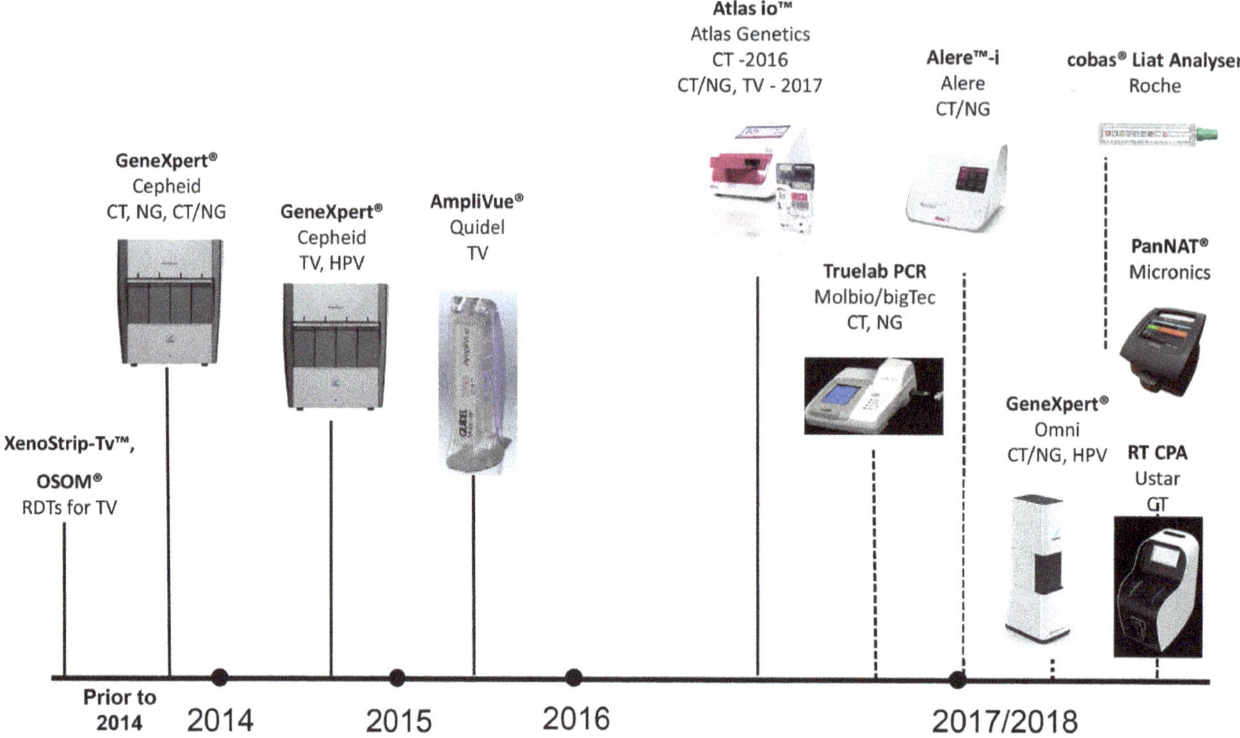


**Fig. 17.1.** Some POC tests for chlamydia, gonorrhoea and trichomonas currently available and in the diagnostic pipeline. (Source: Diagram created by, and used with permission of, Maurine Murtagh)

## ACCEPTABILITY STUDIES OF POINT-OF-CARE TESTING

Acceptability studies on a range of STI POC tests are summarised in Table 17.5, and highlight perceived benefits and barriers. Benefits included improved testing coverage, reduced time to treatment and infectious period, more timely partner notification and more targeted prescribing. Barriers included cost, complexity of the test and unreliability, long turnaround time to result, poor performance, disruption to client flow and time-consuming quality management practices and manual documentation processes. However, as demonstrated by Natoli *et al.* (2015a,b), many perceived barriers do not turn out to be actual barriers in clinical practice. The acceptability studies also highlight factors that should be considered when planning to use STI POC tests routinely, some are specific to STIs and others more general:

- Consider test performance (sensitivity, specificity), ease of use and client flow.
- Review STI clinical guidelines and develop POC procedures.
- Develop systems to maintain or enhance the completeness of communicable disease surveillance and antimicrobial resistance data.
- Develop systems to automate the flow of information between the POC test and medical record systems.
- Identify a funding model to cover equipment, consumables, quality testing and servicing costs to ensure long-term sustainability.
- Develop quality management systems and flexible training models.

## EVIDENCE BASE FOR THE PUBLIC HEALTH EFFECTIVENESS OF POCT FOR CHLAMYDIA, GONORRHOEA AND TRICHOMONIASIS

POC tests have great potential to strengthen existing STI management practices, especially in low-income countries or settings that rely on syndromic management. Also by shortening the test process and enabling earlier diagnosis and treatment, POCT is likely to reduce the infectivity period and enable the process of partner notification to occur without delay, decreasing the likelihood

**Table 17.5.** Acceptability studies of POC tests for chlamydia, gonorrhoea and trichomoniasis

| Type of POC test | Measurement tool | Target group | Setting | POC test | Author | Key acceptability findings |
|---|---|---|---|---|---|---|
| Chlamydia and gonorrhoea | In-depth interviews | Key informants | Australia | Any | Natoli *et al.* 2014, Natoli *et al.* 2015a,b | Participants believed that POC testing could:<br>Reduce the time to treatment and infectious period and expedite partner notification.<br>Improve testing coverage and result in more targeted prescribing, thereby minimising the risk of antibiotic resistance.<br>Participants highlighted there needs to be systems developed to:<br>Maintain the completeness of communicable disease surveillance data given the current dependence on reporting from pathology laboratories.<br>Maintain and improve the flow of NG antibiotic sensitivity data, already compromised by the shift to nucleic acid-based testing.<br>Provide flexible training models.<br>Ensure the quality of testing.<br>Financing of POC testing emerged as an important theme with the cost of POC testing equipment, consumables, proficiency testing and servicing all important considerations. |
| Chlamydia and gonorrhoea | In-depth interviews | Clinical staff | Australia | GeneXpert CT/NG NAAT test (Cepheid) | Natoli *et al.* 2015a,b | After using POC tests routinely, staff indicated the POC test was easy to use and useful in their clinical context.<br>Staff indicated that POC testing had resulted in more timely and targeted treatment, earlier commencement of partner notification, and reduced follow up efforts associated with client recall.<br>Staff expressed confidence in POC test results and treating patients on this basis, and reported greater job satisfaction.<br>For some, challenges included the manual documentation processes and managing positive test results in a shorter timeframe. |
| Gonorrhoea | Informal qualitative feedback from staff | Clinical staff | STI clinic, Brazil | NG Biostar ICT | Benzaken *et al.* 2006 | Staff rated the test as easy to use and results easy to interpret. |
| Trichomoniasis | Survey | Young women – self-testing | Urban hospital emergency department, USA | OSOM® Trichomonas Test (Genzyme Diagnostic) | Huppert *et al.* 2011 | Women initially perceived self-testing as more comfortable but less reliable than clinician testing, and many lacked confidence in their ability to perform a POC test and interpret the results.<br>Allowing a woman to try a POC STI test in the office and review her results with the clinician increased acceptability and trust of self-test results. |

Note: ICT = immunochromatographic test, NAAT = nucleic acid amplification test

of onward transmission (and HIV transmission) and re-infection.

Several modelling studies have been undertaken over the past decade to predict the health impact of POCT on STIs. The earliest modelling studies suggested that POCT for chlamydia and gonorrhoea could have a population health benefit at even moderate levels of sensitivity, especially when there is high potential for further STI transmission in the time between testing and treatment (Vickerman *et al.* 2003). In populations where there are high rates of sexual partner change, high frequency of sexual acts and low condom use, POC tests with sensitivity as low as 20–50% could result in more STIs being averted than when current gold standard tests are used (modelling based on sex workers who had between two and 10 partners per week and one sexual act per partner; condom use was as low as 3%). Gift *et al.* (1999) analysed the potential impact of a two-test algorithm involving a POC test for chlamydia (assumed sensitivity 63%) followed by a more sensitive laboratory test, and found the strategy to be cost-effective where chlamydia prevalence exceeds 9%.

Aledort *et al.* (2006) used mathematical modelling to estimate that use of POC tests for chlamydia and gonorrhoea (sensitivity 85% and specificity 90%) would avert greater than 16.6 million incident gonorrhoea and chlamydia infections, and prevent more than 212 000 new HIV infections (with modelling based on female sex workers in sub-Saharan Africa, China and SE Asia over a 4-year period). Also in Australia, a recent modelling study suggested that a POC test for chlamydia/gonorrhoea with high sensitivity (>95%) could reduce the prevalence of chlamydia and gonorrhoea from 11.9 to 8.9% and 7.1 to 5.7%, respectively, when used in high prevalence settings (Hui *et al.* 2013). If annual STI screening coverage was increased, this impact would be further enhanced. In a country such as Australia, the relative benefits of POC STI testing would be heightened in rural and remote areas, where the burden of chlamydia and gonorrhoea infections is greatest, access to laboratories is limited, and treatment delays and loss to follow up are real-time issues. In contrast, the utility of such tests in the urban context of lower STI rates, shorter treatment delays and minimal loss to follow up is more debatable (Chen *et al.* 2004).

## REFERENCES

Abbai NS, Moodley P, Reddy T, Zondi TG, Rambaran S, Naidoo K, *et al.* (2015) Clinical evaluation of the OneStep gonorrhea RapiCard InstaTest for detection of *Neisseria gonorrhoeae* in symptomatic patients from KwaZulu-Natal, South Africa. *Journal of Clinical Microbiology* **53**, 1348–1350. doi:10.1128/JCM.03603-14

Adeleke SI, Asani MO, Nwokedi EE (2009) Assessment of leukocyte esterase dipstick in diagnosis of childhood urinary tract infection. *African Journal of Clinical and Experimental Microbiology* **10**, 10–14.

Aledort JE, Ronald A, Rafael ME, Girosi F, Vickerman P, Le Blancq SM, *et al.* (2006) Reducing the burden of sexually transmitted infections in resource-limited settings: the role of improved diagnostics. *Nature* **444**(Supplement 1), 59–72. doi:10.1038/nature05447

Australasian Sexual Health Alliance (2015) *Australian STI Management Guidelines For Use in Primary Care*, <http://www.sti.guidelines.org.au/>.

Badman SG, Causer LM, Guy RJ, Tabrizi SN, Francis FDB, Whiley D and on behalf of the TTANGO investigators (2015) A preliminary evaluation of a new GeneXpert (Gx) molecular point-of-care test for the detection of *Trichomonas vaginalis*. *Sexually Transmitted Infections* **0**, 1–3. doi:10.1136/sextrans-2015-052384

Bartelsman M, Van Rooijen MS, Alba S, Vaughan K, Faber WR, Straetemans M, *et al.* (2015) Point-of-care management of urogenital *Chlamydia trachomatis* via Gram-stained smear analysis in male high-risk patients. Diagnostic accuracy and cost-effectiveness before and after changing the screening indication at the STI Clinic in Amsterdam. *Sexually Transmitted Infections* **91**, 479–484. doi:10.1136/sextrans-2014-051941

Benzaken AS, Galban EG, Antunes W, Dutra JC, Peeling RW, Mabey D, *et al.* (2006) Diagnosis of gonococcal infection in high risk women using a rapid test. *Sexually Transmitted Infections* **82**(Supplement 5), v26–v28. doi:10.1136/sti.2006.022566

Bernstein KT, Marcus JL, Nieri G, Philip SS, Klausner JD (2010) Rectal gonorrhea and chlamydia reinfection is associated with increased risk of HIV seroconversion. *JAIDS Journal of Acquired Immune Deficiency Syndromes* **53**, 537–543. doi:10.1097/QAI.0b013e3181c3ef29

Bradford D (2005) Urethral symptoms in males. In *Sexual Health Medicine*. (Eds D Russell, D Bradford and CK Fairley) pp. 59–71. IP Communications, Melbourne.

Brook G (2015) The performance of non-NAAT point-of-care (POC) tests and rapid NAAT tests for chlamydia and gonorrhoea infections. An assessment of currently available assays. *Sexually Transmitted Infections* **91**, 539–544. doi:10.1136/sextrans-2014-051997

Buffardi AL, Thomas KK, Holmes KK, Manhart LE (2008) Moving upstream: ecosocial and psychosocial correlates of sexually transmitted infections among young adults in the United States. *American Journal of Public Health* **98**, 1128–1136. doi:10.2105/AJPH.2007.120451

Buono SA, Watson TD, Borenstein LA, Klausner JD, Pandori MW, Godwin HA (2015) Stemming the tide of drug-resistant *Neisseria gonorrhoeae*: the need for an individualized approach to treatment. *The Journal of Antimicrobial Chemotherapy* **70**, 374–381. doi:10.1093/jac/dku396

Cartwright CP, Lembke BD, Ramachandran K, Body BA, Nye MB, Rivers CA, *et al.* (2013) Comparison of nucleic acid amplification assays with BD affirm VPIII for diagnosis of vaginitis in symptomatic women. *Journal of Clinical Microbiology* **51**, 3694–3699. doi:10.1128/JCM.01537-13

Causer LM, Hengel B, Natoli L, Tangey A, Badman SG, Tabrizi SN, *et al.* (2015) A field evaluation of a new molecular-based point-of-care test for chlamydia and gonorrhoea in remote Aboriginal health services in Australia. *Sexual Health* **12**, 27–33. doi:10.1071/SH14158

CDC (Centers for Disease Control and Prevention) (2011) *2011 Performance measures: Quick Reference Guide.* Centers for Disease Control and Prevention, <http://www.cdc.gov/std/program/2011PerformanceMeasuresQuickGuidel.pdf>.

Chen MY, Tabrizi SN (2015) Challenges to the management of curable sexually transmitted infections. *BMC Infectious Diseases* **15**, 337. doi:10.1186/s12879-015-1061-2

Chen MY, Ryder N, Donovan B (2004) Completeness and timeliness of treatment for chlamydia within a sexual health service. *International Journal of STD & AIDS* **15**, 762–764. doi:10.1258/0956462042395113

Detels R, Green AM, Klausner JD, Katzenstein D, Gaydos C, Handsfield H, *et al.* (2011) The incidence and correlates of symptomatic and asymptomatic *Chlamydia trachomatis* and *Neisseria gonorrhoeae* infections in selected populations in five countries. *Sexually Transmitted Diseases* **38**, 503–509.

Gaydos C, Hardick J (2014) Point of care diagnostics for sexually transmitted infections: perspectives and advances. *Expert Review of Anti-Infective Therapy* **12**, 657–672. doi:10.1586/14787210.2014.880651

Gaydos CA, Hobbs M, Marrazzo J, *et al.* (2015) *Performance of the Amplivue® Trichomonas Assay for the Detection of Trichomonas vaginalis in Women from Vaginal Specimens.* Poster 201. Johns Hopkins University, <http://www.hopkinsmedicine.org/Medicine/std/posters/Gaydos_CVS2015.pdf>.

Geisler WM (2010) Duration of untreated, uncomplicated *Chlamydia trachomatis* genital infection and factors associated with chlamydia resolution: a review of human studies. *The Journal of Infectious Diseases* **201**(Supplement 2), S104–S113. doi:10.1086/652402

Geisler WM, Wang C, Morrison SG, Black CM, Bandea CI, Hook EW 3rd (2008) The natural history of untreated *Chlamydia trachomatis* infection in the interval between screening and returning for treatment. *Sexually Transmitted Diseases* **35**, 119–123. doi:10.1097/OLQ.0b013e318151497d

Gift TL, Pate MS, Hook EW 3rd, Kassler WJ (1999) The rapid test paradox: when fewer cases detected lead to more cases treated: a decision analysis of tests for *Chlamydia trachomatis. Sexually Transmitted Diseases* **26**, 232–240. doi:10.1097/00007435-199904000-00010

Gottlieb SL, Low N, Newman LM, Bolan G, Kamb M, Broutet N (2014) Toward global prevention of sexually transmitted infections (STIs): the need for STI vaccines. *Vaccine* **32**, 1527–1535. doi:10.1016/j.vaccine.2013.07.087

Guy R, Ward JS, Smith KS, Su JY, Huang RL, Tangey A, *et al.* (2012) The impact of sexually transmissible infection programs in remote Aboriginal communities in Australia: a systematic review. *Sexual Health* **9**, 205–212. doi:10.1071/SH11074

Guy R, Natoli L, Ward J, Causer L, Hengel B, Whiley D, *et al.* (2013) A randomised trial of point-of-care tests for chlamydia and gonorrhoea infections in remote communities: Test, Treat And GO – the 'TTANGO' trial protocol. *BMC Infectious Diseases* **13**, 485. doi:10.1186/1471-2334-13-485

Ham JY, Jung J, Hwang BG, Kim WJ, Kim YS, Kim EJ, *et al.* (2015) Highly sensitive and novel point-of-care system, aQcare Chlamydia TRF kit for detecting *Chlamydia trachomatis* by using europium (Eu) (III) chelated nanoparticles. *Annals of Laboratory Medicine* **35**, 50–56. doi:10.3343/alm.2015.35.1.50

Holmes KK, Sparling PF, Stamm WE, Piot P, Wasserheit JN, Corey L, *et al.* (2007) *Sexually Transmitted Diseases.* McGraw-Hill Professional Publishing. New York, USA.

Hui BB, Wilson DP, Ward JS, Guy RJ, Kaldor JM, Law MG, *et al.* (2013) The potential impact of new generation molecular point-of-care tests on gonorrhoea and chlamydia in a setting of high endemic prevalence. *Sexual Health* **10**, 348–356. doi:10.1071/SH13026

Huppert J, Hesse E, Gaydos CA (2010) What's the point? How point of care STI tests can impact infected patients. *Point of Care* **9**, 36–46. doi:10.1097/POC.0b013e3181d2d8cc

Huppert JS, Hesse EA, Bernard MA, Xiao Y, Huang B, Gaydos C, *et al.* (2011) Acceptability of self-testing for trichomoniasis increases with experience. *Sexually Transmitted Infections* **87**, 494–500. doi:10.1136/sextrans-2011-050037

Hurly DSM, Buhrer-Skinner SG, Badman S, Bulu S, Tabrizi N, Tarivonda L, *et al.* (2014) Field evaluation of the CRT and ACON chlamydia point-of-care tests in a tropical, low-resource setting. *Sexually Transmitted Infections* **90**, 179–184. doi:10.1136/sextrans-2013-051246

Jones HE, Pressman EJ, Bell DL, Kerns JL, Lykes ST, Garth J, *et al.* (2011) Managing chlamydia infections in young men: results from an audit of a public men's clinic in New York City. *International Journal of STD & AIDS* **22**, 581–584. doi:10.1258/ijsa.2011.010462

Kirby Institute (2015) 'HIV/AIDS, viral hepatitis and sexually transmissible infections in Australia Annual Surveillance Report'. Sydney, Kirby Institute, University of New South Wales, Sydney.

Kissinger P (2015) Trichomonas vaginalis: a review of epidemiologic, clinical and treatment issues. *BMC Infectious Diseases* **15**, 307. doi:10.1186/s12879-015-1055-0

Krõlov K, Frolova J, Tudoran O, Suhorutsenko J, Lehto T, Sibul H, *et al.* (2014) Sensitive and rapid detection of *Chlamydia trachomatis* by recombinase polymerase amplification directly from urine samples. *The Journal of Molecular Diagnostics* **16**, 127–135. doi:10.1016/j.jmoldx.2013.08.003

Lahra M, Australian Gonococcal Surveillance Programme (2015) 'Australian Gonococcal Surveillance Programme annual report, 2014'. *Communicable Diseases Intelligence Quarterly Report* **39**, E347–E354.

Lahra M, WHO Western Pacific and South East Asian Gonococcal Antimicrobial Surveillance Programmes (2012) 'Surveillance of antibiotic resistance in *Neisseria gonorrhoeae* in the WHO Western Pacific and South East Asian Regions, 2010'. *Communicable Diseases Intelligence Quarterly Report* **36**, 95–100.

Linnes JC, Fan A, Rodriguez NM, Lemieux B, Kong H, Klapperich CM (2014) Paper-based molecular diagnostic for *Chlamydia trachomatis. Royal Society of Chemistry Advances* **4**, 42245–42251.

Ljubin-Sternak S, Mestrovic T (2014) *Chlamydia trachomatis* and genital Mycoplasmas: pathogens with an impact on human reproductive health. *The Journal of Pathology* **2014**, 183167.

Meites E (2013) Trichomoniasis: the 'neglected' sexually transmitted disease. *Infectious Disease Clinics of North America* **27**, 755–764. doi:10.1016/j.idc.2013.06.003

Melendez JH, Huppert JS, Jett-Goheen M, Hesse EA, Quinn N, Gaydos CA, *et al.* (2013) Blind evaluation of the microwave-accelerated metal-enhanced fluorescence ultrarapid and sensitive *Chlamydia trachomatis* test by use of clinical samples. *Journal of Clinical Microbiology* **51**, 2913–2920. doi:10.1128/JCM.00980-13

Natoli L, Maher L, Shephard M, Hengel B, Tangey A, Badman SG, *et al.* (2014) Point-of-care testing for chlamydia and gonorrhoea: implications for clinical practice. *PLoS One* **9**, e100518. doi:10.1371/journal.pone.0100518

Natoli L, Guy RJ, Shephard M, Causer L, Badman SG, Hengel B, *et al.* (2015a) 'I do feel like a scientist at times': a qualitative study of the acceptability of molecular point-of-care testing for chlamydia and gonorrhoea to primary care professionals in a remote high STI burden setting. *PLoS One* **10**, e0145993. doi:10.1371/journal.pone.0145993

Natoli L, Guy RJ, Shephard M, Whiley D, Tabrizi SN, Ward J, *et al.* (2015b) Public health implications of molecular point-of-care testing for chlamydia and gonorrhoea in remote primary care services in Australia: a qualitative study. *BMJ Open* **5**, e006922. doi:10.1136/bmjopen-2014-006922

Newman L, Rowley J, Vander Hoorn S, Wijesooriya NS, Unemo M, Low N, *et al.* (2015) Global estimates of the prevalence and incidence of four curable sexually transmitted infections in 2012 based on systematic review and global reporting. *PLoS One* **10**, e0143304. doi:10.1371/journal.pone.0143304

Owusu-Edusei K Jr, Chesson HW, Gift TL, Tao G, Mahajan R, Ocfemia MC, *et al.* (2013) The estimated direct medical cost of selected sexually transmitted infections in the United States, 2008. *Sexually Transmitted Diseases* **40**, 197–201. doi:10.1097/OLQ.0b013e318285c6d2

Pearce DM, Shenton DP, Holden J, Gaydos CA (2011) Evaluation of a novel electrochemical detection method for *Chlamydia trachomatis*: application for point-of-care diagnostics. *IEEE Transactions on Biomedical Engineering* **58**, 755–758. doi:10.1109/TBME.2010.2095851

Peeling RW (2011) Applying new technologies for diagnosing sexually transmitted infections in resource-poor settings. *Sexually Transmitted Infections* **87**(Supplement 2), ii28–ii30. doi:10.1136/sti.2010.047647

Peeling R (2012) Rapid tests for the detection of sexually transmitted infections. In *Sexually Transmitted Infections.* 2nd edn. (Eds S Gupta and B Kumar) pp. 321–331. Elsevier, New Delhi, India.

Peipert JF (2003) Clinical practice. Genital chlamydial infections. *The New England Journal of Medicine* **349**, 2424–2430. doi:10.1056/NEJMcp030542

Petrin D, Delgaty K, Bhatt R, Garber G (1998) Clinical and microbiological aspects of *Trichomonas vaginalis. Clinical Microbiology Reviews* **11**, 300–317.

Public Health England (2014a) *Sexually Transmitted Infections Annual Data*, <https://www.gov.uk/government/statistics/sexually-transmitted-infections-stis-annual-data-tables>.

Public Health England (2014b) *National Chlamydia Screening Programme (NCSP): Audit Report on Turnaround Times. PHE gateway number: 2014462.* Public Health England, London, UK.

Rani R, Corbitt G, Killough R, Curless E (2002) Is there any role for rapid tests for *Chlamydia trachomatis*? *International Journal of STD & AIDS* **13**, 22–24. doi:10.1258/0956462021924569

Redmond SM, Alexander-Kisslig K, Woodhall S, van den Broek IV, van Bergen J, Ward H, *et al.* (2015) Genital chlamydia prevalence in Europe and non-European high income countries: systematic review and meta-analysis. *PLoS One* **10**, e0115753. doi:10.1371/journal.pone.0115753

Rukh S, Khurana R, Mickey T, Anderson L, Velasquez V, Taylor M (2014) Chlamydia and gonorrhea diagnosis, treatment, personnel cost savings, and service delivery improvements after the implementation of express sexually transmitted disease testing in Maricopa County, Arizona. *Sexually Transmitted Diseases* **41**, 74–78. doi:10.1097/OLQ.0000000000000070

Russell D, Bradford D, Fairley CK (Eds) (2005) *Sexual Health Medicine.* IP Communications, Melbourne.

Ryder N, Woods H, McKay K, Giddings N, Lenton JA, Little C, *et al.* (2012) *Trichomonas vaginalis* prevalence increases with remoteness in rural and remote New South Wales, Australia. *Sexually Transmitted Diseases* **39**, 938–941. doi:10.1097/OLQ.0b013e31826ae875

Sabido M, Hernandez G, Gonzalez V, Valles X, Montoliu A, Figuerola J, *et al.* (2009) Clinic-based evaluation of a rapid point-of-care test for detection of *Chlamydia trachomatis* in specimens from sex workers in Escuintla, Guatemala. *Journal of Clinical Microbiology* **47**, 475–476. doi:10.1128/JCM.01975-08

Samarawickrama A, Alexander S, Ison C (2011) A laboratory-based evaluation of the BioStar Optical ImmunoAssay point-of-care test for diagnosing *Neisseria gonorrhoeae* infection. *Journal of Medical Microbiology* **60**, 1779–1781. doi:10.1099/jmm.0.034116-0

Tabrizi SN, Unemo M, Golparian D, Twin J, Limnios AE, Lahra M, *et al.* (2013) Analytical evaluation of GeneXpert CT/NG, the first genetic point-of-care assay for simultaneous detection of *Neisseria gonorrhoeae* and *Chlamydia trachomatis.*

*Journal of Clinical Microbiology* **51**, 1945–1947. doi:10.1128/JCM.00806-13

Trojian TH, Lishnak TS, Heiman D (2009) Epididymitis and orchitis: an overview. *American Family Physician* **79**, 583–587.

van Dommelen L, van Tiel FH, Ouburg S, Brouwers EE, Terporten PH, Savelkoul PH, *et al.* (2010) Alarmingly poor performance in *Chlamydia trachomatis* point-of-care testing. *Sexually Transmitted Infections* **86**, 355–359. doi:10.1136/sti.2010.042598

Vickerman P, Watts C, Alary M, Mabey D, Peeling RW (2003) Sensitivity requirements for the point of care diagnosis of *Chlamydia trachomatis* and *Neisseria gonorrhoeae* in women. *Sexually Transmitted Infections* **79**, 363–367. doi:10.1136/sti.79.5.363

WHO (World Health Organization) (2007) *Global Strategy for the Prevention and Control of Sexually Transmitted Infections: 2006–2015: Breaking the Chain of Transmission.* WHO, Geneva, Switzerland.

Wong D, Berman SM, Furness BW, Gunn RA, Taylor M, Peterman TA (2005) Time to treatment for women with chlamydial or gonococcal infections: a comparative evaluation of sexually transmitted disease clinics in 3 US cities. *Sexually Transmitted Diseases* **32**, 194–198. doi:10.1097/01.olq.0000154494.95138.70

Workowski KA, Bolan GA (2015) 'Sexually transmitted diseases treatment guidelines'. *MMWR Morbidity and Mortality Weekly Report* **64**, 1–137, <http://www.cdc.gov/mmwr/preview/mmwrhtml/rr6403a1.htm>.

Zhang Y, Agreda P, Kelley S, Gaydos C, Geddes CD (2011) Development of a microwave-accelerated metal-enhanced fluorescence 40 second, <100 cfu/ml point of care assay for the detection of *Chlamydia trachomatis. IEEE Transactions on Biomedical Engineering* **58**, 781–784. doi:10.1109/TBME.2010.2066275

# 18 Point-of-care testing for syphilis

*Igor Toskin, Maurine M Murtagh, James Kiarie and Rosanna W Peeling**

**Summary**

Simple, inexpensive point-of-care (POC) tests for screening maternal syphilis and facilitating treatment before the second trimester of pregnancy have been shown to prevent adverse pregnancy outcomes such as stillbirth and prematurity and save babies from congenital syphilis. Several new POC tests will soon be available and more on the horizon. Although deployment of POC tests can improve access to testing, including screening, case management and surveillance, the introduction of point-of-care testing (POCT) in the developing world has often been hampered by health system constraints as well as political, cultural, socioeconomic and behavioural factors. Implementation of POC tests must focus on advocacy, policy and guideline development, adequate training, quality assurance, data connectivity, supply chain management and monitoring of program effectiveness.

## INTRODUCTION

The World Health Organization (WHO) estimates that in 2012, the most recent year for which such statistics are available, there were ~6 million new cases of syphilis worldwide (Newman *et al.* 2015). The highest disease burden for syphilis is in the WHO African Region.

Syphilis is a sexually transmitted infection (STI) caused by a bacterium called *Treponema pallidum*. It is asymptomatic, but undetected infection has particularly profound consequences for pregnant women and their babies. Maternal syphilis is a significant cause of infant mortality. The WHO estimated that ~1.86 million cases of syphilis occur worldwide among pregnant women each year, many of whom are either untreated or inadequately treated (Gomez *et al.* 2013; WHO 2013). More than 400 000 perinatal deaths (i.e. deaths that occur from 22 weeks gestation through the first 7 days of life) occur each year as a result of untreated maternal syphilis. Without universal testing and treatment of syphilis in pregnancy, as many as 50% of pregnancies in women with syphilis will result in adverse outcomes, including perinatal death, prematurity and low birthweight. Babies born with congenital syphilis in the developing world have a 50% chance of dying within the first 2 years of life. These adverse outcomes could be

*Disclaimer: The authors alone are responsible for the views expressed in this chapter and they do not necessarily represent the views, decisions or policies of the institutions with which they are affiliated. The mention of specific companies or of certain manufacturers' products does not imply that they are endorsed or recommended by the World Health Organization in preference to others of a similar nature that are not mentioned. Errors and omissions excepted, the names of proprietary products are distinguished by initial capital letters.

prevented by screening all pregnant women for syphilis and treating those who are found to be infected with a single dose of penicillin before the third trimester (Berman 2004; Hawkes *et al.* 2011; Watson-Jones *et al.* 2002). Prenatal screening for syphilis is recommended policy in almost every country. According to the latest UNICEF statistics, 75–85% of women attend an antenatal clinic (ANC) at least once during pregnancy, representing an ideal opportunity for screening and treatment.

Since 2007, the WHO and other international partners have been advocating for the elimination of mother-to-child transmission (EMTCT) of HIV and syphilis (Kamb *et al.* 2010; Owiredu *et al.* 2015; WHO 2010). This initiative has been considered a high priority within national HIV/AIDS, STI, and maternal, newborn, and child health (MNCH) programs. Substantial progress has been made in this field, particularly with EMTCT of HIV. The WHO estimates that in 2014 around 73% of the estimated 1.5 million pregnant women living with HIV globally received effective antiretroviral drugs to avoid transmission to their fetus (WHO 2014a).

In order to validate EMTCT at country, regional and national level, the WHO developed minimum targets as follows (WHO 2014b):

- for HIV, <50 new paediatric infections per 100 000 live births and a transmission rate of either <5% in breastfeeding populations or <2% in non-breastfeeding populations
- for syphilis, <50 cases of congenital syphilis per 100 000 live births.

  There are four *process* targets:
- antenatal care coverage (at least one visit) of ≥95%
- coverage of HIV and/or syphilis testing of pregnant women of ≥95%
- antiretroviral treatment coverage of HIV-positive pregnant women of ≥90%
- treatment of syphilis-seropositive pregnant women of ≥95%.

In June 2015, Cuba became the first country in the world that was validated by the WHO as having eliminated MTCT of HIV and syphilis (WHO 2015a).

EMTCT is a realistic public health goal. Screening using POCT and same-day treatment strategy in conjunction with appropriate counselling of women and their partners, as well as encouraging safe delivery and infant feeding practices, plays a pivotal role in achieving the EMTCT impact targets.

In addition to the profound consequences that syphilis has for pregnant women, syphilis can also have serious consequences for individuals in key populations where its prevalence is high: men who have sex with men (MSM) and sex workers (WHO 2015b,c; CDC 2015). The WHO estimates that 5% or more of MSM are infected with syphilis in at least 42 countries, 10% or more in 20 countries and more than 20% in 8 countries. The United States Centers for Disease Control and Prevention (CDC) estimate that 75% of syphilis cases in the USA are among MSM. In addition, the WHO documents a high burden of syphilis in MSM, with 48% of all new syphilis cases in 2012 reported among that population. Untreated syphilis can also increase the risk of acquiring and transmitting HIV.

The WHO estimates that syphilis infects more than 5% of sex workers in 34 countries, more than 10% in 21 countries and more than 20% in 7 countries (WHO 2015c). Sex workers include female, male and transgender individuals who receive money/goods in exchange for sexual services, and they are very vulnerable to HIV and other STIs.

## POINT-OF-CARE TESTS FOR SYPHILIS

Syphilis is usually diagnosed using laboratory-based tests, consisting of both non-*Treponema pallidum* (non-TP) and *Treponema pallidum* (TP) tests (Peeling and Ye 2004). Non-TP tests can be used to detect active syphilis but may give biological false positive results in people with malaria, leprosy and immune disorders. Although non-TP tests can give a result in 8 min, they require centrifugation to obtain serum, a fridge to store the reagents and a shaker for the reaction, making it impossible to use in many antenatal clinic settings. The TP test is technically complex and requires laboratory infrastructure and well-trained technicians and is generally only available at reference laboratories in resource-limited settings. The TP test is highly specific for syphilis but TP antibodies persist. Hence TP tests cannot be used to distinguish between active and past infection. In resource-limited settings, pregnant women who are TP positive by POCT or non-TP positive are treated for syphilis to prevent transmission of the infection. As indicated by Jafari *et al.* (2013) 'This is now accepted practice as the risk of over-treatment due to a past infection or biological false positives which are not syphilis in origin is more acceptable than the risk of

**Table 18.1.** Examples of POC tests for syphilis screening

| POC test | Manufacturer | Specimen | Volume of whole blood or other specimen | Time to result | Storage temperature (°C) | Test type |
|---|---|---|---|---|---|---|
| Alere Determine™ Syphilis TP | Alere, Inc. USA | Whole blood (finger-stick), plasma or serum | 50 µL | 15 min (up to 24 h) | 2–30 | Lateral flow strip |
| SD Syphilis 3.0 | Alere/SD Bioline, South Korea | Whole blood (venous or fingerstick), plasma or serum | 20 µL (whole blood)<br>10 µL (plasma or serum) | 5 to 20 min | 2–30 | Cassette enclosed test card |
| Syphicheck® - WB | The Tulip Group/Qualpro, India | Whole blood (venous or fingerstick), plasma or serum | 25 µL | 15 min | 4–30 | Cassette enclosed test card |
| Visitect® Syphilis | Omega Diagnostics, UK | Whole blood (venous or fingerstick), plasma or serum | 50 µL | 30 min | 4–30 | Cassette enclosed test card |

non-treatment of syphilis.' This is especially true in pregnant women because a single dose of penicillin given before the third trimester can protect the fetus from adverse outcomes.

## POC tests for syphilis screening

In recent years, a range of POC tests that detect TP antibodies for syphilis screening has been developed (Mabey *et al.* 2006). The operational characteristics of four commercially available POC tests that have been evaluated by the WHO are summarised in Table 18.1.

A recent meta-analysis and a systematic review on the performance of TP POC tests demonstrated that their sensitivity and specificity are comparable to laboratory-based tests (Jafari *et al.* 2013; Tucker *et al.* 2010). The point estimates of sensitivity and specificity for each test, using serum and whole blood, around a 95% credible interval (as opposed to a confidence interval) are shown in Table 18.2.

In addition to the four tests that were part of the meta-analysis, other TP RDTs are available. These include, but are not limited to, those listed in Table 18.3.

Of these syphilis POC tests, the Syphilis Health Check™ is FDA-approved and CLIA waived in the USA, and both *OnSite*™ and Uni-Gold™ tests are CE-marked. No regulatory approvals were identified for the Crystal TP Syphilis test, although the company plans to seek CE-IVD marking for the product. There are few peer-reviewed performance evaluations available for these tests.

## Need for additional syphilis POC tests for resource-limited settings

Because of the generally good performance of syphilis RDTs, there is arguably no need for additional 'mono' tests (i.e. detecting TP only). However, there are several important needs for new syphilis 'dual' tests, preferably in the form of POC tests. One of these is for a combination TP/non-TP POC test. Another need is for HIV/syphilis dual tests.

## POC tests for the dual detection of TP and non-TP

Chembio Diagnostic Systems has developed the first dual non-TP and TP syphilis POC test – the DPP® Syphilis Screen & Confirm Assay. The test uses a unique combination of protein A and anti-human IgM antibody, which are conjugated to colloidal gold particles. It also employs a recombinant antigen to TP and synthetic antigens for non-TP, separately bound to the solid phase membrane, enabling the simultaneous, yet separate, detection of both markers.

The DPP® Syphilis Screen & Confirm Assay requires 10 µL of whole blood (capillary or venipuncture). Tests can be stored at room temperature (2–30°C). The turnaround time of the test is 15 to 20 min. The test is highly sensitive and specific, and is useful for the serodiagnosis of syphilis in primary health-care clinics.

Two peer-reviewed publications reported the DPP test performed favourably against laboratory-based reference tests. The first, a laboratory-based evaluation, used 1601

**Table 18.2.** Point estimates for sensitivity and specificity of selected syphilis RDTs (Source: adapted from Jafari *et al.* (2013)

| RDT | Sample | Parameters | Assuming imperfect reference standards (95% CrI) |
|---|---|---|---|
| Alere Determine™ | Serum | Sensitivity | 90.04% (80.45, 95.21) |
| | | Specificity | 94.15% (89.26, 97.66) |
| | Whole blood | Sensitivity | 86.32% (77.26, 91.70) |
| | | Specificity | 95.85% (92.42, 97.74) |
| SD Syphilis 3.0 | Serum | Sensitivity | 87.06% (75.67, 94.50) |
| | | Specificity | 95.85% (89.89, 99.53) |
| | Whole blood | Sensitivity | 84.50% (78.81, 92.61) |
| | | Specificity | 97.95% (92.54, 99.33) |
| Syphicheck® WB | Serum | Sensitivity | 74.48% (56.85, 88.44) |
| | | Specificity | 99.14% (96.37, 100.0) |
| | Whole blood | Sensitivity | 74.47% (63.94, 82.13) |
| | | Specificity | 99.58% (98.91, 99.96) |
| Visitect® Syphilis | Serum | Sensitivity | 85.13% (72.83, 92.57) |
| | | Specificity | 96.45% (91.92, 99.29) |
| | Whole blood | Sensitivity | 74.26% (53.62, 83.68) |
| | | Specificity | 99.43%, (98.22, 99.98) |

Note: CrI = credible interval

banked serum samples. The *Treponema pallidum* particle agglutination (TPPA) assay and a quantitative rapid plasma reagin (RPR) test were used as reference standards for the TP and non-TP components, respectively. Compared with the RPR test, the sensitivity of the DPP® non-TP line was 98.4% when the RPR titres of sera were ≥1:2, and the specificity of the non-TP line was 98.6%. Compared with the TPPA assay, the reactive and

**Table 18.3.** Examples of other syphilis RDTs available on the market

| POC test | Manufacturer | Specimen | Volume of whole blood or other specimen | Time to result | Storage Temperature (°C) | Test type |
|---|---|---|---|---|---|---|
| Crystal TP Syphilis Test | Span Diagnostics (India) | Whole blood (fingerstick), plasma or serum | 1 drop (20 µL) | 15 min | Not available | Cassette enclosed test card |
| OnSite™ Syphilis Ab Combo Rapid Test | CTK Biotech, Inc. (USA) | Whole blood (venous or fingerstick) | 1 drop | 15 min | 2–30 | Cassette enclosed test card |
| Syphilis Health Check™ | Diagnostics Direct (USA) | Whole blood (fingerstick), plasma or serum | 2 drops | 10 min | Room temperature | Cassette enclosed test card |
| Uni-Gold™ Syphilis Treponemal | Trinity Biotech (Ireland) | Whole blood (venous or fingerstick), plasma or serum | ~60 µL | ~15 min | 2–30 | Cassette enclosed test card |

nonreactive concordances of the TP line were 96.5% and 95.5%, respectively (Castro *et al.* 2010).

The second study was a multi-centre field study in China (Yin *et al.* 2013) in which 1323 whole blood (WB), 488 fingerprick blood (FB) and 1323 blood plasma (BP) specimens from 1323 patients were used to evaluate sensitivity and specificity. The TPPA assay and the toluidine red unheated serum test (TRUST) were used as reference standards. Sensitivities of the DPP test versus TPPA were 96.7% for WB, 96.4% for FB, and 94.6% for BP; specificities were 99.3%, 99.1%, and 99.6%, respectively. Compared with TRUST, sensitivities were 87.2% for WB, 85.8% for FB, and 88.4% for BP; specificities were 94.4%, 96.1%, and 95.0%, respectively. Both studies concluded that the DPP® Screen & Confirm Assay could be useful for diagnosing syphilis in primary health-care settings in resource-limited settings.

## POC tests for the dual detection of syphilis and HIV

The greatest need in resource-limited settings now is for a combination test for the screening of syphilis and HIV in MSM, sex workers and pregnant women. A dual test will help EMTCT of HIV and syphilis, which are significant causes of neonatal mortality globally each year. Of the ~2.0 million new HIV infections among adults and children in 2014, it is estimated that ~220 000 are in newborns (UNAIDS 2014). There are effective interventions to prevent MTCT. The CDC estimates that key interventions, including HIV testing and counselling of all pregnant women and provision of antiretroviral drugs to all HIV-positive women during pregnancy, can reduce MTCT of HIV from 35 to 5% (CDC 2012). Programs that include syphilis testing along with timely penicillin treatment for pregnant women who test positive for TP infection can also reduce adverse pregnancy outcomes (Blencowe *et al.* 2011; Hawkes *et al.* 2011). Antenatal screening and treatment has been shown to be cost-effective, even in settings where the prevalence of syphilis in pregnant women is low to moderate (Terris-Prestholt *et al.* 2003).

There are currently five combination HIV/syphilis TP POC tests on the market: the SD Bioline HIV/Syphilis Duo Rapid Test (Alere/Standard Diagnostics, Inc.), the DPP® HIV-Syphilis Assay (Chembio Diagnostics Systems, Inc.), the Multiplo Rapid TP/HIV Antibody Test (MedMira, Inc.), the INSTI™ HIV/Syphilis Multiplex Test (biolytical Laboratories Inc.) and the *OnSite*™ HIV/Syphilis Ab Combo Rapid Test (CTK Biotech Co.).

Three of these tests (SD Bioline HIV/Syphilis Duo Rapid Test, DPP® HIV-Syphilis Assay and Multiplo Rapid TP/HIV Antibody Test) have recently been evaluated in the USA by Humphries *et al.* (2014) and in China and Nigeria by Yin *et al.* (2015). Both evaluations were conducted in laboratory settings with trained users using serum specimens. In the Humphries study ($n$ = 150 samples), POC HIV test results were compared with the Siemens Advia EIA and Western blot; while POC syphilis results were compared with TPPA. Sensitivity for HIV antibody detection by the three RDTs ranged from 98 to 99%; specificity ranged from 94 to 100%. For the detection of TP, sensitivity ranged from 93 to 95% and specificity 97 to 100%.

Yin *et al.* (2015) concluded all three of the HIV/syphilis dual RDTs evaluated had 'acceptable sensitivity and specificity to detect HIV or syphilis, although the sensitivity to detect HIV antibodies (99.0%–99.6%) is generally higher than that for syphilis (94.2%–97.0%)' (Table 18.4). They also suggested that further research on these POC tests is needed to evaluate their performance on whole blood samples in primary health-care settings, in the hands of less well-trained users in target use settings.

The SD Bioline HIV/Syphilis Duo Rapid Test is an easy-to-use, rapid lateral flow assay for the simultaneous detection of HIV-1, including subtype O, and HIV-2 and/or syphilis TP from whole blood (venous or capillary), serum or plasma samples with results produced in ~15–20 min. Three more evaluations, one of which was done in a field setting using centrifuged whole blood, have all found good sensitivity and specificity with respect to both components (HIV and TP) of the test (Bristow *et al.* 2014; Omoding *et al.* 2014; Shimelis and Tadesse 2015).

The DPP® HIV-Syphilis Assay is a single-use immunochromatographic, rapid screening test for the detection of antibodies both to HIV types 1 and 2 (HIV-1/2) and to syphilis TP in capillary or venous whole blood, serum or plasma samples. The test, which requires only 10 μL of sample, includes the Chembio SampleTainer® specimen collection bottle, which is a safe, closed system for handling potentially infectious blood samples. Turnaround time is ~10 min.

The Multiplo Rapid TP/HIV Antibody Test is commercially available in Colombia, and the company is pursuing product registration in several other countries. The combination assay is built on the MedMira Rapid Vertical Flow Technology platform and is sold in in the same packaging formats as the company's rapid HIV antibody test. The Multiplo Rapid TP/HIV Antibody test

**Table 18.4.** Summary of performance of HIV/syphilis dual RDTs

| RDT | Sample n = 1514 | Parameters | Performance (95% CI) HIV antibody[a] | Performance (95% CI) TP antibody[b] |
|---|---|---|---|---|
| SD Bioline HIV/Syphilis Duo Rapid Test | Sera | Sensitivity | 97.9% (92.0–99.6) | 93.0% (84.8–97.1) |
| | | | 99.0% (98.8–99.9) | 96.6% (95.0–97.7) |
| | | Specificity | 100% (91.5–100) | 100% (92.9–100) |
| | | | 99.0% (98.0–99.5) | 99.1% (98.2–99.6) |
| DPP® HIV-Syphilis Assay | Sera | Sensitivity | 98.9% (93.6–99.9) | 95.3% (87.9–98.5) |
| | | Specificity | 99.6% (98.8–99.9) | 97.0% (95.5–98.0 |
| | | | 98.1% (88.6–99.9) | 100% (92.9–100) |
| | | | 97.9% (96.7–98.7) | 99.6% (98.9–99.9) |
| Multiplo Rapid TP/HIV Antibody Test | Sera | Sensitivity | 97.9% (92.0–99.6) | 94.1% (86.3–97.8) |
| | | Specificity | 99.5% (99.4–99.8) | 94.2% (92.3–95.7) |
| | | | 94.2% (83.1–98.5) | 96.9% (88.2–99.5) |
| | | | 98.3% (97.2–99.0) | 99.1% (98.2–99.6) |

[a] This column shows results from an evaluation in the US (Source: Humphries *et al.* 2014)
[b] This column shows results from a laboratory evaluation at three sites, two in Nigeria and one in China (Source: Yin *et al.* 2015)

combines qualitative detection of HIV-1 and HIV-2 with qualitative detection of TP in an immuno-filtration format, with turnaround time ~3 min.

Bristow *et al.* (2015) evaluated this test in a laboratory setting using 200 stored serum specimens collected from MSM and transgender women presenting in STI clinics in Lima, Peru. The estimated sensitivity of the HIV component of the Multiplo test was 100% (95% CI 95.1–100%), and the specificity was 91.9% (CI 85.7–96.1%). The sensitivity and specificity estimates for the TP antibody component were 94.6% (CI 88.5–98.0%) and 92.8% (CI 84.9–97.3%), respectively.

The INSTI™ HIV/Syphilis Multiplex test provides rapid qualitative detection of HIV-1 and HIV-2 and Syphilis TP in a POC test format using immuno-filtration. Turnaround time is ~60 s. No published performance evaluations are available at the time of writing, because the INSTI™ combo test has only recently been introduced onto the market.

The *OnSite*™ HIV/Syphilis Ab Combo Rapid Test is a lateral flow chromatographic immunoassay for the qualitative detection of antibodies to HIV-1, HIV-2 and TP. It is a three-line test that can be used with whole blood, serum or plasma to detect IgG, IgM and IgA to HIV-1 and HIV-2, and TP. Results are available within 15 min. No published studies on performance are available.

Both the SD Bioline and DPP dual assays have been evaluated by the CDC and are on the USAID Waiver List. The SD Bioline and INSTI assays are CE-IVD marked. All but the CTK assay have been submitted to the WHO for prequalification, but to date, only the SD Bioline assay has been prequalified.

## Combined HIV/syphilis tests in the pipeline

Fig. 18.1 provides a timeline showing the market entry of the dual HIV/syphilis tests discussed to date, as well as three more that are in the diagnostic pipeline.

The mChip Assay (Junco Laboratories and Columbia University in collaboration with OPKO Health, Inc.), as well as providing a combination HIV/syphilis TP assay, also intends to include the qualitative detection of non-TP syphilis and the quantitative detection of anaemia (haemoglobin). The device-based format uses a reusable microfluidic mChip and a smart phone for read-out of results. The technology has been evaluated in Rwanda with good results, and the HIV/syphilis TP assay is expected to be available in 2017 (Chin *et al.* 2013).

The ChipCare Corporation is developing a portable, easy-to-use diagnostic platform for laboratory-quality blood testing at the point of care, called ChipCare. The platform uses novel microfluidic and biomarker technologies to provide multiple cell surface and blood analyte tests on a single disposable cartridge. ChipCare's initial assay is for absolute CD4 counting, but the company is developing a combined HIV/syphilis test, which will also provide the option of a third assay (HCV) on the same cartridge. Designed for use by health-care workers in resource-limited settings, the ChipCare device weighs <2 kg and will be sufficiently small and rugged to carry in

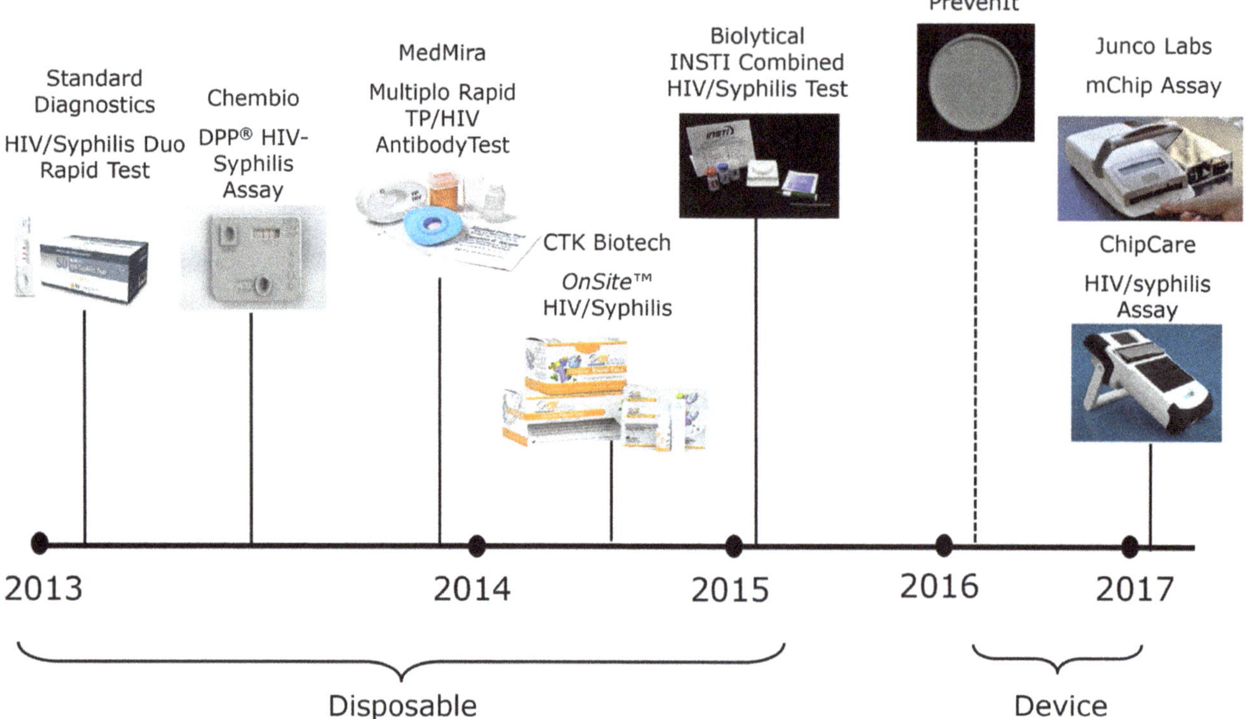


**Fig. 18.1.** Dual point-of-care tests for HIV/syphilis currently available and in the pipeline. (Source: Diagram created by, and used with permission of, Maurine Murtagh)

a backpack. The platform does not require continuous power, cold chain or running water for operation. The ChipCare platform is powered by a lithium ion battery that can be recharged via AC mains, a car battery or solar panel and has built-in connectivity. The combined HIV/syphilis assay is expected to be launched in 2017.

A combination HIV/syphilis assay called PreventIt, funded by the European Union, is under development by a research consortium including the Royal Tropical Institute (The Netherlands), IMAccess (France), Sirigen (UK), CCM (The Netherlands) and the London School of Hygiene & Tropical Medicine (UK). The PreventIt assay is now in the prototype stage of development and will simultaneously diagnose the HIV antigen and syphilis antibody status of individuals.

The test device consists of a circular plate coated at one or more points with immobilised specific analyte and a stabilised reagent. The test is performed by spotting a droplet of sample next to the reagent, which is dissolved, and the mixture is then allowed to react with each of the analytes. Because the plate has a smooth hydrophilic surface, the drop will rapidly flow from one analyte to the next by gravitational force if the plate is tilted back and forth. For optimal strength and sensitivity, the design of the plate ensures the drop will flow in a circle, repeatedly reacting with the bound analyte each time the circular flow is completed.

The diagnostic accuracy of the system is currently under investigation. A digital read-out system is being developed to facilitate reproducibility and easy reading. No commercial launch date has been set for the product.

In conclusion, given the challenges of diagnostic delivery in resource-limited settings, combined HIV/syphilis tests are highly desirable because they make implementation of both tests simpler, and hopefully, more cost-effective. But, not all of the tests in the pipeline meet the desired criteria for such a test. Some tests have multiple steps, several of which require precision timing and/or special technique for adding buffer, for example. The read window, where test results must be read immediately or within a few minutes of the final step in the test process, is inflexible for some tests. In some cases, expected shelf life of reagents is <12 months and environmental tolerances of the tests do not achieve desired specifications. Cost is also a factor for some of the proposed assays. Therefore, continued optimisation of an HIV/syphilis dual test in line with the existing target product profile (IDC 2016) is still required.

## IMPLEMENTATION OF POC TESTS FOR SYPHILIS

POC tests offer an unprecedented opportunity to improve health care and to reduce inequalities in health. However, scientific evidence of good test performance and ease of use often fail to translate into impact due to ineffective implementation and scale up, particularly in fragile or dysfunctional health systems. In Guatemala, a shortage of health-care workers and poor supply chain management limited syphilis screening uptake (Smith *et al.* 2015).

As described in the landscape above, new POC tests for syphilis are now available that do not require electricity and are easy to perform. Several of those on the market meet the ASSURED criteria, being Affordable, Sensitive, Specific, User-friendly, Rapid and robust, Equipment-free and Deliverable to those who need them. It is now possible to advocate for a Same-day Testing and Treatment (STAT) strategy to overcome the barriers to testing. However, if we examine the reasons why syphilis has remained a major cause of stillbirth and neonatal mortality, the barriers faced in implementing POCT are no longer technological, but are often constraints inherent to the health-care system, lack of political will and knowledge of the adverse outcomes of pregnancy associated with syphilis. For effective implementation, it is important for policy makers and program managers to consider the issues discussed in the rest of the chapter.

### Policy and stakeholder consultations

Although prenatal screening for syphilis is recommended policy in almost every country, the implementation of policy has not been effective because program managers do not have the appropriate tools or resources for implementation. In advocating for resources to be allocated to a new technology such as POCT, cost-effectiveness is a top priority. The cost per person screened and treated depends largely on the cost of the test and the prevalence of syphilis. The cost of POC syphilis testing in sub-Saharan Africa can be as low as \$2 per woman screened (Shelley *et al.* 2015). The cost per person treated becomes higher as the prevalence drops.

It is also important to estimate program costs. In models developed based on costs in Tanzania and Haiti, ~50% of the cost of the POC test program is the cost of the tests, with personnel and supplies accounting for <15% of the remaining costs and quality assurance for another 15% (Schackman *et al.* 2007; Terris-Prestholt *et al.* 2012).

Because dual HIV and Syphilis POC tests are commercially available, integrating syphilis screening into prevention of MTCT programs for HIV screening is particularly cost-effective, as personnel time and building space can be considered shared costs, especially in countries that have made a strong commitment for the joint EMTCT of HIV and syphilis.

### Technology assessment and appropriate placement

In countries where Health Technology Assessment has been established, new technologies are reviewed to determine if they meet a public health need for the country. If a technology is deemed useful, decisions need to be made as to where the new technology can be deployed within the health-care system for maximum health impact. The appropriate placement or deployment of the technology should be informed by need, technical capacity, cost-effectiveness, consultation with personnel from all levels of the health-care systems and with civil society.

If more than one POC test with acceptable performance is available, the diagnostic technology assessment panel should consider developing criteria for test selection, including:

- test performance
- ease of use
- conditions of use
- conditions and duration of storage
- requirement for other supplies
- price.

The criteria can be weighted depending on availability of resources, prevalence of infection, technical capacity and existence of co-morbidities. Often, the three As (affordability, accuracy and accessibility) are the most important factors in technology selection. While price and accuracy are often very important considerations, ease of use, which determines how accessible a POC test can be, is also important for maximising test coverage. For remote settings, tests with the longest stability and without the need for refrigeration are preferred by countries in which customs clearance and distribution of commodities to target populations may take a long time.

### Baseline survey and pilot studies to determine health systems failures

Before planning implementation, a baseline survey is critical because policy makers are sometimes not aware of the barriers faced by health facilities around the country. This is especially true when a surveillance system for maternal syphilis screening does not exist or does not function well.

Consultations with the Ministry of Health and other stakeholders on the design and location of pilot projects for test introduction are important. Pilot studies to introduce POC syphilis testing should be conducted in a variety of settings and populations so that results can be generalised to as many countries as possible.

### Acceptability of rapid syphilis tests among health-care workers and communities

Although task shifting has been accepted in recent years, laboratory staff and professional societies are often opposed to the idea of non-laboratory personnel, such as nurses and midwives, performing a task that had traditionally been undertaken by trained laboratory technicians. A new paradigm needs to be created for the role of laboratory staff to be broadened to include the training and supervision of health-care workers conducting POC tests, and in setting up a quality management program to monitor the proficiency of health-care workers in performing the test with corrective action to follow if necessary. Training is also essential to help health-care workers overcome their fear of communicating positive results and improve partner notification. Engagement of community health workers is essential to build local capacity and facilitate community acceptance.

Certificates of competency can provide motivation for health-care workers. It is also important that communities trust the POC test results when delivered by non-laboratory staff.

### Cultural contexts of POCT implementation

In central Haiti, many babies are either stillborn or die in the first year of life. A myth has developed in the communities that a werewolf, the Loup Garou, preys on pregnant women as they sleep, sucking the blood out of the babies in the mother's womb (Fitzgerald and Behet 2002). In introducing syphilis rapid tests, Groupe Haitien d'Etude du Sarcome de Kaposi et des Infections Opportunistes (GHESKIO) and the Ministry of Health worked with health-care workers, traditional healers and voodoo priests to overcome these traditional beliefs. Knowledge of syphilis has empowered pregnant women to understand the importance of syphilis screening in pregnancy and accept treatment to keep their babies healthy.

In working with marginalised populations, understanding their perception of risk, what motivates them to have better health-care-seeking behaviours, and how to gain their trust and make services culturally sensitive and user-friendly are important considerations in increasing the uptake of POCT in populations that are at high risk of both acquiring and transmitting infection.

Cultural issues are also encountered in treatment for STIs. There are cultures in which patients prefer injections to oral therapies. In some countries, health providers are reluctant to give penicillin to syphilis patients because of their fear of allergic reactions.

### Training and site preparations

There is a serious shortage of trained staff in the health sector in many countries and staff turnover is often a problem. Integrated screening for syphilis and HIV in ANCs can reduce the demands on health-care workers, but problems remain in clinics that have a high turnover of staff. Trained health-care workers are often transferred to new facilities and do not always train their counterparts remaining on site, leaving the facility unable to provide testing.

Training materials should be translated into the local language and adapted according to local needs. Courses for trainers and supervisors should be organised, including practical training on how to perform the tests and interpret the results. Since the POC tests are read by eye, visual acuity and colour blindness can lead to misreading of results. Interpretation of a positive result can also be affected by the fear of communicating a positive result to the patient. This is especially true for HIV tests.

Standard operating procedures should be developed for performing a finger-prick, performing a POC test, preparing proficiency panels for quality assurance, performing quality control testing and managing test results, ordering supplies and collecting samples for confirmatory re-testing. Testing algorithms and treatment guidelines should be developed to guide treatment and other patient management decisions. All individuals who test positive should be treated with appropriate drug regimens as recommended in the national guidelines on the same day and requested to refer sexual partners for testing and treatment.

## Supply chain management

Stock outs are the most common reasons for not testing. Health-care workers and their supervisors should receive training in stock management, but problems may remain at national, regional or district levels, especially when there are long delays in clearance through customs. In recent years, simple optical readers or scanners for POC tests have made it possible to transmit test results to a central database (Wedderburn *et al.* 2015). Supply chain problems can be alleviated if test results can be linked to supply chain software, allowing more accurate forecasts based on real-time data on POC test consumption.

## Quality management

For accurate results, it is important to ensure the quality of the tests as well as the testing. A quality management system with connectivity solutions should be developed that includes the development and distribution of standard operating procedures, training of health-care workers and laboratory staff to ensure the quality of the tests and that testing is performed correctly (Ansbro *et al.* 2015).

A simple, low-cost method for proficiency testing has been developed by the CDC to assess the ability of a health-care worker to perform rapid HIV testing correctly and interpret the results (Parekh *et al.* 2010). Dry tube specimen panels are prepared by drying down aliquots of sera with high titre antibodies, and negative control sera. These dry tubes can then be stored and transported at ambient temperature, and reconstituted with buffered saline on arrival at the site of HIV testing. The proficiency panel allows supervisors to identify health-care workers in need of refresher training, motivates health-care workers and reinforces good practice. This is particularly important where there is a rapid turnover of staff.

## Monitoring and evaluation

A checklist for monitoring visits and training for staff is important for POCT programs. Problems can be brought immediately to the attention of the program manager or POCT Coordinator, and solutions tried until a sustainable one is found.

## Impact on other services

Integrating HIV and syphilis screening in prevention of MTCT programs not only avoids the tragedy of babies acquiring HIV and dying of syphilis but is also cost-effective (Peeling and Ye 2004). An essential diagnostic package for prenatal care, which can include diagnostics for both infectious diseases and conditions such as anaemia and pre-eclampsia, should be considered, based on disease prevalence and epidemiological context, to improve the quality of prenatal care in all settings.

## Impact of POCT introduction on health systems

Decentralising testing using POCT puts stress on the health-care system. However, POCT can also strengthen health systems by motivating health-care workers and increasing capacity and efficiency to test and treat, hence reducing the number of return visits required (Garcia *et al.* 2013; Mabey *et al.* 2012). Connectivity solutions for POC test results can be used to further improve supply chain management and quality assurance (Wedderburn *et al.* 2015).

We have conducted a multi-country project to determine feasibility and cost-effectiveness of introducing rapid syphilis screening in prenatal and high-risk populations. Using the STAT strategy, we developed a generic protocol with standardised outcome measures and encouraged all country teams to develop country-specific protocols taking into account the health system infrastructure and the political, cultural and socioeconomic context of their setting (Garcia *et al.* 2013; Mabey *et al.* 2012). In all countries, policy has changed as a result of this demonstration project. What lessons can be learned from this? We learned that, unlike the adoption of new drugs and vaccines, leadership and infrastructure for critical decision making on the adoption of new diagnostic technologies are often fragmented or absent in many countries. The following are critical to the success of POC test implementation:

- engagement of policy makers and stakeholders as peers, throughout the entire study period
- sharing and communication of results
- using clear compelling messages
- identifying champions to promote syphilis screening
- training and technical assistance
- positive feedback to health-care workers
- involving other partners
- making cost-effectiveness analysis user-friendly
- keeping motivation high.

In conclusion, POCT has the potential to improve health outcomes and strengthen health systems. Its introduction and implementation must be culturally sensitive and accompanied by an inter-connected system to monitor appropriate training and quality assurance with supply chain management.

## REFERENCES


Ansbro ÉM, Gill MM, Reynolds J, Shelley KD, Strasser S, Sripipatana T, *et al.* (2015) Introduction of syphilis point-of-care tests, from pilot study to national programme implementation in Zambia: a qualitative study of healthcare workers' perspectives on testing, training and quality assurance. *PLoS One* **10**, e0127728. doi:10.1371/journal.pone.0127728

Berman SM (2004) Maternal syphilis: pathophysiology and treatment. *Bulletin of the World Health Organization* **82**, 433–438.

Blencowe H, Cousens S, Kamb M, Berman S, Lawn JE (2011) Lives saved tool supplement detection and treatment of syphilis in pregnancy to reduce syphilis related stillbirths and neonatal mortality. *BMC Public Health* **11**(Supplement 3), S9. doi:10.1186/1471-2458-11-S3-S9

Bristow CC, Adu-Sarkodie Y, Ondondo RO, Bukusi EA, Dagnra CA, Oo KY, *et al.* (2014) Multi-site laboratory evaluation of a dual HIV/syphilis point-of-care rapid test for simultaneous detection of HIV and syphilis. *Open Forum Infectious Diseases* **1**, ofu015, <http://ofid.oxfordjournals.org/content/1/1/ofu015#xref-fn-1-1. doi:10.1093/ofid/ofu015>.

Bristow CC, Leon SR, Ramos LB, Vargas SK, Flores JA, Konda KA, *et al.* (2015) Laboratory evaluation of a dual rapid immunodiagnostic test for HIV and syphilis infection. *Journal of Clinical Microbiology* **53**, 311–313. doi:10.1128/JCM.02763-14

Castro AR, Esfandiari J, Kumar S, Ashton M, Kikkert SE, Park MM, *et al.* (2010) A novel point-of-care test for the simultaneous detection of non-Treponemal and Treponemal antibodies in patients with syphilis. *Journal of Clinical Microbiology* **48**, 4615–4619. doi:10.1128/JCM.00624-10

CDC (Centers for Disease Control and Prevention) (2012) *Eliminating HIV Infections in Children and Keeping Their Mothers Alive.* Centers for Disease Control and Prevention, Atlanta GA, USA, <http://www.cdc.gov/globalaids/global-hiv-aids-at-cdc/eliminating-hiv-infections.html>.

CDC (2015) *Fact Sheet: Syphilis and MSM.* Centers for Disease Control and Prevention. Atlanta GA, USA, <http://www.cdc.gov/std/syphilis/stdfact-msm-syphilis.htm>.

Chin CD, Cheung YK, Laksanasopin T, Modena MM, Chin SY, Sridhara AA, *et al.* (2013) Mobile device for disease diagnosis and data tracking in resource-limited settings. *Clinical Chemistry* **59**, 629–640. doi:10.1373/clinchem.2012.199596

Fitzgerald D, Behet M (2002) A piece of my mind. Beyond folklore. *Journal of the American Medical Association* **288**, 2791–2792. doi:10.1001/jama.288.22.2791

García PJ, Cárcamo CP, Chiappe M, Valderrama M, La Rosa S, Holmes KK (2013) Rapid syphilis tests as catalysts for health systems strengthening: a case study from Peru. *PLoS One* **8**, e66905. doi:10.1371/journal.pone.0066905

Gomez GB, Kamb ML, Newman LM, Mark J, Broutet N, Hawkes SJ (2013) Untreated maternal syphilis and adverse outcomes of pregnancy: a systematic review and meta-analysis. *Bulletin of the World Health Organization* **91**, 217–226. doi:10.2471/BLT.12.107623

Hawkes S, Matin N, Broutet N, Low N (2011) Effectiveness of interventions to improve screening for syphilis in pregnancy: a systematic review and meta-analysis. *The Lancet Infectious Diseases* **11**, 684–691. doi:10.1016/S1473-3099(11)70104-9

Humphries RM, Woo JS, Chung JH, Sokovic A, Bristow CC, Klausner JD (2014) Laboratory evaluation of three rapid diagnostic tests for dual detection of HIV and *Treponema pallidum* antibodies. *Journal of Clinical Microbiology* **52**, 4394–4397. doi:10.1128/JCM.02468-14

International Diagnostics Centre (IDC) (2016) Target Product Profile: Combined HIV/Syphilis test, <http://www.idc-dx.org/resources/target-product-profile-combined-hivsyphilis-test>.

Jafari Y, Peeling RW, Shivkumar S, Claessens C, Joseph L, Pai NP (2013) Are *Treponema pallidum* specific rapid and point-of-care tests for syphilis accurate enough for screening in resource limited settings? Evidence from a meta-analysis. *PLoS One* **8**, e54695. doi:10.1371/journal.pone.0054695

Kamb ML, Newman LM, Riley PL, Mark J, Hawkes SJ, Malik T, *et al.* (2010) A road map for the global elimination of congenital syphilis. *Obstetrics and Gynecology International* **2010**, 312798. doi:10.1155/2010/312798

Mabey D, Peeling RW, Ballard R, Benzaken AS, Galbán E, Changalucha J, Everett D, Balira R, *et al.* (2006) Prospective, multi-centre clinic-based evaluation of four rapid diagnostic tests for syphilis. *Sexually Transmitted Infections* **82**(Supplement v), v13–v16. doi:10.1136/sti.2006.022467

Mabey D, Sollis K, Kelly H, Benzaken A, Bitarakwate E, Changalucha J, *et al.* (2012) Point-of-care tests to strengthen health systems and save newborn lives: the case of syphilis. *PLoS Medicine* **9**, e1001233. doi:10.1371/journal.pmed.1001233

Newman L, Rowley J, Vander-Hoorn S, Wijesooriya NS, Unemo M, Low N, *et al.* (2015) Global estimates of the prevalence and incidence of four curable sexually transmitted infections in 2012 based on systematic review and global reporting. *PLoS One* **10**, e0143304. doi:10.1371/journal.pone.0143304

Omoding D, Katawera V, Siedner M, Boum IIY (2014) Evaluation of the SD Bioline HIV/syphilis Duo assay at a rural health center in Southwestern Uganda. *BMC Research Notes* **7**, 746. doi:10.1186/1756-0500-7-746

Owiredu MN, Newman L, Nzomo T, Kafando GC, Sanni S, Shaffer N, Bucagu M, Peeling R, *et al.* (2015) Elimination of mother-to-child transmission of HIV and syphilis: a dual approach in the African Region to improve quality of antenatal care and integrated disease control. *International Journal of Gynaecology and Obstetrics: the Official Organ of the International Federation of Gynaecology and Obstetrics* **130**(Supplement 1), S27–S31. doi:10.1016/j.ijgo.2015.04.010

Parekh BS, Kalou MB, Alemnji G, Ou CY, Gershy-Damet GM, Nkengasong JN (2010) Scaling up HIV rapid testing in developing countries: comprehensive approach for implementing quality assurance. *American Journal of Clinical Pathology* **134**, 573–584. doi:10.1309/AJCPTDIMFR00IKYX

Peeling RW, Ye H (2004) Diagnostic tools for preventing and managing maternal and congenital syphilis: an overview. *Bulletin of the World Health Organization* **82**, 439–446.

Peeling RW, Mabey D, Fitzgerald DW, Watson-Jones D (2004) Avoiding HIV and dying of syphilis. *Lancet* **364**, 1561–1563. doi:10.1016/S0140-6736(04)17327-3

Schackman BR, Neukermans CP, Fontain SN, Nolte C, Joseph P, Pape JW, *et al.* (2007) Cost-effectiveness of rapid syphilis screening in prenatal HIV testing programs in Haiti. *PLoS Medicine* **4**, e183.

Shelley KD, Ansbro ÉM, Ncube AT, Sweeney S, Fleischer C, Tembo Mumba G, *et al.* (2015) Scaling down to scale up: A health economic analysis of integrating point-of-care syphilis testing into antenatal care in Zambia during pilot and national rollout implementation. *PLoS One* **13**, e0125675.

Shimelis T, Tadesse E (2015) The diagnostic performance evaluation of the SD Bioline HIV/syphilis Duo rapid test in southern Ethiopia: a cross-sectional study. *BMJ Open* **5**, e007371. doi:10.1136/bmjopen-2014-007371

Smith A, Sabido M, Camey E, Batres A, Casabona J (2015) Lessons learned from integrating simultaneous triple point-of-care screening for syphilis, hepatitis B, and HIV in prenatal services through rural outreach teams in Guatemala. *International Journal of Gynaecology and Obstetrics* **130**, S70–S72. doi:10.1016/j.ijgo.2015.04.009

Terris-Prestholt F, Watson-Jones D, Mugeye K, Kumaranayake L, Ndeki L, *et al.* (2003) Is antenatal syphilis screening still cost effective in sub-Saharan Africa? *Sexually Transmitted Infections* **79**, 375–381. doi:10.1136/sti.79.5.375

Terris-Prestholt F, Vickerman P, Torres-Rueda S, Santesso N, Sweeney S, Mallma P, *et al.* (2015) The cost-effectiveness of 10 antenatal syphilis screening and treatment approaches in Peru, Tanzania, and Zambia. *International Journal of Gynaecology and Obstetrics* **130**(Supplement 1), S73–S80. doi:10.1016/j.ijgo.2015.04.007

Tucker JD, Bu J, Brown LB, Yin YP, Chen XS, Cohen MS, *et al.* (2010) Accelerating worldwide syphilis screening through rapid testing: a systematic review. *The Lancet Infectious Diseases* **10**, 381–386. doi:10.1016/S1473-3099(10)70092-X

UNAIDS (2014) *How AIDS Changed Everything.* Fact sheet. The Joint United Nations Programme on HIV/AIDS, Geneva, Switzerland, <http://www.unaids.org/sites/default/files/media_ asset/20150714_FS_MDG6_Report_en.pdf>.

Watson-Jones D, Gumodoka B, Weiss H, Changalucha J, Todd J, Mugeye K, *et al.* (2002) Syphilis in pregnancy in Tanzania. II. The effectiveness of antenatal syphilis screening and single-dose benzathine penicillin treatment for the prevention of adverse pregnancy outcomes. *Journal of Infectious Diseases* **186**, 948–957.

Wedderburn CJ, Murtagh M, Toskin T, Peeling RW (2015) Using electronic readers to monitor progress toward elimination of mother-to-child transmission of HIV and syphilis: an opinion piece. *International Journal of Gynaecology and Obstetrics* **130**, S81–S83. doi:10.1016/j.ijgo.2015.04.006

WHO (World Health Organization) (2010) *PMTCT Strategic Vision 2010–2015: Preventing Mother-to-Child Transmission of HIV to Reach the UNGASS and Millennium Development Goals.* WHO, Department of Reproductive Health and Research, Geneva, Switzerland, <http://www.who.int/hiv/pub/mtct/strategic_vision.pdf?ua=1>.

WHO (2013) *Sexually Transmitted Infections.* Fact Sheet 110. WHO, Geneva, Switzerland, <http://www.who.int/mediacentre/factsheets/fs110/en/>.

WHO (2014a) *HIV/AIDS.* Fact Sheet N360. WHO, Geneva, Switzerland, <http://www.who.int/mediacentre/factsheets/fs360/en/>.

WHO (2014b) *Elimination of Mother-to-Child Transmission (EMTCT) of HIV and Syphilis. Global Guidance on Criteria and Processes for Validation.* WHO, Geneva, Switzerland, <http://www.who.int/hiv/pub/emtct-validation-guidance/en/>.

WHO (2015a) *WHO Validates Elimination of Mother to Child Transmission of HIV and Syphilis in Cuba.* News Release. WHO Media Centre, Geneva, Switzerland and Washington DC, USA, <http://www.who.int/mediacentre/news/releases/2015/mtct-hiv-cuba/en/>.

WHO (2015b) *Men Who Have Sex With Men and Syphilis.* WHO, Global Health Observatory (GHO) data, Geneva, Switzerland, <http://www.who.int/gho/sti/sex_msm/en>.

WHO (2015c) *Sex Workers with Active Syphilis.* WHO, Global Health Observatory (GHO) data, Geneva, Switzerland, <http://www.who.int/gho/sti/sex_workers/en>.

Yin YP, Chen XS, Wei WH, Gong KL, Cao WL, Yong G, *et al.* (2013) A dual point-of-care test shows good performance in simultaneously detecting nontreponemal and treponemal antibodies in patients with syphilis: a multisite evaluation study in China. *Clinical Infectious Diseases* **56**, 659–665. doi:10.1093/cid/cis928

Yin YP, Ngige E, Anyaike C, Ijaodola G, Oyelade TA, Vaz RG, *et al.* (2015) Laboratory evaluation of three dual rapid diagnostic tests for HIV and syphilis in China and Nigeria. *International Journal of Gynaecology and Obstetrics* **130**(Supplement 1), S22–S26. doi:10.1016/j.ijgo.2015.04.004

# 19 Point-of-care testing for HIV

*Damian Conway*, Phillip Keen* and Rebecca Guy*

**Summary**

The human immunodeficiency virus (HIV) and acquired immune deficiency syndrome (AIDS) epidemics have been recognised by the United Nations as a global emergency, requiring an exceptional response to reduce new HIV transmissions and to diagnose and treat people with HIV and AIDS. Worldwide, half of the people with HIV remain undiagnosed, and less than half of those who have been diagnosed receive treatment. Point-of-care (POC) tests for screening, diagnosis and monitoring of HIV infection can greatly expand access to and uptake of HIV testing, and support clinical management, especially in low and middle income countries with limited laboratory infrastructure and high HIV prevalence. Most HIV POC tests for screening and diagnosis are relatively simple devices that can be used in clinical, community and outreach settings, and some can be self-administered. Molecular-based POC test platforms with laboratory-equivalent analytical performance are now available for some HIV monitoring tests, and more such devices are in the development pipeline.

## CLINICAL INTRODUCTION

### Global and regional burden

Since the beginning of the HIV epidemic, an estimated 78 million people worldwide have been infected with HIV and there have been 39 million deaths related to AIDS (UNAIDS 2014a). In 2014, an estimated 2 million people were newly infected, 37 million people were living with HIV infection, and there were 1.2 million AIDS-related deaths worldwide (UNAIDS 2015). Globally, AIDS-related deaths have fallen in the last decade (from 2 million in 2005 to 1.2 million in 2014), mainly due to the effects of treatment with antiretroviral therapy (ART) and by June 2015, ~16 million people worldwide were being treated with ART (Maartens *et al.* 2014; UNAIDS 2015).

Global HIV incidence has decreased by 35% from 3.1 million per year in 2000 to 2 million in 2014, largely due to reductions in heterosexual transmission and access to ART (UNAIDS 2015). Global HIV prevalence among adults aged 15–49 years is estimated to be 0.8%, though this varies considerably between countries and regions of the world (UNAIDS 2014a). The median HIV prevalence is highest in sub-Saharan Africa where 25.8 million people live with HIV infection (66% of the global total) (UNAIDS 2015). In this region, HIV infection rates are estimated at 5% of adults aged 15–49 years, 8% of young women aged 15–24 years, 37% of female sex workers, and 19% of gay, bisexual and other men who have sex with men (MSM) (UNAIDS 2014a).

Generalised HIV epidemics are those where HIV is established in the general population and HIV prevalence in pregnant women is consistently over 1%. Concentrated epidemics are those where HIV prevalence is consistently over 5% in at least one sub-population but is below 1% in pregnant women attending antenatal clinics (WHO 2015b). The HIV epidemic in sub-Saharan Africa and in some Caribbean countries is generalised with heterosexual and vertical transmission as the main modes of transmission.

*joint first authors

The main risk factors for HIV transmission in most other regions of the world are male-to-male sexual contact, injecting drug use and sex work (Fettig *et al.* 2014).

### Risk factors

Risk factors for HIV vary by population. Among heterosexually acquired HIV cases, risk factors can be biological (the risk of getting HIV during vaginal sex without a condom is much higher for women than it is for men) and there are a range of individual and social risk factors. These include the number of lifetime and concurrent sexual partners, poverty, level of education, gender inequality and violence, lack of male circumcision and health system factors, such as limited access to HIV prevention or treatment programs (Dunkle *et al.* 2004; Gcis *et al.* 2011; Tanser *et al.* 2011). In people who inject drugs, the main mode of HIV acquisition is use of contaminated injecting equipment. Factors that increase the risk of HIV acquisition include younger age, frequency of injecting, type of drugs used and poly-drug use. Social determinants predict needle-sharing behaviour (Strathdee *et al.* 1997). Among people involved in sex work, inconsistent condom use is the main mode of exposure, but the degree of exposure to HIV risk and sex work harm varies across different physical environments, types of sex services and legal situation (Harcourt and Donovan 2005). Often these risk groups overlap. Sex workers who inject drugs often have much higher HIV incidence and prevalence than non-injecting sex workers (Baral *et al.* 2013). In MSM, the main mode of HIV acquisition is condomless anal intercourse (CLAI), which represents a spectrum of behaviours with different HIV risk strata (Mao *et al.* 2006; Jin *et al.* 2009; Guy *et al.* 2011).

### Pathophysiology and complications of HIV

HIV is currently an incurable infection that increases the risk of certain cancers and requires lifelong drug treatment that is associated with cumulative metabolic toxicity (Deeks *et al.* 2013; Maartens *et al.* 2014). Without treatment, HIV infection causes a spectrum of clinical disorders, leading to progressive immune dysfunction, AIDS and death. During HIV seroconversion illness (also called primary HIV infection or acute retroviral syndrome), antibodies to HIV develop and there are high levels of viraemia. The clinical syndrome of acute HIV infection, which develops in 50–90% of people during the first few weeks after infection, is characterised by fever, malaise, arthralgia/myalgia, headache and erythematous maculopapular skin rash. Patients may also experience lymphadenopathy, pharyngitis, anorexia, mucosal ulceration and diarrhoea, although severe manifestations (such as meningoencephalitis or myelitis) are rare (Chu and Selwyn 2010). Progression of HIV infection impairs immune function and causes a median decline in CD4 cell count per year of 67 cells/mm$^3$ (range 64–69 cells/mm$^3$) (Lodi *et al.* 2010). The median CD4 cell count in healthy HIV-negative people is 952 cells/mm$^3$ (range 771–1109 cells/mm$^3$) and the median time taken to develop AIDS without treatment is 11 years after seroconversion (Collaborative Group on AIDS 2000; Le *et al.* 2013).

## HIV TESTING

In 2015, new HIV testing guidelines were released by the World Health Organization (WHO 2015b), including specific recommendations for offering testing and re-testing by service and epidemic type (concentrated, generalised) and for key populations (groups at increased risk for HIV due to specific higher risk behaviours; these include MSM, people who inject drugs, people in prisons and other closed settings, sex workers and transgender people).

- *In all settings*, testing should be considered for malnutrition clinics, sexually transmissible infections (STIs), hepatitis, tuberculosis (TB) and antenatal care services, and all services for key populations. Re-testing of all people newly and previously diagnosed with HIV should be undertaken before they enrol in care and initiate ART. Re-testing should be offered at least annually to people from key populations and people in serodiscordant couples, or more frequently depending on client risk behaviours.
- *In generalised epidemics*, testing should be offered to all clients and in all services and re-testing offered to all HIV-negative pregnant women in their third trimester, and to HIV negative partners in serodiscordant couples at least annually, or more frequently depending on risk behaviours.
- *In concentrated epidemics*, testing should be offered to all patients presenting with HIV indicator conditions, including presumed and confirmed TB cases, and re-testing offered to HIV-negative partners in serodiscordant couples or those from key population groups.

Increased access to HIV testing and more frequent testing is essential for earlier HIV diagnosis, which leads to improved health outcomes and life expectancy for HIV-infected individuals (Branson *et al.* 2013). Cohort studies have estimated the increased survival and life expectancy of HIV-infected people who are diagnosed, engaged in clinical care, and treated with antiretroviral therapy (May *et al.* 2014; van Sighem *et al.* 2010). Life expectancy of those with HIV infection in the UK was found to be normal compared with the general population, provided they were virally suppressed on ART with a CD4 count greater than 350 cells/mm$^3$, and had no history of injecting drug use (May *et al.* 2014).

## UPTAKE OF HIV POINT-OF-CARE TESTING

HIV POC tests have been used in a range of countries and for differing purposes. HIV POC tests have expanded access to testing, especially in resource poor high burden settings where access to laboratory services is limited (Peeling and Mabey 2010). Efforts to improve access to HIV point-of-care testing (POCT) have also been strengthened through better integration of HIV testing with sexual and reproductive health, maternal and child health programs (Chamla *et al.* 2014; Tudor Car *et al.* 2012) and recently with the policy focus on early diagnosis and treatment of HIV for prevention (WHO 2015a).

In developed countries, HIV POC tests have largely been used where patients interact with the health system (such as emergency and obstetric departments and STI clinics) but also through outreach, especially targeted to those at greatest risk of infection (Gaydos and Hardick 2014). HIV POC tests are useful for hard-to-reach populations (e.g. homeless or marginalised), and in clinical situations where prompt treatment decisions must be made, such as for pregnant women in labour where their HIV status is unknown (Sturenburg and Junker 2009). Studies involving HIV POCT in a range of settings suggest this approach can improve uptake of HIV testing and receipt of results, and that it is preferable to conventional testing for many client groups (Pai *et al.* 2007; Pottie *et al.* 2014; Thornton *et al.* 2012; Turner *et al.* 2013).

Although HIV POCT has expanded access to testing in many settings, barriers to testing uptake and implementation have been documented (Pai *et al.* 2015). Test coverage remains low in many parts of the world and UNAIDS estimate more than half of all people (54%) living with HIV globally do not know their HIV status (UNAIDS 2014a). Additionally, only 42% of infants born to HIV-infected mothers in low and middle income countries received a test within the first 2 months of life, as recommended by the WHO (UNAIDS 2014a). The global push to improve access to diagnostics so that 90% of people with HIV know their status by 2020 will provide impetus to improve these statistics.

## HIV MONITORING TESTS

Monitoring clinical status in HIV infection includes assessing CD4 cell count (surrogate marker of immune function) and HIV viral load (quantitative measurement of HIV ribonucleic acid [RNA] in the blood). HIV viral load test and CD4 cell test results are used to monitor the status of HIV disease and the effectiveness of therapy, and help detect drug resistance. Previously, these tests were also used to determine when to begin ART; however, recent studies have shown that starting ART early both improved health outcomes for individuals (The INSIGHT START Study Group 2015) and had public health benefits (Cohen *et al.* 2011). Hence, in 2015 the WHO recommended that ART should be commenced immediately after diagnosis, irrespective of viral load and CD4 count (WHO 2015a).

HIV viral load is an important tool to evaluate the efficacy of the HIV 'treatment as prevention (TasP)' strategy, which involves increased HIV testing and treating people diagnosed with HIV with ART earlier to reduce community viral load and the risk of HIV transmission (Cohen *et al.* 2011). The efficacy of TasP depends on the extent to which all people with HIV infection in a population are engaged in the spectrum of HIV care, and the way in which engagement with care progressively falls along this spectrum is called the HIV care and treatment cascade (Gardner *et al.* 2011). The WHO 90:90:90 targets recommend 90% of those with HIV-infection are diagnosed, 90% of those diagnosed are on ART, and 90% of those on ART are virally suppressed (UNAIDS 2014b). Deficiencies in the components of the spectrum of HIV care prevent the best clinical and TasP outcomes being achieved (Gardner *et al.* 2011).

The recent change in WHO guidelines to recommend ART for all HIV-infected people and viral load testing to monitor treatment success and identify treatment failure (WHO 2015a) requires scaling up capacity for monitoring HIV viral load, including using POC viral load tests in settings with limited or no access to laboratory infrastructure (Cogswell *et al.* 2016). Another application for POC HIV viral load tests is their use in HIV diagnosis among infants born to HIV-positive mothers – antibody testing being unsuitable due to the passive transfer of maternal antibodies across the placenta (WHO 2015b).

In settings where universal access to treatment is not yet possible, measuring CD4 will remain an important strategy to prioritise decisions regarding ART initiation, and CD4 cell count informs clinical assessment regarding starting and stopping prophylaxis for AIDS-related opportunistic infections (UNITAID 2015). Increased access to quality-assured POC tests for HIV viral load, early infant diagnosis and CD4 testing has the greatest potential to improve HIV care and treatment globally. (UNITAID 2015).

## HIV POC SCREENING DEVICES

HIV POC tests are designed to detect anti-HIV antibodies rapidly (ideally within 20 min) so results are available during the clinical consultation. HIV POC tests are commonly qualitative immunoassays for detection of HIV antibody in either immunochromatographic test (ICT) strip or flow-through formats. Most POC tests use whole blood (from finger-pricks or venipuncture), plasma or serum specimens, and a small number use oral fluid. Although a single HIV POC test cannot be used to diagnose HIV infection, in settings with limited or no laboratory infrastructure, algorithms with POC tests used sequentially or in parallel are used to identify cases of HIV infection; the most sensitive POC test is used for first-line screening and other highly specific POC tests selected to verify the reactive test results of first-line assays (WHO 2015b). Evaluation of the performance of the POC tests selected for the algorithm is important, because false positives have been reported using this method (Baveewo *et al.* 2012). In settings with good laboratory infrastructure, confirmation of HIV infection is achieved using laboratory testing algorithms involving HIV immunoassays and Western Blot.

HIV POC tests can have sensitivity and specificity >99%, though variations occur depending on which test, reference standard and sampling method (oral fluid, whole blood, plasma or serum) are used (Pavie *et al.* 2010; Pai *et al.* 2012).

In 2006, there were four US Food and Drug Administration (FDA) approved rapid HIV tests with sensitivity in package inserts of 99.6–100% on serum, plasma and finger-prick whole blood specimens: OraSure OraQuick Advance Rapid HIV test, MedMira Reveal G-2 Rapid HIV test, Trinity Biotech Uni-Gold Recombigen HIV test, and Bio-Rad Multispot HIV-1 & HIV-2 test. The Multispot test was unique in terms of its ability to differentiate between HIV-1 and HIV-2, but, due to its relative complexity with dilution of specimens and the reagent and wash steps, was unsuitable for use outside laboratories. Sensitivity reported for the OraQuick test was lower if used with oral fluid specimens at 99.3%, and reported specificity ranged from 99.1% for the Reveal test to 100% for the OraQuick test (Franco-Paredes *et al.* 2006; Greenwald *et al.* 2006).

A large evaluation at two clinical sites in Los Angeles examined the performance of six rapid HIV tests using oral fluid, finger-prick whole blood, and venipuncture whole blood, serum or plasma specimens collected from 6282 patients (69% MSM) between 2003 and 2008 (Delaney *et al.* 2011). Four tests (Clearview Complete, Clearview Stat-Pak, Orasure OraQuick Advance and Reveal G-3) were evaluated using fresh specimens and two tests were evaluated using stored serum and plasma specimens in the laboratory (Multispot HIV 1 & 2 and Uni-Gold Recombigen). Sensitivity was 100% for all methods when used to test patients with known HIV infection who were ART-naïve; but, when used to test patients with HIV infection who were taking ART, sensitivity ranged from 97.7 to 100%, being lowest for the OraSure test using oral fluid specimens and highest for the Multispot, Reveal and Uni-Gold tests with serum and plasma specimens. The reference assay for these sensitivity analyses was a first-generation laboratory immunoassay (BioMerieux Vironostika HIV-1 Microelisa System). Specificity ranged from 99.3% for plasma specimens used with the Multispot to 100% for most of the other methods and specimen types.

Three commonly used HIV POC tests (OraSure OraQuick, Abbott Determine and Trinity Uni-Gold) were evaluated in 2003–2004 using patient serum, plasma and whole blood specimens from five countries (US, Malawi, Zimbabwe, Zambia and South Africa) and referenced to second and third generation laboratory HIV immunoassays (Piwowar-Manning *et al.* 2010). The sensitivity reported for OraSure OraQuick, Abbott Determine, and Trinity Uni-Gold assays was 99.3%, 99.8% and 98.5%, respectively, while specificity was 99.3%, 99.4% and 99.5%, respectively.

In a systematic review of the performance of oral fluid versus blood-based specimens with the OraSure OraQuick Advance assay, the pooled sensitivity was nearly 2% lower for oral fluid specimens: 98.0% for oral fluid specimens versus 99.7% for blood-based specimens. Specificity was similar for both specimen types: 99.7% for oral fluid versus 99.9% for blood-based (Pai *et al.* 2012).

The difference in sensitivity may be due to the concentration of IgG antibody in plasma being four to five times larger than that in oral mucosal transudate (i.e. gingival crevicular fluid) (Mortimer and Parry 1994).

Despite their ability to expand access to HIV testing, if POC tests that detect HIV antibody only are used for screening, then their longer window period may result in acute HIV infections being missed in some populations (Patel *et al.* 2012; Stekler *et al.* 2009). A robust POC test that can reliably detect cases of acute HIV infection is therefore needed, given the risk of inadvertent onward HIV transmission and the potential public health implications involved if a positive case is missed (Patel *et al.* 2012; Pilcher *et al.* 2010).

The Alere Determine HIV Combo assay was introduced in 2009 as the first HIV POC assay containing both HIV antibody and antigen components and specifically designed to increase test sensitivity in patients recently infected with HIV (Guidasci 2009). In 2010, an evaluation of this assay in a Belgian reference laboratory reported sensitivity of the antibody component in chronic infection as 100% and specificity in negative specimens as 100% (Beelaert and Fransen 2010). However, subsequent studies demonstrated poor sensitivity of the antigen component in acute infection. In a large field evaluation using finger-prick specimens for screening in a high prevalence population in Malawi, the antigen component failed to detect any of the eight antigen-positive cases of acute HIV infection (HIV viral load range 45 000–750 000 copies/mL) and demonstrated disappointing specificity of 98.3% (Rosenberg *et al.* 2012). An evaluation involving 3195 finger-prick blood specimens in sexual health clinics in Sydney found that sensitivity of the test in early HIV infection (within the last 6 months) was 66.7%, the antigen component did not detect any of nine HIV p24 antigen positive specimens, and the median viral load of the cases of HIV infection that were missed was 238 025 copies/mL (Conway *et al.* 2014). In a field evaluation in Swaziland involving over 18 000 subjects tested via venepuncture-collected whole blood specimens in their homes, 12 individuals were falsely identified as having acute HIV infection by the antigen component and 13 who had acute infection detected by HIV RNA testing (viral load range 300 to >10 000 000 copies/mL) were missed by the antigen component (Duong *et al.* 2014). Further published evaluations of the Determine HIV Combo assay are summarised in Table 19.1 and the difference in the test's performance in the laboratory versus in the field demonstrates the importance of evaluating POC assays using fresh specimens in the hands of typical users.

When the Determine HIV Combo assay has been evaluated head-to-head with other POC tests in the same patient population, it has, however, been shown to be the most sensitive assay in acute infection. In a laboratory evaluation in the US, the Determine HIV Combo and other assays were compared with pooled HIV RNA testing in San Francisco from 2003 to 2008 (Pilcher *et al.* 2013). In 57 specimens classified as acute infections, the sensitivity of Determine HIV Combo assay was 54%, compared with 87% for the Abbott Architect fourth generation immunoassay, 35% for the Genetic Systems third generation immunoassay, 26% for the Trinity Biotech Uni-Gold Recombigen HIV rapid test, and 5% for the OraSure OraQuick Advance HIV rapid test.

## NEW DEVELOPMENTS IN HIV POC SCREENING DEVICES

Recently, POC tests for the dual detection of HIV and syphilis have become available that may increase access to testing for both HIV and syphilis, especially in antenatal settings (Bristow *et al.* 2014). POC platforms that enable self-testing have also become available. HIV self-testing (HIVST) enables a person who wants to know his or her HIV status to collect a specimen, perform a test and interpret the test result privately. HIVST has been legalised in the US, UK, France, Australia, Brazil, Kenya, Hong Kong, Malawi and Rwanda, and in several other countries policies are under development and devices for HIVST are available informally (WHO and UNITAID 2015) (Table 19.2).

There are several HIV POC tests that can be used for self-testing but only a limited number specifically packaged for HIVST. Three HIV POC tests for self-testing are formally available and approved by a stringent regulatory authority: the OraQuick In-Home HIV Test (OraSure Technologies Inc., Bethlehem PA, USA); Autotest VIH (AAZ Laboratories) and BioSure HIV Self Test (BioSURE, UK, Ltd) (WHO and UNITAID 2015).

The OraQuick In-Home HIV Test was approved in the USA on public health grounds despite its relatively lower sensitivity in the field trials in an effort to increase testing and reduce the pool of undiagnosed HIV (Myers *et al.* 2013). OraQuick In-Home HIV test is a second generation test that detects HIV 1/2 antibodies in oral fluid. The specimen is obtained by swabbing the upper and lower gums using a collector device, which is transferred to a solution and the results are read in 20–40 min (OraSure Technologies 2012). The sensitivity and specificity of the OraQuick HIVST in the hands of untrained users is

**Table 19.1.** Determine HIV Combo assay performance evaluations published between 2010 and 2014

| Citation | Setting (testers) | Specimen | Population | Study size | Reference tests | Performance |
|---|---|---|---|---|---|---|
| Beelaert and Fransen 2010 | Belgium, laboratory (laboratory technician) | Serum, plasma, VWB, CCS | Not reported, non-B subtype 13% | 179 CHI<br>67 AHI<br>50 CCS<br>200 Neg | Vironostika 4G IA<br>Innotest p24Ag IA<br>Inno-Lia Confirmation | Sensitivity Ab 100%<br>Specificity Ab 100%<br>Sensitivity Ag 86.6% |
| Pavie *et al.* 2010 | France, clinic/ laboratory (doctors/ laboratory technicians) | FSB, Serum | HIV Clinic, known Pos 69% on ART, 83% male, subtype B 63% | 199 CHI<br>2 RHI<br>20 Neg | Abbott Architect 4G IA<br>VIDAS p24Ag IA<br>Roche Cobas Taqman VL<br>Biorad WB | Sensitivity 95.8% FSB v. 100% serum<br>Sensitivity 95.1% subtype B<br>Sensitivity 96.1% non-B subtype<br>Specificity 100%<br>Invalid 15% |
| Fox *et al.* 2011 | UK, laboratory (laboratory scientist) | Serum | Not reported | 36 AHI Ag Pos (10 Ab Pos, 26 Ab Neg) | Abbott Architect and five other 4G IAs<br>Immunocomb Bispot 3G IA<br>VIDAS p24Ag IA | Sensitivity Ag 50% all samples<br>Sensitivity Ag 62% Ab Neg samples<br>Sensitivity Ag 20% Ab Pos samples<br>Sensitivity Ab 80% Ab Pos samples |
| Naylor *et al.* 2011 | UK, HIV clinic (not reported) | FSB | HIV Clinic, Known Pos 61% on ART | 142 CHI<br>5 AHI | Abbott Architect 4G IA<br>Immunocomb Bispot 3G IA<br>VIDAS p24Ag IA | Sensitivity Ag 60% AHI<br>Specificity Ag 98.6%<br>Invalid 13% |
| Bhowan *et al.* 2012 | South Africa, laboratory (laboratory technician) | VWB, plasma | Pregnant and post partum women | 345 antenatal<br>674 post partum | Advance Quality and Acon Triline RHTs (referenced to less sensitive Ab only RHTs) | Sensitivity Ab 100% plasma<br>Sensitivity Ab 100% VWB<br>Specificity Ab 99.8% plasma<br>Specificity Ab 99.3% VWB |
| Rosenberg *et al.* 2012 | Malawi, STI clinic/HTC centre (counsellors) | FSB | High HIV risk (prevalence 17%) | 163 CHI<br>8 AHI<br>838 Neg | AHI: Roche Monitor VL<br>CHI: Determine HIV (Ab only) and Trinity Unigold RHTs | Sensitivity Ab CHI 99.4%<br>Specificity Ab 99.2%<br>Sensitivity Ag AHI 0%<br>Specificity Ag 98.3%<br>Sensitivity overall AHI 25%<br>Specificity overall 97.9% |

**Table 19.1.** *(continued)*

| Citation | Setting (testers) | Specimen | Population | Study size | Reference tests | Performance |
|---|---|---|---|---|---|---|
| Kilembe *et al.* 2012 | Rwanda/Zambia, laboratory (laboratory staff) | Plasma | Cohort study, subtype C 85% | 34 AHI<br>18 RHI<br>28 CHI<br>55 Neg | Coulter & Vironostika p24Ag IAs<br>Roche Amplicor VL | Sensitivity Ag 1.9%<br>Sensitivity Ab 100% |
| Patel *et al.* 2012 | US, laboratory (laboratory technicians) | Plasma | CDC AHI study | G1: 33 AHI<br>G2: 40 AHI<br>44 CHI, 30 Neg | Abbott Architect 4G IA<br>Genetic Systems 3G IA<br>Siemens Versant VL | G1: Sensitivity overall AHI 76%<br>G2: Sensitivity overall 88%<br>G2: Specificity overall 100% |
| Chetty *et al.* 2012 | South Africa, laboratory (not reported) | Plasma | Pregnant women (HIV incidence cohort study) | 32 AHI Ag Pos (14 Ab Neg, 18 Ab Pos)<br>189 CHI<br>32 Neg | Roche Elecys 4G IA<br>Vironostika 3G IA<br>Roche p24Ag IA | Sensitivity overall 94%<br>Sensitivity CHI 100%<br>Sensitivity AHI Ag 0%<br>Sensitivity AHI Ab 59%<br>Specificity Ag 96.9%<br>Specificity Ab 100% |
| Laperche *et al.* 2012 | France, laboratory (not reported) | Plasma, CCS | Not reported | 119 CCS<br>20 plasma AHI | Innotest p24Ag IA, WHO/French p24Ag reference standards | Limit of detection Ag 40–50 pg/mL<br>Sensitivity Ag CCS 21% all subtypes<br>Sensitivity Ag CCS 62% subtype B<br>Sensitivity Ag AHI 60% all subtypes<br>Sensitivity Ag AHI 56% subtype B |
| Jones *et al.* 2012 | UK, clinic (not reported) | FSB | High HIV risk (prevalence 2.3%) | 985 | Abbott Architect 4G IA<br>Unspecified VIDAS IA | Sensitivity overall 90.5%<br>Specificity overall 99.8%<br>Invalid 0.6% |
| Faraoni *et al.* 2013 | Italy, laboratory (not reported) | Serum | MSM, PWID, heterosexual | 17 AHI<br>124 Neg | Abbott Architect 4G IA<br>Roche COBAS Taqman VL<br>Biorad WB | Sensitivity Ab 59% AHI<br>Sensitivity Ag 29% AHI<br>Sensitivity overall 88% AHI<br>Specificity Ab 100%<br>Specificity Ag 100%<br>Specificity overall 100% |

| Citation | Setting (testers) | Specimen | Population | Study size | Reference tests | Performance |
|---|---|---|---|---|---|---|
| Brauer *et al.* 2013 | South Africa, laboratory (not reported) | Serum | Routine testing, blood donors | 30 AHI Ag Pos (16 Ab Neg, 14 Ab Pos) | Abbott AxSYM/ Architect | Sensitivity Ab 90.7% |
| | | | | | Roche Combi 4G IAs Innotest | Specificity Ab 100% |
| | | | | | Roche p24Ag IAs | Sensitivity Ag 10% AHI |
| | | | | 29 CHI | Abbott Prism 3G IA | Specificity Ag 100% |
| | | | | 20 Neg | Procleix VL | |
| Conway *et al.* 2014 | Australia, clinic (doctors and nurses) | FSB | MSM | 3 AHI | Abbott Architect | Sensitivity overall 87.2% |
| | | | | 9 RHI | Roche Combi 4G IAs | Sensitivity Ab 94.4% |
| | | | | 32 CHI | Biorad p24Ag IA | Sensitivity Ag 0% |
| | | | | 3151 Neg | Biorad, Fujirebio 3G IAs | Sensitivity early infection 66.7% |
| | | | | | MP Diagnostics WB | Specificity overall 99.4% |
| | | | | | | Invalid 0.2% |
| Duong *et al.* 2014 | Swaziland, household survey (nurses) | VWB | High HIV risk (prevalence 32%) | 13 AHI | Biorad, Vironostika 4G IAs | Sensitivity overall 99.8% |
| | | | | 5802 CHI | Roche COBAS Taqman VL | Sensitivity CHI 100% |
| | | | | 12 357 Neg | Trinity Uni-Gold RHT | Sensitivity AHI 0% |
| | | | | | | Specificity overall 99.7% |

Note: 3G = 3rd generation; 4G = 4th generation; Ab = antibody; Ag = p24 antigen; AHI = acute HIV infection; ART = antiretroviral therapy; CHI = chronic HIV infection; CCS = cell culture supernatant; FSB = fingerstick whole blood; G1 = group 1; G2 = group 2; HTC = HIV testing and counselling; IA = immunoassay; MSM = men who have sex with men; Neg = negative; Pos = positive; PWID = people who inject drugs; RHI = recent HIV infection; RHT = rapid HIV test; STI = sexually transmitted infection; VL = HIV viral load; VWB = venous whole blood; WB = HIV Western blot

**Table 19.2.** HIV self-testing (HIVST) policy tracking by country (Source: WHO and UNITAID 2015)

| Country and year HIVST approved | Policies explicitly allowing HIVST | Policies under development | HIVST available informally |
|---|---|---|---|
| USA 2012 | Australia | South Africa | China |
| UK 2015 | Brazil | Zimbabwe | Namibia |
| France 2015 | Kenya | Zambia | South Africa |
| | Hong Kong; Macau | Peru | Russian Federation |
| | Malawi | Thailand | Tanzania |
| | Rwanda | Namibia | Nigeria |
| | | Switzerland | Ukraine |

91.7% (95% CI: 84.2–96.3%) and 99.9% (95% CI: 99.9–100.0%), respectively (OraSure Technologies 2012). More recently, finger-prick based HIV self-tests have become available including the BioSure HIV Self Test – the first approved HIVST in the UK – and the Autotest VIH® (AAZ Laboratories), available in pharmacies in France. Several observational studies in different settings and populations have shown users find self-testing highly acceptable and easy to perform (Figueroa *et al.* 2015; Krause *et al.* 2013) and there is little or no evidence of harm associated with self-testing (Brown *et al.* 2014).

## HIV VIRAL LOAD DEVICES

Current formats for POC and near-POC viral load tests include nucleic acid amplification tests (NAAT), which detect and quantify viral RNA, and non-NAAT-based technologies, which detect and quantify HIV viral proteins (p24) and enzymes (reverse transcriptase; RT) that correlate with the level of HIV viral RNA (Haleyur Giri Setty and Hewlett 2014). Near-POC systems generally require slightly higher laboratory infrastructure, such as electricity and a clean sample processing room, and greater technician training than POC sites. Test platforms use either whole blood or plasma, or both (Haleyur Giri Setty and Hewlett 2014).

Only a small number of HIV viral load test devices are commercially available for POC and near-POC use, but many new platforms are in development. As of October 2015, the Cepheid (Xpert HIV-1 Viral Load), and Diagnostics for the Real World Ltd (SAMBA I/II) were available (Table 19.3). The Xpert HIV-1 Viral Load test is a polymerase chain reaction (PCR) based NAAT assay, with a portable version (GeneXpert Omni) that can

**Table 19.3.** Summary of analytical performance of HIV viral load tests

| Author | Test name (manufacturer) | POC test method | Specimen type | Sensitivity | Specificity |
|---|---|---|---|---|---|
| UNITAID 2015 | Xpert HIV-1 VL (Cepheid) | RT–PCR | Plasma | LOD: 18.3 cp/mL<br>LOQ: 40 cp/mL | 100% (95% CI: 96.7–100) |
| UNITAID 2015 | SAMBA I (Diagnostics for the Real World) | NAAT | EID: 100 µL whole blood<br>VL: 200 µL plasma | EID: 95.7–100%<br>VL concordance: 94.8–98%[a] | EID: 99.2–100% |
| UNITAID 2015 | SAMBA II (Diagnostics for the Real World) | NAAT | EID: 100 µL whole blood<br>VL: 200 µL plasma or 120 µL whole blood | Equivalent to SAMBA I (EID and VL)[c] | Equivalent to SAMBA I (EID)[b] |

Note: VL = viral load; RT–PCR = real-time quantitative reverse-transcription PCR; EID = early infant diagnosis; LOD = limit of detection; cp/mL = copies per millilitre; LOQ = limit of quantification; NAAT = nucleic acid amplification test

[a]Range from several evaluations

[b]From in-house testing

[c]From in-house testing and a field evaluation in Uganda

operate via AC-DC power, or battery power alone. The SAMBA 1/II system are NAAT-based HIV tests that perform: (i) a semiquantitative test with a cut-off of 1000 copies/mL for monitoring ART using plasma; (ii) a semiquantitative test with a cut-off of 1000 copies/mL for monitoring ART using whole blood; (iii) a semiquantitative test based on plasma or whole blood for the detection of acute HIV infection during the window period before the appearance of antibodies and (iv) an early infant diagnosis (EID) test based on whole blood (UNITAID 2015). In an assessment based on the WHO HIV RNA genotype panel, the SAMBA assay detected all HIV-1 subtypes (UNITAID 2015). The Alere q HIV 1/2 VL, the Northwestern Global Health Foundation Savanna p24 and the Cavidi RT were expected to be available later in 2015 and 2016 (UNITAID 2015).

Challenges in the development of POC and near-POC viral load platforms include over-estimation of viral load by platforms using whole blood samples and the high cost of devices and reagents. Future developments in HIV viral load POC tests are likely to include POC platforms that support both EID and quantitative viral load testing, and POC plasma separation systems (UNITAID 2015).

## CD4 TEST DEVICES

Most CD4 tests use flow cytometry to differentiate and count cells. Several POC CD4 test devices are on the market and in the development pipeline. Most are portable bench-top electronic devices (e.g. Alere Pima CD4 Test), but one disposable lateral flow device to qualitatively measure above and below 350 cells/mm$^3$ (Omega Diagnostics Group/Burnet Institute VISITECT CD4) is also available (UNITAID 2015).

## EVIDENCE BASE FOR THE PUBLIC HEALTH EFFECTIVENESS OF POC SCREENING FOR HIV

An emerging body of literature suggests that HIV POCT may increase the detection of undiagnosed infections, facilitate earlier treatment and care (reducing morbidity), and help prevent the onward transmission of HIV. A recent systematic review showed that community-based HIV testing across multiple countries (many using HIV POC tests) has increased the uptake of HIV testing, the proportion of first-time testers and the proportion of participants with CD4 counts above 350 cells/mm$^3$ compared with facility-based (clinic-based) approaches. Community-based services were defined as testing outside of health facilities, such as door-to-door testing, mobile services, self-testing and testing in workplaces, churches and schools. At community-based services, HIV positivity was lower than facility-based approaches but this may have been a consequence of people testing at clinics being higher risk, having STI symptoms or being tested because they were a contact of a sexual partner (Suthar *et al.* 2013).

A cluster randomised trial involving 34 communities in Africa and 14 communities in Thailand found community-based HIV POCT with support services increased testing rates by 25% overall, by 45% in men and 15% in women, while HIV incidence was significantly reduced in women older than 24 years (Coates *et al.* 2014). A Malawian study also found that community-based HIV POCT and counselling dramatically improved case finding and enrolment into care of HIV-infected infants and children; this is an important finding because early diagnosis of HIV is critical to ensure prompt initiation of ART, which is associated with lower mortality in HIV-infected children (Ahmed *et al.* 2015).

In regards to HIV self-tests, a recent analysis based on the Australian epidemic demonstrated that there would be a public health benefit (detection of HIV infections that would have otherwise remained undiagnosed) from self-testing if higher-risk MSM complemented their existing testing at clinics with the OraQuick self-test or previously untested MSM tested themselves for the first time using a self-test (UNSW-AMR HIV HTAG 2015). There is evidence from a randomised controlled trial in Seattle showing that access to HIV self-testing increases HIV testing frequency among MSM (Katz *et al.* 2015). A cluster-randomised trial in Malawi had 84% population-level uptake of community-based HIVST: just under half (44%) were first-time testers, the majority were adolescents and 12% were found to be HIV-positive by self-testing (Choko *et al.* 2015).

## REFERENCES


Ahmed S, Kim MH, Dave AC, Sabelli R, Kanjelo K, Preidis GA, *et al.* (2015) Improved identification and enrolment into care of HIV-exposed and -infected infants and children following a community health worker intervention in Lilongwe, Malawi. *Journal of the International AIDS Society* **18**, 19305. doi:10.7448/IAS.18.1.19305

Baral S, Todd CS, Aumakhan B, Lloyd J, Delegchoimbol A, Sabin K (2013) HIV among female sex workers in the Central Asian Republics, Afghanistan, and Mongolia: contexts and convergence with drug use. *Drug and Alcohol*

*Dependence* **132**(Supplement 1), S13–S16. doi:10.1016/j.drugalcdep.2013.07.004

Baveewo S, Kamya MR, Mayanja-Kizza H, Fatch R, Bangsberg DR, Coates T, *et al.* (2012) Potential for false positive HIV test results with the serial rapid HIV testing algorithm. *BMC Research Notes* **5**, 154. doi:10.1186/1756-0500-5-154

Beelaert G, Fransen K (2010) Evaluation of a rapid and simple fourth-generation HIV screening assay for qualitative detection of HIV p24 antigen and/or antibodies to HIV-1 and HIV-2. *Journal of Virological Methods* **168**, 218–222. doi:10.1016/j.jviromet.2010.06.002

Bhowan K, Kalk E, Khan S, Sherman G (2012) Identifying HIV infection in South African women: how does a fourth generation HIV rapid test perform? *African Journal of Laboratory Medicine* **1**, 1–5.

Branson BM, Viall A, Marum E (2013) Expanding HIV testing: back to the future. *JAIDS Journal of Acquired Immune Deficiency Syndromes* **63**, S117–S121. doi:10.1097/QAI.0b013e3182986f25

Brauer M, De Villiers JC, Mayaphi SH (2013) Evaluation of the Determine™ fourth generation HIV rapid assay. *Journal of Virological Methods* **189**, 180–183. doi:10.1016/j.jviromet.2013.01.017

Bristow CC, Adu-Sarkodie Y, Ondondo RO, Bukusi EA, Dagnra CA, Oo KY, *et al.* (2014) Multisite laboratory evaluation of a dual human immunodeficiency virus (HIV)/Syphilis point-of-care rapid test for simultaneous detection of HIV and Syphilis infection. *Open Forum Infectious Diseases* **1**, ofu015. doi:10.1093/ofid/ofu015

Brown A, Djimeu E, Cameron D (2014) A review of the evidence of harm from self-tests. *AIDS and Behavior* **18**, 445–449. doi:10.1007/s10461-014-0831-y

Chamla D, Luo C, Adjorlolo-Johnson G, Vandelaer J, Young M, Costales MO, *et al.* (2014) Integration of HIV infant testing into immunization programmes: a systematic review. *Paediatrics and International Child Health*. doi:10.1179/2046905514Y.0000000169

Chetty V, Moodley D, Chuturgoon A (2012) Evaluation of a 4th generation rapid HIV test for earlier and reliable detection of HIV infection in pregnancy. *Journal of Clinical Virology* **54**, 180–184. doi:10.1016/j.jcv.2012.02.021

Choko AT, MacPherson P, Webb E, Willey BA, Feasy H, Sambakunsi R, *et al.* (2015) Uptake, accuracy, safety, and linkage into care over two years of promoting annual self-testing for HIV in Blantyre, Malawi: a community-based prospective study. *PLoS Medicine* **12**, e1001873. doi:10.1371/journal.pmed.1001873

Chu C, Selwyn PA (2010) Diagnosis and initial management of acute HIV infection. *American Family Physician* **81**, 1239–1244.

Coates TJ, Kulich M, Celentano DD, Zelaya CE, Chariyalertsak S, Chingono A, *et al.* (2014) Effect of community-based voluntary counselling and testing on HIV incidence and social and behavioural outcomes (NIMH Project Accept; HPTN 043): a cluster-randomised trial. *The Lancet. Global Health* **2**, e267–e277. doi:10.1016/S2214-109X(14)70032-4

Cogswell HA, Ohadi E, Avila C (2016) Viral-load point-of-care technologies to achieve an AIDS-free generation. *Future Microbiology* **11**, 5–9. doi:10.2217/fmb.15.121

Cohen MS, Chen YQ, McCauley M, Gamble T, Hosseinipour MC, Kumarasamy N, *et al.* (2011) Prevention of HIV-1 infection with early antiretroviral therapy. *The New England Journal of Medicine* **365**, 493–505. doi:10.1056/NEJMoa1105243

Collaborative Group on AIDS (2000) Time from HIV-1 seroconversion to AIDS and death before widespread use of highly-active antiretroviral therapy: a collaborative reanalysis. *Lancet* **355**, 1131–1137.

Conway DP, Holt M, McNulty A, Couldwell DL, Smith DE, Davies SC, *et al.* (2014) Multi-centre evaluation of the Determine HIV Combo assay when used for point of care testing in a high risk clinic-based population. *PLoS One* **9**, e94062. doi:10.1371/journal.pone.0094062

Deeks SG, Lewin SR, Havlir DV (2013) The end of AIDS: HIV infection as a chronic disease. *Lancet* **382**, 1525–1533. doi:10.1016/S0140-6736(13)61809-7

Delaney KP, Branson BM, Uniyal A, Phillips S, Candal D, Owen SM, *et al.* (2011) Evaluation of the performance characteristics of 6 Rapid HIV antibody tests. *Clinical Infectious Diseases* **52**, 257–263. doi:10.1093/cid/ciq068

Dunkle KL, Jewkes RK, Brown HC, Gray GE, McIntryre JA, Harlow SD (2004) Gender-based violence, relationship power, and risk of HIV infection in women attending antenatal clinics in South Africa. *Lancet* **363**, 1415–1421. doi:10.1016/S0140-6736(04)16098-4

Duong YT, Mavengere Y, Patel H, Moore C, Manjengwa J, Sibandze D, *et al.* (2014) Poor performance of the Determine HIV-1/2 Ag/Ab Combo Fourth-Generation rapid test for detection of acute infections in a national household survey in Swaziland. *Journal of Clinical Microbiology* **52**, 3743–3748. doi:10.1128/JCM.01989-14

Faraoni S, Rocchetti A, Gotta F, Ruggiero T, Orofino G, Bonora S, *et al.* (2013) Evaluation of a rapid antigen and antibody combination test in acute HIV infection. *Journal of Clinical Virology* **57**, 84–87. doi:10.1016/j.jcv.2013.01.007

Fettig J, Swaminathan M, Murrill CS, Kaplan JE (2014) Global epidemiology of HIV. *Infectious Disease Clinics of North America* **28**, 323–337. doi:10.1016/j.idc.2014.05.001

Figueroa C, Johnson C, Verster A, Baggaley R (2015) Attitudes and acceptability on HIV self-testing among key populations: a literature review. *AIDS and Behavior* **19**, 1949–1965. doi:10.1007/s10461-015-1097-8

Fox J, Dunn H, O'Shea S (2011) Low rates of p24 antigen detection using a fourth-generation point of care HIV test. *Sexually Transmitted Infections* **87**, 178–179. doi:10.1136/sti.2010.042564

Franco-Paredes C, Tellez I, del Rio C (2006) Rapid HIV testing: a review of the literature and implications for the clinician. *Current HIV/AIDS Reports* **3**, 169–175. doi:10.1007/s11904-006-0012-3

Gardner EM, McLees MP, Steiner JF, del Rio C, Burman WJ (2011) The spectrum of engagement in HIV care and its relevance to test-and-treat strategies for prevention of HIV Infection. *Clinical Infectious Diseases* **52**, 793–800. doi:10.1093/cid/ciq243

Gaydos C, Hardick J (2014) Point of care diagnostics for sexually transmitted infections: perspectives and advances. *Expert Review of Anti-Infective Therapy* **12**, 657–672. doi:10.1586/14787210.2014.880651

Geis S, Maboko L, Saathoff E, Hoffmann O, Geldmacher C, Mmbando D, *et al.* (2011) Risk factors for HIV-1 infection in a longitudinal, prospective cohort of adults from the Mbeya Region, Tanzania. *JAIDS Journal of Acquired Immune Deficiency Syndromes* **56**, 453–459. doi:10.1097/QAI.0b013e3182118fa3

Greenwald JL, Burstein GR, Pincus J, Branson B (2006) A rapid review of rapid HIV antibody tests. *Current Infectious Disease Reports* **8**, 125–131. doi:10.1007/s11908-006-0008-6

Guidasci T (2009) Fourth generation point of care HIV screening. *Clinical Laboratory International* **33**, 26–28.

Guy R, Wand H, Wilson D, Prestage G, Jin F, Templeton D, *et al.* (2011) Using population attributable risk to choose HIV prevention strategies in gay men. *BMC Public Health* **11**, 247. doi:10.1186/1471-2458-11-247

Haleyur Giri Setty MK, Hewlett IK (2014) Point of care technologies for HIV. *AIDS Research and Treatment* **2014**, 497046. doi:10.1155/2014/497046

Harcourt C, Donovan B (2005) The many faces of sex work. *Sexually Transmitted Infections* **81**, 201–206. doi:10.1136/sti.2004.012468

Jin F, Crawford J, Prestage GP, Zablotska I, Imrie J, Kippax SC, *et al.* (2009) Unprotected anal intercourse, risk reduction behaviours, and subsequent HIV infection in a cohort of homosexual men. *AIDS (London, England)* **23**, 243–252. doi:10.1097/QAD.0b013e32831fb51a

Jones CB, Kuldanek K, Muir D, Phekoo K, Black A, Sacks R, Smith A, Jones CB, K (2012) Clinical evaluation of the Determine HIV-1/2 Ag/Ab Combo test. *Journal of Infectious Diseases* **206**, 1947–1949; author reply 1949–1950.

Katz D, Golden M, Hughes J, Farquhar C, Stekler J (2015) HIV self-testing increases HIV testing frequency among high-risk men who have sex with men: a randomized controlled trial. In *Journal of the International AIDS Society.* 8th IAS Conference on HIV Pathogenesis, Treatment & Prevention. 19–22 July, Vancouver, Canada.

Kilembe W, Keeling M, Karita E, Lakhi S, Chetty P, Price MA, *et al.* (2012) Failure of a novel, rapid antigen and antibody combination test to detect antigen-positive HIV infection in African adults with early HIV infection. *PLoS One* **7**, e37154. doi:10.1371/journal.pone.0037154

Krause J, Subklew-Sehume F, Kenyon C, Colebunders R (2013) Acceptability of HIV self-testing: a systematic literature review. *BMC Public Health* **13**, 1–9. doi:10.1186/1471-2458-13-735

Laperche S, Leballais L, Ly TD, Plantier JC (2012) Failures in the detection of HIV p24 antigen with the Determine HIV-1/2 Ag/Ab Combo rapid test. *Journal of Infective Diseases* **206**, 1946–1947; author reply 1949–1950.

Le T, Wright EJ, Smith DM, He W, Catano G, Okulicz JF, *et al.* (2013) Enhanced CD4+ T-cell recovery with earlier HIV-1 antiretroviral therapy. *The New England Journal of Medicine* **368**, 218–230. doi:10.1056/NEJMoa1110187

Lodi S, Phillips A, Touloumi G, Pantazis N, Bucher HC, Babiker A, *et al.* (2010) CD4 decline in seroconverter and seroprevalent individuals in the precombination of antiretroviral therapy era. *AIDS (London, England)* **24**, 2697–2704. doi:10.1097/QAD.0b013e32833ef6c4

Maartens G, Celum C, Lewin SR (2014) HIV infection: epidemiology, pathogenesis, treatment, and prevention. *Lancet* **384**, 258–271. doi:10.1016/S0140-6736(14)60164-1

Mao L, Crawford JM, Hospers HJ, Prestage GP, Grulich AE, Kaldor JM, *et al.* (2006) 'Serosorting' in casual anal sex of HIV-negative gay men is noteworthy and is increasing in Sydney, Australia. *AIDS (London, England)* **20**, 1204–1206. doi:10.1097/01.aids.0000226964.17966.75

May MT, Gompels M, Delpech V, Porter K, Orkin C, Kegg S, *et al.* (2014) Impact on life expectancy of HIV-1 positive individuals of CD4+ cell count and viral load response to antiretroviral therapy. *AIDS (London, England)* **28**, 1193–1202. doi:10.1097/QAD.0000000000000243

Mortimer PP, Parry JV (1994) Detection of antibody to HIV in saliva: a brief review. *Clinical and Diagnostic Virology* **2**, 231–243. doi:10.1016/0928-0197(94)90048-5

Myers JE, El-Sadr WM, Zerbe A, Branson BM (2013) Rapid HIV self-testing: long in coming but opportunities beckon. *AIDS (London, England)* **27**, 1687–1695. doi:10.1097/QAD.0b013e32835fd7a0

Naylor E, Axten D, Makia F, Tong C, White J, Fox J (2011) Fourth generation point of care testing for HIV: validation in an HIV-positive population. *Sexually Transmitted Infections* **87**, 311. doi:10.1136/sextrans-2011-050056

OraSure Technologies (2012) *Final Advisory Committee Briefing Materials: Available for Public Release.* OraSure Technologies Inc., Bethlehem PA, USA.

Pai NP, Tulsky JP, Cohan D, Colford JM Jr, Reingold AR (2007) Rapid point-of-care HIV testing in pregnant women: a systematic review and meta-analysis. *Tropical Medicine & International Health* **12**, 162–173. doi:10.1111/j.1365-3156.2006.01812.x

Pai NP, Balram B, Shivkumar S, Martinez-Cajas JL, Claessens C, Lambert G, *et al.* (2012) Head-to-head comparison of accuracy of a rapid point-of-care HIV test with oral versus whole-blood specimens: a systematic review and meta-analysis. *The Lancet Infectious Diseases* **12**, 373–380. doi:10.1016/S1473-3099(11)70368-1

Pai NP, Wilkinson S, Deli-Houssein R, Vijh R, Vadnais C, Behlim T, *et al.* (2015) Barriers to implementation of rapid and point-of-care tests for human immunodeficiency virus infection: findings from a systematic review (1996–2014). *Point of Care* **14**, 81–87. doi:10.1097/POC.0000000000000056

Patel P, Bennett B, Sullivan T, Parker MM, Heffelfinger JD, Sullivan PS (2012) Rapid HIV screening: missed opportunities for HIV diagnosis and prevention. *Journal of Clinical Virology* **54**, 42–47. doi:10.1016/j.jcv.2012.01.022

Pavie J, Rachline A, Loze B, Niedbalski L, Delaugerre C, Laforgerie E, *et al.* (2010) Sensitivity of five rapid HIV tests on oral fluid or finger-stick whole blood: a real-time comparison in a healthcare setting. *PLoS One* **5**, e11581. doi:10.1371/journal.pone.0011581

Peeling RW, Mabey D (2010) Point-of-care tests for diagnosing infections in the developing world. *Clinical Microbiology and Infection* **16**, 1062–1069. doi:10.1111/j.1469-0691.2010.03279.x

Pilcher CD, Christopoulos KA, Golden M (2010) Public health rationale for rapid nucleic acid or p24 antigen tests for HIV. *The Journal of Infectious Diseases* **201**(Supplement 1), S7–S15. doi:10.1086/650393

Pilcher CD, Louie B, Facente S, Keating S, Hackett J Jr, Vallari A, *et al.* (2013) Performance of rapid point-of-care and laboratory tests for acute and established HIV infection in San Francisco. *PLoS One* **8**, e80629. doi:10.1371/journal.pone.0080629

Piwowar-Manning EM, Tustin NB, Sikateyo P, Kamwendo D, Chipungu C, Maharaj R, *et al.* (2010) Validation of rapid HIV antibody tests in 5 African countries. *Journal of the International Association of Providers of AIDS Care* **9**, 170–172. doi:10.1177/1545109710368151

Pottie K, Medu O, Welch V, Dahal GP, Tyndall M, Rader T, *et al.* (2014) Effect of rapid HIV testing on HIV incidence and services in populations at high risk for HIV exposure: an equity-focused systematic review. *BMJ Open* **4**, e006859. doi:10.1136/bmjopen-2014-006859

Rosenberg NE, Kamanga G, Phiri S, Nsona D, Pettifor A, Rutstein SE, *et al.* (2012) Detection of acute HIV infection: a field evaluation of the Determine HIV-1/2 Ag/Ab Combo test. *The Journal of Infectious Diseases* **205**, 528–534. doi:10.1093/infdis/jir789

Stekler J, Swenson P, Coombs R, Dragavon J, Thomas K, Brennan C, *et al.* (2009) HIV testing in a high incidence population: is antibody testing alone good enough? *Clinical Infectious Diseases* **49**, 444–453. doi:10.1086/600043

Strathdee SA, Patrick DM, Archibald CP, Ofner M, Cornelisse PG, Rekart M, *et al.* (1997) Social determinants predict needle-sharing behaviour among injection drug users in Vancouver, Canada. *Addiction (Abingdon, England)* **92**, 1339–1347. doi:10.1111/j.1360-0443.1997.tb02852.x

Sturenburg E, Junker R (2009) Point-of-care testing in microbiology: the advantages and disadvantages of immunochromatographic test strips. *Deutsches Ärzteblatt International* **106**, 48–54.

Suthar AB, Ford N, Bachanas PJ, Wong VJ, Rajan JS, Saltzman AK, *et al.* (2013) Towards universal voluntary HIV testing and counselling: a systematic review and meta-analysis of community-based approaches. *PLoS Medicine* **10**, e1001496. doi:10.1371/journal.pmed.1001496

Tanser F, Barnighausen T, Hund L, Garnett GP, McGrath N, Newell ML (2011) Effect of concurrent sexual partnerships on rate of new HIV infections in a high-prevalence, rural South African population: a cohort study. *Lancet* **378**, 247–255. doi:10.1016/S0140-6736(11)60779-4

The INSIGHT START Study Group (2015) Initiation of antiretroviral therapy in early asymptomatic HIV infection. *The New England Journal of Medicine* **373**, 795–807. doi:10.1056/NEJMoa1506816

Thornton AC, Delpech V, Kall MM, Nardone A (2012) HIV testing in community settings in resource-rich countries: a systematic review of the evidence. *HIV Medicine* **13**, 416–426. doi:10.1111/j.1468-1293.2012.00992.x

Tudor Car L, Van Velthoven MH, Brusamento S, Elmoniry H, Car J, Majeed A, *et al.* (2012) Integrating prevention of mother-to-child HIV transmission programs to improve uptake: a systematic review. *PLoS One* **7**, e35268. doi:10.1371/journal.pone.0035268

Turner SD, Anderson K, Slater M, Quigley L, Dyck M, Guiang CB (2013) Rapid point-of-care HIV testing in youth: a systematic review. *The Journal of Adolescent Health* **53**, 683–691. doi:10.1016/j.jadohealth.2013.07.029

UNAIDS (United Nations Programme on HIV and AIDS) (2014a) *The Gap Report.* Joint United Nations Programme on HIV and AIDS, Geneva, Switzerland, <http://www.unaids.org/en/resources/documents/2014/20140716_UNAIDS_gap_report>.

UNAIDS (2014b) *90–90–90 An Ambitious Treatment Target to Help End the AIDS Epidemic.* Joint United Nations Programme on HIV and AIDS. Geneva, Switzerland, <http://www.unaids.org/sites/default/files/media_asset/90-90-90_en_0.pdf>.

UNAIDS (2015) *2015 World AIDS Day Report: Fact Sheet 2015.* Joint United Nations Programme on HIV and AIDS, Geneva, Switzerland, <http://www.unaids.org/en/resources/campaigns/HowAIDSchangedeverything/factsheet>.

UNITAID (2015) *HIV/AIDS Diagnostics Technology Landscape.* 5th edn. World Health Organization, Geneva, Switzerland, <http://unitaid.org/images/marketdynamics/publications/UNITAID_HIV_Nov_2015_Dx_Landscape.PDF>.

UNSW-AMR HIV HTAG (University of New South Wales and St Vincent's Centre for Applied Medical Research HIV Home Testing Assessment Group) (2015) Potential public health benefits of HIV testing occurring at home in Australia. *The Medical Journal of Australia* **202**, 529–531.

van Sighem AI, Gras LA, Reiss P, Brinkman K, de Wolf F, ATHENA National Observational Cohort Study (2010) Life expectancy of recently diagnosed asymptomatic HIV-infected patients approaches that of uninfected individuals. *AIDS (London, England)* **24**, 1527–1535. doi:10.1097/QAD.0b013e32833a3946

WHO (World Health Organization) (2015a) *Guideline on When to Start Antiretroviral Therapy and on Pre-Exposure Prophylaxis for HIV.* WHO, Geneva, Switzerland, <http://apps.who.int/iris/bitstream/10665/186275/1/9789241509565_eng.pdf?ua=1>.

WHO (2015b) *Consolidated Guidelines on HIV Testing Services.* WHO, Geneva, Switzerland, <http://apps.who.int/iris/bitstream/10665/179870/1/9789241508926_eng.pdf?ua=1&ua=1>.

WHO and UNITAID (2015) *Landscape for HIV rapid diagnostic tests for HIV self-testing.* WHO, Geneva, Switzerland, <http://unitaid.org/images/marketdynamics/publications/HIV_ST_Landscape_Nov_2015-_UNITAID_WHO.pdf>.

# 20 Point-of-care testing for hepatitis

*Nitika Pant Pai, Paul Baum and Robert Luo*

**Summary**

In this chapter, we provide an overview of the burden of the global silent epidemics of hepatitis C and hepatitis B infections, quantifying the problem by region, and reviewing risk factors and modes of transmission. We provide a macro- and micro-perspective of their pathophysiology to understand the development of diagnostics better and to appreciate the distinction between screening and staging of hepatitis infections. Point-of-care (POC) diagnostic methods for hepatitis B and hepatitis C are then reviewed. Point-of-care testing (POCT), if effectively combined with improved combination treatment regimens, can potentially herald a turning point in the epidemic history of both these infections.

## INTRODUCTION, RISK FACTORS AND TRANSMISSION

Hepatitis B and C are diseases of the liver and are caused by viruses. Hepatitis B virus belongs to the Hepadnavirus family and hepatitis C virus belongs to the Hepacivirus family. Hepatitis B virus (HBV DNA) is more infectious than HIV; it is spread through contact with blood and infectious body fluids, while hepatitis C virus (HCV RNA) is primarily blood borne.

Hepatitis B and C viruses cause hepatitis B and C infections, respectively. Both infections present in two phases: an acute infection phase and a chronic infection phase. In the acute infection phase, non-specific symptoms dominate; therefore these infections remain undiagnosed for long periods of time. Long-term sequelae for both infections include cirrhosis, liver failure and end-stage liver disease. Most adults (95%) who are exposed to the hepatitis B virus clear the infection spontaneously while only ~5% go on to develop chronic disease (PHAC 2014). In contrast, ~15–25% of individuals infected with hepatitis C clear the infection spontaneously, but a vast majority (75–85%) may develop chronic hepatitis C infection (PHAC 2015).

Hepatitis B and C infections also share common risk factors for transmission. These include: (i) injection drug use; (ii) high-risk sexual activities (e.g. unprotected sex, multiple sexual partners); (iii) being born in regions where HBV/HCV is endemic; (iv) exposure to contaminated blood/blood products, medical or dental devices; (v) sharing of personal articles with an infected person; (vi) exposure in the workplace by infected needles or sharp equipment; (vii) tattooing, body piercing or acupuncture when unsterile equipment or techniques are used; and (viii) organ donation (PHAC 2014, 2015). Burden of hepatitis B is a huge concern in pregnant women who do not get screened in time for it. Screening women in the first trimester for hepatitis B, and linking them to treatment pathways, is a natural step towards prevention of transmission of hepatitis B in their infants. Hepatitis C infection is majorly associated with unsafe injection practices, unsafe blood transfusions and unscreened donor transplants (WHO 2014).

According to the World Health Organization (WHO), ~39 countries do not routinely screen for blood-borne viruses (WHO 2014). For example, in Egypt, unsafe injection practices account for a majority of the HCV burden; while in Asia, 50% of 12 billion injections administered annually are unsafe and carry a substantial risk of hepatitis transmission (WHO 2014).

## DISEASE BURDEN, PREVALENCE AND INCIDENCE

Hepatitis C and B infections together constitute a substantial disease burden exceeding the burden contributed by HIV/AIDS (33 million) and other sexually transmitted and blood-borne infections (137 million) (Pai and Daher 2015). Worldwide, the combined total burden of hepatitis C and hepatitis B infection is estimated to be ~550 million, of which 350 million individuals are living with hepatitis B (Pai and Daher 2015) and ~185 million are living with hepatitis C infection (WHO 2014). Both infections are asymptomatic and prone to misdiagnosis, and there is delayed presentation of patients in care; as a consequence, their true burden remains underestimated. About 350 000 people die from HCV infection each year (WHO 2014), while approximately 1 million die from HBV infection each year (Khuroo *et al.* 2014).

Globally, the prevalence of hepatitis C infection varies across regions. The burden of disease remains highest in Asia (Central, East Asia, South Asia and the Asia Pacific) with 115 million infections (WHO 2014). Europe and the African subcontinent account for 20 million and North Africa/Middle East for 19 million infections, respectively. In North America, the burden of disease is estimated to be 4.4 million (WHO 2014). In the USA, an estimated 2.7 million people are currently living with chronic hepatitis C infection. A further 30 000 individuals are living with undiagnosed hepatitis C infection (CDC 2015a).

Hepatitis C often is accompanied by co-infections. Globally, an estimated 5 million people are living with HIV/HCV co-infections (WHO 2014). PHAC estimates that, while ~33% of HIV infected adults are co-infected with HCV (PHAC 2015), in contrast only ~5% are co-infected with hepatitis B. About 25% of HCV infected persons are estimated to be co-infected with HBV (WHO 2014). Co-infections carry a substantial burden; hence, focussed efforts to screen, treat and vaccinate populations can help bring down the disease burden.

Acute hepatitis C and B infections are less well documented. Further, the acute infectious phase lasts for only a brief period and patients typically do not show up in health-care facilities to seek care and get tested in time. As with any disease, early and timely action that includes early screening, vaccination and prophylaxis for hepatitis B, and timely treatment for hepatitis C, is the key to controlling both these infections. Hepatitis B is a vaccine-preventable disease. In the USA, a 1991 plan for elimination of hepatitis B with vaccinations in children has brought down the total number of infections by ~82% (CDC 2015b). This is a promising statistic that demonstrates that a good plan can generate meaningful results.

## SIGNIFICANCE: GLOBAL AND LOCAL

Hepatitis C infection is more of a concern today more than ever before. Fortunately, there is an ever-increasing repertoire of medications that can cure HCV and an impressive array of emerging diagnostic technologies that can detect HCV quite accurately in minutes–hours. Patients do not have to wait for months to get an HCV diagnosis. Although vaccines are not available for hepatitis C, newer direct acting antiviral (DAA) treatments are very effective. Therefore, the global enthusiasm to control this infection has never been so strongly felt. This is not entirely surprising. For once in history, we stand at the threshold of making a dent in the trajectory of the epidemic (chronic hepatitis C infection) in high-income settings.

The current need is to take an informed timely action – this entails screening the undiagnosed, staging preliminary positives, treating the confirmed and retaining them in care to cure. We also need to educate them about the possibility of re-infection.

Timely screening, staging and actionable treatment plans will, in many instances, cure many infections. This scenario is a reality for the high-income settings. However, DAA therapies that are available in North America and Europe remain unaffordable to many low- and middle-income (LMIC) settings. And, sadly, a bulk of the infection resides in marginalised populations – in LMIC settings of Asia and Africa – where people traditionally lack access to care and receive sub-optimal health-care services (WHO 2014).

In many LMIC settings, even though initial screening tests are accurate and moderately priced (US$5–10), the cost of algorithms needed to confirm, stage, treat and monitor hepatitis C and B infections remains very high (US$30–40 and above). These expenses involved in controlling a chronic infection can deter many from seeking treatment. In future, it is hoped that a combination of hepatitis C antibody and relatively inexpensive hepatitis C core antigen screening tests that screen and confirm chronic infection will be more cost effective (Cohn *et al.* 2015).

The available diagnostics and treatment package for hepatitis C is expensive even for US and Canadian populations – US$171–360 (Cohn *et al.* 2015). This package is an exorbitant one for Asian, East European and African populations that carry the bulk of the disease burden. A high cost of medicines, the need for universal screening and regular monitoring, the need for expensive confirmatory nucleic acid tests, and health facilities with trained hepatologists and infectious disease specialists will increase the cost of treatment substantially (Cohn *et al.* 2015). Perhaps, in future, primary care practitioners will step in to improve disease management.

In conclusion, in addition to prevention, screening and treatment guidelines, we will also need subsidised POC screening tests, and treatment plans for all at risk populations. These plans will make an affordable screen, treat and retain strategy for hepatitis C and B patients a reality (Cohn *et al.* 2015).

## PATHOPHYSIOLOGY

The term hepatitis refers to inflammation of the liver. This can be due to many causes, including infection, alcohol and other toxins, medication side effects and autoimmune and genetic disorders (reviewed in Pratt and Kaplan 2000). Severe cases of hepatitis can lead to death through acute liver failure, chronic liver scarring (cirrhosis) or liver cancer (hepatocellular carcinoma).

Viruses are major causes of hepatitis. The five most common liver-specific (hepatocyte-tropic) viruses are listed in Table 20.1.

Hepatitis B and C are the primary focus for POC diagnostic testing, because they are common infections that

**Table 20.1.** Overview of the major hepatitis viruses

| Virus | Type | Epidemiology | Syndrome | Treatment | Prevention tools |
|---|---|---|---|---|---|
| Hepatitis A | DNA | Faecal-oral transmission through food or sex | Acute hepatitis | Supportive | Vaccine; immunoglobulin |
| Hepatitis B | DNA | Childhood, blood-borne or sexual transmission | Acute hepatitis; asymptomatic carriage; chronic hepatitis, cirrhosis, hepatocellular carcinoma | Rarely curative; drugs include: interferon, ribavirin, reverse transcriptase inhibitors | Vaccine; immunoglobulin |
| Hepatitis C | RNA | Blood-borne transmission | Spontaneous clearance; asymptomatic carriage; chronic hepatitis, cirrhosis, hepatocellular carcinoma | Usually curative; drugs include: interferon, ribavirin, multiple classes of direct acting agents (DAAs) | None |
| Hepatitis D | DNA | A defective virus that can accompany HBV | Exacerbation of HBV infection | Hepatitis B treatment | Hepatitis B vaccine |
| Hepatitis E | RNA | Contaminated water | Usually self-limited but may cause severe hepatitis in immunocompromised patients | Supportive | None |

**Table 20.2.** Interpretation of hepatitis B serologic tests

| HBsAg surface antigen | Anti-HBs surface antibody | Anti-HBc core antibody | Interpretation |
|---|---|---|---|
| – | – | – | Susceptible to future infection |
| – | + | + | Immune due to previous natural infection |
| – | + | – | Immune due to immunisation |
| + | – | + | Hepatitis B infected |
| – | – | + | Four interpretations: resolved infection; false positive anti-HBc; low-level chronic infection; or resolving acute infection ('window period') |

cause significant disability and death, and they are now treatable with specific antiviral drug regimens.

## HEPATITIS B PATHOGENESIS

Hepatitis B virus may cause acute hepatitis followed by clearance, or it may cause chronic infection. Chronic infection is more likely to result if the hepatitis B infection occurs during childhood, as is common in East Asia. The virus itself does not cause hepatocyte damage (cytopathic effect), but in some patients the body's immune response to the virus can cause chronic inflammation, eventually leading to fibrosis (cirrhosis) and a loss of liver function. The virus can also lead to hepatocellular carcinoma, and is the major cause of liver cancer worldwide.

A surface-antigen-based vaccine can prevent hepatitis B infection. Hepatitis B can also be treated with interferon, ribavirin and reverse transcriptase inhibitors (WHO 2015). Chronic hepatitis B infection is difficult to eradicate because the virus can be stored in hepatocytes as covalently closed circular DNA (cccDNA), forming a latent reservoir. The goals of treatment are to suppress inflammation and improve immune control of the virus. This can be assessed through seroconversion of viral e antigen to anti-e antibody or, rarely but more significantly, surface antigen to anti-surface antibody. The interpretation of hepatitis B serologic tests is detailed in Table 20.2.

In patients who are hepatitis B infected (HBsAg+), further testing can be performed. The presence of IgM antibodies against HBc indicates acute infection. Lack of IgM antibodies against HBc indicates chronic infection. The presence of e antigen (HBeAg) indicates high levels of viral replication and high infectivity. The loss of HBeAg and development of anti-HBe antibodies can be an indication of a partial response to antiviral therapy.

## HEPATITIS C PATHOGENESIS

Hepatitis C virus is typically spread through blood, but its transmission routes are not completely characterised. Hepatitis C infection is spontaneously cleared during the acute infection in 10–20% of patients, but most patients proceed to chronic infection. Although many chronically infected individuals will not experience clinically significant liver injury, a significant proportion will progress to cirrhosis if untreated. There has been a revolution in the ability to cure hepatitis C, due to new direct acting antiviral drugs that have been developed (Kohli *et al.* 2014). The hepatitis C virus has six genotypes, and certain therapies are only indicated for certain genotypes. One factor underlying the success of treatment is that, unlike hepatitis B, there is no reservoir for the virus, so if replication can be completely suppressed the virus can be fully eradicated.

Despite the fact that hepatitis viruses are infecting the liver, viral nucleic acids and protein antigens are abundantly detectable in the blood, forming the basis for monitoring assays (including those by POCT) (Table 20.3).

## CURRENT HEPATITIS B POCT METHODS

Current POCT options for HBV focus on the diagnosis of chronically infected individuals from blood samples. HBV diagnostic algorithms rely on the detection of hepatitis B surface antigen (HBsAg), hepatitis B surface antibody (anti-HBs), and hepatitis B core antibody (anti-HBc) (CDC 2005; WHO 2015). Hepatitis B e antigen (HBeAg) is also used as a marker for active HBV replication and infectivity. Rapid immunoassays use antigens and/or antibodies to detect one or more of these biomarkers, typically through a colourimetric indicator that is visible to the test user. Although HBV DNA viral load testing is recommended for treatment initiation and monitoring,

Table 20.3. Use of HCV viral load monitoring in HCV seropositive patients

| Timing | Interpretation |
|---|---|
| Baseline before treatment | If negative, patient has spontaneously cleared virus and does not need treatment; patients with detectable viral loads are chronically infected. Viral load can predict likelihood of response to therapy. |
| 4 weeks into treatment | Rapid virological response (RVR), an indication of whether therapy is working |
| Typically 12 or 24 weeks after treatment is completed | Sustained virological response (SVR) or cure |

no POCT methods are currently available and molecular testing must be done in sophisticated centralised laboratories. This section will review the literature on currently available HBV POCT diagnostic methods.

The majority of POCT for HBV detect HBsAg by rapid immunoassay. Although the Determine™ test (Alere, Waltham, MA) is one of the most popular tests worldwide, many other manufacturers have developed HBsAg tests, including: Acon Laboratories, San Diego CA, USA; Asan Pharmaceutical, Seoul, South Korea; Atlas Medical, Cambridge, UK (One Check, Accurate, and Atlas tests); Blue Cross, Beijing, China; Cortez Diagnostics, Calabasas CA, USA; Cypress Diagnostics, Langdorp, Belgium; Daewoong Biotech, Daejeon, South Korea; Diagnostics for the Real World, Cambridge, UK; Fujirebio, Tokyo, Japan (Serodia test); Geseeschaft fur Diagnostika mbH, Gottingen, Germany (DIMA test); Green Cross, Yongin, South Korea (Genedia test); Human Diagnostics Worldwide, Wiesbaden, Germany (Hexagon test); Hybritech (San Diego CA, USA); Intec Products (Xiamen, China); Inverness Medical, Waltham MA, USA (Dainascreen test); J. Mitra & Co, New Delhi, India (Hepacard test); Orchid Biomedical Systems, Goa, India (Virucheck); Trinity Biotech, Bray, Ireland (Uni-Gold) and Standard Diagnostics, Daejeon, South Korea (SD Bioline) (Shivkumar *et al.* 2012b). Table 20.4 summarises the specifications of selected HBV (and HCV) POC tests.

The Determine test is a lateral flow immunoassay for the detection of HBsAg in serum, plasma or whole blood that is simple to perform and provides results in 15 min. Multiple studies have evaluated its performance in countries around the world, primarily in Asia, Africa and Latin America (Bottero *et al.* 2013; Davies *et al.* 2010; Franzeck *et al.* 2013; Lien *et al.* 2000; Lin *et al.* 2008; Randrianirina *et al.* 2008). These studies have demonstrated a sensitivity between 92.7% and 99.6% and specificity between 96.0% and 100%, when compared with reference enzyme immunoassays. Two panel-based studies comparing the performance of different HBsAg tests, including the Determine test, were also done by the WHO and the International Consortium for Blood Safety, demonstrating 99.0% and 97.6% sensitivity, respectively, and 99.4% and 99.8% sensitivity, respectively (ICBS 2007; WHO 2001). A meta-analysis reviewing the Determine test calculated a pooled sensitivity of 96.7% (95% CI: 95.3–97.7%) and pooled specificity of 99.7% (95% CI: 98.6–99.9%) across all published studies (Khuroo *et al.* 2014).

Compared with the high sensitivity and specificity of the Determine test, results from evaluations of other HBV POCT devices have been quite varied. Some tests have shown sensitivities of <60%, although the specificity of all tests was still >95% (Chameera *et al.* 2013; Khan *et al.* 2010; Torane and Shastri 2008). Overall, however, HBsAg tests have performed quite well in published evaluations. One systemic review of the literature examining studies of over 15 different tests showed a pooled sensitivity of 94.7% (95% CI: 93.7–95.6%) and pooled specificity of 99.4% (95% CI: 99.2–99.6%) (Shivkumar *et al.* 2012b). Because testing programs have been shown to vary widely, HBV programs should research the performance of any tests they are considering using as well as conduct their own evaluation of a new test whenever possible.

Certain manufacturers also produce anti-HBs and HBeAg tests, including Alere, Asan, Daewoong Biotech, Green Cross and Standard Diagnostics. Use of these tests is less common, and fewer evaluations have been conducted and published on them. However, the available literature suggests that anti-HBs performance is typically not as robust as HBsAg tests, particularly with regards to specificity. For anti-HBs tests, reported sensitivities have ranged between 85 and 96%, with specificities between 74 and 100% (Cha *et al.* 2006; Oh *et al.* 1999; Whang and Um 2005). The pooled sensitivity and specificity of these tests were 92.7% (95% CI: 89.7–95.0%) and only 87.4% (95% CI: 83.5–90.7%), respectively (Shivkumar *et al.* 2012b). For the Binax NOW (Binax, Scarborough ME, USA)

**Table 20.4.** Specifications of selected HBV and HCV POC tests (Source: Table prepared by Nadia Lapczak)

| Infection | Test name | Manufacturer | Target | Sample type | Sample volume | Time to result (minutes) |
|---|---|---|---|---|---|---|
| Hepatitis B | Determine | Alere, Waltham, MA, USA | Hepatitis B Surface antigen | Serum, plasma, whole blood | 50 µL | 15 |
| Hepatitis B | SD Bioline HBsAg | Standard Diagnostics, Daejon, South Korea | Hepatitis B Surface antigen | Serum, plasma, whole blood | 100 µL | 20 |
| Hepatitis B | Uni-Gold HBsAg | Trinity Biotech plc, Bray, Ireland | Hepatitis B Surface antigen | Serum, plasma, whole blood | 100 µL | 15 |
| Hepatitis C | Bioeasy HCV Rapid Test | Bioeasy Diagnostica Ltda, Belo Horizonte, Minas Gerais, Brazil | Hepatitis C antibodies | Serum, plasma, whole blood | 10 µL | 5–20 |
| Hepatitis C | Genedia HCV Rapid LF | Green Cross Life Science Corp., Chungbuk, South Korea | Hepatitis C antibodies | Serum, plasma, whole blood | 20 µL | 20–30 |
| Hepatitis C | Hexagon HCV | Human Diagnostics Worldwide, Wiesbaden, Germany | Hepatitis C antibodies | Serum, plasma, whole blood | 10 µL | 5–20 |
| Hepatitis C | OraQuick HCV Rapid Antibody Test | OraSure Technologies, Bethlehem PA, USA | Hepatitis C antibodies | Serum, plasma, whole blood, oral fluids | 1 drop | 20–40 |
| Hepatitis C | SD Bioline HCV | Standard Diagnostics Inc., Yongin-si, Kyonggi-do, South Korea | Hepatitis C antibodies | Serum, plasma, whole blood | 10 µL | 5–20 |

combined HBsAg/HBeAg test, sensitivities ranged between 93.8% and 99.8% and specificities were between 98.4% and 100%, for a pooled sensitivity of 97.9% (95% CI: 95.4–99.7%) and pooled specificity of 99.7% (95% CI: 97.8–100%) (Khuroo *et al.* 2014).

In addition to sensitivity and specificity, several studies also used panels of known HBsAg concentration to examine the analytical sensitivity of tests. Despite claimed limit of detections of ~0.5 IU/mL in many package inserts, 19 tests that were evaluated could not detect samples with concentrations <4 IU/mL (ICBS 2007; Lin *et al.* 2008). Furthermore, 17 of these tests displayed variable analytical sensitivity for different HBV mutants. These tests should be used with caution in patients who may already be on antiviral therapy, in patients who are recovering from acute HBV infection, and in populations with a low prevalence of HBV.

Finally, when studies of the Determine HBV POC test in developing countries were compared with those in developed countries, no significant differences in sensitivity or specificity were seen, demonstrating the ability of the test to perform well across all different settings (Khuroo *et al.* 2014). For example, a study in Tanzania in HIV-infected patients demonstrated high sensitivity and specificity of the Determine test compared with a reference laboratory immunoassay. Not only was a high prevalence of HBV co-infection identified, but the diagnosis of hepatitis B also enabled clinicians to optimise antiviral therapy to treat both HIV and HBV, whenever possible (Franzeck *et al.* 2013). Notably however, other HBV POCT have shown variability between developed and developing country settings, highlighting the importance of using tests that have been validated in the settings where they will be implemented (Khuroo *et al.* 2014).

In summary, HBV POCT benefits from several rapid serologic tests that are inexpensive, accurate and easy to use. Although not all tests perform similarly, the majority of tests have high sensitivity and specificity. HBV POCT has been successfully deployed in both developed and developing countries, and can be found in a variety of different settings, including in clinical care for the diagnosis of acute and chronic HBV infections, for screening of blood donors and blood products before blood transfusion, and in epidemiologic and surveillance research.

## CURRENT HEPATITIS C POCT METHODS

The most common HCV POCT methods are rapid immunoassays, which cover the first step of recommended diagnostic algorithms for HCV: detection of anti-HCV antibody (CDC 2015c; WHO 2014). Although these tests cannot distinguish between HCV exposure and chronic infection, they are typically inexpensive, easy to use and do not require advanced laboratory equipment or skills. Sample types for these tests include whole blood, serum, plasma and, more recently, oral fluid. The following section will examine the reported performance of anti-HCV tests.

Several manufacturers produce rapid anti-HCV tests, including: Acon San Diego CA, USA; Axiom, Bierstadt, Germany; Bhat Biotech, Bangalore, India (Hepa-Scan HCV Card); Bioeasy (Belo Horizonte, Brazil); Bionike, San Francisco, CA (Advanced Quality One Step HCV Test); Chembio Diagnostic Systems, Medford NY, USA (Dual Path Platform test); CORE (Birmingham, UK); FirstVue, Woodbury NY, USA (AT First Diagnostics); Fuji Rebio, Tokyo, Japan (Serodia HCV); Green Cross, Yongin, South Korea (Genedia HCV Rapid LF); Human Diagnostics Worldwide, Wiesbaden, Germany (Hexagon HCV); Inverness Medical Innovations, Waltham MA, USA (ImmunoComb); J. Mitra, New Delhi, India (HCV Bi-Dot, HCV Tri-Dot); MedMira, Halifax, Nova Scotia, Canada (Multiplo Rapid HIV/HCV Antibody Test); MP Biomedical, Burlingame CA, USA (Assure HCV Rapid Test, HCV Spot); OraSure Technologies, Bethlehem PA, USA (OraQuick HCV Rapid Antibody Test); SEROMed, Pollenfeld, Germany (SM-HCV Rapid Test); Standard Diagnostics, Yongin, South Korea (SD Bioline HCV); Tema Ricerca, Bologna, Italy (Anti-HCV Ab rapid test) and Trinity Biotech, Bray, Ireland (SeroCard HCV) (Khuroo *et al.* 2015; Shivkumar *et al.* 2012a). Specifications of some of these anti-HCV POC tests are shown in Table 20.4.

The largest number of studies on HCV POCT has been done on tests using serum. A meta-analysis of the literature calculated a pooled sensitivity of 96.5% (95% CI: 93.9–98.0%) and pooled specificity of 99.0% (98.4–99.4%) compared with reference immunoassay (Khuroo *et al.* 2015). Although most tests performed quite well, there were a few outliers with sensitivities below 90%, and as low as 22% for the HCV Spot test (Nyirenda *et al.* 2008; Smith *et al.* 2011). Additionally, false-positive results have been seen in HIV co-infected patients, and false-negatives may be possible as well, due to alterations of the immune response (Smith *et al.* 2011; Soriano *et al.* 2010). Less is known about the role of other co-infections, and the effect of different genotypes on test performance has also not been well characterised.

With regards to other sample types, no significant differences have been found between the pooled performances of tests using serum, and those using whole blood, plasma or oral fluid (Khuroo *et al.* 2015; Shivkumar *et al.* 2012b). Although not statistically significant, oral fluid did have the lowest point estimates for pooled sensitivity in meta-analyses compared with other sample types; this may be due to: dilution of sample in collection buffer, as opposed to direct application of blood, serum or plasma onto the test; antibody binding differences in oral fluid versus whole blood; or a lower concentration of anti-HCV antibodies in oral fluid compared with blood. Oral fluid tests enable non-invasive testing, which can help improve access to, and acceptability of, HCV screening. One oral fluid test, OraQuick, has shown superior sensitivity to other oral fluid tests, with a pooled specificity of 95.9% (95% CI: 92.1–97.9%) and pooled specificity of 99.4% (95% CI: 98.1–99.8%). This test was also the only test in eight different studies to identify acute HCV at the same time as a reference immunoassay in seroconversion panel studies, while other tests lagged behind by a few days to a few weeks (Khuroo *et al.* 2015).

With the availability of new direct-acting antivirals, there has been a renewed emphasis on HCV screening and treatment. However, anti-HCV POCT cannot identify which patients need treatment. HCV RNA testing is

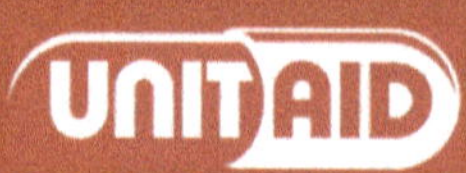


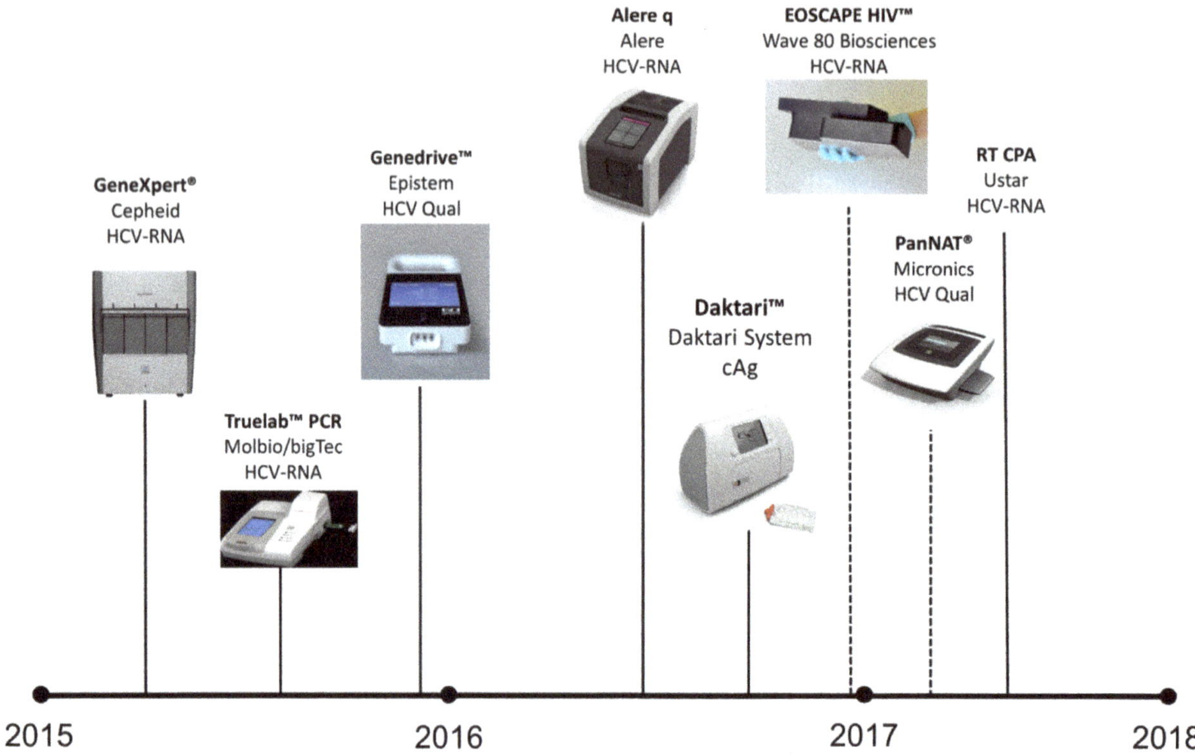


**Fig. 20.1.** Hepatitis C POCT technology 'in the diagnostic pipeline'. (Source: Reprinted with permission from UNITAID 2015; ©World Health Organization)

recommended for all patients with positive anti-HCV results, but currently this test requires a molecular testing laboratory with trained personnel (CDC 2015c; WHO 2014). Companies such as Alere (Waltham MA, USA), Cepheid (Sunnyvale CA, USA), Epistem (Manchester, UK), Molbio (Goa, India) and UStar (Hangzhou, China) are currently working on molecular POCT for HCV RNA testing (UNITAID 2015). Alternatively, hepatitis C core antigen is also being explored as a marker of chronic HCV infection, and companies such as Daktari (Cambridge MA, USA) are looking to make such a POC test. However, core antigen is not currently recommended in HCV diagnosis guidelines. Finally, dried blood spots have been examined as an alternative to POCT. Although they enable simple sample collection and transport of samples to a centralised laboratory, they still require further validation and lack the rapidity and ease of use benefits seen with POCT (Greenman *et al.* 2015).

In summary, HCV POCT can be conducted using rapid anti-HCV tests with high levels of sensitivity and specificity, even in non-invasive samples such as oral fluid. Similar to HBV, some tests have shown quite poor performance in evaluations, and caution should be observed whenever implementing a new test. More research is needed on the impact of co-infections, particularly HIV co-infection, and across geographic settings to evaluate the performance of the tests across different HCV genotypes. New tests in the pipeline also have the potential to enable both diagnosis and treatment of HCV through POCT (UNITAID 2015) (Fig. 20.1). Molecular POCT platforms can enable confirmation of chronic HCV infection, as well as treatment monitoring through quantitative HCV RNA viral load testing. Such platforms may eventually be used for HBV treatment monitoring as well if further tests are developed.

## IMPLEMENTATION OF HEPATITIS POCT

Several recent studies have reported the successful implementation of hepatitis POCT for identifying new cases. For example, the introduction of HBV POCT has increased testing uptake in difficult to reach populations, such as rural villages in Guatemala and undocumented immigrants in Italy (El-Hamad *et al.* 2015; Smith *et al.* 2015). Testing not only improved linkage to clinical care, but also enabled identification of HBV-negative patients eligible for HBV vaccination. Similarly for HCV, numerous studies around the world have shown willingness to use and uptake of rapid POCT in a diversity of settings, including correctional facilities, urban health clinics and other high-risk locations (Beckwith *et al.* 2016; Jewett *et al.* 2013; Parisi *et al.* 2014; Sharma *et al.* 2015). Notably, POCT implementation was seen as useful when test performance was poor, highlighting the importance of using high-quality POCT (Kant *et al.* 2013).

POCT has also been used to screen for HBV, HCV, and other infectious diseases in blood donors and blood products in resource limited settings where centralised laboratory testing is not available. Although some studies showed good performance with POCT, many showed sensitivities far below those claimed in package inserts, particularly for HBV (Pruett *et al.* 2015). Therefore, testing should be conducted only with tests with validated performance and in conjunction with rigorous quality control systems and risk-based donor screening wherever possible. The WHO has been working with many countries on developing blood-screening guidelines and national policies, including appropriate use of rapid POCT in emergency settings or health-care settings without access to a centralised blood-screening laboratory (WHO 2010).

The cost effectiveness of hepatitis POCT has been examined in one study comparing the use of the OraQuick test on whole blood with laboratory-based anti-HCV tests in the USA, followed by HCV RNA testing for all positive results. Both POCT and laboratory-based anti-HCV screening were found to be cost-effective, although OraQuick was actually less expensive overall, primarily driven by its low rate of false positives, resulting in fewer unnecessary HCV RNA tests (Chapko *et al.* 2015). More research is needed on the cost-effectiveness of POCT for both hepatitis B and C, particularly on other sample types such as oral fluid, in settings outside the USA and using other tests.

Overall, POCT for hepatitis has shown excellent performance compared with reference laboratory tests. These tests are not sufficient to complete the entire diagnostic algorithm for HBV and HCV, but they do provide a simple, rapid and cost-effective way to screen patients, especially in populations without ready access to centralised laboratory testing. Furthermore, the real-world performance of tests may differ significantly from the package insert. Similar to any laboratory test, new POC tests should be validated and monitored through relevant quality management systems. Additional tests are also in development, including molecular POCT, which can enable confirmation of chronic infection and treatment monitoring. As POCT continues to expand worldwide, additional research will provide further lessons about test performance and implementation. POCT will also enable testing programs to reach more patients, contributing to global efforts towards controlling the HBV and HCV epidemics.

## CASE PRESENTATION – A LOOK TO THE FUTURE

A 54-year-old man attends his family medical clinic for a check-up. He has hypertension but no other medical problems. Because he experimented with intravenous drugs while in college, he is screened for hepatitis C with a POC antibody test. He is hepatitis C seropositive, which means that he was exposed to hepatitis C infection. He is then tested with a POC hepatitis C nucleic acid test to determine whether he is among the 10% of patients who spontaneously clear HCV and do not need treatment. The nucleic acid test detects hepatitis C RNA in the patient's blood, so he is offered treatment for hepatitis C. The patient embarks on a 12-week treatment program. His HCV viral load is tested after 4 weeks of treatment and it is below the limit of detection of the test, so he continues the remaining 8 weeks of the program. He is tested 12 weeks after finishing the treatment and still has no detectable HCV viral load, so he is deemed cured.

In this example, the initial POCT reduced the risk that the patient would not be followed up, because he learned he needed treatment at the same clinic visit. The POC monitoring during his treatment eliminated the problems of communicating and following up on laboratory results, and the immediate availability of the results was gratifying for the patient and the physician.

## REFERENCES


Beckwith CG, Kurth AE, Bazerman LB, Patry EJ, Cates A, Tran L, *et al.* (2016) A pilot study of rapid hepatitis C virus testing in the Rhode Island Department of Corrections. *Journal of Public Health* **38**, 130–137. doi:10.1093/pubmed/fdv023

Bottero J, Boyd A, Gozlan J, Lemoine M, Carrat F, Collignon A, *et al.* (2013) Performance of rapid tests for detection of HBsAg and anti-HBsAb in a large cohort, France. *Journal of Hepatology* **58**, 473–478. doi:10.1016/j.jhep.2012.11.016

CDC (Centers for Disease Control and Prevention) (2005) A comprehensive immunization strategy to eliminate transmission of hepatitis B virus infection in the United States: recommendations of the Advisory Committee on Immunization Practices. Part I: immunization of infants, children, and adolescents. Centers for Disease Control and Prevention. *MMWR Morbidity and Mortality Weekly Report* **54**, 1–31.

CDC (2015a) *Viral Hepatitis – Hepatitis C Information.* Centers for Disease Control and Prevention, US Department of Health & Human Services, Atlanta GA, USA, <http://www.cdc.gov/hepatitis/hcv/>.

CDC (2015b) *Viral Hepatitis – Hepatitis B Information.* Centers for Disease Control and Prevention, US Department of Health & Human Services. Atlanta GA, USA, <http://www.cdc.gov/hepatitis/hbv/>.

CDC (2015c) *Testing Recommendations for Hepatitis C Virus Infection.* Centers for Disease Control and Prevention. CDC, Atlanta GA, USA, <http://www.cdc.gov/hepatitis/hcv/guidelinesc.htm>.

Cha YJ, Yang JS, Chae SL (2006) Evaluation of indigenously manufactured immunochromatographic assay systems for rapid detection of hepatitis B surface antigen and antibody. *The Korean Journal of Laboratory Medicine* **26**, 52–57. doi:10.3343/kjlm.2006.26.1.52

Chameera EWS, Noordeen F, Pandithasundara H, Abeykoon AMSB (2013) Diagnostic efficacy of rapid assays used for the detection of hepatitis B virus surface antigen. *Sri Lankan Journal of Infectious Diseases* **3**, 21–27. doi:10.4038/sljid.v3i2.5172

Chapko MK, Dufour DR, Hatia RI, Drobeniuc J, Ward JW, Teo CG (2015) Cost-effectiveness of strategies for testing current hepatitis C virus infection. *Hepatology (Baltimore, Md.)* **62**, 1396–1404. doi:10.1002/hep.27966

Cohn J, Roberts T, Amorosa V, Lemoine M, Hill A (2015) Simplified diagnostic monitoring for hepatitis C, in the new era of direct-acting antiviral treatment. *Current Opinion in HIV and AIDS* **10**, 369–373. doi:10.1097/COH.0000000000000180

Davies J, van Oosterhout JJ, Nyirenda M, Bowden J, Moore E, Hart IJ, *et al.* (2010) Reliability of rapid testing for hepatitis B in a region of high HIV endemicity. *Transactions of the Royal Society of Tropical Medicine and Hygiene* **104**, 162–164. doi:10.1016/j.trstmh.2009.10.010

El-Hamad I, Pezzoli MC, Chiari E, Scarcella C, Vassallo F, Puoti M, *et al.* (2015) Point-of-care screening, prevalence, and risk factors for hepatitis B infection among 3,728 mainly undocumented migrants from non-EU countries in northern Italy. *Journal of Travel Medicine* **22**, 78–86. doi:10.1111/jtm.12176

Franzeck FC, Ngwale R, Msongole B, Hamisi M, Abdul O, Henning L, *et al.* (2013) Viral hepatitis and rapid diagnostic test based screening for HBsAg in HIV-infected patients in rural Tanzania. *PLoS One* **8**, e58468. doi:10.1371/journal.pone.0058468

Greenman J, Roberts T, Cohn J, Messac L (2015) Dried blood spots in the genotyping, quantification and storage of HCV RNA: a systematic literature review. *Journal of Viral Hepatitis* **22**, 353–361. doi:10.1111/jvh.12345

ICBS (International Consortium for Blood Safety) (2007) *HBV Test Kit Evaluation Results.* ICBS, New York, USA and ICBS-Europe, Düsseldorf, Germany, <http://www.icbs-web.org/page31.html>.

Jewett A, Al-Tayyib AA, Ginnett L, Smith BD (2013) Successful integration of hepatitis C virus point-of-care tests into the Denver Metro Health Clinic. *AIDS Research and Treatment* **2013**, Article ID 528904. doi:10.1155/2013/528904

Kant J, Möller B, Heyne R, Herber A, Böhm S, Maier M, *et al.* (2013) Evaluation of a rapid on-site anti-HCV test as a screening tool for hepatitis C virus infection. *European Journal of Gastroenterology & Hepatology* **25**, 416–420.

Khan J, Lone D, Hameed A (2010) Evaluation of the performance of two rapid immunochromatographic tests for detection of hepatitis B surface antigen and anti HCV antibodies using ELISA tested samples. *Annals of King Edward Medical University Journal* **16**, 84–87.

Khuroo MS, Khuroo NS, Khuroo MS (2014) Accuracy of rapid point-of-care diagnostic tests for hepatitis B surface antigen – a systematic review and meta-analysis. *Journal of Clinical and Experimental Hepatology* **4**, 226–240. doi:10.1016/j.jceh.2014.07.008

Khuroo MS, Khuroo NS, Khuroo MS (2015) Diagnostic accuracy of point-of-care tests for hepatitis C virus infection: a systematic review and meta-analysis. *PLoS One* **10**, e0121450. doi:10.1371/journal.pone.0121450

Kohli A, Shaffer A, Sherman A, Kottilil S (2014) Treatment of Hepatitis C: a systematic review. *Journal of the American Medical Association* **312**, 631–640. doi:10.1001/jama.2014.7085

Lien TX, Tien NTK, Chanpong GF, Cuc CT, Yen VT, Soderquist R, *et al.* (2000) Evaluation of rapid diagnostic tests for the detection of human immunodeficiency virus types 1 and 2, hepatitis B surface antigen, and syphilis in Ho Chi Minh City, Vietnam. *The American Journal of Tropical Medicine and Hygiene* **62**, 301–309.

Lin YH, Wang Y, Loua A, Day GJ, Qiu Y, Nadala EC, Jr, *et al.* (2008) Evaluation of a new hepatitis B virus surface antigen rapid test with improved sensitivity. *Journal of Clinical Microbiology* **46**, 3319–3324. doi:10.1128/JCM.00498-08

Nyirenda M, Beadsworth MB, Stephany P, Hart CA, Hart IJ, Munthali C, *et al.* (2008) Prevalence of infection with hepatitis B and C virus and coinfection with HIV in medical inpatients in Malawi. *The Journal of Infection* **57**, 72–77. doi:10.1016/j.jinf.2008.05.004

Oh J, Kim TY, Yoon HJ, Min HS, Lee HR, Choi TY (1999) Evaluation of Genedia HBsAg rapid and Genedia anti-HBs rapid for the screening of HBsAg and anti-HBs. *Korean Journal of Clinical Pathology* **19**, 114–117.

Pai NP, Daher J (2015) Multiplexed testing for HIV and related bacterial and viral co-infections at the point-of-care: quo vadis? *Expert Review of Molecular Diagnostics* **15**, 463–469. doi:10.1586/14737159.2015.1021335

Parisi MR, Soldini L, Vidoni G, Mabellini C, Belloni T, Brignolo L, *et al.* (2014) Point-of-care testing for HCV infection: recent advances and implications for alternative screening. *The New Microbiologica* **37**, 449–457.

PHAC (Public Health Agency of Canada) (2014) *Hepatitis B – Get the Facts.* Public Health Agency of Canada, <http://www.phac-aspc.gc.ca/hcai-iamss/bbp-pts/hepatitis/hep_b-eng.php>.

PHAC (2015) *Hepatitis C – Get the Facts.* Public Health Agency of Canada, <http://www.phac-aspc.gc.ca/hepc/pubs/get-facts-informezvous/index-eng.php>.

Pratt DS, Kaplan MM (2000) Evaluation of abnormal liver-enzyme results in asymptomatic patients. *The New England Journal of Medicine* **342**, 1266–1271. doi:10.1056/NEJM200004273421707

Pruett CR, Vermeulen M, Zacharias P, Ingram C, Tayou Tagny C, Bloch EM (2015) The use of rapid diagnostic tests for transfusion infectious screening in Africa: a literature review. *Transfusion Medicine Reviews* **29**, 35–44. doi:10.1016/j.tmrv.2014.09.003

Randrianirina F, Carod JF, Ratsima E, Chretien JB, Richard V, Talarmin A (2008) Evaluation of the performance of four rapid tests for detection of hepatitis B surface antigen in Antananarivo, Madagascar. *Journal of Virological Methods* **151**, 294–297. doi:10.1016/j.jviromet.2008.03.019

Sharma M, Al Kaabi S, John AK, Al Dweik N, Ullah Wani H, Babu Thandassary R, *et al.* (2015) Screening for hepatitis C in average and high-risk populations of Qatar using rapid point-of-care testing. *United European Gastroenterology Journal* **3**, 364–370. doi:10.1177/2050640615580725

Shivkumar S, Peeling R, Jafari Y, Lawrence J, Pai NP (2012a) Accuracy of rapid and point-of-care screening tests for Hepatitis C: a systematic review and meta-analysis. *Annals of Internal Medicine* **157**, 558–566. doi:10.7326/0003-4819-157-8-201210160-00006

Shivkumar S, Peeling R, Jafari Y, Lawrence J, Pai NP (2012b) Rapid point-of-care first-line screening tests for hepatitis B infection: a meta-analysis of diagnostic accuracy (1980–2010). *The American Journal of Gastroenterology* **107**, 1306–1313. doi:10.1038/ajg.2012.141

Smith BD, Drobeniuc J, Jewett A, Branson BM, Garfein RS, Teshale E, *et al.* (2011) Evaluation of three rapid screening assays for detection of antibodies to hepatitis C virus. *The Journal of Infectious Diseases* **204**, 825–831. doi:10.1093/infdis/jir422

Smith A, Sabidó M, Camey E, Batres A, Casabona J (2015) Lessons learned from integrating simultaneous triple point-of-care screening for syphilis, hepatitis B, and HIV in prenatal services through rural outreach teams in Guatemala. *International Journal of Gynaecology and Obstetrics* **130**, S70–S72. doi:10.1016/j.ijgo.2015.04.009

Soriano V, Vispo E, Labarga P, Medrano J, Barreiro P (2010) Viral hepatitis and HIV co-infection. *Antiviral Research* **85**, 303–315. doi:10.1016/j.antiviral.2009.10.021

Torane VP, Shastri JS (2008) Comparison of ELISA and rapid screening tests for the diagnosis of HIV, hepatitis B and hepatitis C among healthy blood donors in a tertiary care hospital in Mumbai. *Indian Journal of Medical Microbiology* **26**, 284–285. doi:10.4103/0255-0857.42071

UNITAID (2015) *Hepatitis C Diagnostics Technology Landscape.* World Health Organization, Geneva, Switzerland, <http://unitaid.org/images/marketdynamics/publications/UNITAID-HCV Diagnostic_Landscape-1st_edition.pdf>.

Whang DH, Um T (2005) Comparison of immunochromatography assays and quantitative immunoassays for detecting HBsAg and anti-HBs. *The Korean Journal of Laboratory Medicine* **25**, 186–191.

WHO (World Health Organization) (2001) *Hepatitis B Surface Antigen Assays: Operational Characteristics (Phase I).* WHO, Geneva, Switzerland, <http://www.who.int/diagnostics_laboratory/evaluations/en/hep_B_rep1.pdf>.

WHO (2010) *Screening Donated Blood for Transfusion-Transmissible Infections: Recommendations.* WHO, Geneva, Switzerland, <http://www.who.int/bloodsafety/ScreeningDonatedBloodforTransfusion.pdf>.

WHO (2014) *Guidelines for the Screening, Care and Treatment of Persons with Hepatitis C Infection.* WHO, Geneva, Switzerland, <http://www.who.int/hiv/pub/hepatitis/hepatitis-c-guidelines/en/>.

WHO (2015) *Guidelines for the Prevention, Care and Treatment of Persons with Chronic Hepatitis B Infection.* WHO, Geneva, Switzerland, <http://apps.who.int/iris/bitstream/10665/154590/ 1/9789241549059_eng.pdf?ua=1>.

# 21 Rapid influenza diagnostic tests: clinical usage and significance

*Caroline Chartrand, Christian Renaud and Nicolas Tremblay*

**Summary**

Influenza is a viral infection of the lower respiratory tract, which can afflict 5–10% of the world's population each year. Rapid influenza diagnostic test (RIDT) kits are widely available and can detect both influenza A and B, although some do not distinguish between the two. These rapid tests have highly variable sensitivity due to a range of factors such as the type of influenza virus, the patient age, the duration of illness and the quality of specimen tested. Nonetheless, they occupy an important place in the diagnostic arsenal for influenza. Rapid portable molecular testing devices for influenza are now appearing on the diagnostic market.

## GLOBAL BURDEN OF INFLUENZA

Influenza is a viral infection that accounts for a large proportion of lower respiratory tract infections (LRTI) worldwide. It affects almost anybody from infants and children to young and older adults. According to the World Health Organization (WHO), 5–10% of the adult population and 20–30% of children will get the flu each year (WHO 2014). Although an influenza infection commonly resolves on its own, it can have tremendous consequences in select 'at-risk' population that develop a severe form of illness resulting in an estimated 1 million deaths each year. As such, influenza is a global health concern regarding human life, medical resources, public health and associated cost.

Influenza spreads during the cold months (December to March) in the northern regions of the globe and year round in the moderate or warmer climate zones. Despite a considerable amount of epidemiological data streaming from local and regional surveillance programs, it remains a challenge, to this day, to predict potential influenza outbreaks, dissemination patterns or prevalence (Bresee and Hayden 2013). Moreover, the 2009 pandemic episode of influenza reminded the world's medical and political community that novel strains of influenza are always ready to start their global dissemination of illness and that all countries should have a plan to manage an overwhelming number of influenza cases. As such, local, regional and global surveillance programs are essential to gather and analyse epidemiological data about seasonal influenza and to inform public health policies on prevention and treatment strategies.

## HEALTH AND ECONOMIC BURDEN OF INFLUENZA IN HIGH-INCOME COUNTRIES

In high-income countries (HIC), influenza surveillance networks are well established and provide valuable information about the health and economic burden of the seasonal flu. In the USA, there are ~100 000 hospitalisations (ranging from 50 000 to 200 000) per year due to laboratory-confirmed influenza (CDC 2015a). A recent retrospective study estimated that direct medical cost attributable to influenza was US$16.3 billion with up to US$87.1 billion of economic strain when indirect costs were factored in the analysis (Molinari *et al.* 2007). In plain terms, this US$87.1 billion represents ~$1 in each $20 spent on medical care in the USA, notwithstanding the enormous amount of over-the-counter medications that are used to alleviate influenza's associated symptoms and that account for an additional US$102 billion annually (Klepser 2014). In Germany, the same kind of analysis showed that almost 82% of the costs were attributable to absenteeism from work because of the illness (Ehlken *et al.* 2015).

## HEALTH AND ECONOMIC BURDEN OF INFLUENZA IN LOW–MIDDLE-INCOME COUNTRIES

In low- or middle-income countries (LMIC), the lack of adequate medical infrastructure (intensive care unit, antiviral drugs, diagnostic and monitoring equipment or vaccination) combines with underlying LMIC comorbidities (e.g. malnutrition and tuberculosis) to result in a disproportionate disease burden from influenza compared with HIC (Fischer *et al.* 2014). Infants and elders from LMIC are more likely to be admitted to hospital for an influenza-like illness, up to 5 to 10-fold for Kenyan children compared with American children. They also have a far worse prognosis than in HIC, with mortality rates rising to almost 50% (Fischer *et al.* 2014; Fuller *et al.* 2013; Katz *et al.* 2014; Kyeyagalire *et al.* 2014; McMorrow *et al.* 2015). On the economic front, a recent meta-analysis of the cost of seasonal influenza in LMIC showed that total cost per capita accounted for 2–8% of their gross domestic product (GDP) compared with 0.04–0.13% of high-income countries' GDP (de Francisco Shapovalova *et al.* 2015). As such, it is clear that seasonal influenza accounts for a significant economic and medical burden in countries that are already plagued by a disproportionate health burden. Although there is no quick fix to this situation, health-care policy makers should reflect on a solution to increase surveillance, prevention and treatment of seasonal influenza.

## PATHOPHYSIOLOGY OF INFLUENZA ILLNESS

Influenza is an enveloped negative-strand RNA virus of the Orthomyxoviridae family. Two types, influenza A and B, cause the majority of human cases. Influenza A is further classified into subtypes based on the hemagglutinin (H) and the neuraminidase (N) glycoproteins present on its membrane, with H1N1 and H3N2 being the most common circulating subtypes. Each subtype encompasses many different strains that are the products of minor antigenic variations, called antigenic drift. Although both influenza A and B are subject to antigenic drift that gives rise to the annual influenza epidemics, only influenza A can cause global pandemics through antigenic shift: a significant change in the hemagglutinin or neuraminidase glycoproteins, producing novel infectious subtypes for which individuals may not have prior immunological protection.

## CLINICAL PRESENTATION

The influenza virus is mainly transmitted from person to person through large-particle respiratory droplets produced by coughing or sneezing. Influenza illness, or flu, typically begins with the sudden onset of fever and constitutional symptoms (such as headache, malaise and myalgia), followed by respiratory tract symptoms such as a sore throat, rhinitis and cough. Although the majority of infected individuals exhibit a self-limited illness, or are even asymptomatic, severe disease and complications can occur, including viral or bacterial pneumonia, ear and sinus infections and exacerbation of underlying medical conditions. Though severe illness can occur even in young, previously healthy individuals, those at greatest risk are the elderly, young children (younger than 5 years old) and individuals with chronic pulmonary, cardiac, renal or hepatic disease or metabolic disorders. Increased severity and medical complications attributable to influenza have also been described among immunosuppressed persons, pregnant women, Indigenous people and the morbidly obese (BMI ≥40).

Unfortunately, respiratory illness caused by influenza is difficult to distinguish on clinical grounds alone from illnesses caused by other respiratory viruses (respiratory syncytial virus, adenovirus, rhinovirus and parainfluenza) or bacterial agents (*Chlamydophila pneumoniae*, *Mycoplasma pneumoniae*, *Streptococcus pneumoniae*, and *Legionella* sp.) that often co-circulate during the same period. For this reason, the physicians often turn to laboratory diagnostics tests when the diagnosis of influenza is likely to impact patient management.

## DIAGNOSTICS OPTIONS

### Conventional cell culture and rapid culture

Isolation and identification of circulating strains are critical to the preparation of annual vaccines. Influenza virus isolation has long been considered the gold standard, but expertise in traditional culture methods is variable and disappearing. Rhesus monkey kidney (RhMK) or Madin-Darby canine kidney (MDCK) cell cultures are examined microscopically for 10–14 days for influenza cytopathic effects and screened by haemadsorption. Influenza virus isolates are identified as type A or B by immunofluorescence. Time to detection ranges from 2 to 14 days, with a median of 3–5 days. Conventional culture may be less affected by genetic and antigenic changes in influenza virus strains, but safety is a concern when influenza virulence is high or unknown. Cell culture relies on infectious viruses and is less sensitive than most reverse-transcription polymerase chain reaction (RT–PCR) tests. RT–PCR does not require infectious virus, is less affected by delays in transport and processing, and also remains positive longer than culture. Rapid cultures have replaced conventional cell cultures in many laboratories because they are simpler and faster to complete. In one report, rapid cultures detected 98.6% of influenza conventional culture positives (Leonardi *et al.* 2010). Samples are centrifuged onto cell monolayers to enhance infectivity, incubated for 1–2 days, then fixed and stained by immunofluorescence with a pool of monoclonal antibodies to seven or eight targeted respiratory viruses, including influenza types A and B.

### Immunofluorescence

Immunofluorescence assays are performed directly on clinical samples and detect viral antigens in exfoliated respiratory epithelial cells applied to microscope slides. They allow assessment of sample quality. These assays gained popularity in clinical virology laboratories in the past decade due to high-quality pooled monoclonal antibodies (Mab) that detect respiratory syncytial virus (RSV), influenza A and B, parainfluenza types 1, 2, 3, and adenovirus in a single cell spot. Samples can be tested on demand, with results available within 2 h and detection rates 85–95% of culture. Use of a cytospin to prepare slides enhances sensitivity and allows accurate identification of as few as one to two virus-positive cells. However, immunofluorescence is a demanding, manual test that requires significant expertise and judgment for accurate interpretation. Thus, its sensitivities and specificities are highly variable between laboratories.

### Nucleic acid detection

RT–PCR is the most common molecular amplification method for RNA viruses used by laboratories. Automated extraction instruments simplify the purification of nucleic acids from clinical samples. Real-time assays combine the amplification and detection steps, shorten assay time, reduce cross-contamination and provide an indicator of viral load. No assay is 100% sensitive, including RT–PCR. Although multiplex assays are more efficient and cost-effective, they may be less sensitive than monoplex RT–PCR assays. Laboratories must be alert to the fact that even small changes in nucleic acid sequences of circulating viruses can affect the sensitivity of molecular methods. Laboratory-developed tests can be more rapidly adapted than commercial kits to accommodate these changes. Falsely negative RT–PCR results have been reported in patients when upper, instead of lower, respiratory tract samples were tested. Because of lower viral loads, false-negative RT–PCR results may be more common in adults than young children, but they can occur at any age.

## TREATMENT AND PREVENTION

Two classes of antiviral drugs are available for treatment: adamantanes (amantadine and rimantadine) and neuraminidase inhibitors (zanamivir, oseltamivir and peramivir).

As of now, the burden of evidence shows that adamantanes are not more effective than a placebo to decrease symptoms length or severity in children and the elderly, suggesting a limited use in an evidence-based medical practice (Alves Galvão *et al.* 2014). While there is a limited correlation between the use of neuraminidase inhibitors and clinical improvement (shortened duration of illness by <1 day), there is no evidence that they are effective in decreasing hospitalisation rate or limiting complications in healthy adults and children (Jefferson *et al.* 2014). As such, they are recommended in patients with severe, complicated or progressive illness or at high-risk for influenza complications (Fiore *et al.* 2011; Harper *et al.* 2009). However, antiviral therapy needs to be started within 24–48 h of onset of symptoms to be effective.

As an error-prone virus, resistance of influenza to direct acting antiviral drugs is an increasing concern and vaccination stands as the best way to prevent influenza. Vaccine efficacy varies each year, depending on how well the vaccine strains match circulating strains. The development of vaccines that could provide broad protection against antigenically variant influenza viruses has long been the ultimate goal, and such vaccines may now be within reach. However, vaccination uptake remains low in the general population, as well as in exposed (healthcare workers) and at-risk populations (Black *et al.* 2015; Lu *et al.* 2015, 2016).

## POINT-OF-CARE TESTING FOR INFLUENZA

Rapid influenza diagnostic tests (RIDTs) emerged on the diagnostic scene in the early 1990s to overcome the shortcomings of the conventional diagnostic modalities for influenza, namely in providing clinicians with an answer to the question 'Does this patient have influenza?' in a clinically relevant timeframe.

### Description of rapid influenza diagnostic tests

RIDTs are usually immunoassays that detect the viral nucleoprotein antigens of influenza A and/or B. These internal structural proteins tend to be highly conserved among the different strains of influenza A and B viruses, making these tests useful regardless of the circulating seasonal strains. They also differ between influenza A and B, allowing distinction between the two. All commercially available RIDTs can detect both influenza A and B, although some do not distinguish between the two. However, there is currently no RIDT that can identify distinct influenza strains, be it pandemic 2009 H1N1 or other new emerging strains (e.g. avian flu).

In general, RIDTs are made of bound or eluted dye-labelled proprietary antibodies, attached to a nitrocellulose strip (presented either as a dipstick, a cassette or a card), that recognise specific influenza nucleoprotein peptides (WHO 2011). They are designed to be used with respiratory secretions collected from the upper respiratory tract of patients with influenza-like illness. Specimen can be obtained either through swabbing of the respiratory passages (nasal, nasopharyngeal or throat swab) or through aspiration of secretions with a sterile suction catheter before (nasal or nasopharyngeal aspirate) or after instillation of several drops of normal saline (nasal or nasopharyngeal washings). Although most tests can be used with more than one type of specimen, acceptable specimens vary from test to test. If influenza nucleoproteins are present in the specimen being tested, the binding of the peptides present in the sample to the anti-influenza antibodies on the test strip will produce a colour change to signal positivity. As per the manufacturer's recommendation, even a slight colour change should be interpreted as positive, adding an element of subjectivity to the interpretation of an otherwise dichotomous (yes/no) test.

To facilitate the analysis of barely positive RIDTs, manufacturers have introduced a new generation of tests that uses a small bench-top reader designed to return a positive or negative result. Although they rely on the same basic principle as their first generation counterparts, they remove the need for a qualitative visual assessment of the test by giving an instrument-based objective digital readout of the results.

Dozens of different RIDTs are currently commercialised throughout the world. Although the amount of hands-on time and the number of required steps vary among the different brands of RIDTs, results can be available within 15 min of sample collection. Most are simple enough to be used by non-laboratory personnel after minimal training and, as such, can be employed in a point-of-care (POC) setting such as physician offices, emergency departments or even at the bedside. In the USA, most RIDTs are given a waiver from the 1988 *Clinical Laboratory Improvement Act* (CLIA), meaning that they are deemed, by the Federal Food and Drug Administration (FDA), simple, safe and accurate enough to be used outside of a formal laboratory setting.

### Accuracy of rapid influenza diagnostic tests

The main drawback of these rapid, simple, POC tests is their limited and highly variable sensitivity. A recent comprehensive meta-analysis of 119 articles assessing RIDT accuracy found an overall modest sensitivity of 62.3% (95% CI: 57.9–66.6%), with reports ranging from as little as 5% to as high as a 100%, and a high specificity of 98.2% (95% CI: 97.5–98.7%), consistent across studies (Chartrand *et al.* 2012). This means that, although false positive tests are rare, a false negative test is likely to happen and negative results should be interpreted with caution because a patient who tested negative is predicted to have influenza four times out of 10.

Many factors might account for the variability in sensitivity across different studies. Most of them influence accuracy through their effect on the amount of viruses present in the sample being tested. Detection of influenza by rapid testing requires relatively high virus titres in the submitted sample, and their performance drops significantly and rapidly with decreasing virus concentration (CDC 2012). Thus, every effort should be made, when using these tests, to maximise the amount of virus in the sample, by collecting adequate specimens early in the course of the disease, and transporting and storing them adequately.

In that regard, duration of illness at the time of sample collection is of paramount importance and specimens should be collected within 3–4 days of symptoms onset, because viral shedding in influenza peaks at 48–72 h of illness with few to no virus detectable in respiratory secretions after 5 days (Fiore *et al.* 2011). Of note, samples taken too early might also negatively affect test performances, because reports have found lower accuracy of RIDTs on the first day of illness, compared with the second or third day (Chartrand *et al.* 2012). Thus, there is a very narrow window of opportunity for the optimal use of RIDTs, which fortunately corresponds to the time where the patient is the sickest and so the more likely to seek medical attention.

The type of specimen will also influence the amount of virus collected. Nasopharyngeal specimens are expected to yield a higher amount of virus than nasal or throat specimens (Fiore *et al.* 2011; Harper *et al.* 2009), and swabbing, while collecting fewer secretions than aspiration, will collect more epithelial cells that contain the influenza virus (Daley *et al.* 2006). However, the selection of a collection method over another is most often dictated by practical reasons. Although the optimal respiratory specimen for influenza, nasopharyngeal swabs cannot be collected from infants and their discomfort might interfere with adequate sample collection in even the most cooperative adult. Interestingly, a recent meta-analysis of RIDTs did not show any statistically significant differences between the different types of specimen (Chartrand *et al.* 2012), leaning in favour of more 'patient-accepted' modes of specimen collection.

The age of the patient, though not amenable to modification, will also impact RIDT performance through the concentration of viral antigens in the collected sample. Children have a higher viral load, owing in part to their immature immune defences, and longer viral shedding than adults (up to 10 days) (Fiore *et al.* 2011). RIDTs consequently perform significantly better in children than in adults, with an increase of ~13% in their sensitivity (Chartrand *et al.* 2012). With five to seven influenza-related outpatient visits per 100 children annually (CDC 2015b), children also bear the brunt of the influenza infection and are thus more likely to benefit from rapid testing.

The circulating types and subtypes of influenza might also affect test accuracy. Although, the antibodies used in these immunoassays target highly conserved viral nucleoproteins, these antigens might vary slightly in structure and expression from strains to strains affecting their capture by the test antibodies. Ease of detection of a given strain will also vary from test to test, depending on their proprietary antibodies (CDC 2012). Periodic re-evaluation of RIDT performance in detecting currently circulating influenza viruses is thus highly advisable. Although the analytical performance of RIDTs is comparable for influenza A and B in laboratory testing, they are in practice significantly less sensitive for detecting influenza B (Chartrand *et al.* 2012), owing to the milder disease caused. As such, seasons in which influenza B is the predominant virus type will be associated with overall poor test performance.

Lastly, the context in which these tests are performed can have an impact on their accuracy. Although most of these tests are licenced for POC use, they have mostly been validated under rigorous laboratory conditions, by trained professionals, with strict adherence to manufacturer instructions. It is then difficult to extrapolate their real accuracy at the bedside, where the demands of a busy clinical environment might mean slight protocol deviations and usage of the tests by inexperienced staff. Although a review of the existing literature has not shown a significant difference in terms of accuracy between studies in which RIDTs were performed at the POC versus in a laboratory (Chartrand *et al.* 2012), it is good to bear in mind that the context of a study, where everything is scrutinised and recorded, differs significantly from real life. To ensure optimal test performance, a detailed protocol and sufficient training should be provided before the implementation of RIDTs in clinical settings. If, however, the rapid test is performed in a laboratory setting, it is likely that the turnover time will be more than 30 min and that the principal advantage of a rapid test – namely to inform clinical practice through prompt diagnostics – will be mitigated. In that circumstance, serious consideration should be given to using more accurate, and time-consuming, conventional laboratory diagnosis methods such as RT–PCR or immunofluorescence.

## Impact of rapid influenza diagnostic tests

Though the sensitivity of RIDTs varies widely, depending on factors such as the type of influenza virus, the patient age, the duration of illness and the quality of the specimen being tested, they have demonstrated consistently high specificity. For the clinician, this means that a positive test in a patient presenting with symptoms compatible with an influenza-like illness is unlikely to be erroneous. In the presence of a positive RIDT result, a clinician can confidently diagnose influenza without any additional laboratory confirmation and manage the patient accordingly.

A negative test, as previously mentioned, does not reliably exclude influenza, especially when the prevalence of influenza is high, such as in the middle of the influenza season. Although this is an important shortcoming of RIDTs, it is not in itself a definite argument against their use. The unaided clinical diagnosis of influenza suffers from the same low sensitivity compounded by an equally low specificity. Cough and fever, the two primary symptoms of the case definition of influenza-like illness, have a sensitivity of 64–65% and a specificity of 67% for the diagnosis of influenza (Call *et al.* 2005; Petrozzino *et al.* 2010). Thus, the addition of a positive RIDT to a clinical suspicion of influenza, based on the presence of fever and cough, tremendously improves the likelihood that a patient indeed has influenza (D'Heilly *et al.* 2008; Petrozzino *et al.* 2010). If the RIDT is negative, then the clinician is left, without undue delays, with the same choice as before: to rely solely on uncertain clinical judgment to guide patient management or to wait for the results of more expensive conventional tests with a turnaround time of at least a few hours.

Because of the void they fill at the patient bedside by giving clinicians a confirmation of a diagnosis of influenza in a clinically relevant time frame, RIDTs are in a unique position to influence patient-important outcomes. They could enable clinicians to institute prompt infection control measures during an influenza outbreak, start antiviral treatment in high-risk populations while they are still likely to impact the course of illness, and make informed decisions concerning further diagnostic investigations and the empirical start of antibiotics in ill patients with fever.

Successful management of institutional outbreaks depend on the prompt identification of the causing agent and timely establishment of adequate control measures. A RIDT can point to influenza as the likely culprit in mere minutes, rather than waiting hours or days for the results of conventional diagnosis methods while allowing further spread of the infection. Because of their high specificity, a positive result, especially if present in multiple subjects, makes influenza a near certainty. Studies conducted in nursing homes have shown that access to rapid diagnosis for influenza indeed reduces the duration and the final attack rate of institutional outbreaks (Church *et al.* 2002; Leonardi *et al.* 1994). Outbreak control is, therefore, one of the usages of RIDTs endorsed by the CDC and the WHO (CDC 2015c; WHO 2011).

Current antiviral treatments for influenza – adamantanes and neuraminidases inhibitors – can reduce the duration and severity of influenza illness and decrease associated complications, but they must be started within 48 h of symptoms onset to produce maximum benefits (Harper *et al.* 2009). Most patients are likely to present for medical attention towards the end of this time frame, leaving the clinician with little time to make the appropriate diagnosis and start antiviral treatment. Because conventional testing is unlikely to provide the answer in time, this has often led to empirical treatment of suspected influenza cases. Although this strategy might be sound in an epidemic context, where negative RIDT results are likely to be false negatives, and in high-risk patients, because of their higher morbidity and mortality rate, it comes at a high cost not only in terms of unnecessary medication cost, but also in terms of the potential side effects of medication and the danger of emerging antiviral resistance. In fact, the cost associated with antiviral overuse and their possible side effects exceed the cost of testing by RIDTs (Sintchenko *et al.* 2002) and a strategy of antiviral treatment based on RIDT results cost around CAN$7500 less per 100 000 person-years than empirical treatment (Nshimyumukiza *et al.* 2016). Moreover, antiviral treatment decisions based on RIDT results have a higher expected utility in low-risk patients than empirical treatment (Nshimyumukiza *et al.* 2016; Sintchenko *et al.* 2002) and could result in approximately two lives saved per 100 000 person-years because of quicker treatment (Nshimyumukiza *et al.* 2016).

The impact of rapid testing for influenza on ancillary tests and antibiotic prescriptions has mostly been studied in children. The influenza season is associated with a 10–30% increase in the number of courses of antibiotics prescribed to children (AAP 2015), which far exceeds the prevalence of secondary bacterial infection associated with influenza. As such, medical care encounters for children with influenza are an important cause of inappropriate antimicrobial use: an alarming fact in an era of increasing antibiotic resistance. Because the decision to prescribe antibiotics is made during the patient's visit and is unlikely to be changed by results that would become available hours after the patient left the office or was discharged from the emergency, the RIDT is the only diagnostic test for influenza likely to influence antibiotic usage. Although most studies have shown a trend towards fewer antibiotic prescriptions in the emergency department with the use of RIDTs, sometimes by more than half (Noyola and Demmler 2000), a recent Cochrane review (Doan *et al.* 2014) did not find a statistically significant difference in prescribing patterns between clinicians given access to RIDT results and those that relied solely on clinical judgement. Similarly, although they reduce the number of chest X-rays, rapid testing did not change the number of blood or urine test conducted in the emergency department (Doan *et al.* 2014). This could be partly explained by the insidious reverse effect of a negative test: while a positive test will reassure the clinician that a child has a viral condition that does not necessitate antibiotics or further testing, a negative test might alarm the clinician into thinking a serious bacterial condition has been missed when he/she was previously considering influenza as the most likely diagnosis. A clear understanding by clinicians that, because of its limited sensitivity, a negative RIDT result is compatible with a diagnosis of influenza is therefore necessary for these tests to positively impact patient management at the POC.

### The recommended use of rapid influenza diagnostic tests

If correctly interpreted, RIDTs have a role to play in clinical decision making and can serve important public health purposes. Decisions concerning patient management are usually made right at the bedside, or soon after that. The confirmation that influenza is currently circulating in a given patient population can significantly enhance the accuracy of a clinical diagnosis by raising the pre-test probability of influenza (WHO 2011). In the community setting, where laboratory access is limited, RIDTs are probably the best tools to document influenza activity in real time, especially to signal the start of the yearly influenza epidemic. During peak activity, however, testing every patient with influenza-like illness would likely be a waste of resources since a positive test would only confirm clinical suspicions and a negative test would have a high probability of being a false negative. At the height of the epidemic, testing should, therefore, be reserved for situations where it can influence timely patient management (WHO 2011).

Although influenza testing is recommended for every hospitalised patient with influenza-like illness, RIDTs should not be encouraged where RT–PCR and immunofluorescence are available (CDC 2015c; Harper *et al.* 2009; WHO 2011). In their absence, such as in remote settings or when the specialised laboratory is overwhelmed (pandemic), RIDTs could be considered to assist in patient management, although antiviral treatment for a hospitalised patient should not be delayed, withheld or stopped based on a negative RIDT result.

Although most national and international organisations give RIDTs a limited place in clinical management of individual patients, they all agree that these tests can serve important public health purposes, especially to identify influenza as the cause of a respiratory outbreak in closed or semi-closed settings (such as nursing homes, chronic care facilities, cruise ships, schools and summer camps) and assist in the prompt institution of infection control measures (CDC 2015c; WHO 2011). Although these tests can also assist in influenza surveillance efforts, and might in fact reflect the extent of the spread of influenza in the community better than hospital-centred laboratory testing, they should not be used alone for surveillance purposes because they do not provide isolates for identification of circulating strains and determination of strain characteristics, such as antiviral susceptibilities and relatedness to vaccine strains.

## CONCLUSIONS

Despite their limited recommended uses, RIDTs are in practice occupying an important place in the diagnostic arsenal for influenza. In the USA, between 2007 and 2009, they were used in 46% of emergency department visits in which a diagnosis of influenza was made and in 2% of all visits to the emergency department (Blaschke *et al.* 2013). They have the potential to directly impact patient management by promoting the appropriate and early use of antiviral treatment while decreasing antibiotic overuse and unnecessary ancillary testing. Furthermore, the usage of RIDTs in LMIC, where access to advanced diagnostic tools is limited, could contribute to improving the treatment and outcome of influenza patients as part of a comprehensive plan to decrease the health burden of the flu.

Although RT–PCR is by all account the preferred diagnostic modality for influenza (CDC 2015c; WHO 2011), its longer turn-around time, prohibitive cost and the expertise required to perform it, have so far limited its use to specialised settings, thus leaving an empty place at the POC that only RIDTs have been able to fill. However, this might be about to change. In the past couple of years, rapid isothermal nucleic acid amplification tests (e.g.

Alere™ i influenza A&B) have appeared on the market. These self-contained, partially automated, easy-to-use devices can qualitatively detect viral RNA in respiratory specimens within 15 min. Because there is no need for separate RNA extraction and purification, these devices are appropriate for POC use, though they are more cumbersome, technology-dependent and costly than simple dipstick RIDTs. Compared with conventional RT–PCR, these rapid, portable versions have thus far demonstrated adequate, though reduced sensitivity (75–95%), with high specificity 99–100% (Hazelton *et al.* 2015; Hurtardo *et al.* 2015). By transporting the accuracy of RT–PCR at the patient bedside, these devices might eventually bridge the gap between accurate and definitive laboratory testing and fast and easy POCT.

## PATIENT CASE STUDY

On a chilly winter night, you are working your usual shift as a paediatric physician attending at a busy inner-city emergency department. You are called to consult on a 3-month-old girl who was brought by her mother to ER after 2 days of fever (>39.5°C), vomiting and mild rhinorrhoea. On physical examination, the child is alert but irritable. The rest of the exam is unremarkable. Because of the height and duration of the fever, you are concerned that this child might have a serious bacterial infection. You order a chest X-ray, complete blood count (CBC), urinalysis and blood and urine cultures. As you are discussing your differential diagnosis with your senior resident, you note that you are in the middle of the seasonal influenza epidemic and that your patient could have an atypical presentation of influenza illness with gastrointestinal symptoms that is more common in infants. You also know that a secondary bacterial infection is unlikely in an infant with a confirmed viral infection. As such, you want to test for an influenza infection as soon as possible to determine whether or not to start prophylactic antibiotherapy pending the results of the blood and urine cultures. Although your hospital is equipped with cutting edge multiplex RT–PCR for viral diagnosis, the tests are run in batches during the day shift. Thus, it would not provide the answer you are looking for in a clinically relevant timeframe. Luckily, the ER department has recently put in place a protocol for POCT of influenza and respiratory syncytial virus. The RIDT is positive for influenza A in your patient and, because of this test's high specificity and the current high prevalence of influenza in your region, you know that the result is unlikely to be a false positive. Thus, you decide to withhold prophylactic antibiotherapy and promptly start the patient on a course of oseltamivir, because she is at high-risk of complications from influenza illness because of her young age. You decide to keep her under observation because of her vomiting and her mother's concerns about inadequate fluid intake. Because the emergency department is overcrowded, the nurse asks you if she can put your patient in the same room as a 5-year-old boy with similar symptoms of fever and vomiting, accompanied by diarrhoea. Because your patient has confirmed influenza, you decided it would be best to keep her isolated or to cohort her with other influenza patients to prevent nosocomial transmission of the virus.

## REFERENCES


AAAP (American Academy of Pediatrics) (2015) *Influenza in Red Book*. (Eds W Kimberlin, M Brady, MA Jackson and S Long) pp. 477–493. AAP Publishing, Elk Grove Village IL, USA.

Alves Galvão MG, Rocha Crispino Santos MA, Alves da Cunha AJ (2014) Amantadine and rimantadine for influenza A in children and the elderly. *Cochrane Database of Systematic Reviews* **4**, CD002745.

Black CL, Yue X, Ball SW, Donahue SM, Izrael D, de Perio MA, *et al.* (2015) Influenza vaccination coverage among health care personnel–United States, 2014–15 Influenza Season. *MMWR Morbidity and Mortality Weekly Report* **64**, 993–999. doi:10.15585/mmwr.mm6436a1

Blaschke AJ, Shapiro DJ, Pavia AT, Byington CL, Ampofo K, Stockmann C, *et al.* (2013) A national study of the impact of rapid influenza testing on clinical care in the emergency department. *Journal of the Pediatric Infectious Diseases Society* **3**, 112–118. doi:10.1093/jpids/pit071

Bresee J, Hayden FG (2013) Epidemic influenza – responding to the expected but unpredictable. *The New England Journal of Medicine* **368**, 589–592. doi:10.1056/NEJMp1300375

Call SA, Vollenweider MA, Hornung CA, Simel DL, McKinney WP (2005) Does this patient have influenza? *Journal of the American Medical Association* **293**, 987–997. doi:10.1001/jama.293.8.987

CDC (Centers for Disease Control and Prevention) (2012) Evaluation of 11 commercially available rapid influenza diagnostic tests–United States, 2011–2012. Centers for Disease Control and Prevention. *MMWR Morbidity and Mortality Weekly Report* **61**, 873–876.

CDC (2015a) *Fluview Database - US Virologic Surveillance*. Center for Disease Control and Prevention, <http://www.cdc.gov/flu/weekly/fluviewinteractive.htm>.

CDC (2015b) *Influenza in Epidemiology and Prevention of Vaccine-Preventable Diseases*. (Eds J Hamborsky, A Kroger, S

Wolfe) pp. 187–208. Public Health Foundation, Atlanta GA, USA.

CDC (2015c) *Guidance for Clinicians on the Use of Rapid Influenza Diagnostic Tests.* Centers for Disease Control and Prevention, <http://www.cdc.gov/flu/professionals/diagnosis/clinician_guidance_ridt.htm>.

Chartrand C, Leeflang MM, Minion J, Brewer T, Pai M (2012) Accuracy of rapid influenza diagnostic tests: a meta-analysis. *Annals of Internal Medicine* **156**, 500–511. doi:10.7326/0003-4819-156-7-201204030-00403

Church DL, Davies HD, Mitton C, Semeniuk H, Logue M, Maxwell C, *et al.* (2002) Clinical and economic evaluation of rapid influenza A virus testing in nursing homes in Calgary, Canada. *Clinical Infectious Diseases* **34**, 790–795. doi:10.1086/338960

Daley P, Castriciano S, Chernesky M, Smieja M (2006) Comparison of flocked and rayon swabs for collection of respiratory epithelial cells from uninfected volunteers and symptomatic patients. *Journal of Clinical Microbiology* **44**, 2265–2267. doi:10.1128/JCM.02055-05

de Francisco Shapovalova N, Donadel M, Jit M, Hutubessy R (2015) A systematic review of the social and economic burden of influenza in low- and middle-income countries. *Vaccine* **33**, 6537–6544. doi:10.1016/j.vaccine.2015.10.066

D'Heilly SJ, Janoff EN, Nichol P, Nichol KL (2008) Rapid diagnosis of influenza infection in older adults: influence on clinical care in a routine clinical setting. *Journal of Clinical Virology* **42**, 124–128.

Doan Q, Enarson P, Kissoon N, Klassen TP, Johnson DW (2014) Rapid viral diagnosis for acute febrile respiratory illness in children in the emergency department. *Cochrane Database of Systematic Reviews* **5**, CD006452.

Ehlken B, Anastassopoulou A, Hain J, Schröder C, Wahle K (2015) Cost for physician-diagnosed influenza and influenza-like illnesses on primary care level in Germany – results of a database analysis from May 2010 to April 2012. *BMC Public Health* **15**, 578. doi:10.1186/s12889-015-1885-0

Fiore AE, Fry A, Shay D, Gubareva L, Bresee JS, Uyeki TM, Centers for Disease Control and Prevention (CDC) (2011) Antiviral agents for the treatment and chemoprophylaxis of influenza – recommendations of the Advisory Committee on Immunization Practices (ACIP). *MMWR Morbidity and Mortality Weekly Report* **60**, 1–24.

Fischer WA, II, Gong M, Bhagwanjee S, Sevransky J (2014) Global burden of influenza as a cause of cardiopulmonary morbidity and mortality. *Global Heart* **9**, 325–336. doi:10.1016/j.gheart.2014.08.004

Fuller JA, Summers A, Katz MA, Lindblade KA, Njuguna H, Arvelo W, *et al.* (2013) Estimation of the national disease burden of influenza-associated severe acute respiratory illness in Kenya and Guatemala: a novel methodology. *PLoS One* **8**, e56882. doi:10.1371/journal.pone.0056882

Harper SA, Bradley JS, Englund JA, File TM, Gravenstein S, Hayden FG, *et al.* (2009) Seasonal influenza in adults and children – diagnosis, treatment, chemoprophylaxis, and institutional outbreak management: clinical practice guidelines of the Infectious Diseases Society of America. *Clinical Infectious Diseases* **48**, 1003–1032. doi:10.1086/598513

Hazelton B, Gray T, Ho J, Ratnamohan VM, Dwyer DE, Kok J (2015) Detection of influenza A and B with the Alere™ i Influenza A & B: a novel isothermal nucleic acid amplification assay. *Influenza and Other Respiratory Viruses* **9**, 151–154. doi:10.1111/irv.12303

Hurtado JC, Mosquera M, de Lazzari E, Martínez E, Torner N, Isanta R, *et al.* (2015) Evaluation of a new, rapid, simple test for the detection of influenza virus. *BMC Infectious Diseases* **15**, 44. doi:10.1186/s12879-015-0775-5

Jefferson T, Jones MA, Doshi P, Del Mar CB, Hama R, Thompson MJ, *et al.* (2014) Neuraminidase inhibitors for preventing and treating influenza in healthy adults and children. *Cochrane Database of Systematic Reviews* **1**, CD008965.

Katz MA, Muthoka P, Emukule GO, Kalani R, Njuguna H, Waiboci LW, *et al.* (2014) Results from the first six years of national sentinel surveillance for influenza in Kenya, July 2007-June 2013. *PLoS One* **9**, e98615. doi:10.1371/journal.pone.0098615

Klepser ME (2014) Socioeconomic impact of seasonal (epidemic) influenza and the role of over-the-counter medicines. *Drugs* **74**, 1467–1479. doi:10.1007/s40265-014-0245-1

Kyeyagalire R, Tempia S, Cohen AL, Smith AD, McAnerney JM, Dermaux-Msimang V, Cohen C (2014) Hospitalizations associated with influenza and respiratory syncytial virus among patients attending a network of private hospitals in South Africa, 2007–2012. *BMC Infectious Diseases* **14**, 694. doi:10.1186/s12879-014-0694-x

Leonardi GP, Leib H, Birkhead GS, Smith C, Costello P, Conron W (1994) Comparison of rapid detection methods for influenza A virus and their value in health-care management of institutionalized geriatric patients. *Journal of Clinical Microbiology* **32**, 70–74.

Leonardi GP, Mitrache I, Pigal A, Freedman L (2010) Public hospital-based laboratory experience during an outbreak of pandemic influenza A (H1N1) virus infections. *Journal of Clinical Microbiology* **48**, 1189–1194. doi: 10.1128/JCM.01657-09

Lu PJ, O'Halloran A, Williams WW, Lindley MC, Farrall S, Bridges CB (2015) Racial and ethnic disparities in vaccination coverage among adult populations in the U.S. *Vaccine* **33**, D83–D91. doi:10.1016/j.vaccine.2015.09.031

Lu PJ, O'Halloran A, Ding H, Srivastav A, Williams WW (2016) Uptake of influenza vaccination and missed opportunities among adults with high-risk conditions, United States, 2013. *The American Journal of Medicine* **129**, 636.e1–636.e11. doi:10.1016/j.amjmed.2015.10.031

McMorrow ML, Emukule GO, Njuguna HN, Bigogo G, Montgomery JM, Nyawanda B, *et al.* (2015) The unrecognized burden of influenza in young Kenyan children, 2008–2012. *PLoS One* **10**, e0138272. doi:10.1371/journal.pone.0138272

Molinari NA, Ortega-Sanchez IR, Messonnier ML, Thompson WW, Wortley PM, Weintraub E, *et al.* (2007) The annual impact of seasonal influenza in the US: measuring disease burden and costs. *Vaccine* **25**, 5086–5096. doi:10.1016/j.vaccine.2007.03.046

Noyola DE, Demmler GJ (2000) Effect of rapid diagnosis on management of influenza A infections. *The Pediatric Infectious Disease Journal* **19**, 303–307. doi:10.1097/00006454-200004000-00008

Nshimyumukiza L, Douville X, Fournier D, Duplantie J, Daher R, Charlebois I, *et al.* (2016) Cost effectiveness analysis of antiviral treatment in the management of seasonal influenza A: point-of-care rapid test versus clinical judgment. *Influenza and Other Respiratory Viruses* **10**, 113–121. doi:10.1111/irv.12359

Petrozzino JJ, Smith C, Atkinson MJ (2010) Rapid diagnostic testing for seasonal influenza: an evidence-based review and comparison with unaided clinical diagnosis. *The Journal of Emergency Medicine* **39**, 476–490. doi:10.1016/j.jemermed.2009.11.031

Sintchenko V, Gilbert GL, Coiera E, Dwyer D (2002) Treat or test first? Decision analysis of empirical antiviral treatment of influenza virus infection versus treatment based on rapid test results. *Journal of Clinical Virology* **25**, 15–21. doi:10.1016/S1386-6532(00)00182-7

WHO (World Health Organization) (2011) *Use of Influenza Rapid Diagnostic Tests.* World Health Organization, Geneva, Switzerland.

WHO (2014) *Influenza (Seasonal) – Fact Sheet No. 211.* World Health Organization, Geneva, Switzerland, <http://www.who.int/mediacentre/factsheets/fs211/en/>.

# 22 Point-of-care testing for malaria

*David Bell and Jane Cunningham*

**Summary**

Malaria, caused by *Plasmodium* spp. and carried by *Anopheles* spp. mosquitoes, is endemic in 97 countries. It is a major cause of mortality due to infectious disease, and disproportionally affects children. Clinically malaria is indistinguishable from the early stages of other co-endemic diseases, but presumptive treatment was standard practice for decades in high burden settings, largely due to lack of quality point-of-care testing (POCT). Over the last 15 years, the availability of accurate and affordable antigen-detecting malaria lateral flow assays/rapid diagnostic tests (RDTs) coupled with effective treatment has revolutionised malaria case management.

## GLOBAL AND REGIONAL PREVALENCE

Despite being preventable and curable, malaria remains one of the major causes of mortality due to infectious disease. In 2014, there were an estimated 214 million malaria cases (with an uncertainty range of 149–303 million) and an estimated 438 000 deaths (with an uncertainty range of 236 000–635 000); 306 000 of these are under-5s, including 292 000 children in the African Region.

Although these figures remain staggering, they represent a 37% global decrease in malaria incidence and a 60% decrease in global malaria mortality rates between 2000 and 2015. In this same 15-year period, malaria death rates among children aged under 5 years have fallen, impressively, by 65% worldwide and by 71% in Africa (WHO 2015a). Although malaria is no longer the leading cause of death among children in sub-Saharan Africa, it remains a major killer of children, taking the life of a child every 2 min.

Although progress has been made in all regions, the burden of disease is still concentrated in the African Region, which accounted for 88% of cases in 2014, followed by the South-East Asia Region with 10% of cases and the Eastern Mediterranean Region (2%). (For listing of countries in WHO region groupings, see http://www.who.int/about/regions/en/.) Fewer than 0.5% of cases are in the Americas (390 000 cases in 2014) and the European Region reported zero indigenous cases of malaria in 2015. Malaria remains endemic in 97 countries.

## COST BURDEN TO THE HEALTH SYSTEMS

Malaria is a disease of poverty; the burden of malaria is greatest where there is low spending per capita on health. Effective malaria control requires significant investment in health facilities and training of health and field workers who must be equipped with commodities for prevention of infection and appropriate case management. Patient care delivery costs generally outstrip the costs of commodities, and donors invest primarily in commodities, leaving the endemic country governments and patients themselves to finance health-care services. WHO analysis estimates that, since 2001, average annual cost of malaria case management in sub-Saharan Africa was nearly US$300 million (WHO 2015a). When indirect costs, such as time lost from work, and severity of illness are taken into consideration, additional costs are incurred. A cost-of-illness approach in India revealed that the total economic burden from malaria in India could be around US$1940 million (Gupta and Chowdhury 2014). From a macroeconomic perspective, the available evidence indicates that the presence of malaria may have reduced economic growth by 1–2% a year in affected countries during recent decades (Gallup and Sachs 2001).

## EFFECT ON THE HOST

According to the latest WHO global estimates, 3.2 billion people remain at risk of infection by one or more malaria species infecting humans, including *Plasmodium falciparum*, found in tropical and subtropical areas of Central and South America, Africa and South East Asia, *P. vivax* prevalent in Central and South America, Asia and parts of Africa, *P. ovale* (two species) mainly in sub-Saharan Africa, and *P. knowlesi* in forested areas of South-East Asia (WHO 2015a).

### Aetiology/pathophysiology

Malaria infection in humans is caused by infection with one or more *Plasmodium* species, including *P. falciparum, P. vivax, P. ovale* (two species), *P. malariae and P. knowlesi* and is transmitted during the blood meal of 30 predominant species of *Anopheles* mosquitoes. The life cycle begins when a female *Anopheles* spp. mosquito infected with malaria parasites takes a blood meal, where it injects haploid sporozoites from its salivary glands into the vertebrate host. The sporozoites swiftly invade hepatocytes where they undergo asexual multiplication, producing thousands of merozoites. In *P. vivax* or *P. ovale* infection, some sporozoites become hypnozoites: a dormant stage within hepatocytes. Merozoites are released from infected hepatocytes into the circulation where they invade new erythrocytes. Within the erythrocyte, they multiply asexually and evolve from ring-stage parasites to trophozoites to schizonts. Erythrocytes eventually rupture every 42–48 h, releasing 8–32 merozoites that can infect new erythrocytes and releasing haemozoin and other toxic factors that activate macrophages and release cytokines responsible for the periodic cycles of fever, muscle aches, chills, vomiting and diarrhoea. These symptoms typically last 6–10 h and begin after a 7–30-day incubation period. The shorter periods are observed most frequently with *P. falciparum* and the longer with *P. malariae.*

Some blood stage parasites enter a process of gametocytogenesis, male and female gametocytes develop and it is the mature forms of these that are taken up by the mosquito when it feeds on an infected human. Sexual reproduction and formation of oocysts subsequently takes place in the insect's midgut. Sporozoites are released from the oocyst and migrate to the mosquito's salivary glands, ready for onward transmission with the next blood meal (Fig. 22.1).

### Clinical presentation

Infection with malaria parasites results in a clinical picture ranging from asymptomatic infection to severe disease and death. A constellation of non-specific symptoms including fever, rigours, headache and body pains can be indistinguishable from the early stages of other co-endemic diseases (Armstrong-Schellenberg and Smith 1994; Chandramohan *et al.* 2002; Reyburn *et al.* 2004). Even in its severe form, symptoms and signs of malaria are not pathognomonic, but merge with those of meningitis, encephalitides and sepsis (Reyburn *et al.* 2004).

### Risk factors

Humans with low levels of acquired, protective immunity are at highest risk of having clinically significant malaria. This group includes infants and young children (<5 years), pregnant women and non-immune travellers. Risk factors for severe *falciparum* malaria and death include high parasitaemia (~2.5% parasitaemia in low transmission areas or parasitaemia >20% in any setting), second and third trimesters of pregnancy, HIV/AIDS and splenectomy. The risk of severe vivax malaria is greatest among young children and individuals with co-morbidities (WHO 2015b).

### Complications

When appropriate antimalarial treatment is administered promptly, malaria infection resolves without any serious complications. However, *P. falciparum* and rarely, *P. vivax* can cause vital organ dysfunction over a period of hours to days if undiagnosed and/or inappropriately treated. Severe

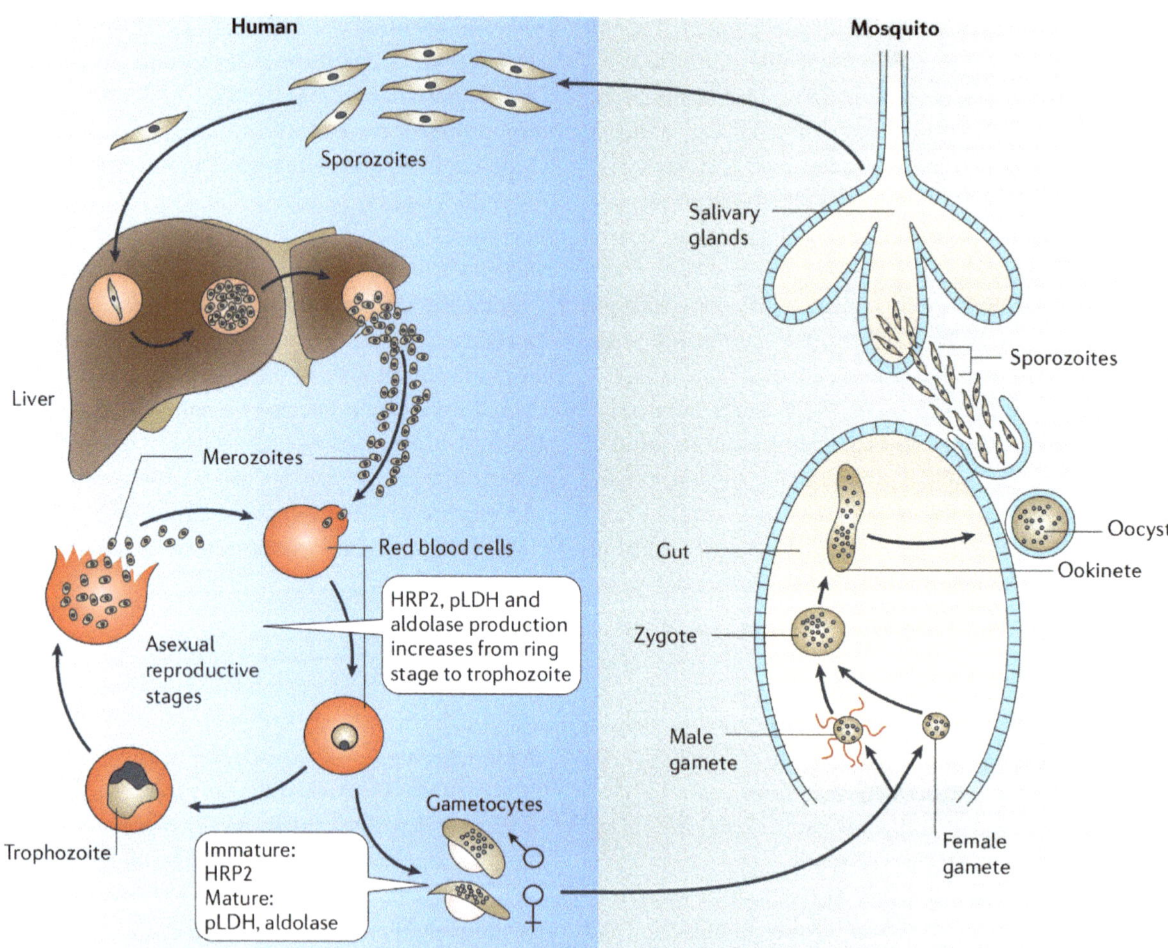


In the erythrocytic cycle, production of histidine-rich protein 2 (HRP2) and Plasmodium lactate dehydrogenase (pLDH), and probably aldolase, increases throughout trophozoite development after the invasion of red blood cells by merozoites, and reduces on development of further merozoites and cell rupture. HRP2 is also found in immature gametocytes and pLDH (and probably aldolase) is found in mature gametocytes.

**Fig. 22.1.** Stages of development of *Plasmodium falciparum* at which antigens detected by malaria rapid diagnostic tests are produced. (Source: Figure modified with permission from Bell *et al.* (2006). Permission was also granted by Macmillan Publishers Ltd to use the original figure from *Nature Reviews Microbiology*.)

malaria usually presents with one or more of impaired consciousness, seizures, metabolic acidosis, hypotension/shock, severe anaemia, hypoglycaemia, acute renal failure, pulmonary oedema, jaundice and abnormal bleeding (WHO 2015b). Those who survive cerebral malaria may be left with neurological deficits. Malaria during pregnancy can result in premature delivery and/or infants with low birthweight.

Recurrent and untreated infections with malaria can lead to severe anaemia, especially in young children and also to a rare condition known as hyper-reactive malarial syndrome (previously referred to as tropical splenomegaly syndrome), characterised by an enlarged spleen, weight loss, high levels of antibodies to *Plasmodium* spp., elevated immunoglobulin M, serum cryoglobulin and autoantibody levels and increased risk of skin and respiratory infections. *P. vivax* infection has been associated with splenic rupture and repeat or longstanding *P. malariae* infections with nephrotic syndrome.

## CASE MANAGEMENT AND POINT-OF-CARE TESTING

Despite the lack of specificity of symptoms and signs, acute fever has been presumptively treated as malaria throughout much of recent history. Reflecting a lack of alternative management options, this resulted in poor and delayed treatment for other potentially severe illness, and ignorance of the true burden of malaria across much of its range. During the past decade, the scale-up of POCT for malaria has begun to dramatically change this picture.

In view of the recently pervasive emphasis on presumptive treatment of fever with anti-malarial drugs, malaria point-of-care (POC) tests can be viewed in low-resource health systems as essentially POC tests for acute fever rather than malaria (Fig. 22.2). This has important implications for understanding their cost–benefits and programmatic implications of their use. In sub-Saharan Africa where incidence and mortality is high, the use of a parasite-based test for malaria serves mainly to guide the *withholding* of antimalarial therapy in cases of a negative test result, raising awareness of the likely presence of other potentially life-threatening disease. In highlighting the burden of non-malaria febrile disease, the scale-up of access to POC parasite-based testing for malaria has raised both challenges and opportunities for health services. It has forced a revolution in thinking both in the management of acute illness at the POC, and the supply lines, human resources and information systems required to support their use. The benefits and costs of this are already extending well beyond management of the target disease.

## Diagnosis of malaria and parasite screening

Diagnosis of 'malaria' implies the requirement for demonstration of parasitaemia above a certain parasite

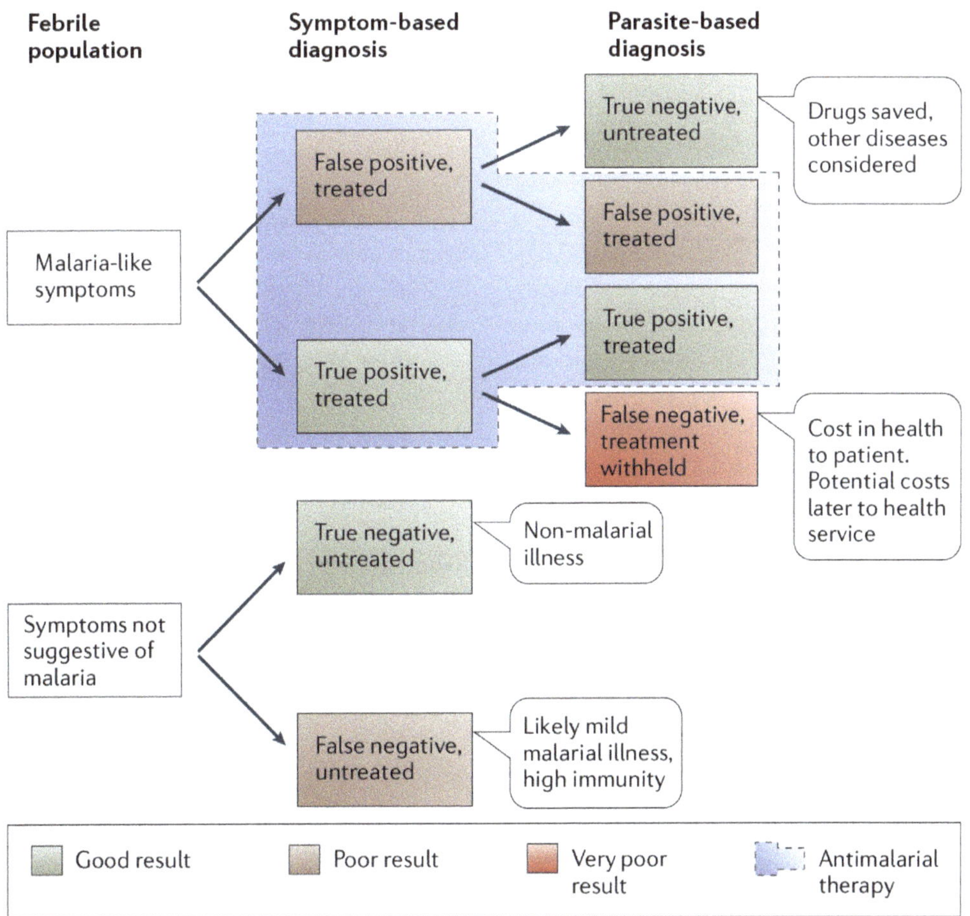


It is assumed that the criteria for using parasite-based diagnosis (for example, a rapid diagnostic test (RDT)) are identical to those on which the allocation of antimalarial drugs is currently made. The inclusion of RDTs in disease management solutions that are currently reliant on symptoms and signs will only reduce diagnostic sensitivity for malaria. However, as this figure illustrates, the advantages accrue elsewhere in the process, including improved management of non-malarial fever, savings in drug costs and also improved adherence to therapy and healthworker morale by improving diagnostic accuracy.

**Fig. 22.2.** The effect of adding parasite-based diagnosis to malaria case management based on symptoms and signs. (Source: Figure modified with permission from Bell *et al.* (2006). Permission was also granted by Macmillan Publishers Ltd to use the original figure from *Nature Reviews Microbiology*.)

density – symptoms commonly occur at a parasite density above ~100 parasite/µL, similar to the lower limit of detection of field-level light microscopy and visually read lateral flow assays (LFAs, commonly known as rapid diagnostic tests [RDTs]) (WHO 2010a). Although parasitaemia is always worth eliminating with antimalarial therapy to prevent onward transmission or later evolution of symptoms, the demonstration of parasites is not necessarily conclusive evidence of causality of disease and the probability of causality.

Definitions are important when referring to POCT: 'care' being the operative word and implying the presence of illness. Thus, when using the term 'POCT' for malaria, we refer primarily to tests that are used to identify malarial illness – detecting parasite densities commonly associated with symptoms of the disease in a person who is ill. The threshold of detection of malaria parasites by currently available RDTs appears to be safe for purposes of case management, as a basis for withholding anti-malarial therapy on a negative result (Mtove *et al.* 2011; Senn *et al.* 2011). Tests intended to detect parasitaemia irrespective of the presence of symptoms – 'parasite-screening tests' – require far lower limits of detection and the current candidates are nucleic acid amplification tests, though LFAs may theoretically reach these densities with sample concentration and digital readers.

The importance of recognition of these very low-level parasitaemia has gained increasing importance with the rising emphasis of malaria programs on elimination of malaria transmission. The contribution of sub-clinical low density infectious reservoir in host populations to maintenance of transmission in areas with low malaria prevalence has been increasingly recognised (Cheng *et al.* 2015; Imwong *et al.* 2015; Okell *et al.* 2009). An ideal parasite screening test would operate in a similar situation to a POC test, enabling rapid testing and return of results with minimal equipment at a village or household level (malERA 2011). The likelihood of wrongly identifying low-density malaria parasitaemia as a cause of fever will complicate their role in case management.

## Options for point-of-care testing

Because malaria can progress rapidly to severe disease, a test must be close to the POC – readily accessible to a sick individual – to be effective. Because it is frequently associated with relatively remote populations in low-resource settings (a disease of poverty), tests must be of low cost and simple enough for operation by relatively low-trained and supervised health workers. For this reason, though being the primary mode of diagnosis since the identification of parasites by Laveran in 1880, light microscopy remains relatively limited to centralised clinics with sufficient laboratory capacity, and requires considerable training and quality assurance, good optical equipment protected from environmental exposure, and good slide preparation (reagents and skill). Microscopy could be considered a POC test where the patient is in close proximity to a laboratory and technicians and equipment are readily available, and ~200 million cases were still reported as diagnosed by microscopy in 2014. However, delivery of results is frequently delayed and so cannot influence immediate treatment.

Other assay platforms, including methods for fluorescent staining, nucleic acid amplification tests (NAAT) and detection of haemozoin, a by-product of parasite haem metabolism, have failed to make great inroads (Delahunt *et al.* 2014). Modifications of microscopy including digitising of images through adaptions of smart phones have not reached scale, having failed to demonstrate equivalent performance of traditional microscopy and RDTs.

RDTs are currently the only assay with potential to offer accessible diagnosis to all populations in malaria-risk areas, since they displaced microscopy as the predominant test for malaria (WHO 2015a). RDTs have been dramatically extending the accessibility of accurate malaria diagnosis at the POC, and are the focus of the remainder of this chapter.

## Treatment

The WHO recommends confirmation of malaria diagnosis by quality microscopy or malaria rapid diagnostic testing, before administration of antimalarials. These results should be available within 2 h of patient presentation; otherwise, a decision should be taken on clinical grounds. Furthermore, if severe malaria is suspected, parasitological diagnosis should not delay initiation of antimalarial treatment. Treatment regimens vary between species and have changed greatly in the last two decades, with much emphasis now placed on monitoring and managing the emergence of resistance.

In the absence of any signs of severe disease, *P. falciparum* infection in children and adults (except pregnant women in their first trimester) should be treated with an appropriate dose of artemisinin-based combination therapy (ACT) for 3 days. Recently, a single low dose of primaquine was recommended for all patients (except pregnant women, infants aged <6 months and women breastfeeding infants aged <6 months) in low transmission settings to reduce transmissibility (WHO 2015b).

In most areas, infections with *P. vivax, P. ovale, P. malariae or P. knowlesi* can still be treated with chloroquine, although ACT is also recommended in adults and in children. However, in areas where there are chloroquine-resistant parasites, infections with *P. vivax* should be treated with ACT (except pregnant women in the first trimester).

Treatment with ACT kills only blood stage infections and therefore, in the case of *P. vivax* and *P. ovale* malaria, another medicine is required to kill the liver stage (hypnozoites), which are the source of relapse infections. Only one medicine is currently available to treat the liver stage, primaquine, and it can cause haemolysis in individuals with G6PD. Therefore, G6PD testing is recommended where available before administration of primaquine to prevent relapsing *P. vivax* and *P. ovale* (WHO 2015b).

Adults and children with any form of severe malaria are given at least 24 h of parental therapy, preferably with artesunate; otherwise artemether or quinine can be administered. This should be followed by a full 3-day course of ACT. If parenteral therapy is delayed, a pre-referral dose of rectal artesunate or intramuscular artesunate, artemether or quinine and broad-spectrum antibiotic are recommended (WHO 2015b). Supportive management of complications (anaemia, hypoglycaemia, shock and seizures) is essential.

## INTRODUCTION AND SCALE-UP OF MALARIA RAPID DIAGNOSTIC TESTS

Malaria RDTs were the first diagnostic pathogen-specific assays widely available in the peripheral centres of many health systems in low-resource countries. On their initial introduction in the early 1990s (Premji *et al.* 1994; Shiff *et al.* 1993, 1994), malaria RDTs were relatively slow to achieve significant programmatic use. Aside from scattered field trials, use for routine diagnostic testing was essentially limited to programs in South-East Asia. A 1999 WHO consultation laid out a plan to clarify the role of LFAs in case management (WHO 2000), leading to a series of WHO consultations from 2003 to develop guidance on malaria RDT implementation and a quality control program to provide assurance of reliability (WHO/WPRO 2003; WHO 2004; WHO-TDR-FIND 2010; WHO-FIND-CDC-HTD 2013). An associated increase in available products led to over 21 manufacturers requesting testing on 41 products for the first round of WHO product testing in 2008. The WHO evaluation program, conducted at the US Centers for Disease Control and Prevention (CDC) and involving various institutions in malaria endemic and non-endemic countries, formed a basis for procurement recommendations of WHO (WHO-FIND-CDC-HTD 2013; WHO-FIND-CDC 2015).

Procurement and use of malaria RDTs increased rapidly after 2005, with 314 million RDTs sold in 2014 (WHO 2015a). The drivers of this uptake extend beyond the positive WHO recommendations. Financial support for malaria programs expanded rapidly from 2002, with large-scale funding by The Global Fund followed by the United States Agency for International Development through the US President's Malaria Initiative. Increased funding coincided with other WHO recommendations on replacement of chloroquine by ACT in the face of rapidly increasing resistance of *P. falciparum* to various antimalarial drugs. The cost-effectiveness of presumptive treatment on the basis of fever alone became a potentially more expensive option than pathology-guided treatment.

Although parasite-based diagnosis had been more commonly practiced in Asia and South America, presumptive therapy had been routine in much of sub-Saharan Africa despite evidence from the field indicating that tests are safe when of adequate quality and well prepared (Mtove *et al.* 2011; Senn *et al.* 2011). The high level of confidence required with malaria test introduction in part explains their relatively slow initial uptake in sub-Saharan countries. However, as tests were rolled out, the inadequacy of previous symptom-based treatment became apparent, with a dramatic reduction in reported malaria in many cases (Thiam *et al.* 2011; Yukich *et al.* 2012). Thus, as the cost of ACT reduced and the direct cost-driven imperative of parasite-based diagnosis became less clear, evidence of the need for improved diagnosis of acute fever continued to drive ACT use, with the WHO formally recommending parasite-based diagnosis (by RDTs or microscopy) in 2010 (WHO 2010a).

As the availability of more accurate diagnosis has demonstrated that most acute febrile disease is not malaria, the burden of non-malarial febrile disease has been highlighted. Acute febrile disease arises from a broad range of pathogens (Black *et al.* 2010; Crump *et al.* 2013; Mayxay *et al.* 2013; Reyburn *et al.* 2004), many of which impart significant mortality; as a result, resources are then required for further diagnosis and a range of management options.

There is much interest in multiplexing malaria tests, including detecting of markers for other pathogens, but this adds cost and pathogen prevalence varies widely across geography and time (Black *et al.* 2010; Crump *et al.* 2013; Mayxay *et al.* 2013). Addition of a biomarker for disease severity, or to identify broad classes of pathogen susceptible to a particular therapy, would reduce complexity while keeping costs down. Suitable biomarkers with sufficient specificity are yet to be identified.

Beyond the need for action on negative test results, malaria RDTs have raised the need for efficient supply lines to the periphery of health service reach in often difficult geography, for effective supervision and training, and for improved tracking and use of diagnostic results in health sector planning. Although most malaria LFAs are relatively stable at moderate temperatures (WHO-FIND-CDC 2015), supply lines need to maintain adequate stock and protect this stock against extremes of temperature at which biological assays can degrade.

These are considerable challenges for health systems that are poorly resourced and have many competing priorities. Early introductions have often seen relatively poor outcomes, with prevalent stock-outs and poor training probably contributing to poor test performance and poor compliance with results (Bisoffi *et al.* 2009; Reyburn *et al.* 2007). However, success has also been well demonstrated at scale, and while considerable time is required to develop the necessary structures for quality control, training, communications and confidence-building (D'Acremont *et al.* 2010, 2011; Masaninga *et al.* 2012; Thiam *et al.* 2011; Yukich *et al.* 2012), the improvement in access to accurate malaria diagnosis has brought dramatic changes in malaria management and stimulated a broad reassessment of acute febrile disease management overall.

## LATERAL FLOW ASSAYS AS MALARIA RAPID DIAGNOSTIC TESTS – TARGETS AND FORMATS

RDTs used in malaria case management are lateral flow assays: sandwich assays, capturing malaria parasite-specific antigen between a capture antibody bound to a nitrocellulose (NC) membrane and a signal antibody conjugated to a signalling agent, commonly a gold nanoparticle (Fig. 22.3).

A blood sample, generally capillary blood from a finger-prick, is placed on a pad containing the signal antibody and a lysing agent. A chase buffer then flushes the

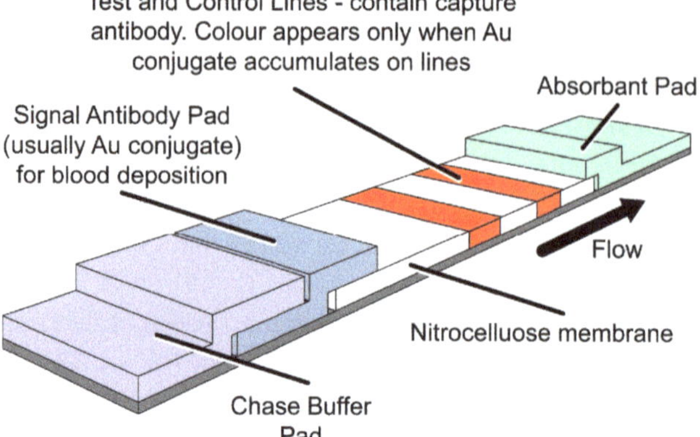


**Fig. 22.3.** Basic components of a lateral flow assay. (Source: Reproduced with permission from Kevin Nichols, Intellectual Ventures Laboratory)

antigen-signal antibody complex along the NC membrane and across the test lines. A positive result is obtained when sufficient signalling agent to be visually detectable has accumulated on the test line (capture antibody). A further flow control line binds conjugated antibody (usually other than the signal antibody) to indicate flow of reagent along the length of the strip (Fig. 22.4). Certain reader technologies can detect below the limit of human vision, but are not currently widely used.

### Target antigens

Target antigens for malaria tests fall into three major classes: histidine-rich protein-2 (HRP2), plasmodium lactate dehydrogenase (pLDH) and plasmodium aldolase. Although aldolase was employed in several early products, currently available tests almost exclusively target HRP2 and/or pLDH, with aldolase tests having frequently demonstrated poorer sensitivity in comparative trials (WHO-FIND-CDC 2015).

HRP2 is produced exclusively by *P. falciparum*, so HRP2-detecting tests are specific for this species. The protein varies considerably in primary structure between parasite isolates. Although thought to be involved in detoxification of haem, HRP2 is non-essential for parasite survival, as hrp2-deleted populations can survive and expand in the wild (Gamboa *et al.* 2010). Aldolase and pLDH, being enzymes involved in the glycolytic pathway and essential for cell survival, are present in all species. Little or no intra-species variability occurs, but limited structural variation is seen between species (Lee *et al.* 2006; Mariette *et al.* 2008; Talman *et al.* 2007). Although anti-aldolase antibodies in commercial tests have targeted

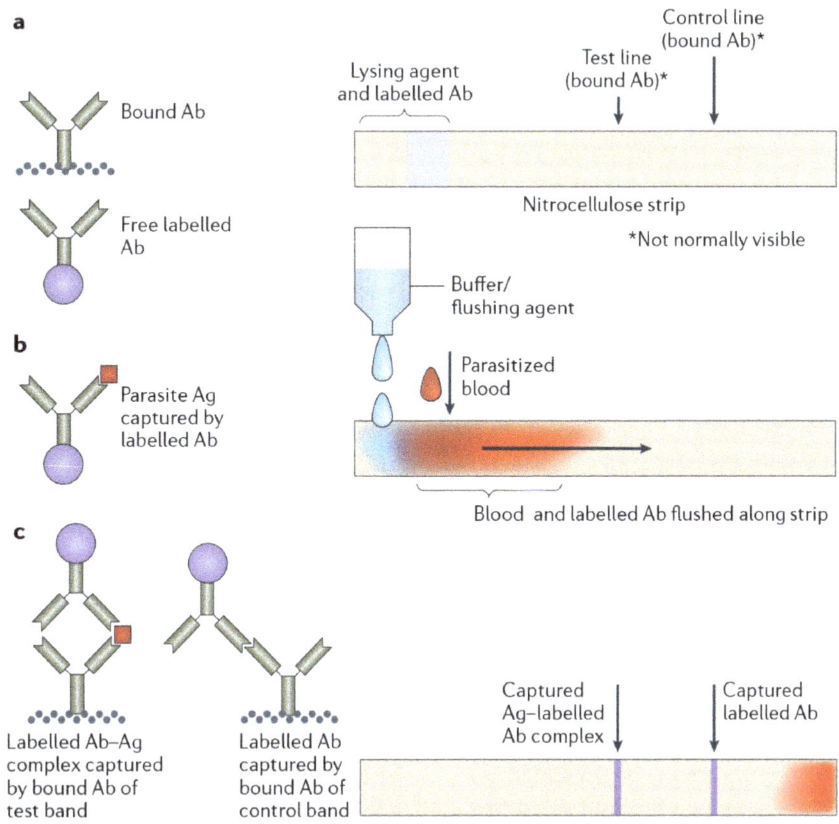


**Fig. 22.4.** Mode of action of antigen-detecting malaria rapid diagnostic tests. (Source: Figure modified with permission from Bell *et al.* (2006). Permission was also granted by Macmillan Publishers Ltd to use the original figure from *Nature Reviews Microbiology*.)

epitopes common to the main human malaria species infecting humans (*P. falciparum, P vivax, P. ovale* and *P. malariae)*, antibodies binding pLDH in commercial tests variously target all species ('pan-specific'), or have relative specificity to one or more species. Thus, multiple assays combining capture (test) lines for HRP2 and pan-specific and/or species-specific pLDH antibodies can enable differentiation between the infecting malaria parasite species. The range of such combinations is considerable (WHO-FIND-CDC 2015), and the usefulness of differentiation between species varies with drug regimens and program requirements.

## Test formats

Commercially available tests come in several physical formats, most commonly as a cassette, with the strip enclosed in a plastic housing, with wells for placement of blood and buffer and a results window to view test and control lines. The added cost of the plastic cassette is generally considered to outweigh the added risks of user-error in using a simple dipstick format, because tests are commonly performed by relatively untrained health workers with limited supervision or laboratory support. Less commonly, a cardboard backing (card) has been used to support the NC membrane and hybrid cassette and dip-stick formats also exist (WHO-FIND-CDC 2015).

All commercially available tests are designed for whole blood, most commonly 5 μL. A blood transfer device incorporating some form of volume restriction or guide is usually required to transfer blood from finger-prick to the test cassette, while certain cassettes are designed for direct deposition of blood and are intended to limit volume through other means. While performing essentially the same job in all cases, the design of blood transfer devices differs widely. Because simplicity and accuracy of volume are important to overall test performance, this variety is somewhat surprising and perhaps reflects a lack of optimisation, as clear differences in performance have been noted (Hopkins *et al.* 2011).

## RDT ANALYTICAL AND CLINICAL PERFORMANCE

Like other antigen-capture LFAs, the sensitivity of malaria RDTs is dependent on the antigen concentration in the sample being above a certain threshold, on adequate sample volume and buffer being placed on the strip, and on sufficient time for passage of reagent up the strip. They require the signal antibody to remain conjugated to the signalling mechanism (e.g. nanoparticle), the capture antibody to remain bound to the NC membrane, and the affinity of both antibodies for the target antigen to be preserved. As with any LFA, the intensity of the test line is dependent on the density of nanoparticles accumulated, with the test sensitivity therefore being dependent to some extent on the density of capture antibody and width of this adherent antibody line, the rate of flow across the line (providing time for binding events to occur and reducing flow-related dissociation), and the concentration of antigen. The last implies a somewhat linear relationship between antigen concentration and line intensity within certain bounds, providing a limited degree of quantitation. However, at high antigen density, the intensity of the test line can peak and then reduce, because binding of free antigen on the test line can block binding events involving the antigen-signal antibody complex on which visualisation relies – a high-dose hook, or prozone-like, effect. Although this tends to occur with antigen concentrations that approach biological implausibility in commercially available tests (Luchavez *et al.* 2011), it may be an occasional cause of false-negative test results and more often faint lines (Gillet *et al.* 2009). The clinical significance of this is limited by its rarity, and by existing case management guidelines that require anti-malarial therapy irrespective of diagnosis in suspected severe malaria (into which cases with such high antigen concentration (parasitaemia >10%) are expected to fall) (WHO 2010b).

Although there is significant variation between products, lower limits of detection of around 1–2 ng/mL are attained by several products detecting both HRP2 and pLDH (WHO-FIND-CDC 2015). This delivers potentially high sensitivities for detection of parasitaemia in blood samples of around 100–200 parasites/μL in clinical samples (WHO-FIND-CDC 2015). Although the relationship between parasite density and clinical malaria varies with host immunity and other factors, this level is fairly consistent with the lower limits of parasite density commonly associated with symptoms (WHO 2015b). Extensive studies in children to establish safety of RDTs in the field consistently show that the use of tests detecting this threshold provide a safe basis for withholding antimalarial therapy, at least in children in areas with moderate to high transmission (Mtove *et al.* 2011; Senn *et al.* 2011). Although it is possible that some clinical malaria may remain undiagnosed and untreated, infections likely to progress to severe disease and death appear to be well detected. As noted above, this level of detection, while sufficient for managing most clinical malaria, is insufficient to detect all infectious individuals (Cheng *et al.* 2015; Imwong *et al.* 2015; Okell *et al.* 2009).

Specificity of LFAs is imperfect due to such mechanisms as non-specific binding of antibody to proteins with similar epitopes and to the affinity of certain host antibodies to the capture system (e.g. human anti-mouse antibodies). A background false positivity rate of 1–5% is typical in laboratory studies of malaria LFAs (WHO-FIND-CDC 2015). Although this has limited direct clinical impact in fever case management – antimalarial drugs have few adverse effects – it is of potential consequence in that a mis-diagnosis of malaria may result in other potentially severe diseases being overlooked. In situations of very low malaria incidence, a low false positive rate may dominate true positives in cases of acute fever, rendering data unreliable.

A further specificity issue arises due to the persistence of HRP2 in circulation for up to weeks after treatment (Humar *et al.* 1997). This is not technically a false-positive result because the test is detecting the antigen to which it is targeted, but is false positive from a clinical perspective. Thus, testing a febrile person within a few weeks of treatment may falsely suggest treatment failure or re-infection. The importance of this to case management depends on the epidemiological context. Where transmission is very low, re-infection soon after definitive treatment is unlikely and the probability of false diagnosis is correspondingly greater. In an area of high transmission, re-infection may occur frequently, thus making an assumption of false positivity more hazardous.

Management protocols commonly recommend an alternative test more directly demonstrating parasitaemia, such as microscopy, for confirmation of diagnosis after recent treatment.

Despite the apparent simplicity of the tests, sensitivity (and specificity) are highly dependent on correct preparation and interpretation. The published literature provides extensive evidence of poor preparation and interpretation (Jelinek *et al.* 2000; Rennie *et al.* 2007), but also the potential to achieve high-quality diagnosis with appropriate training and instruction, including in the hands of health personnel with relatively little prior training (Counihan *et al.* 2012; Mayxay *et al.* 2004).

Provider and patient adherence to results, although not strictly an issue of diagnostic quality, is obviously critical to the overall usefulness of malaria RDTs. As with the introduction of any significant new intervention, effective uptake can be affected by training and communication, peer influence, prior experience, and time to achieve confidence and trust in the technology. Consistent with this, poor adherence is well documented in relatively small-scale implementation or when monitored over a short period of time, while dramatic reductions in anti-malarial drug use have been achieved when training and quality control mechanisms have been considered and sufficient time allowed for behaviour change among health personnel (Odaga *et al.* 2014; Thiam *et al.* 2011; Yukich *et al.* 2012).

## PROGRAMMATIC IMPACT AND COST-EFFECTIVENESS

The impact and difficulty of introducing malaria RDTs into health systems has been largely dependent on the pre-existing emphasis on parasite-based diagnosis. Where microscopy had been extensively used as a near POC tool, such as certain countries in South-East Asia and South America, RDTs have provided a method to extend reach of rapid parasite-based diagnosis to more remote populations and to those presenting out-of-hours, while experience with the support structures for parasite-based diagnosis was to some extent in place. By contrast, in much of sub-Saharan Africa, the introduction of malaria RDTs has forced a greater rethink of health systems management. Because malaria RDTs were one of the first broadly used community level POC tests in low-resource settings, malaria programs have had to deal with the requirements of moving biohazard risk (finger-prick), waste-disposal, stock management, quality control and new levels of training and supervision to far more peripheral health staff than were previously deemed appropriate for such procedures (FIND 2013). In turn, the availability of new data on parasite prevalence and relative risk has placed pressure on central levels of health systems to cater for data transfer and the incorporation of data into health planning and strategy development. Budgeting for RDT implementation extends well beyond commodity procurement. The benefits accrued through this development should extend beyond malaria, because systems requirements for malaria diagnosis are common to a range of emerging diagnostics.

The program management and logistics systems required to implement RDT-based diagnosis also come at considerable cost. The cost–benefits of malaria RDT implementation are therefore complex. Although one of the early drivers of malaria RDT roll-out was the rising costs of drug therapy on ACT introduction, ACT costs can now be similar to those of RDTs when total costs of implementation are considered. Direct cost-effectiveness will therefore vary with test positivity rates. In very high transmission areas, the additional cost of a diagnostic will add less benefit, because most will go on to treatment. Where transmission is low, savings in drug costs will be far greater (Lubell *et al.* 2008; Shillcutt *et al.* 2008). These costs are sensitive to the threshold of clinical information on which a decision to test is based, as well as diagnostic and therapeutic costs, and to the costs that result from a negative diagnosis (i.e. management costs of non-malarial fever that would otherwise not have been incurred). The latter is difficult to quantify – both the causes of non-malarial fever and the ability to act on it vary across populations, as does the prior action that was undertaken before RDT introduction.

In many malaria endemic countries, a large proportion of management of acute fever takes place in the private sector. Although formal private sector clinics and hospitals can sometimes be well incorporated into public sector mechanisms, the informal private sector prevalent in many malaria-endemic countries – consisting of informal dispensaries and retail outlets – presents great challenges in management of diagnostic quality, biohazard and data management. A disincentive to parasite-based diagnosis and adherence to result is present when drug sales constitute a large proportion of the income of the provider. Although significant private sector diagnosis programs exist (Ansah *et al.* 2015; Khin *et al.* 2015;

Mbonye *et al.* 2015; Poyer *et al.* 2015), the requirements for quality control and oversight in the provision of a safe diagnostic program are perhaps more likely to stimulate efforts to reduce informal private sector involvement in malaria management and strengthening of alternative points of access.

Modelling of cost-effectiveness suggests that RDT introduction is beneficial in areas of low and medium prevalence (Lubell *et al.* 2008; Shillcutt *et al.* 2008), though these models cannot accurately reflect the less quantifiable costs of immediate non-malaria fever management, and still less tangible costs of failure to treat non-malarial fever and management of its sequelae. The WHO policy of parasite-based diagnosis is perhaps best justified not on an issue of direct costs, but on the assumed public-health good of identifying non-malaria cases for further investigation, provision of accurate data for planning and resource allocation, and the human right of people to have access to health and have control over it. None of these are to be under-estimated; while many health systems struggle to address diagnosis of other diseases or act on large datasets emerging from increased diagnostic use, the failure to provide the information on which appropriate management can be based will perpetuate poor management. The availability of accurate information is a necessary catalyst for change.

## CASE STUDY. CHANGING A DIAGNOSTIC CULTURE: THE INTRODUCTION OF POCT FOR MALARIA IN SENEGAL

Like most sub-Saharan countries with endemic malaria, Senegal had long practised presumptive diagnosis for malaria, treating cases of acute fever with antimalarial drugs on the basis of symptoms alone. Microscopy was limited to hospitals, and used in only 3.1% of suspected malaria cases in 2006. With a strong public health sector serving an estimated 75% of the population, over 1.5 million cases of malaria were reported that year, almost solely based on non-specific clinical diagnosis. The majority were treated with artimesinin-based combination therapy at a small fee to the patient, and significant burden to the malaria control program.

After a successful pilot, a systematically executed plan of RDT introduction was commenced in 2007, based around extensive training and a tightening of the clinical definition of suspected malaria, and use of RDTs that were quality controlled before distribution to more than 2500 health facilities across the country. By the end of 2009, 96% of suspected malaria cases were being tested, and only 31% of fever cases were now classified as malaria.

As RDT use was ramped up and provider and patient confidence built, ACT consumption in the public sector dropped from 68% of the total rate of malaria-like fever to closely track the frequency of positive test results 18 months into the roll-out. Total ACT consumption declined from ~625 000 courses in the 8 months of 2007 immediately preceding RDT introduction, to only 184 000 throughout the entire year of 2009, with reported malaria mortality also declining in the same period. Savings in antimalarial drug costs were estimated at more than US$1.5 million.

The program demonstrated what is possible at scale when introduction of a POC test is approached in a systematic manner and health worker and community confidence built. In doing so, it opened up both a challenge and an opportunity by revealing the hitherto overlooked burden of non-malarial febrile illness (Thiam *et al.* 2011).

## REFERENCES

Ansah EK, Narh-Bana S, Affran-Bonful H, Bart-Plange C, Cundill B, Gyapong M, *et al.* (2015) The impact of providing rapid diagnostic malaria tests on fever management in the private retail sector in Ghana: a cluster randomized trial. *British Medical Journal* **350**, h1019. doi:10.1136/bmj.h1019

Armstrong-Schellenberg JRM, Smith T, Alonso PL, Hayes RJ (1994) What is clinical malaria? Finding case definitions for field research in highly endemic areas. *Parasitology Today (Personal Ed.)* **10**, 439–442. doi:10.1016/0169-4758(94)90179-1

Bell D, Wongsrichanalai C, Barnwell JW (2006) Ensuring quality and access for malaria diagnosis: how can it be achieved? *Nature Reviews. Microbiology* **4**, S7–S20. doi:10.1038/nrmicro1525

Bisoffi Z, Sirima BS, Angheben A, Lodesani C, Gobbi F, Tinto H, *et al.* (2009) Rapid malaria diagnostic tests vs. clinical management of malaria in rural Burkina Faso: safety and effect on clinical decisions. A randomized trial. *Tropical Medicine & International Health* **14**, 491–498. doi:10.1111/j.1365-3156.2009.02246.x

Black RE, Cousens S, Johnson HL, Lawn JE, Rudan I, Bassani DG, *et al.* (2010) Global, regional, and national causes of child mortality in 2008: a systematic analysis. *Lancet* **375**, 1969–1987. doi:10.1016/S0140-6736(10)60549-1

Chandramohan D, Jaffar S, Greenwood B (2002) Use of clinical algorithms for diagnosing malaria. *Tropical Medicine & International Health* **7**, 45–52. doi:10.1046/j.1365-3156.2002.00827.x

Cheng Q, Cunningham J, Gatton ML (2015) Systematic review of sub-microscopic *P. vivax* infections: prevalence and determining factors. *PLoS Neglected Tropical Diseases* **9**, e3413. doi:10.1371/journal.pntd.0003413

Counihan H, Harvey SA, Sekeseke-Chinyama M, Hamainza B, Banda R, Malambo T, *et al.* (2012) Community health workers use Malaria Rapid Diagnostic Tests (RDTs) safely and accurately: results of a longitudinal study in Zambia. *The American Journal of Tropical Medicine and Hygiene* **87**, 57–63. doi:10.4269/ajtmh.2012.11-0800

Crump JA, Morrissey AB, Nicholson WL, Massung RF, Stoddard RA, Galloway RL, *et al.* (2013) Etiology of severe non-malaria febrile illness in Northern Tanzania: a prospective cohort study. *PLoS Neglected Tropical Diseases* **7**, e2324. doi:10.1371/journal.pntd.0002324

D'Acremont V, Lengeler C, Genton B (2010) Reduction in the proportion of fevers associated with *Plasmodium falciparum* parasitaemia in Africa: a systematic review. *Malaria Journal* **9**, 240. doi:10.1186/1475-2875-9-240

D'Acremont V, Kahama-Maro J, Swai N, Mtasiwa D, Genton B, Lengeler C (2011) Reduction of anti-malarial consumption after rapid diagnostic tests implementation in Dar es Salaam: a before-after and cluster randomized controlled study. *Malaria Journal* **10**, 107. doi:10.1186/1475-2875-10-107

Delahunt C, Horning MP, Wilson BK, Proctor JL, Hegg MC (2014) Limitations of haemozoin-based diagnosis of *Plasmodium falciparum* using dark-field microscopy. *Malaria Journal* **13**, 147.

FIND (Foundation for Innovative New Diagnostics) (2013) *Malaria Rapid Diagnostic Tests - An Implementation Guide*. Foundation for Innovative New Diagnostics, Geneva, Switzerland.

Gallup JL, Sachs JD (2001) The economic burden of malaria. *American Journal of Tropical Medicine and Hygiene* **64** (Supplement 1–2), 85–96.

Gamboa D, Ho MF, Bendezu J, Torres K, Chiodini PL, Barnwell JW, *et al.* (2010) A large proportion of *P. falciparum* isolates in the Amazon region of Peru lack *pfhrp2* and *pfhrp3*: implications for malaria rapid diagnostic tests. *PLoS One* **5**, e8091. doi:10.1371/journal.pone.0008091

Gillet P, Mori M, Van Esbroeck M, Van den Ende J, Jacobs J (2009) Assessment of the prozone effect in malaria rapid diagnostic tests. *Malaria Journal* **8**, 271. doi:10.1186/1475-2875-8-271

Gupta I, Chowdhury S (2014) Economic burden of malaria in India: the need for effective spending. *WHO South-East Asia Journal of Public Health* **3**, 95–102.

Hopkins H, Oyibo W, Luchavez J, Mationg ML, Asiimwe C, Albertini A, *et al.* (2011) Blood transfer devices for malaria rapid diagnostic tests: evaluation of accuracy, safety and ease of use. *Malaria Journal* **10**, 30. doi:10.1186/1475-2875-10-30

Humar A, Ohrt C, Harrington MA, Pillai D, Kain KC (1997) Parasight F test compared with the polymerase chain reaction and microscopy for the diagnosis of *Plasmodium falciparum* malaria in travelers. *The American Journal of Tropical Medicine and Hygiene* **56**, 44–48.

Imwong M, Nguyen T, Tripura R, Peto TJ, Lee SJ, Lwin KM, *et al.* (2015) The epidemiology of subclinical malaria infections in South-East Asia: findings from cross-sectional surveys in Thailand-Myanmar border areas, Cambodia, and Vietnam. *Malaria Journal* **14**, 381. doi:10.1186/s12936-015-0906-x

Jelinek T, Grobusch MP, Nothdurft HD (2000) Use of dipstick tests for the rapid diagnosis of malaria in nonimmune travelers. *Journal of Travel Medicine* **7**, 175–179. doi:10.2310/7060.2000.00055

Khin HS, Chen I, White C, Sudhinaraset M, McFarland W, Littrell M, *et al.* (2015) Availability and quality of anti-malarials among private sector outlets in Myanmar in 2012: results from a large, community-based, cross-sectional survey before a large-scale intervention. *Malaria Journal* **14**, 269. doi:10.1186/s12936-015-0778-0

Lee N, Baker J, Bell D, McCarthy J, Cheng Q (2006) Assessing the genetic diversity of the aldolase genes of *Plasmodium falciparum* and *Plasmodium vivax* and its potential effect on performance of aldolase-detecting rapid diagnostic tests. *Journal of Clinical Microbiology* **44**, 4547–4549. doi:10.1128/JCM.01611-06

Lubell Y, Reyburn H, Mbakilwa H, Mwangi R, Chonya S, Whitty CJ, Mills A (2008) The impact of response to the results of diagnostic tests for malaria: cost-benefit analysis. *British Medical Journal* **336**, 202–205. doi:10.1136/bmj.39395.696065.47

Luchavez J, Baker J, Alcantara S, Belizario V, Jr, Cheng Q, McCarthy JS, *et al.* (2011) Laboratory demonstration of a prozone-like effect in HRP2-detecting malaria rapid diagnostic tests: implications for clinical management. *Malaria Journal* **10**, 286.

malERA (Malaria Eradication Research Agenda) (2011) A research agenda for malaria eradication: diagnoses and diagnostics. *PLoS Medicine* **8**, e1000396.

Mariette N, Barnadas C, Bouchier C, Tichit M, Menard D (2008) Country-wide assessment of the genetic polymorphism in *Plasmodium falciparum* and *Plasmodium vivax* antigens detected with rapid diagnostic tests for malaria. *Malaria Journal* **7**, 219. doi:10.1186/1475-2875-7-219

Masaninga F, Sekeseke-Chinyama M, Malambo T, Moonga H, Babaniyi O, Counihan H, *et al.* (2012) Finding parasites and finding challenges: improved diagnostic access and trends in reported malaria and anti-malarial drug use in Livingstone district, Zambia. *Malaria Journal* **11**, 341. doi:10.1186/1475-2875-11-341

Mayxay M, Newton PN, Yeung S, Pongvongsa T, Phompida S, Phetsouvanh R, *et al.* (2004) Short communication: an assessment of the use of malaria rapid tests by village health volunteers in rural Laos. *Tropical Medicine & International Health* **9**, 325–329. doi:10.1111/j.1365-3156.2004.01199.x

Mayxay M, Castonguay-Vanier J, Chansamouth V, Dubot-Peres A, Paris D-H, Phetsouvanh R, *et al.* (2013) Causes of non-malarial fever in Laos: a prospective study. *The Lancet. Global Health* **1**, e46–e54. doi:10.1016/S2214-109X(13)70008-1

Mbonye AK, Clarke SE, Lal S, Chandler CI, Hutchinson E, Hansen KS, *et al.* (2015) Introducing rapid diagnostic tests for malaria into registered drug shops in Uganda: lessons learned and policy implications. *Malaria Journal* **14**, 448. doi:10.1186/s12936-015-0979-6

Mtove G, Hendriksen IC, Amos B, Mrema H, Mandia V, Manjurano A, *et al.* (2011) Treatment guided by rapid diagnostic tests for malaria in Tanzanian children: safety and alternative bacterial diagnoses. *Malaria Journal* **10**, 290. doi:10.1186/1475-2875-10-290

Odaga J, Sinclair D, Lokong JA, Donegan S, Hopkins H, Garner P (2014) Rapid diagnostic tests versus clinical diagnosis for managing people with fever in malaria endemic settings. *Cochrane Database of Systematic Reviews* **4**, CD008998.

Okell LC, Ghani AC, Lyons E, Drakeley CJ (2009) Submicroscopic infection in *Plasmodium falciparum*-endemic populations: a systematic review and meta-analysis. *The Journal of Infectious Diseases* **200**, 1509–1517. doi:10.1086/644781

Premji Z, Minjas JN, Shiff CJ (1994) Laboratory diagnosis of malaria by village health workers using the rapid manual ParaSight-F test. *Transactions of the Royal Society of Tropical Medicine and Hygiene* **88**, 418.

Poyer S, Shewchuk T, Tougher S, Ye Y, Mann AG, Willey BA, *et al.* (2015) Availability and price of malaria rapid diagnostic tests in the public and private health sectors in 2011: results from 10 nationally representative cross-sectional retail surveys. *Tropical Medicine & International Health* **20**, 744–756. doi:10.1111/tmi.12491

Rennie W, Phetsouvanh R, Lupisan S, Vanisaveth V, Hongvanthong B, Phompida S, *et al.* (2007) Minimising human error in malaria rapid diagnosis: clarity of written instructions and health worker performance. *Transactions of the Royal Society of Tropical Medicine and Hygiene* **101**, 9–18. doi:10.1016/j.trstmh.2006.03.011

Reyburn H, Mbatia R, Drakeley C, Carneiro I, Mwakasungula E, Mwerinde O, *et al.* (2004) Overdiagnosis of malaria in patients with severe febrile illness in Tanzania: a prospective study. *British Medical Journal* **329**, 1212. doi:10.1136/bmj.38251.658229.55

Reyburn H, Mbakilwa H, Mwangi R, Mwerinde O, Olomi R, Drakeley C, *et al.* (2007) Rapid diagnostic tests compared with malaria microscopy for guiding outpatient treatment of febrile illness in Tanzania: randomised trial. *British Medical Journal* **334**, 403. doi:10.1136/bmj.39073.496829.AE

Senn N, Rarau P, Manong D, Salib M, Siba P, Robinson LJ, *et al.* (2011) Rapid diagnostic test-based management of malaria: an effectiveness study in Papua New Guinean infants with Plasmodium falciparum and Plasmodium vivax malaria. *Clinical Infectious Diseases* **54**, 644–651. doi:10.1093/cid/cir901

Shiff CJ, Premji Z, Minjas JN (1993) The rapid manual ParaSight-F test. A new diagnostic tool for Plasmodium falciparum infection. *Transactions of the Royal Society of Tropical Medicine and Hygiene* **87**(6), 646–648.

Shiff CJ, Minjas J, Premji Z (1994) The ParaSight(R)-F test: A simple rapid manual dipstick test to detect Plasmodium falciparum infection. *Parasitology Today (Personal Ed.)* **10**, 494–495. doi:10.1016/0169-4758(94)90164-3

Shillcutt S, Morel C, Goodman C, Coleman P, Bell D, Whitty CJ, *et al.* (2008) Cost-effectiveness of malaria diagnostic methods in sub-Saharan Africa in an era of combination therapy. *Bulletin of the World Health Organization* **86**, 101–110. doi:10.2471/BLT.07.042259

Talman AM, Duval L, Legrand E, Hubert V, Yen S, Bell D, *et al.* (2007) Evaluation of the intra- and inter-specific genetic variability of Plasmodium lactate dehydrogenase. *Malaria Journal* **6**, 140. doi:10.1186/1475-2875-6-140

Thiam S, Thior M, Faye B, Ndiop M, Diouf ML, Diouf MB, *et al.* (2011) Major reduction in anti-malarial drug consumption in Senegal after nation-wide introduction of malaria rapid diagnostic tests. *PLoS One* **6**, e18419. doi:10.1371/journal.pone.0018419

WHO (World Health Organization) (2000) 'New perspectives: malaria diagnosis'. Report of a joint WHO/USAID informal consultation 25–27 October 1999. WHO, Geneva, Switzerland.

WHO (2004) *The Use of Malaria Rapid Diagnostic Tests.* WHO Regional Office for the Western Pacific, Manila, Philippines.

WHO (2010a) *Guidelines for the Treatment of Malaria.* 2nd edn. WHO, Geneva, Switzerland.

WHO (2010b) 'Parasitological confirmation of malaria diagnosis'. Report of a WHO technical consultation Geneva, 6–8 October 2009. WHO, Geneva, Switzerland.

WHO (2015a) 'World malaria report, 2015'. WHO, Geneva, Switzerland.

WHO (2015b) *Guidelines for the Treatment of Malaria.* 3rd edn. WHO, Geneva, Switzerland.

WHO-FIND-CDC (2015) *Malaria Rapid Diagnostic Test Performance: Results of WHO Product Testing of Malaria RDTs: Round 6 (2014–2015).* WHO, Geneva, Switzerland.

WHO-FIND-CDC-HTD (2013) *Methods Manual for Product Testing of Malaria Rapid Diagnostic Tests (Version 5).* WHO, Geneva, Switzerland.

WHO-TDR-FIND (2010) *Methods Manual for Laboratory Quality Control Testing of Malaria Rapid Diagnostic Tests, (Version 6).* WHO, Geneva, Switzerland.

WHO-WPRO (2003) *Malaria Rapid Diagnosis: Making it Work.* Meeting report, 20–23 January. Report No. RS/2003/GE/05(PHL). WHO Regional Office for the Western Pacific, Manila, Philippines.

Yukich JO, Bennett A, Albertini A, Incardona S, Moonga H, Chisha Z, *et al.* (2012) Reductions in artemisinin-based combination therapy consumption after the nationwide scale up of routine malaria rapid diagnostic testing in Zambia. *The American Journal of Tropical Medicine and Hygiene* **87**, 437–446. doi:10.4269/ajtmh.2012.12-0127

# 23 Point-of-care testing for active tuberculosis

*Catherine Hogan and Madhukar Pai*

**Summary**

The incidence of tuberculosis declined throughout the 20th century but there has been a resurgence of the disease and it remains a significant cause of morbidity and mortality that disproportionately affects the poor. The recent introduction of molecular testing on the Cepheid GeneXpert® has facilitated a paradigm shift in tuberculosis diagnostics by allowing same-day diagnosis of tuberculosis with very high sensitivity, as well as simultaneous detection of rifampicin resistance; it has also inspired the development of new molecular tests that are likely to be affordable in decentralised settings. Tuberculosis point-of-care testing (POCT) alone will not have a clinical impact, unless rapid treatment is also ensured. Tuberculosis POCT must be delivered as part of an integrated package of 'test and treat' and not as a standalone test.

## INTRODUCTION

Infection with *Mycobacterium tuberculosis* has afflicted mankind for centuries. The incidence of tuberculosis progressively declined throughout the 20th century; however, lack of sustained control efforts has led to a resurgence of the disease. Major challenges to the control of the disease include proper diagnosis and management of multidrug-resistant tuberculosis (MDR-TB) as well as TB-HIV co-infection.

### Global burden of tuberculosis

Despite improvements in diagnosis and treatment modalities in the last decades, tuberculosis remains a significant cause of morbidity and mortality that disproportionately affects the poor. Tuberculosis ranks second only to HIV as the leading cause of death due to a single infectious agent. In 2014, an estimated 9.6 million people were infected with tuberculosis, of whom 1.1 million were co-infected with HIV (WHO 2015a). Despite the reduction in mortality rates since 1990, 1.5 million deaths were attributable to tuberculosis in 2014. This figure remains unacceptably high, given that most of these are preventable deaths.

The highest burden of tuberculosis in absolute numbers is concentrated in two countries: India and China, with 24% and 11% of the total burden, respectively. Diagnosis of MDR-TB, defined as resistance to isoniazid and rifampicin, is on the rise, with 480 000 incident cases diagnosed in 2014. However, 3.6 of the 9.6 million new cases a year are considered 'missing', owing to either lack of diagnosis or lack of reporting of diagnosed cases. Moreover, of the 4.9 million cases of pulmonary tuberculosis reported in 2014, only 58% were confirmed microbiologically (smear or culture-positive, or positive with a World Health Organization (WHO)-endorsed test such as Xpert® MTB/RIF); the remainder were either diagnosed empirically or with chest X-ray.

## Pathophysiology

*Mycobacterium tuberculosis* is an acid-fast bacillus that is acquired by the inhalation of airborne droplet nuclei. Transmission occurs when an individual inhales *M. tuberculosis* droplet nuclei that traverse the respiratory tract and are deposited in the alveoli. In immunocompetent individuals, the bacilli are then engulfed by macrophages, where they may or not be destroyed depending on host and bacterial factors (Canadian Thoracic Society 2013).

Following primary infection, ~5% of exposed individuals will develop primary disease within a few months. The bacilli may then spread through the lymphatic and circulatory systems, with resultant metastatic spread. In the remaining 95%, the organism will remain dormant as latent tuberculosis infection (LTBI). It is estimated that one-third of the world's population is latently infected with tuberculosis. Overall, an estimated 5% of people infected with LTBI will reactivate in their lifetime. This risk is greatest in the first 18 months after primary infection. These risks vary widely according to several host factors that are discussed below.

It is widely thought that cell-mediated immunity is responsible for maintaining latency, mainly through its T-cell (Th1) and macrophage responses. The immune response results in the formation of granulomas (well circumscribed collections of inflammatory cells) that serve to contain the organism and prevent its further spread. This mechanism falters in those with depressed immune responses, such as those with HIV co-infection and deficient CD4 T lymphocytes (Lawn and Zumla 2011).

## Risk factors

There are many risk factors for the acquisition of tuberculosis. They can be broadly divided into the major social determinants of health (e.g. poverty, education, access to health care and housing), as well as host, pathogen and environmental factors. Increased risk of transmission has been documented with crowded living conditions, poor ventilation, air pollution and smoking. Similarly, HIV, malnutrition, diabetes and alcohol consumption have also been linked to an increased risk of tuberculosis transmission (Canadian Thoracic Society 2013).

There are now many risk factors identified for the progression of latent to active tuberculosis, most of which depend on the host's immune status. The strongest risk factor for reactivation is AIDS, with a disease risk of up to 10% per year.

## Symptoms

The most common site of predilection for tuberculosis is the lung (pulmonary tuberculosis, which accounts for ~80% of all TB cases), whereby symptoms of cough, dyspnoea and haemoptysis dominate the clinical picture. These are often accompanied by constitutional symptoms with fever, weight loss and night sweats. However, tuberculosis may affect practically any other organ (extrapulmonary tuberculosis), leading to a wide variety of symptoms, depending on the affected site. Among extrapulmonary presentations, TB lymphadenitis and pleural TB are the most common. Moreover, there has been increasing recognition through active case-finding of a category of early sub-clinical active disease that is asymptomatic, especially in people living with HIV (Agizew *et al.* 2010). These cases represent a greater challenge for the recognition and diagnosis of tuberculosis.

## Treatment

Treatment for tuberculosis invariably involves a combination of antimicrobials to prevent emergence of drug resistance and limit onward transmission of the infection. According to WHO guidelines, standard first-line therapy for drug-susceptible tuberculosis consists of an intensive phase of 2 months of isonazid, rifampicin, pyrazinamide and ethambutol, followed by a maintenance phase of 4 months of isoniazid and rifampicin. Treatment success rates of new drug-susceptible tuberculosis reach ≥85%. Drug regimens for multidrug-resistant tuberculosis are complex, and treatment duration can exceed 24 months.

As advocated by the WHO End TB Strategy, universal drug-susceptibility testing should be performed in all patients at the time of diagnosis to quickly identify resistance and tailor therapy (WHO 2015b). Unfortunately, in many low-income settings, patients with resistant tuberculosis are only diagnosed as such once they fail first-line therapy, which contributes to mounting drug resistance and lower treatment success rates.

## Diagnosis

Smear microscopy remains the most widely used diagnostic test worldwide in the evaluation of suspected tuberculosis, despite its important performance limitations. There have been improvements in the tuberculosis diagnostic strategies in the last decade, including fluorescence microscopy (10% increase in sensitivity over conventional Ziehl-Neelsen smear microscopy method), and automated liquid culture (faster and increased yield compared to solid culture). However, smear microscopy has limited sensitivity, and most programs require at least two sputum samples to be analysed by smears. Liquid cultures have a 2–3 week turnaround time, which limits the clinical impact. Moreover, higher costs associated with cultures and requirement for biosafety level 3 (BSL-3) laboratories reduce access in low-income settings.

There is a pressing need to develop point-of-care (POC) tests that can rapidly make the diagnosis of tuberculosis and identify drug resistance, at the time of diagnosis, to ensure rapid initiation of treatment that is guided by drug-susceptibility testing (DST) results.

## POCT OPTIONS TO DIAGNOSE ACTIVE TUBERCULOSIS

POCT has already been defined in this book as 'testing performed in a clinical setting at the time of patient consultation, generating a rapid test result that enables timely clinical action for patient care.' Moreover, desirable characteristics for POCT have so far largely been 'product-dominated' as detailed in the 'ASSURED' acronym: affordable, sensitive, specific, user-friendly, rapid/robust, equipment-free and deliverable (WHO 2004).

Some have advocated for a more goal-oriented definition of POCT, whereby the test would be evaluated against its intended purpose and ability to enable completion of the 'test-and-treat' loop in a short timeframe (ideally, in the same clinical encounter) as opposed to the sole characteristics of the technology (Pai *et al.* 2015). As such, POCT should be viewed as a spectrum that integrates testing within an enabling health system, and POC testing can be carried out in a variety of settings (Fig. 23.1).

Despite significant effort and investment, there is currently no tuberculosis test that satisfies all of the POCT criteria listed above. Nonetheless, there are technologies that partially fulfil this description. For example, smear microscopy is an affordable, specific and relatively

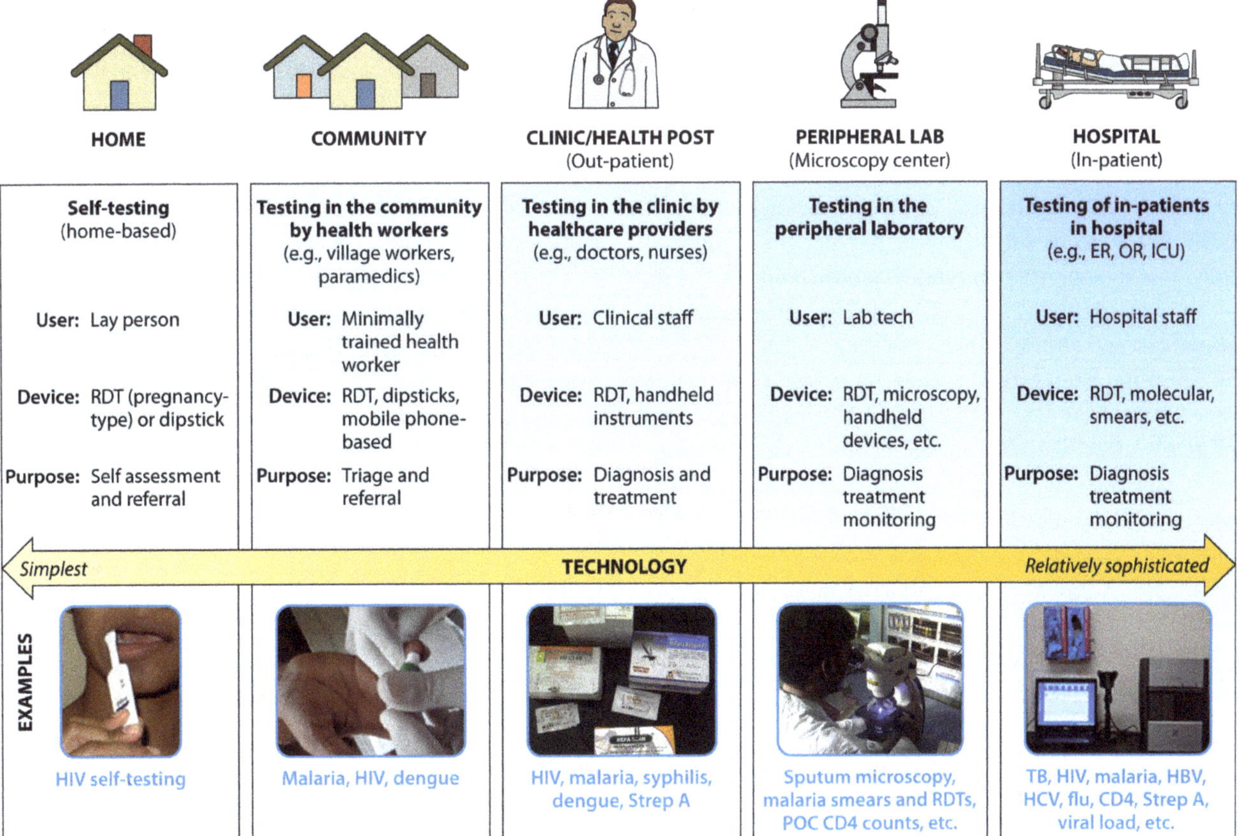


**Fig. 23.1.** The spectrum of test-and-treat as applied to tuberculosis and other infectious diseases. (Source: adapted from Pai *et al.* 2012)

user-friendly technique that can be used to diagnose a patient with smear-positive tuberculosis on the first clinical encounter, prompting same-day start of therapy. However, its poor sensitivity requires at least two smears to be performed. This usually means that a patient has to come back the next day, and pre-treatment losses to follow-up are well documented (MacPherson *et al.* 2014). To overcome this issue, the WHO published a policy in 2011 that allows for same-day smear microscopy (WHO 2011a). So, this policy allows health systems to collect two spot samples that can be subjected to microscopy, and a patient could potentially be initiated on treatment on the same day. In practice, most health-care systems have not managed to implement and scale-up same-day smear microscopy. Thus, the POCT potential of smear microscopy is not fully realised.

Similarly, the recent introduction of the Xpert® MTB/RIF assay (Cepheid Inc., Sunnyvale CA, USA) enabled a major paradigm shift in tuberculosis diagnostics in allowing same-day diagnosis of tuberculosis with greater sensitivity than smear as well as simultaneous detection of rifampicin resistance. However, it remains a test that is much more expensive than smear microscopy. In addition, infrastructural requirements, such as continuous power and temperature control, have largely confined its use to district-level or reference laboratories. Some projects have attempted the use of the Xpert MTB/RIF as POC tests to permit same-day diagnosis and treatment (Hanrahan *et al.* 2015; Schumacher *et al.* 2015; Theron *et al.* 2014; Van Rie *et al.* 2013). These projects suggest that it is feasible in some settings to implement the Xpert as a POC test to support same-day diagnosis and treatment. However, such POCT implementation requires additional resources, and clinical impact has been variable.

There has been greatly renewed interest in developing new tuberculosis diagnostics in the last decade in the area of POCT as evidenced by a very active product development pipeline (Fig. 23.2). Evidence-based target product profiles (TPPs) have been published for many types of diagnostic tests to guide product developers (Denkinger *et al.* 2015; Kik *et al.* 2014). This chapter will discuss the main POC tests available as well as technologies currently in the developmental pipeline.

## METHOD PRINCIPLE – POCT

### Smear microscopy

The most basic POCT for tuberculosis, smear microscopy, has been in use for over a century and remains the most widely used test for the diagnosis of tuberculosis worldwide. The patient's sputum is collected, spread on a slide, stained and examined under the microscope for the detection of mycobacteria. The Ziehl-Neelsen staining technique is quick, inexpensive and specific. However, low sensitivity (50–60%) means that almost half of the cases of tuberculosis are missed. Sensitivity is even lower in children and cases of HIV-TB co-infection and extrapulmonary tuberculosis due to the low number of bacilli in the sputum. Another major limitation of microscopy is the inability to detect drug resistance.

Where available, WHO-endorsed light-emitting diode (LED) microscopy with auramine staining offers a 10% increment in sensitivity (with preserved specificity) and up to four times faster reading than conventional smear microscopy (Steingart *et al.* 2006). It is recommended that at least two sputum samples be collected to increase sensitivity; this implies the patient must return for the collection of repeat sputum samples. Front-loaded microscopy, another WHO-endorsed approach, has provided an advantage in allowing two spot sputum sample collections to take place on the same day. This provides an important advantage in reducing loss to follow-up at the cost of slightly reduced sensitivity. Automated microscopy systems are also in development for use in peripheral settings. Regardless of the specific technique employed, smear microscopy needs to be followed by culture and drug-susceptibility testing. The current reference standard for the diagnosis of tuberculosis is liquid culture, which takes 2–3 weeks to produce results.

Delay in tuberculosis diagnosis and loss to follow-up of active tuberculosis cases spur onward transmission of the organism and contribute to disease burden. Even in smear-positive cases, there can be an important delay in the start of treatment, as documented in India (Sreeramareddy *et al.* 2014) and South Africa (Claassens *et al.* 2013). The objective of a POC test for tuberculosis is to provide same-day diagnosis with upfront drug susceptibility testing and rapid initiation of treatment – goals that currently cannot be met with microscopy alone, or with liquid cultures.

### Nucleic acid amplification tests

The nucleic acid amplification tests (NAAT) are most commonly based on polymerase chain reaction (PCR) technology. There are now many such tests commercially available for the diagnosis of tuberculosis; however, only three have been endorsed by the WHO: GenoType

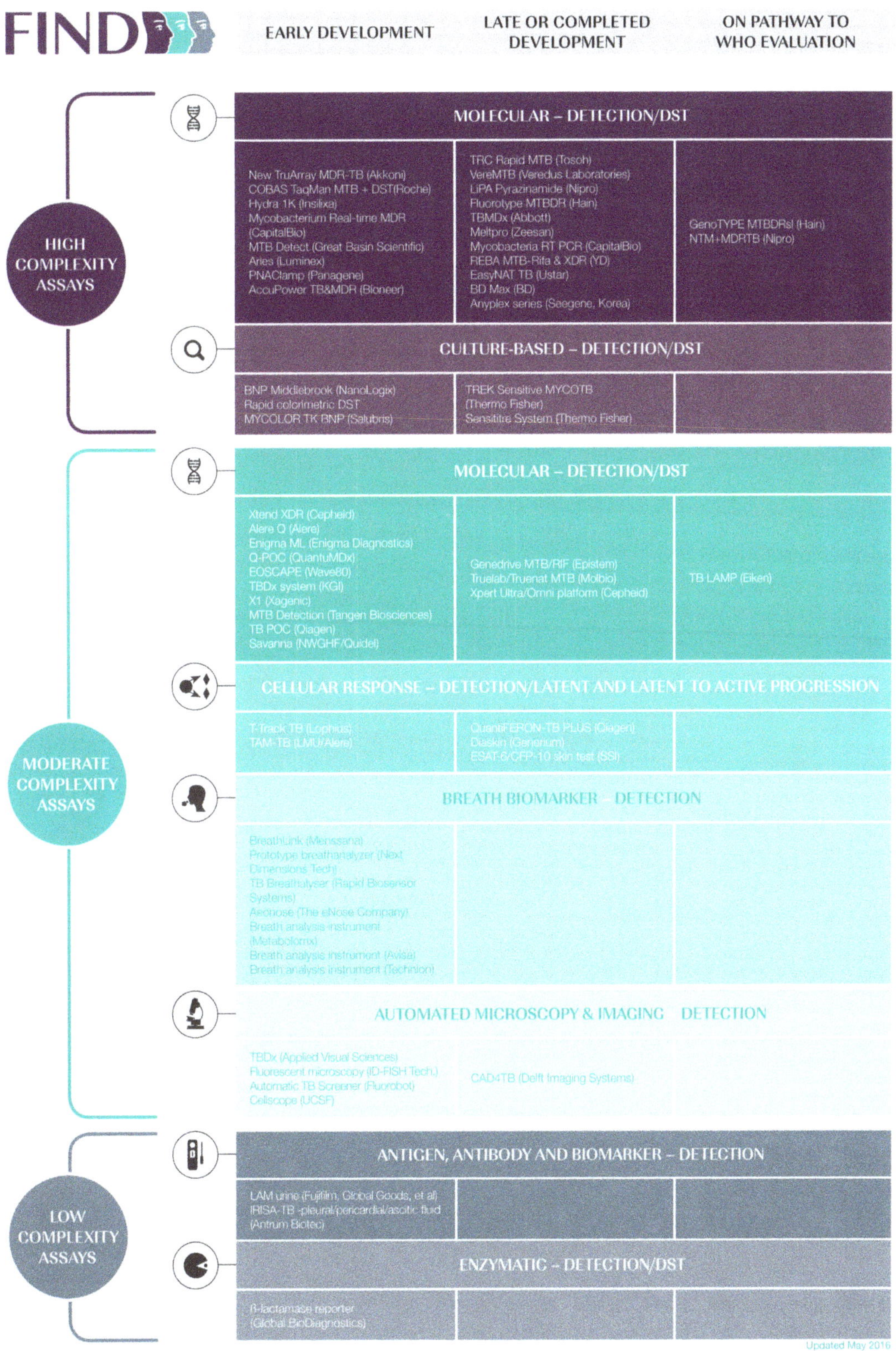


**Fig. 23.2.** Global tuberculosis diagnostic pipeline by level of complexity (as defined by US Food and Administration criteria for similar diagnostics) and stage of development. Early development refers to product development after the proof of concept, whereas late development refers to a product ready for manufacture. (Source: UNITAID 2015. Reproduced with permission).

MTBDR*plus* (Hain Lifesciences, Germany), Nipro NTM +MDRB assay (Nipro Corporation, Japan), and Xpert® MTB/RIF (Cepheid Inc., USA). Of these, the GenoType MTBDR*plus* and Nipro assay are line-probe assays that are intended for the rapid detection of rifampicin conferring mutations in acid-fast bacilli (AFB) smear-positive samples and positive cultures. The WHO does not recommend the use of line probe assays (LPAs) in AFB smear-negative samples. In contrast, Xpert® MTB/RIF can be used on all persons with suspected TB, and can be used for detection, as well as rifampicin resistance screening. Also, although LPAs are intended for sophisticated, reference laboratories, Xpert can be used in more decentralised settings (i.e. closer to POC).

NAATs have revolutionised the diagnosis of tuberculosis and other infectious diseases, with rapid turnaround time owing to the detection of even small quantities of DNA of organisms present in the sample (Dheda *et al.* 2013). The current NAAT tuberculosis diagnostics pipeline is quite robust and reflects the dynamic interest in the field; however, there are very limited options geared towards peripheral microscopy centres (Fig. 23.3).

#### Xpert® MTB/RIF

The Xpert® MTB/RIF assay was endorsed by the WHO in 2010 and has since been rolled out worldwide, changing the landscape of tuberculosis diagnostics. The technology is based on an automated, nested polymerase chain reaction (PCR) platform that detects *M. tuberculosis* DNA and resistance to rifampicin with a turnaround time of <2 h. The Xpert® MTB/RIF detects rifampicin resistance through the use of nucleic acid probes termed molecular beacons that can detect the presence of the rifampicin susceptible *rpoB* gene of tuberculosis (Lawn and Nicol 2011). Expectorated sputum is first homogenised and incubated with a sample buffer that homogenises the mixture and inactivates viable mycobacterium bacilli within 15 min. A 2-mL volume of the mixture is then pipetted into the single-use cartridge and loaded onto the platform for run initiation.

The WHO now estimates that over 21 000 modules and 16 million cartridges have been procured by concessional pricing since its approval. The system has proven particularly interesting because it does not require highly skilled technicians and is geared towards the more peripheral centres. Nonetheless, its use in the field has predominantly been based in district-level and reference laboratories.

*Evidence base*

A 2014 Cochrane systematic review synthesised the large evidence base on the accuracy of the Xpert® MTB/RIF (Steingart *et al.* 2014). When used as an initial diagnostic test for tuberculosis diagnosis, Xpert® MTB/RIF achieved a pooled sensitivity of 88% and specificity of 98% compared with culture. The pooled sensitivity was lower in smear-negative, culture-positive cases (68%) and in people living with HIV (80%), and was higher in smear-positive, culture-positive cases (98%). The performance for the detection of rifampicin resistance through the *rpoB* mutation in the same meta-analysis showed a pooled sensitivity of 95% and specificity of 98%. Sensitivity was more prone to variability at low levels of rifampicin resistance. The evidence on Xpert MTB/RIF has also been summarised in systematic reviews for extrapulmonary TB (Denkinger *et al.* 2014) and paediatrics (Detjen *et al.* 2015).

Recent studies have considered the use of Xpert® MTB/RIF in decentralised settings, an advantage made possible through the lack of need of highly skilled users to operate the technology. In southern Africa, implementation of the technology at the primary-care health-care level resulted in a greater number of patients on treatment and reduced the time to treatment (Hanrahan *et al.* 2015; Theron *et al.* 2014). However, these benefits were not associated with improvements in tuberculosis-related morbidity or mortality, largely owing to empiric treatment regardless of the test result. The drivers of such empiric treatment are complex and stem from multiple factors at the provider and infrastructure levels (Engel *et al.* 2015).

*Cost-effectiveness*

Cost-effectiveness analyses of the implementation of Xpert® MTB/RIF have been conducted in both high- and low-burden settings. Based on decision analytic modelling from India, South Africa and Uganda, Xpert® MTB/RIF was found to be cost-effective as an add-on test to smear microscopy and clinical diagnosis (Vassall *et al.* 2011). In the USA, tuberculosis diagnostics algorithms that included Xpert® MTB/RIF were considered highly cost-effective compared with testing with smear microscopy and culture alone, and improved health outcomes (Choi *et al.* 2013).

#### Line-probe assays

The line-probe assay (LPA) is a NAAT technology that was endorsed by the WHO in 2008 (and reviewed in 2015)

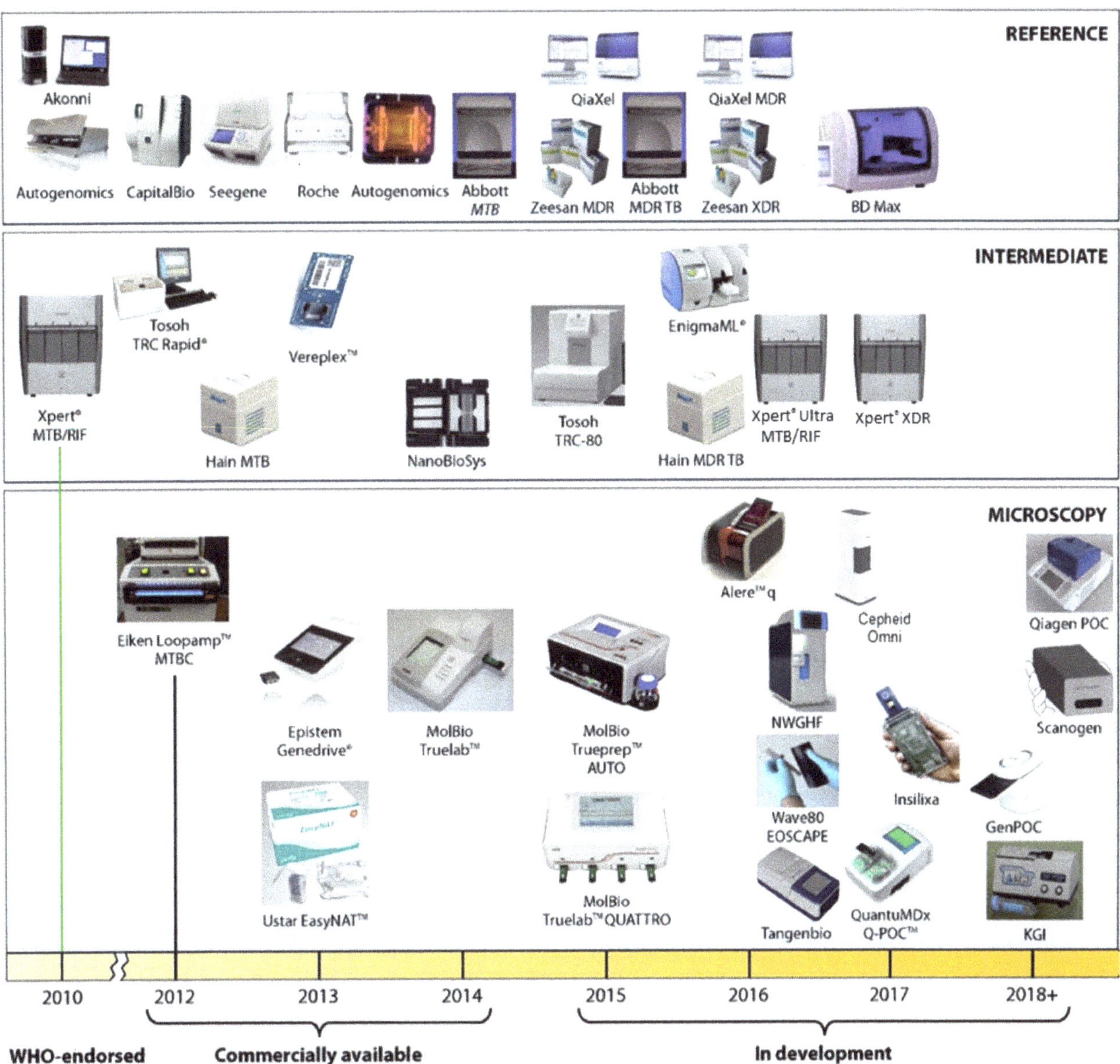


**Fig. 23.3.** Global tuberculosis nucleic acid amplification test (NAAT) diagnostic pipeline by target laboratory level of use and predicted time of market entry. (Source: UNITAID 2015. Reproduced with permission)

and that is suited for use by reference laboratories. The first-line drug LPA (GenoType MTBDR*plus*®, HAIN Lifescience, Germany) uses a DNA strip test that can detect both *M. tuberculosis* as well as the most common resistance genes for rifampicin and isoniazid, with a turnaround time of <5 h. The WHO recently recommended the two versions of the GenoType MTBDRplus assay, as well as another LPA called Nipro NTM+MDRB assay by Nipro Corporation, Japan. A second-line drug LPA (GenoType MTBDR*sl*®, HAIN Lifescience, Germany) designed to differentiate extensively drug resistant (XDR)-TB from MDR-TB is also under study, although it has not been recommended as a replacement for conventional drug susceptibility testing.

#### LAMP (loop-mediated isothermal amplification)

The Loopamp™ MTBC assay (Eiken Chemical Co., Japan) is a tuberculosis-specific NAAT that uses a fluorescent visual readout with high-throughput and a <2-h turnaround time. *M. tuberculosis* is identified when LED-read samples turn fluorescent green, indicating DNA amplification. It requires minimal instrumentation, and sample processing and analysis is not automated the way Xpert MTB/RIF is. However, user training takes 2 days because important user contribution is required for sample preparation and interpretation of the test result. The performance of the LAMP assay compared to LED microscopy and to Xpert MTB/RIF® was investigated in 14 countries in collaboration with the Foundation for Innovative New Diagnostics (FIND). Data from these studies were reviewed by a WHO expert group in June 2015; recommendations regarding its use are forthcoming.

### Biomarker-based tests

Antibody-based assays for TB (ELISA, as well as lateral flow assays) are commercially available, but none of them are accurate enough for clinical use (Steingart *et al.* 2011). In a 2011 policy, the WHO discouraged their use, but encouraged R&D in this area because of the potential to develop a simple, instrument-free rapid test (WHO 2011b).

Antigen-detection-based tests are appealing because they can be rapid, inexpensive and easier to perform. However, finding the optimal biomarker and cut-off values have represented a significant challenge in developing these tests.

#### Urine LAM assay

LAM (lipoarabinomannan) is an immunogenic glycolipid component of the *M. tuberculosis* cell wall. As part of the lateral flow urinary LAM assay, it has been the most studied tuberculosis antigen so far and represents the only available biomarker-based commercial test (Alere Determine™ TB LAM Ag, USA). Its utility has been hampered by limited sensitivity, with values ranging from 23 to 84%, with specificity ranging from 75 to 99% (WHO 2015c). It performs best in detecting smear-negative tuberculosis in individuals with HIV and advanced immunosuppression. In 2015, the WHO published its policy on urine LAM lateral flow tests (WHO 2015c) in which it recommended the test for persons with HIV with a CD4 count <100 or who are seriously ill, a subgroup a patients that is difficult to diagnose with existing methods. In contrast, it recommended against the use of urine LAM as a screening test for TB.

#### β-lactamase detection

The *M. tuberculosis* complex almost universally possesses β-lactamase, which might have some potential as a triage test for tuberculosis (Cheng *et al.* 2014). Global Bio Diagnostics (GBDbio, USA) and partners are currently developing a sputum-based assay that detects TB blaC as a biomarker for active tuberculosis, the GBD TB REaD™ POC test. This assay is meant for use at the community level and prospective studies are underway to evaluate its performance.

A comparison of some of the diagnostic test options for tuberculosis is provided in Table 23.1.

Other methods for detecting tuberculosis include breath testing and digital chest X-rays.

### Breath test

A rapid breath test based on the detection of labelled volatile organic compounds represents another potential approach to the rapid screening of tuberculosis (Choi *et al.* 2014). There are many breath tests in development including the eNose (eNose Co., the Netherlands and Nanosynth, USA) and TB Breathalyser (Rapid Biosensor Systems Ltd, UK). Validation studies are underway for the eNose device in many countries. Similarly, a non-governmental organisation (APOPO, Belgium) has trained giant-pouched rats to screen sputum samples to detect tuberculosis with reasonable accuracy (Reither *et al.* 2015). Work is underway in Tanzania and Mozambique to evaluate potential use of this detection system.

### Digital chest X-ray

The use of computer-aided digital chest X-ray interpretation has been proposed as a new means to screen for tuberculosis with decreased reliance on infrastructure and highly trained personnel to interpret the images. Chest X-rays have high sensitivity for TB, but modest specificity. Thus, their role is to triage patients who will benefit from confirmatory testing. Currently, there is only one tuberculosis-specific software platform available, the CAD4TB (DIAG and Delft Imaging Systems, Netherlands). This software analyses abnormalities consistent with tuberculosis and assigns a score ranging from 0 to 100 in 1 min. The technology in this field remains expensive and relatively complex in design (FIND 2015). Ongoing work in this area will have to focus on the development of a solid, portable and completely digital chest X-ray solution to fully leverage the potential of this diagnostic test.

## DISCUSSION

The past decade has seen considerable progress in the development and use of new TB diagnostics, and rapid

Table 23.1. Comparison of diagnostic tests for tuberculosis

| Technology | LED fluorescence smear microscopy | Liquid culture with DST (BACTEC 960/ MGIT) | Xpert® MTB/ RIF | Line probe assay (GenoType MTBDRplus) | Loopamp™ MTBC assay | LAM lateral flow assay |
|---|---|---|---|---|---|---|
| Method principle | Direct visualisation of mycobacteria | Conventional mycobacterial culture | NAAT (qPCR) | NAAT (LPA) | NAAT (LAMP) | Antigen detection |
| Use | MTB diagnosis | MTB diagnosis and rif resistance | MTB diagnosis and rif resistance | MTB diagnosis and rif and INH resistance | MTB diagnosis | MTB diagnosis |
| Sensitivity | 52–97% (SSM+/C+) | 89% (SSM+/C+) 73% (SSM-/C+) | 98% (SSM+/C+) 67% (SSM-/C+) Rif resistance: 95% | 98% (rif resistant); 84% (INH resistant) | 80% (pooled) | 44% (pooled) (C+/Xpert+); 54% (HIV+ inpatients) |
| Specificity | 94–100% (SSM-/C-) | >99% (SSM-/C-) | 99% (SSM-/C-) Rif resistance: 98% | 99% (rif resistant); >99% (INH resistant) | 96% (pooled) | 92% (pooled) (C-/ Xpert-); 90% (HIV+ inpatients) |
| Endorsed by WHO (year) | Yes (2009) | Yes (2007) | Yes (2010) | Yes (2008) | No | Conditional recommendations (2015) |
| Target setting of use | Peripheral/ reference laboratory | Reference laboratory | District or sub-district laboratory | Reference laboratory | Peripheral laboratory | Peripheral laboratory |
| Turnaround time | 10 min[a] | 10–21 days | <2 h | 5 h[a] | <2 h | 25 min |
| Amenable to rapid test-and-treat? | Yes | No | Yes | No | Yes | Yes |
| Reference | Steingart *et al.* 2006 | Cruciani *et al.* 2004 | Steingart *et al.* 2014 | Ling *et al.* 2008 | Yuan *et al.* 2014 | WHO 2015c |

Note: LED: light-emitting diode; MGIT: mycobacteria growth indicator tube; DST: drug susceptibility testing; LAM: lipoarabinomannan; NAAT: nucleic acid amplification test; PCR: polymerase chain reaction; LPA: line probe assay; LAMP: loop amplification; MTB: Mycobacterium tuberculosis; rif: rifampicin; INH: isoniazid; SSM: Sputum smear microscopy; C: culture; HIV: human immunodeficiency virus; WHO: World Health Organization [a]May require longer turnaround time due to batching of specimens

molecular tests such as Xpert and LPA have greatly improved the detection of drug-resistant TB. However, the TB community is still waiting for a rapid, simple, instrument-free test that can be done in a primary care setting.

The success of Xpert MTB/RIF has inspired the development of several new molecular tests, including those aimed at microscopy centres (UNITAID 2015). Unfortunately, the development of new molecular tests has not been accompanied by the high-quality validation field studies that are essential to justify policy endorsements. Developers are often small companies that lack the funding and support to ensure proper evaluation and subsequent scale-up of their technology. By contrast, larger companies such as Cepheid have marketed their technology for tuberculosis as a test that fits onto an existing PCR platform; future use of these tests may thus be envisioned as multiplex panels including combined rapid testing for HIV and TB.

Better tools are needed to tackle the challenge of diagnosis of MDR-TB and paucibacillary disease. For example, the Xpert® MTB/RIF assay is being improved to increase the sensitivity of its detection (Xpert MTB/RIF Ultra) and to add detection of resistance to other drugs (Xpert XDR). A more portable, battery-powered version of the GeneXpert device, called GeneXpert OMNI, is also being released in 2017 to facilitate use in peripheral settings. Many other PCR-based platforms are also in development to increase throughput, integrate reflexive drug-susceptibility testing to first-line drugs and to expand drug-susceptibility testing to second-line drugs. These tests need to be developed in convergence with the new tuberculosis drugs, including delamanid and bedaquiline, and drug regimens under trial (e.g. PaMZ). In parallel, although not covered specifically in this chapter, better diagnostic methods are also needed for the detection of latent tuberculosis infection.

Finally, a major concern of the POCT applied to tuberculosis is that testing alone will not have a clinical impact, unless rapid treatment is also ensured. It is essential that treatment capacity be scaled-up in parallel to the use of new technologies to ensure diagnosis translates to better clinical outcomes for patients. More specifically, as argued by some in the field, the time has come to look beyond accuracy measures alone (Schumacher and Pai 2015). Tuberculosis POCT must be delivered as part of an integrated package of 'test and treat' and not as a stand-alone test.

## CONCLUSION

The tuberculosis pipeline has been reinvigorated by the global roll-out of the Xpert® MTB/RIF assay and is now in full expansion with multiple new technologies set to hit the market in the coming years. However, despite the emergence of a variety of new tests, we have yet to find a molecular test that is truly applicable and affordable for use in the decentralised setting. Moreover, there are critical unmet needs that range from a simple, triage test for use in the community, to DST tools that can detect a range of mutations for several important drugs that will make up future drug regimens. For the development of rapid triage tests, non-sputum based tests for active TB and highly predictive latent TB tests, we need validated biomarkers.

## PATIENT CASE STUDY FOR TUBERCULOSIS POCT: SOUTH AFRICA

South Africa has played a leading role in the roll-out of the Xpert® MTB/RIF assay as a replacement test for smear microscopy. Here, we present two scenarios that illustrate the working field models of POCT (adapted from Hanrahan *et al.* 2015).

### Scenario 1: Xpert® MTB/RIF in the primary care setting

A patient with cough for 3 weeks and unintentional weight loss presents to a local Johannesburg clinic for evaluation. On initial interview, the patient is tested for HIV and screens positive by questionnaire for suspected tuberculosis. He is requested to produce two spontaneous sputum samples: one for the clinic Xpert® MTB/RIF test and the other to be sent to the Johannesburg NHLS laboratory for LED microscopy and liquid culture. He is also referred to a nearby hospital for a chest X-ray as per the clinic physician.

Within 2 h, the patient receives a positive Xpert® MTB/RIF result: *M. tuberculosis* is detected with absence of rifampicin resistance. The patient is thus started on a standard four-line drug regime for tuberculosis on the same day. Proper culture and phenotypic drug-susceptibility testing is then performed at the reference laboratory to guide further treatment.

*Comment:* Assuming the Xpert® MTB/RIF platform is used frequently enough and the patient is willing to wait, diagnosis and start of treatment can be completed on the same day, including appropriate treatment for suspected MDR-TB. Data suggest Xpert® MTB/RIF use is similar in the primary care and reference laboratory settings, and that the test can be run by people with a high school level of education or less.

### Scenario 2: Xpert® MTB/RIF in an off-site laboratory

The same patient presents to a local Johannesburg clinic for evaluation and screens positive by questionnaire for suspected tuberculosis. Two sputum samples are collected and sent off to the NHLS laboratory: one for the Xpert® MTB/RIF test and the other for LED microscopy and liquid culture. Turnaround time for the Xpert® at the laboratory is between 1 and 2 days after sputum collection, with the results made available online to the provider. In the meantime, most clinicians will wait for the Xpert® MTB/RIF result before beginning therapy. However, a certain proportion will begin empiric treatment for tuberculosis before the result becomes available.

*Comment:* The impact of the introduction of a new technology such as Xpert® MTB/RIF depends on where and how it is placed. Standard empiric therapy may be inappropriate in the context of an MDR-TB strain and contribute to mounting resistance if there is significant delay in acting on the results or if the patient is lost to follow-up after the first clinical encounter.

*Discussion:* This case study favoured placement of Xpert® MTB/RIF in the primary care setting, whereby a greater proportion of patients were started on treatment in a shorter timeframe. However, as in previous studies, there was no benefit seen on either morbidity or mortality from the quicker and/or more accurate diagnosis afforded by Xpert® MTB/RIF. This seems to be largely driven by high rates of empiric treatment in high-burden settings and possibly by lack of control of significant co-morbidities including HIV.

## REFERENCES


Agizew TB, Arwady MA, Yoon JC, Nyirenda S, Mosimaneotsile B, Tedla Z, *et al.* (2010) Tuberculosis in asymptomatic HIV-infected adults with abnormal chest radiographs screened for tuberculosis prevention. *The International Journal of Tuberculosis and Lung Disease* **14**, 45–51.

Canadian Thoracic Society (2013) *Canadian Tuberculosis Standards.* 7th edn. Canada, <http://www.respiratory-guidelines.ca/tb-standards-2013>.

Cheng Y, Xie H, Sule P, Hassounah H, Graviss EA, Kong Y, *et al.* (2014) Fluorogenic probes with substitutions at the 2 and 7 positions of cephalosporin are highly BlaC-specific for rapid Mycobacterium tuberculosis detection. *Angewandte Chemie International Edition* **53**, 9360–9364. doi:10.1002/anie.201405243

Choi HW, Miele K, Dowdy D, Shah M (2013) Cost-effectiveness of Xpert® MTB/RIF for diagnosing pulmonary tuberculosis in the United States. *The International Journal of Tuberculosis and Lung Disease* **17**, 1328–1335. doi:10.5588/ijtld.13.0095

Choi SW, Maiga M, Maiga MC, Atudorei V, Sharp ZD, Bishai WR, *et al.* (2014) Rapid in vivo detection of isoniazid-sensitive *Mycobacterium tuberculosis* by breath test. *Nature Communications* **5**, 4989. doi:10.1038/ncomms5989

Claassens MM, du Toit E, Dunbar R, Lombard C, Enarson DA, Beyers N, *et al.* (2013) Tuberculosis patients in primary care do not start treatment. What role do health system delays play? *The International Journal of Tuberculosis and Lung Disease* **17**, 603–607. doi:10.5588/ijtld.12.0505

Cruciani M, Scarparo C, Malena M, Bosco O, Serpelloni G, Mengoli C (2004) Meta-Analysis of BACTEC MGIT 960 and BACTEC 460 TB, with or without solid media, for detection of Mycobacteria. *Journal of Clinical Microbiology* **42**, 2321–2325. doi:10.1128/JCM.42.5.2321-2325.2004

Denkinger CM, Schumacher SG, Boehme CC, Dendukuri N, Pai M, Steingart KR (2014) Xpert MTB/RIF assay for the diagnosis of extrapulmonary tuberculosis: a systematic review and meta-analysis. *The European Respiratory Journal* **44**, 435–446. doi:10.1183/09031936.00007814

Denkinger CM, Dolinger D, Schito M, Wells W, Cobelens F, Pai M, *et al.* (2015) Target product profile of a molecular drug-susceptibility test for use in microscopy centers. *The Journal of Infectious Diseases* **211**(Supplement 2), S39–S49. doi:10.1093/infdis/jiu682

Detjen AK, DiNardo AR, Leyden J, Steingart KR, Menzies D, Schiller I, *et al.* (2015) Xpert MTB/RIF assay for the diagnosis of pulmonary tuberculosis in children: a systematic review and meta-analysis. *The Lancet. Respiratory Medicine* **3**, 451–461. doi:10.1016/S2213-2600(15)00095-8

Dheda K, Ruhwald M, Theron G, Peter J, Yam WC (2013) Point-of-care diagnosis of tuberculosis: past, present and future. *Respirology* **18**, 217–232. doi:10.1111/resp.12022

Engel N, Ganesh G, Patil M, Yellappa V, Pant Pai N, Vadnais C, *et al.* (2015) Barriers to point-of-care testing in India: results from qualitative research across different settings, users and major diseases. *PLoS One* **10**, e0135112. doi:10. 1371/journal.pone.0135112

FIND (Foundation for Innovative New Diagnostics) (2015) *Tuberculosis.* FIND, Geneva, Switzerland, <http://www.finddiagnostics.org/export/sites/default/resource-centre/reports_brochures/docs/digital-radiology-solutions-for-TB-dx-report2015.pdf>.

Hanrahan CF, Clouse K, Bassett J, Mutunga L, Selibas K, Stevens W, Scott L, *et al.* (2015) The patient impact of point-of-care vs. laboratory placement of Xpert® MTB/RIF. *The International Journal of Tuberculosis and Lung Disease* **19**, 811–816. doi:10.5588/ijtld.15.0013

Kik SV, Denkinger CM, Chedore P, Pai M (2014) Replacing smear microscopy for the diagnosis of tuberculosis: what is the market potential? *The European Respiratory Journal* **43**, 1793–1796. doi:10.1183/09031936.00217313

Lawn SD, Nicol MP (2011) Xpert® MTB/RIF assay: development, evaluation and implementation of a new rapid molecular diagnostic for tuberculosis and rifampicin resistance. *Future Microbiology* **6**, 1067–1082. doi:10.2217/fmb.11.84

Lawn SD, Zumla AI (2011) Tuberculosis. *Lancet* **378**, 57–72. doi:10.1016/S0140-6736(10)62173-3

Ling DI, Zwerling AA, Pai M (2008) GenoType MTBDR assays for the diagnosis of multidrug-resistant tuberculosis: a meta-analysis. *The European Respiratory Journal* **32**, 1165–1174. doi:10.1183/09031936.00061808

MacPherson P, Houben RM, Glynn JR, Corbett EL, Kranzer K (2014) Pre-treatment loss to follow-up in tuberculosis patients in low- and lower-middle-income countries and high-burden countries: a systematic review and meta-analysis. *Bulletin of the World Health Organization* **92**, 126–138. doi:10.2471/BLT.13.124800

Pai NP, Vadnais C, Denkinger C, Engel N, Pai M (2012) Point-of-care testing for infectious diseases: diversity, complexity, and barriers in low- and middle-income countries. *PLoS Medicine* **9**, e1001306. doi:10.1371/journal.pmed.1001306

Pai M, Ghiasi M, Pant Pai N (2015) Point-of-care diagnostic testing in global health: what is the point? *Microbe* **10**, 103–107.

Reither K, Jugheli L, Glass TR, Sasamalo M, Mhimbira FA, Weetjens BJ, *et al.* (2015) Evaluation of giant African pouched rats for detection of pulmonary tuberculosis in patients from a high-endemic setting. *PLoS One* **10**, e0135877. doi:10.1371/journal.pone.0135877

Schumacher SG, Pai M (2015) Xpert® MTB/RIF for extra-pulmonary tuberculosis: time to look beyond accuracy. *The International Journal of Tuberculosis and Lung Disease* **19**, 2. doi:10.5588/ijtld.14.0850

Schumacher SG, Thangakunam B, Denkinger CM, Oliver AA, Shakti KB, Qin ZZ, *et al.* (2015) Impact of point-of-care implementation of Xpert® MTB/RIF: product vs. process innovation. *The International Journal of Tuberculosis and Lung Disease* **19**, 1084–1090. doi:10.5588/ijtld.15.0120

Sreeramareddy CT, Qin ZZ, Satyanarayana S, Subbaraman R, Pai M (2014) Delays in diagnosis and treatment of pulmonary tuberculosis in India: a systematic review. *The International Journal of Tuberculosis and Lung Disease* **18**, 255–266. doi:10.5588/ijtld.13.0585

Steingart KR, Henry M, Ng V, Hopewell PC, Ramsay A, Cunningham J, *et al.* (2006) Fluorescence versus conventional sputum smear microscopy for tuberculosis: a systematic review. *The Lancet Infectious Diseases* **6**, 570–581. doi:10.1016/S1473-3099(06)70578-3

Steingart KR, Flores LL, Dendukuri N, Schiller I, Laal S, Ramsay A, *et al.* (2011) Commercial serological tests for the diagnosis of active pulmonary and extrapulmonary tuberculosis: an updated systematic review and meta-analysis. *PLoS Medicine* **8**, e1001062. doi:10.1371/journal.pmed.1001062

Steingart KR, Schiller I, Horne DJ, Pai M, Boehme CC, Dendukuri N (2014) Xpert® MTB/RIF assay for pulmonary tuberculosis and rifampicin resistance in adults. *Cochrane Database of Systematic Reviews* **1**, CD009593. doi:10.1002/14651858.CD009593.pub3

Theron G, Zijenah L, Chanda D, Clowes P, Rachow A, Lesosky M, *et al.* (2014) Feasibility, accuracy, and clinical effect of point-of-care Xpert® MTB/RIF testing for tuberculosis in primary-care settings in Africa: a multicentre, randomised, controlled trial. *Lancet* **383**, 424–435. doi:10.1016/S0140-6736(13)62073-5

UNITAID (2015) *Tuberculosis Diagnostics Technology and Market Landscape*. 4th edn. World Health Organization, Geneva, Switzerland.

Van Rie A, Page-Shipp L, Hanrahan CF, Schnippel K, Dansey H, Bassett J, *et al.* (2013) Point-of-care Xpert® MTB/RIF for smear-negative tuberculosis suspects at a primary care clinic in South Africa. *The International Journal of Tuberculosis and Lung Disease* **17**, 368–372. doi:10.5588/ijtld.12.0392

Vassall A, van Kampen S, Sohn H, Michael JS, John KR, der Boon S, *et al.* (2011) Rapid diagnosis of tuberculosis with the Xpert® MTB/RIF assay in high burden countries: a cost-effectiveness analysis. *PLoS Medicine* **8**, e1001120. doi:10.1371/journal.pmed.1001120

WHO (World Health Organization) (2004) *Mapping the Landscape of Diagnostics for Sexually Transmitted Infections*. WHO and Special Program for Research and Training in Tropical Diseases, Geneva, Switzerland, <http://www.who.int/tdr/publications/documents/mapping-landscape-sti.pdf?ua=1>.

WHO (2011a) *Same-day Diagnosis of Tuberculosis by Microscopy*. WHO, Geneva, Switzerland, <http://apps.who.int/iris/bitstream/10665/44603/1/9789241501606_eng.pdf>.

WHO (2011b) *Commercial Serodiagnostic Tests for Diagnosis of Tuberculosis Policy Statement*. WHO, Geneva, Switzerland, <http://apps.who.int/iris/bitstream/10665/44652/1/9789241502054_eng.pdf>.

WHO (2015a) *Global Tuberculosis Report 2015*. WHO, Geneva, Switzerland, <http://www.who.int/tb/publications/global_report/en/>.

WHO (2015b) *The END TB Strategy*. WHO, Geneva, Switzerland, <http://www.who.int/tb/End_TB_brochure.pdf?ua=1>.

WHO (2015c) *The Use of Lateral Flow Urine Lipoarabinomannan Assay (LF-LAM) for the Diagnosis and Screening of Active Tuberculosis in People Living with HIV*. WHO, Geneva, Switzerland, <http://apps.who.int/iris/bitstream/10665/193633/1/9789241509633_eng.pdf>.

Yuan LY, Li Y, Wang M, Ke ZQ, Xu WZ (2014) Rapid and effective diagnosis of pulmonary tuberculosis with novel and sensitive loop-mediated isothermal amplification (LAMP) assay in clinical samples: a meta-analysis. *Journal of Infection and Chemotherapy* **20**, 86–92. doi:10.1016/j.jiac.2013.07.003

# 24 Point-of-care testing for Ebola and other highly infectious threats: principles, practice, and strategies for stopping outbreaks

*Gerald J Kost*

**Summary**

This chapter identifies key principles of point-of-care testing (POCT) for Ebola patients and others exposed to highly contagious diseases. It assesses evidence from recent crises: Ebola in West Africa and MERS in South Korea. Hospitals that admitted Ebola patients mitigated risk by using POCT for critical care support in isolation units. Principle-based strategies comprise: needs assessment; the SCP™; FAST•POC™; POCT•POD™; diagnostic centres; matrix education; point-of-care (POC) culture; and enhanced POC technologies for diagnosis, triage, de-risking, monitoring and stopping outbreaks. Epidemics incur huge economic penalties. POCT helps avoid these costs through early detection and accurate diagnosis, while preventing needless suffering and unnecessary loss of human life. Impactful medical outcomes plus significant return on investment (ROI) warrant substantial funding, anticipatory planning, and comprehensive training. Ebola and MERS proved unequivocally the importance of POCT. Countries should produce national POC testing policies and guidelines, so that POCT is properly supported, quality controlled and cleverly adapted to cultural expectations.

## INTRODUCTION

This chapter presents imaginative, dynamic and spatially innovative strategies for dealing with outbreaks of highly infectious diseases by: (i) detecting them quickly using optimised point-of-care testing (POCT); (ii) providing a strategic planning tool for enhancing public health resilience, the Spatial Care Path™ (SCP™); (iii) preparing individual communities to limit the spread of disease through facilitated-access self-testing at the POC (FAST•POC™); and (iv) facilitating screening, diagnosis, monitoring and support for patients as they progress along SCPs™ in community small-world networks (SWNs).

We must think globally *and act globally*, while performing POCT in the context of local community culture, so that medical intervention is welcome. This POC culture (Kost *et al.* 2015a) means people expect rapid diagnosis of high-risk viruses, accomplished using disposable test strips, self-contained automated technologies, and mobile cartridge-, cassette- or cuvette-based instruments, as well as innovations in molecular diagnostics such as detection of viruses in exhaled breath when screening for highly transmissible influenza. In the next decade, POC diagnostics that fulfil these popular expectations, while also delivering ultrahigh sensitivity, specificity and predictive values, will help stifle outbreaks in vulnerable countries.

Defined as medical testing at or near the site of patient care, POCT is driving this cultural revolution. Even if the

WHO and CDC had responded more quickly to Ebola in West Africa and its dissemination to other world regions, POC diagnostics were not, and still are not, readily available – a stunning flaw that needs correcting worldwide. FAST•POC™ can interrupt the rapid spread of outbreaks. POCT personal outcome (outbreak) devices (detection) (POCT•PODs™) could be implemented in primary care on SCPs™.

Multiplex PCR assays and flexible test menus are beneficial when samples are difficult to collect or short on volume, because different pathogens may create similar clinical constellations of symptoms and signs. Traceability of infected individuals by knowing POC test results, geospatial locations, physical movements and trends over time and across borders can help contain highly infectious threats. A clear understanding of POC principles will help transform the practice of public health to immediate diagnosis at points of need.

## FUNDAMENTAL PRINCIPLES

Table 24.1 lists underlying principles. POC technologies could be used to detect and intercept viruses at initial points of animal origin in zoonotic reservoirs, as well as in food (A). Recent epidemics and disasters demonstrated the value of assessing outcomes and needs, which set future directions (B). Past encounters show clearly the role of POCT in preventing spread of disease (C). Entrepreneurial gaps in instrumentation are filled by invention and innovation (D). Optimising strategic planning (E), enhancing resilience (F), and creating policy and guidelines (G) inspire future problem solving (Table 24.2).

## SPREAD OF OUTBREAKS

In early 2015, a NIH Clinical Center patient improved from critical to serious condition and was discharged. In late 2015 before being diagnosed, a New York City physician created alarm by circulating among his 'social network nodes', such as family and friends. Treated with the experimental antiviral drug, Brincidofovir (http://www.chimerix.com/) and donor-immune plasma from an Ebola survivor, he was discharged well from Bellevue Hospital Center after 21 days. Subsequently, people returning to the USA from West Africa were monitored for 21 days. New treatment options, such as the Cerus Intercept blood system (http://www.intercept-usa.com/), which treats pathogens in Ebola survivors before giving plasma to patients, have been cleared by the US Food and Drug Administration (FDA). Advanced treatment and adaptive response in the USA has limited deaths.

However, if unabated, infectious diseases spread in patterns characteristic of SWNs (Kost 2015). Okeke *et al.* (2014) stated, 'By collating and analysing epidemiological data from documented outbreaks, we observed that diagnostic delay contributes to epidemic size for Ebola … hemorrhagic fever outbreaks. Even greater reductions in outbreak size were seen when all febrile patients were tested for endemic infections or when febrile health-care workers were tested.' Oleś *et al.* (2012) found that '… the required extent of prevention … depends on the time till detection…,' a very clear indication for the use of rapid POCT. Thus, it is not conjecture that POCT will work, but instead a matter of planning, funding and implementing.

## TRANSFORMING PUBLIC HEALTH

POCT has blossomed into an innovative, ubiquitous and rapidly evolving resource. It is transforming crisis medicine and public health practice. However, striking gaps in preparedness generate uncertainty and unpredictability. Suppose that Ebola or MERS becomes more contagious, albeit less deadly, in a genetic give and take. Then, distributing resources will enhance resilience. A benefit of POCT rests with its '24/7' utility. That is, once used regularly by well-trained operators, POCT can meet the needs of emergency, urgent and routine care simultaneously. Public health practitioners can be integrated into this scheme to reduce dependence on distant reference laboratories and non-dedicated hospital laboratories.

In fact, faced with extraordinary risk, need for speed and epidemiological containment, hospitals admitting patients with Ebola rapidly implemented POCT directly within isolation areas, rather than depending on clinical laboratories (Kost *et al.* 2015b,c). The Ebola crisis demonstrated the intrinsic value of testing at points of contact in isolation units and diagnostic centres, which can include mobile ones placed within or near hospitals, next to or inside alternate care facilities (ACFs), or along SCPs™ in regional SWNs. POCT•PODs™ can provide controlled environments for isolated individual patient testing positioned at portals of entry and immigration.

These strategies will create a new POC public health framework. The WHO, organisations such as the CDC in the USA, and public health practitioners everywhere should anticipate points of first critical need by

**Table 24.1.** Point-of-care principles, practice and strategies for Ebola and other threats

| Principles | Practice and strategies |
|---|---|
| A. Intercepting disease at points of origin | Develop portable field devices for rapid detection and monitoring of viruses in zoonotic animal reservoirs, map temporal trends and use geospatial analysis to determine the risks of animal to human transmission. |
| | Use handheld and disposable food assays to find viruses in animal sources (e.g. Ebola in fruit bats linked with bush meat consumed by humans: the West Africa index case where a 2-year-old child in south-eastern Guinea played with infected bats in 2014, and a 2015 recrudescence in Liberia where three villagers shared a meal of contaminated dog meat). |
| | Detect transmissible viruses in exhaled breath when screening for high-risk airborne contagions. |
| B. Assessing needs and outcomes | Published evidence proves unequivocally that POCT is needed at initial points of contact, in patient isolation units and, logically, for other purposes, such as immigration screening and quarantine. |
| | POC devices should be simplified, integrated, standardised and harmonised for worldwide use. |
| | Basic test clusters must cover molecular detection, whole-blood analysis for critical care, detection of coagulopathy and disseminated intravascular coagulation (DIC), and ruling out of confounding infections. |
| | Viral load assays must be implemented, because blood levels of Ebola (and most likely, other highly contagious viruses) are predictive of death and relapse. |
| | Diagnostic testing at first points of contact must be implemented in a culturally acceptable manner to optimise usefulness, acceptability, outcomes and value. |
| C. Preventing spread and stopping outbreaks | Practice donning personal protective equipment (PPE), performing testing, then doffing the PPE. |
| | Design alternate care facilities for patient diagnosis, triage, segregation and critical care. |
| | Separately and individually isolate patients, health-care staff, and the environment. |
| | Plan for prolonged (21-day) observation (quarantine) of exposed subjects, including health-care personnel. |
| | Implement diagnostic centres. |
| | Detect onset and relapse in humans using viral load assays, haematology tests and temporal trend mapping of phases in the immunological response. |
| D. Inventing and innovating | New cost-effective approaches (e.g. FAST•POC™ and POCT•POD™) are needed so that patients, public health practitioners and primary health-care staff can perform testing quickly, easily and safely. |
| | Instruments must have flexible multiplex test clusters, detect novel new threats, and cover both acute diagnosis and chronic relapse, both of which have been observed for Ebola. |
| | The sensitivity and specificity of pathogen detection must be improved to ultrahigh levels to minimise false negatives during the interval when patients are first encountered and may be asymptomatic. |
| E. Optimising strategic planning | FAST•POC™ will help stop outbreaks by moving decision making upstream on the SCP™. |
| | POCT•PODs™ in mobile and built settings will help assure that molecular diagnostics can be implemented effectively. |
| | International mobility and spread of epidemics warrant significant support of geospatial optimisation of POC sites in SWNs. |
| F. Enhancing resilience | Public health must shift focus and resources to early detection of Ebola and other threats before patients spread disease, rather than relying on transporting and shipping dangerous specimens to reference laboratories. |
| | Comprehensive planning for community resilience must be improved by systematically identifying resources and alternative care facilities in advance. |
| | ER staff must re-educate, re-tool and refresh to avoid missing diagnoses and discharging highly contagious patients while sick and contagious. |
| G. Developing national policy and guidelines | POCT will help stop outbreaks, and therefore, limit regional epidemics, while also preventing uncontrolled growth into global 'newdemics' plagued with recrudescence, patient relapses, chronic side effects and vicious cycles of waste. |
| | Overwhelming economic losses associated with outbreaks justify funding substantial POC technology development. |
| | In view of international population mobility, responsibility for preparedness falls on all nations, each of which should develop and implement national POCT policy and guidelines, including training POC coordinators in adequate numbers and sufficient competence to be able to respond to crises. |

**Table 24.2.** Cybermedicine, robots, automation and mobile strategies for Ebola and other highly infectious threats.

- Smartphones and apps with remote bidirectional videoconferencing to health-care professionals can be used to deliver FAST•POC™ to patients efficiently and effectively, and to operate POCT•PODs™.
- Robots serving as facilitators can replace health workers, hold instruction placards for FAST•POC™, talk patients through testing, and obviate risks of contracting Ebola or other infections.
- Bank-like automated testing machines could process specimens, communicate via hands-off voice recognition, and use light sensors to read out assay results from disposable kit reagents.
- Automated self-cleaning and self-sterilising POCT•PODs™ can automatically process blood samples in isolated conditions, read reagent strip lines and other types of end points, and/or perform actual assays under suitable ambient conditions, while communicating recited history, patient interactions and test results.
- Mobile laboratories could move to 'hot spots' specifically to stop outbreaks.
- Cybermedical, robotic and automated laboratories can be installed in alternative care facilities to reduce health personnel risks of initial contact and exposure to highly contagious viruses.

assimilating POC know-how and technologies in order to acquire knowledge bases of sensitivity, specificity and predictive values while epidemics are underway. These data will help refine evidence-based medicine for target diseases, prepare first responders for future outbreaks, and improve real-world diagnostics by refining design criteria/device specifications.

## DESIGN CRITERIA/DEVICE SPECIFICATIONS

Extensive formal needs assessment surveys have defined specifications – namely high sensitivity, safety and user-friendliness – for portable molecular pathogen detection with biohazard containment (Kost and Curtis 2015). In October 2014, the WHO published an urgent call with acceptance criteria and priority features for Ebola diagnostics in a 'target product profile' (http://www.who.int/medicines/publications/target-product-profile.pdf). The WHO features comprise high clinical sensitivity in the first 10 days of patient presentation (>98% desired, >95% acceptable), extremely high analytical specificity (>99% desired, >99% acceptable), and minimally invasive and validated sample types (e.g. fingerstick capillary blood, saliva or buccal). However, the WHO target population, 'Patients presenting with fever to health care facilities for assessment,' presents high risk of contagion. To stop an outbreak, POC detection should be upstream at the first point of contact before sick patients spread the disease to others. Implicit in the WHO specifications is low cost. However, our global field experience has shown that cost-effectiveness is attained by assessing the overall *value* of POC diagnostics, not just the prices charged for instruments, reagents and quality control materials.

WHO specifications emphasise efficient process steps performed by the operator (<3 desired, <10 acceptable, preferably with no, or a maximum of one, timed steps), no or facilitated transfer of a precise volume of sample, quick analysis (<30 min desired, <3 h acceptable), internal controls, no or automated sample preparation, and several operational characteristics, such as robust operating conditions (0–50°C desired, 0–40°C acceptable; both up to 90% relative humidity), durable reagents and minimal training requirements.

The WHO temperature upper limit of 50°C for reagent storage may lead to bubble formation in reagent cassettes and other physical aberrations in the sample, but temperature can be controlled in a diagnostic centre or POCT•POD™. The WHO format is a small handheld (<2 kg, desired) or tabletop portable (acceptable) instrument with 30–60 min time limits for using opened reagents. Ideally, it uses solar, alternative or rechargeable battery power operating up to 8 h. Such well-configured, portable, robust and ergonomic POC devices would be ideal for isolation units, ACFs, mobile venues, SCPs™ and POCT•PODs™.

## RISK MITIGATION

Construction of 1400 isolation units in Hong Kong was motivated by SARS, which infected 1800 people and killed 299, and by Avian Influenza. In Guangzhou, SARS killed 8000. At Emory University Medical Center, samples from patients with Ebola were not sent to the clinical laboratory for fear of breakage, contamination and prolonged shutdowns for cleaning mainframe instruments. Testing was moved to the POC. No centrifugation was permitted when processing samples within the isolation area established 12 years previously with the CDC. Samples were allowed to settle and clot passively: a time-consuming step. Commercial carriers refused to pick up properly packaged (category A) containers labelled as containing Ebola and destined for the CDC.

This reluctance creates a serious logistics gap in communities needing rapid screening and diagnosis, although World Carrier (http://www.worldcourier.com/) may ship, if properly documented. Thus, the Emory '... strategy was to establish near-patient testing within the quarantine facility itself ...' and '... (to do so for) approximately three weeks of inpatient care.' The '... approach exceeded CDC requirements for the safe management of patients infected with Ebola.' Centrifugation and automated stopper removal, which produce dangerous aerosols, were avoided at the University of Nebraska Medical Centre (MC) in favour of closed-tube sampling in the core laboratory and performing POCT, including blood gases, within a biocontainment unit.

Dallas Ebola cases proved high-risk for patients and nurses exposed through inadvertent body fluid transmission or direct contact. Estimated viral inoculum is 1 nL. Two infected nurses from Dallas survived. Unfortunately, a physician in the Nebraska MC, who had volunteered in West Africa, died. These events motivated preparedness measures in the USA, China, the Philippines, Thailand and other countries. In China, emphasis was placed on immigration screening. Travellers from Guinea, Liberia and Sierra Leone were forced into limited quarantine in 'Little Africa' in Guangzhou. The Philippines and Taiwan are planning national guidelines for POCT. In 2014, the Thai MOPH sponsored a convocation on POCT national guidelines and a special presentation on Ebola preparedness (by GK). Several hospitals in Bangkok have implemented isolation areas and diagnostic centres with embedded POC instruments.

Table 24.3 lists POC technologies selected for the isolation area at Emory (A), used in the biocontainment unit at Nebraska MC (B), and designed for other Ebola containments and suites (C/D).

Additional POC tests can be selected from web sources and Clinical Laboratory Improvement Amendments (CLIA)-waived POC lists. Be aware of which tests are FDA-cleared for critically ill Ebola patients and identify test clusters that fulfil needs cost-effectively on as few instruments as possible. POC staff and other POC device operators must be trained in use of personal protective equipment (PPE), sample handling procedures and the care of Ebola patients. Multi-disciplinary 'matrix education' should cover all dimensions of learning, validation and annual certification of competency.

Novel new technologies exist, such as surface acoustic wave detection, a recombinase polymerase amplification panel and multicoloured silver nanoparticles. Manufacturers should respond to future outbreaks by producing user-friendly POC cassettes/cartridges/cuvettes with flexible test clusters designed specifically for Ebola patients. Coagulation tests on handheld devices (cleared by the FDA for anticoagulation warfarin monitoring) are not intended for diagnosing disseminated intravascular coagulation, one of the most serious complications of Ebola. These gaps must be closed to improve survival of Ebola patients who develop rampant bleeding, septic shock, multi-organ failure and acute hepatic necrosis leading to fatal outcomes.

## EBOLA ALTERNATE CARE FACILITY

ACFs and diagnostic centres can be implemented in large regional hospitals; placed in free standing facilities, such as in Seattle-King County, Washington State; used during disaster response; and transported in mobile venues (Kost and Curtis 2015). The ACF should consolidate functions essential for Ebola care (Fig. 24.1). This design is modular and expandable by moving wall partitions to increase the number of isolation beds, by adding to the overall gross dimensions for greater usable square footage, and/or by replicating the facility according to community needs and SWN topography.

A suitable ACF can serve several communities. Climate-controlled facilities (e.g. tents) and temporary hospitals can be placed next to ACFs that have staff trained to deal with patients with Ebola. The ACF concept shortens virtually all measurable metrics for care, such as patient and specimen transport times, service walking distances and therapeutic turnaround times for diagnostic tests, because it spatially compresses dispersed process steps and multiple sites into one centralised configuration.

The ACF integrates POCT devices and near-patient testing performed directly within isolation. When fully developed, emerging Ebola molecular diagnostic tests will be performed safely by means of instruments with self-contained cartridges, automatic specimen processing and biohazard disposal not requiring BSL-4 capability, which is scarce throughout the world. Manual processes

**Table 24.3.** Point-of-care tests implemented for Ebola-secured settings

A. Emory University Hospital Specialised Isolation Area

| Manufacturer website | Instrument | Tests/status |
|---|---|---|
| Abaxis<br>www.abaxis.com | Piccolo Express | Chemistry profiles, magnesium, phosphate, liver enzyme assays, others available |
| Instrumentation Laboratory<br>www.instrumentationlaboratory.com | GEM Premier 4000 | pH, $pCO_2$, $pO_2$, electrolytes, calcium, lactate, haematocrit, haemoglobin, co-oximetry, bilirubin |
| Siemens<br>www.healthcare.siemens.com | CLINITEK Status automated urinalysis | Albumin, bilirubin, creatinine, glucose, ketones, leukocytes, nitrite, pH, protein, specific gravity, urobilinogen, others available |
| Roche Diagnostics<br>www.coaguchek.com | CoaguChek | PT/INR |
| Sysmex<br>www.sysmex.com | pocH-100i | CBC: WBC (3-part differential), RBC, haemoglobin, haematocrit, MCV, MCH, MCHC, platelets |
| Alere<br>www.alere.com | BinaxNOW | Malaria |
| BioFire Diagnostics<br>www.biofiredx.com | FilmArray | Infectious diseases including Ebola [FDA Ebola EUA 10/25/14, reissue 3/2/15] |

B. University of Nebraska MC Biocontainment BSL-3 Laboratory

| Manufacturer website | Instrument/method | Tests |
|---|---|---|
| Abbott<br>www.Abbott.com | i-Stat | G3+ cartridge (pH, $pCO_2$, $pO_2$) and Chem8+ cartridge (electrolytes, total $CO_2$, calcium, glucose, urea, creatinine, haematocrit) |
| International Technidyne Corp.<br>www.itcmed.com | Hemochron Signature Elite | Citrate prothrombin time (PT), citrate-activated partial thromboplastin time (aPTT) |
| Slide agglutination | Manual | Blood and serum antibody typing (for transfusion) |
| Slide preparation | Manual | Malaria—modified for the slide to be fixed in methanol 15 min before delivering to Core Laboratory for staining and interpretation |
| Not specified | Rapid manual assay | HIV Ab/Ag |
| Urine dipstick | Manual dipstick | For tests not on strip, specimen transferred with precautions to Core Laboratory for non-decapped DxI800 & DXC800i analysis |
| Not specified | RPR | Syphilis (card assay) |

C. Ebola Holding Units (4) in Sierra Leone, West Africa

| Developer website | Method | Performance |
|---|---|---|
| United Kingdom's Defence Science & Technology Laboratory<br>https://www.gov.uk/government/organisations/defence-science-and-technology-laboratory | Rapid diagnostic antigen test | Sensitivity: 100% (95% CI: 78.2–100).<br>Specificity: 96.6% (95% CI: 91.3–99.1).<br>Positive and negative predictive values: 79.0% (95% CI: 54.4–93.8) and 100% (95% CI: 96.7–100). |

D. Suite Environment, ARUP Institute for Clinical and Experimental Pathology

| Manufacturer website | Instrument/method | Tests, evaluation study objectives |
|---|---|---|
| Abaxis<br>www.abaxis.com | Piccolo Express | Liver Panel Plus using disposable exact volume transfer pipettes and BSL-2 cabinet in BSL-3 suite environment for Ebola patient workup. Checked device air flow characteristics are suitable. |

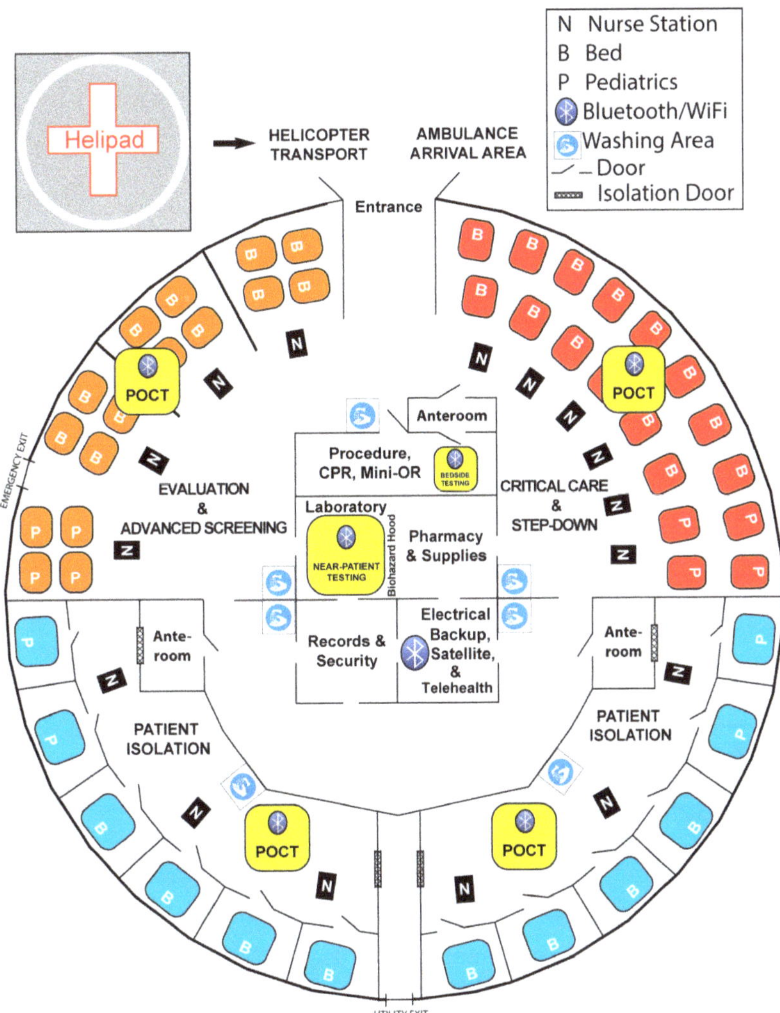


**Fig. 24.1.** Alternative care facility. This design serves as an integrated community resource that increases efficiency and decreases risk, while using POCT to accelerate diagnosis and decision making. PPE-trained staff oversee diagnostic instruments. Modular partitions can be moved to increase the number of individual isolation rooms for suspected, but not confirmed, patients. The overall gross dimensions can be enlarged to increase capacity. ACFs can be replicated to meet triage needs.

prove awkward for personnel donning PPE, so instruments operated in a biosafety cabinet should be automated and easy to operate. The CDC recommended working in a BSL-2 environment. We designed a diagnostic centre that can be placed in an ACF, hospital, or other site (Fig. 24.2). POC devices (top left) are operated in a BSL-3 biosafety cabinet, but in some cases, built diagnostic centres use BSL-2. This type of diagnostic centre has been installed in several Bangkok hospitals.

As reported in December 2015 by the WHO, Ebola had a case fatality rate (CFR) of 40% (11 315 deaths, 28 637 cases). By avoiding delays in specimen transport, rapid evidence-based decision making within the ACF will enhance community resilience should patients with Ebola appear with increasing frequency and demand more isolation beds, efficient patient workflow and epidemiological confinement. The ACF is selective in regard to community response and internal rearrangements that can flexibly adjust to the relative proportions of suspected persons under investigation versus confirmed. If desired, ACFs can be dedicated to one group or the other. POC tests performed in association with the ACFs and diagnostic centres should also be capable of ruling in and out other febrile infectious diseases, such as malaria.

Rudimentary structures are observed outside the USA, such as a segregated high-risk zone and basic quarantine facility used in Liberia, where historically the CFR has approached 70%. According to the user stated needs yet

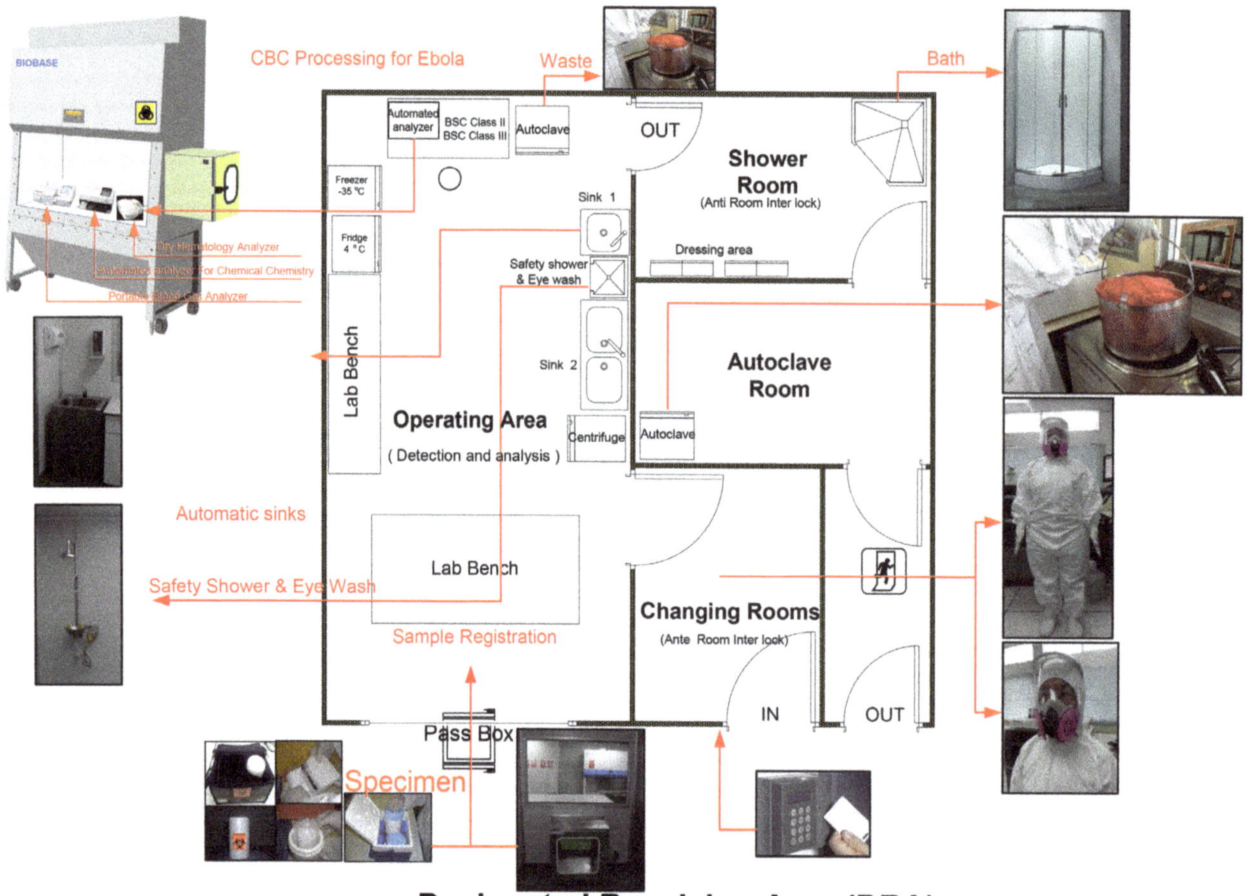


**Fig. 24.2.** Ebola diagnostic centre. This diagnostic centre has been deployed in Bangkok, Thailand. The left area is at negative pressure (22°C, RH 55%), a clean room class 10K. On the right, the shower and changing rooms are at positive pressure, the latter with an interlocking anteroom. The top left inset shows POC testing in the biosafety cabinet (BSL-3). Specimen preparation, then routing through a pass box are shown along the bottom, and PPE used in SE Asia, on the right. A diagnostic centre on a mobile vehicle could move to hotspots to break the log jam of slow or no diagnostic testing.

to be met, '... point-of-service laboratory testing is likely to significantly improve outcomes.' West Africa style treatment centres would be difficult to implement in affluent communities and also unlikely to meet standards of care, OSHA general safety requirements and biohazard containment thresholds. Selective and targeted resources provided by ACFs have already been shown to be feasible in Seattle-King County and North Carolina, albeit not yet for Ebola. When limited numbers of CDC-approved treatment centres face increased caseloads, community ACFs can provide early surveillance, rapid POCT and treatment to prevent spread in local and regional SWNs.

## THE SPATIAL CARE PATH™

### Definition

An SCP™ is the most efficient route taken by the patient when receiving definitive care in a SWN. SCP™ principles include: (i) start diagnosis immediately wherever the patient is located; (ii) implement POC technologies according to needs in homes, ambulances, primary care, SWN hubs and critical care; (iii) thereby, achieve timely evidence-based decision making based on POC test results as the patient progresses through the SWN; (iv) coordinate access to critical elements and scarce specialists to achieve a continuum of care; and (v) optimise medical resources for the problem at hand, especially when the SWN becomes compromised by disasters or patients are quarantined.

### Rationale

In South Korea, health-care workers did not place the MERS index case patient in isolation. Some people who became infected occupied the same room. Others had been in the same ward from 5 min to several hours. Prime Minister Park Geun-hye said, '... there were (sic) some insufficiency in the initial response, including the judgment on its contagiousness.' How many times will this scenario repeat, at what cost, and to whom, before local and national responses are properly restructured and enabled at first points of contact? Well-designed SCP™ vectors of medical care can help.

## Vector concept

*Spatial* refers to shrewd positioning of POCT, elimination of unnecessary process steps and use of geographic information systems (GISs) to identify effective and efficient routes from population clusters to the nearest care. SCPs™ consolidate SWN dispersion into one or more community sites with diagnostic centres where useable space and workflow are optimised. Isolation beds can be augmented to house patients suspected, but not confirmed, thereby avoiding patient-to-patient spread of disease. Besides spatial attributes, the SCP™ is a multi-functional vector that integrates operational elements, such as optimised POCT, connections to conventional care paths, and enhanced resilience.

## Strategy

Fig. 24.3 illustrates an Ebola SCP™ with ACF and embedded POCT connected to the expedient of an individual isolation area with limited beds within a hospital. An SCP™ will deploy the best available molecular diagnostic testing at the point of initial contact and eliminate time-consuming steps in the care sequence, such as transporting high-risk patients with Ebola from one community to another, or sending hazardous samples to distant reference laboratories, assuming couriers will pick up and transport high-risk containers labelled as Ebola.

Other SCP™ research currently underway is determining the most efficient uses of POCT for expedited medical problem solving in limited-resource settings for patients with acute myocardial infarction, prediabetes and diabetes, anticoagulation and snake-bite coagulopathies, and infectious diseases and sepsis, with the objective of empowering care teams, public health practitioners, and industry to understand how best to position POC testing. Designing SCPs™ facilitates prevention, intervention and

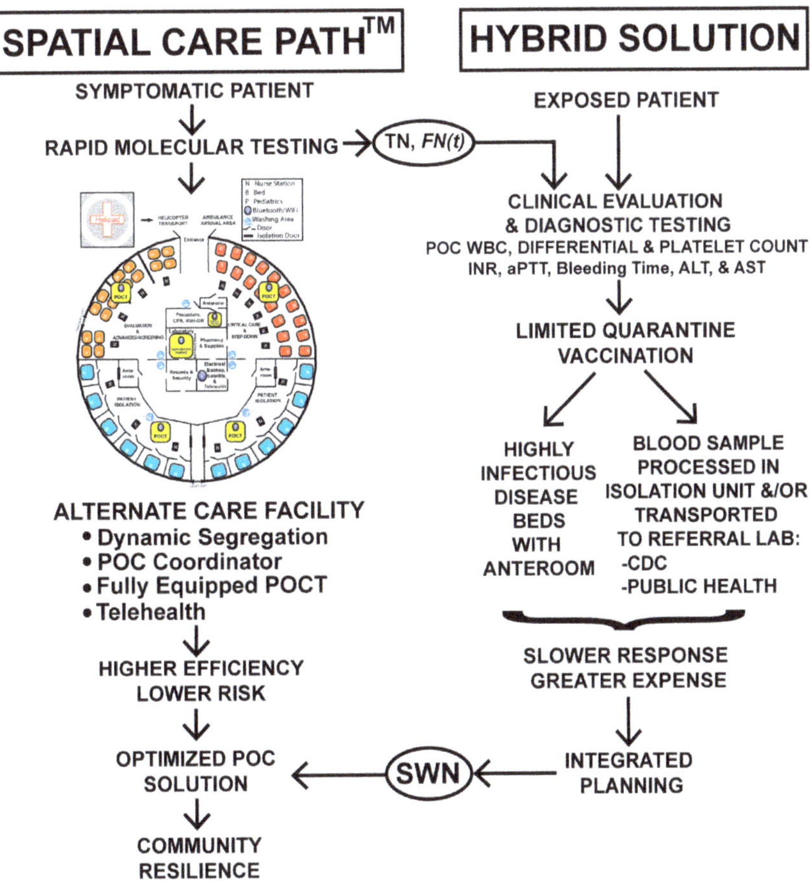


**Fig. 24.3.** Ebola Spatial Care Path (SCP™). The Ebola SCP™ starts wherever the patient is first encountered. Rapid molecular diagnostic testing begins as close to the point of contact as possible. The ACF accelerates evaluation and advanced screening. Diagnostic centres can be placed along SCPs™, outside ACFs, or inside. Optimised POC testing, spatial consolidation, telehealth and fewer process steps enhance community SWN resilience – a valuable and cost-effective outcome.

resilience in the event of wider presence of Ebola in regional SWNs and simultaneously fulfils community recommendations of the CDC.

Ebola SCPs™ will help stop future spread of disease within health-care delivery systems and their community SWNs when isolation beds in treatment centres become overwhelmed because of high case burden, whether patients are under observation or receiving treatment. SCPs™ must be tailored to local geography, population demographics, community culture and referral patterns. County, state and federal agencies must endorse community-based response. Thus, each regional SWN should ready its own SCPs™ with POCT, to avoid the reactive, presumptive, and arguably illegal, general quarantines that were enacted in some states in the USA, such as New York and New Jersey.

## DIAGNOSTIC CENTRES

Fig. 24.2 shows a diagnostic centre designed for Ebola care. POCT within the biosafety cabinet comprises:

- the Spotchem EZ (Arkray, http://www.arkrayusa.com/) for glucose, total protein, albumin, alanine aminotransferase, aspartate aminotransferase, alkaline phosphatase, cholesterol, triglycerides, high-density lipoprotein cholesterol, urea, creatinine, calcium and total bilirubin, or combinations thereof (this instrument has been used for support of patients with viral haemorrhagic fever in Ghana)
- the Opti CCA-TS2 whole-blood analyser (http://www.optimedical.com/products-services/opti-CCA-TS2.html) for pH, $pCO_2$, $pO_2$, total haemoglobin, oxygen saturation, sodium, potassium, chloride, calcium, glucose, urea and lactate, but only eight analytes at one time using a directly loading syringe cartridge that minimises contamination
- a haematology instrument, such as the QBC Star (http://www.druckerdiagnostics.com/hematology/qbc-star/qbc-star-centrifugal-hematology-analyzer.html), a dry reagent analyser that produces a nine-component complete blood count (haematocrit, haemoglobin, mean corpuscular haemoglobin concentration, platelet count, WBC, granulocyte count/percentage, and lymphocyte/monocyte count/percentage) from a specialised sample tube with stains and float separator inside, or the HemoCue WBC-DIFF (http://www.hemocue.com/en/products/white-blood-cell-count/wbc-diff), which provides a five-part differential
- a vital signs monitor (e.g. VTrust TD-2300) at the bedside.

The containment level in the diagnostic centre should match the intended purpose of the ACF, free-standing facility, mobile transportable application or treatment centre. Diagnostics on mobile vehicles are effective in epidemics for '… rapid TAT (that) provides an important role in the support of patient management.' In fact, the first public health mobile laboratory appeared in 1930. Instruments in our diagnostic centre have connectivity to the electronic medical record by means of the LINK data management system implemented by Connect Diagnostics (http://connectdiagnostics.com/) in Bangkok. LINK allows wireless ordering of tests and facilitates test performance by either laboratory staff or nurses according to ISO 22870.

## TEST CLUSTERS

Premonitory POC test results, such as initial leukopaenia, suppressed lymphocyte count on the differential, increased percentage of granulocytes, and thrombocytopaenia help confirm the diagnosis of Ebola. Later, patients have increased WBC, immature granulocytes and atypical lymphocytes. West Africa should be replete with POCT and diagnostic centres, but is not, thereby handicapping expeditious detection of premonitory signs in villages and evidence-based critical care support in treatment centres.

Striking electrolyte changes need monitoring to support repletion. Unfortunately, there is no small FDA-cleared handheld device for monitoring coagulation (except PT/INR when adjusting warfarin anticoagulant). Filoviral haemorrhagic fever is accompanied by prolonged PT, aPTT and bleeding time, potentially progressing to disseminated intravascular coagulation (DIC) with elevated D-dimer. D-dimer is available on the handheld cobas h232 (Roche Diagnostics, http://www.cobas.com/home/ product/point-of-care-testing/cobas-h-232.html) available outside the USA. Platelets are consumed rapidly early in the course of the infection and should be trend mapped to see recovery, along with platelet function.

Fatally infected patients fail to develop an antibody response. Thus, detection of virus-specific IgM and IgG is a good prognostic sign. In critically ill patients with Ebola, plasma loss and bleeding affect haemoglobin and the haematocrit, both of which should be monitored. A recent case of relapse in the UK (http://time.com/4074377/pauline-cafferkey-ebola-nurse-critically-ill/), apparently missed upon primary care follow-up, illustrated just how evasive Ebola can be, and that we must have available POC technologies, both direct and indirect, for determining recurrence.

## FUTURE CHALLENGES

Future challenges include:

- reduction in initial false negatives, FN = *FN(t)*, as a function of time, to ramp up sensitivity, {TP/[TP + *FN(t)*]}, to ultrahigh levels in infected patients during the first 72 h, when symptoms may be mild or absent, in order to avoid shunting false negative cases to community hospitals ill prepared to receive high-risk patients
- automation of totally self-contained and sealable specimen cassettes and cartridges to eliminate need for expensive high-level biosafety cabinets
- proof of effectiveness in controlling internal contamination in portable instruments
- sustained ultrahigh specificity [TN/(TN + FP)] to minimise false positives that place non-infected people at risk if confined near infected patients, and as more sophisticated compact technologies become available
- determination of quantitative viral titres for: (i) detecting exposure and onset in small volumes of specimen; (ii) de-escalating the level of care and quarantine: (iii) trend monitoring to spot relapses; (iv) avoiding sexual transmission; and (v) predicting outcomes.

The FDA has been accelerating approval of new diagnostic tests for Ebola by issuing emergency use authorisations (EUAs) continuously since late 2014 (http://www.fda.gov/EmergencyPreparedness/Counterterrorism/MedicalCountermeasures/MCMLegalRegulatoryandPolicyFramework/ucm182568.htm#ebola). When performed properly with biohazard precautions in the near-patient testing area of an isolation unit or diagnostic centre, POC results are available more quickly than results obtained by sending specimens to a public health laboratory or the CDC. Speed facilitates screening, focussed triage and effective workflow. These efficiencies help offset professional shortages in countries with extraordinarily large numbers of people per physician, such as in Liberia, Sierra Leone and Guinea.

Several organisations have pleaded urgently for rapid diagnostics to help make up for these personnel shortfalls. Self-contained cartridge/cassette-based rapid molecular tests available on small portable platforms, such as the Alere i and Roche Diagnostics cobas Liat (both CLIA-waived), that test for infectious diseases forecast the feasibility of introducing Ebola assays on existing light-weight platforms. These operator-friendly designs are simple to operate, require minimal or no quality control, and are suitable for FAST•POC™ when industry progresses EUAs to inexpensive, portable and safe detection of Ebola, MERS, and other threats in capillary blood (Strecker *et al.* 2015).

## FAST•POC™ AND POCT•POD™

FAST•POC™ (Fig. 24.4) means the patient obtains his or her own capillary blood (or other) specimen with an automatic retractable lancet (or other sampling device) built into a self-aspirating and self-contained microcassette/microcuvette/cartridge, which then seals for automated processing and automatic testing on an integrated POC instrument, while another person, the 'facilitator,' instructs and guides, so there is extremely limited or no

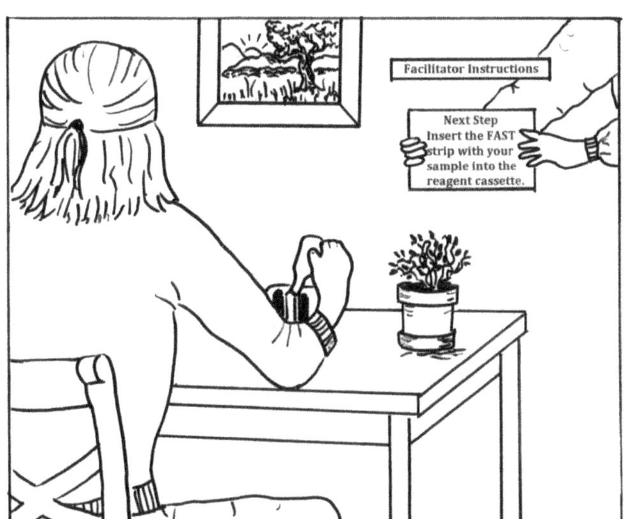


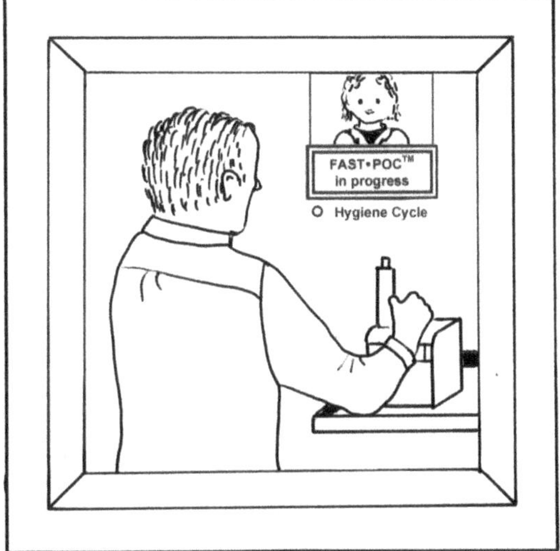


**Fig. 24.4.** FAST•POC™: The patient on the left is performing self-testing at home with the help of a facilitator. POCT•POD™: The patient on the right in an isolation pod is following instructions for testing. After the patient exits, the pod begins a hygiene cycle and self-cleans.

exposure to infectious agents. FAST•POC™ will help stop future outbreaks because of minimal exposure to others, or of oneself, to infected patients. Technological developments in POCT and molecular diagnostics indicate that FAST•POC™ soon will become a reality.

Similar to self-monitoring of blood glucose by patients with diabetes, family members can instruct each other in homes and obtain results without actually contacting blood or other specimens. FAST•POC™ could be performed in a POCT•POD™ installed in an ACF, primary care, urgent care clinic or emergency room. Visiting local public health workers can educate, instruct, guide and facilitate self-testing without necessarily touching the patient or assay components. In limited-resource settings, FAST•POC™ will help eliminate fear of going to treatment centres, being separated from family, and assigning loved ones to lonely deaths, when they may have Dengue, hepatitis, HIV, influenza, malaria, syphilis, tuberculosis or other common illnesses, but not Ebola. In West Africa, POCT•PODs™ would enable treatment centres to be sought out as sites for speed of diagnosis and excellence of care with improved chances of survival.

## TREATMENT CENTRES

In treatment centres in hot and humid West Africa, health-care workers are pressed for time because heat accumulates rapidly inside PPE. Only a few minutes are available for patient evaluation. In the absence of diagnostic testing, it may not be clear which patients have, or do not have, Ebola. Adequate restoration of electrolyte balance and management of other basic critical care support was virtually impossible, because, 'no ancillary testing (was) available…'. Patients fear contracting Ebola in treatment centres that do not provide a quick and definitive diagnosis and either rule in (high specificity) or rule out (high sensitivity) differential diagnoses.

West African treatment centres helped stop Ebola, but poor outcomes stigmatised them as terminal palliation. Patients sought help only when their symptoms were severe. Meanwhile, they spread the virus. Delays in diagnostic results were capricious, and the diagnostic centre, as described here, generally was overlooked. POCT in diagnostic centres properly positioned along SCPs™ will improve logistics, evidence-based decision making, patient outcomes, and therefore, cultural acceptance where hope of recovery becomes a reality.

CDC-approved hospital treatment centres are distributed unevenly. The new National Ebola Training and Education Center (CDC, HHS ASPR – http://www.hhs.gov/about/news/2015/07/01/hhs-launches-national-ebola-training-and-education-center.html), comprising Emory, Nebraska MC, and the Bellevue Hospital Center in New York City, recently launched the development of knowledge management. Nine current centres will have enhanced capabilities, but CDC online plans appear to omit POCT as a core strategy and POC coordinators for professional competency – serious deficits that must be corrected.

## HUMAN LOSS AND ECONOMIC PENALTIES

Outbreaks wreak havoc on national economies. The World Bank estimates the financial burden of the West Africa Ebola epidemic at US$32.6 billion by 2017. Loss of life is staggering, because of the high death rate and lack of critical care support. By late 2015, the Ebola toll was 11 299 deaths/28 598 cases (40% CFR). Collateral deaths in Sierra Leone resulted from poor maternity care, lack of support of childbirth, unaffordable bribes for delivering babies, scarcity of childhood vaccines, closed facilities, bacterial and parasitic infections, inadequate nurses and doctors, and a 165-fold increase in newborn mortality when birthing at home (Hongoltz-Hetling 2015). The disease is smouldering, not eradicated, with relapse reported. Eye infections and uveitis require clinical treatment. Sequelae include visual blurriness, arthralgias, hearing loss, palpitations and shortness of breath, while only one of 10 in the USA had none.

Health-care system decimation was reported to be killing people who are not infected with Ebola in a ratio of 1:1 with those who died from the disease. Sierra Leone, plagued with these secondary effects, has received US$2 billion from the US alone, but still has only three doctors per 500 000 persons and virtually the worst medical statistics of any country in the world. The CDC listed 55 Ebola treatment centres (http://www.cdc.gov/vhf/ebola/healthcare-us/preparing/current-treatment-centers.html), but the centres are unevenly distributed, fixed in location and, for some states, simply not there. Better planning will avoid the harsh human and economic penalties resulting from lack of preparedness.

In June 2015, MERS, for which a feasible rapid POC molecular diagnostic and FDA EUA exist, was spreading throughout South Korea – 1369 in quarantine, 30 cases confirmed, 540 schools closed, public facilities closed, two dead, one who travelled sick to China exposed all on an airplane, and, according to the Korean Health

Minister, not enough was done to detect the first wave, stop spread and end the outbreak. By late 2015, tallies stood at 37 deaths/186 cases (20% CFR) in South Korea and 579 deaths/1618 cases (36% CFR) in Saudi Arabia, where MERS originated. This respiratory disease spreads like a cold or flu to other countries. Little is known because cultural barriers prohibit autopsies and few scientific reports have been published. We can predict heavy economic impact from future highly infectious diseases in ASEAN+6 countries.

## DIGITAL DOCTORS

The West Africa epidemic need not be repeated elsewhere if more emphasis is placed on POCT and correct strategy for enhancing capacity to investigate outbreaks in remote areas. Vaccines require substantial time for development, clinical evaluation and distribution. An Ebola solution must therefore tackle very quickly the lack of diagnostic centres, late detection and rapid spread through SWNs to cities with high population densities, exacerbated by fragile regional and national health-care systems devastated by deaths among local health-care nurses and physicians.

In a 2015 issue of *Point of Care*, authors provided viewpoints of POC technologies and testing modalities at institutions, but none adequately dealt with the future global scope of the POC field. The practice of medicine has become a shared societal enterprise. Now, primary care can be practiced cost-effectively by 'digital doctors.' Widespread inexpensive online consultations using smartphones, i-pads, and other mobile technologies will be embraced rapidly by NGOs, third-party payers and insurers who will fund cheaper bidirectional mobile venues and distributed diagnostic testing. This telehealth approach can be used with FAST•POC™ and POCT•PODs™ to achieve timeliness of detection and diagnosis.

## POINT OF CARE CULTURE/'POINT OF CAREOLOGY'

Recent field evaluations for Ebola demonstrated interesting POC results (Broadhurst *et al.* 2015) and support the feasibility of enhancing POC culture to stop outbreaks. POC culture is defined as medical empowerment of the individual and family nucleus integrated with norms, behaviours, beliefs, attitudes, expectations, POC technology and outcomes (Kost *et al.* 2015a). POCT crosses cultural barriers unobtrusively. Education, guided tutorials and step-by-step instructions conveyed by public health workers (e.g. for FAST•POC™) can be tailored to local settings, spoken dialects and cultural expectations. Aided by smartphone-enabled POCT advances, results can be made available in community geographical information systems (GISs) to speed rescue, isolation and treatment. Immediate empowerment without the risks of waiting days for diagnostic test results will reduce the fear of foreign intervention in limited-resource countries. Importantly, quelling hotspots will prevent spread of disease within family and social SWNs. The quicker an outbreak is found, before it regenerates exponentially, the smaller it will be. That is the promise of culturally tuned POCT.

Global society, not institutions, should be where we focus our future vision. Ebola and MERS have driven that vision into a reality demanding POCT (Chua *et al.* 2015). Should there be a large-scale epidemic, care will quickly shift into the community where people are quarantined. Diagnostic testing will follow the most efficient SCP™. Now is the time to empower people with POC tools, so they can build chains of resilience, stop outbreaks and resolve demographically endemic health problems. Geospatially optimised POCT is needed to empower challenging SWNs where transportation is difficult and air rescue generally is not available. Besides potential infectious disease threats, prediabetes and other serious health problems, especially those plaguing burgeoning populations (e.g. in China), will propel POC culture forward. We call this new field of medicine and the POC culture it embodies, '*Point-of-Careology*' (Liu *et al.* 2016).

## VISION FOR THE FUTURE – 10 EVIDENCE-BASED CONCLUSIONS

1. POCT is improving global health, and now global health problems and threats of new viruses are propelling POCT and its cultural assimilation worldwide. Recent revelations of accidents, secrecy and adverse outcomes from highly infectious diseases made public by investigative journalists highlight potential for outbreaks locally within the USA and other countries. Zoonotic reservoirs sustain major virus threats while enabling jumps to humans. Because animal reservoirs generally cannot be eliminated, innovative strategies for human detection are necessary.
2. Financial losses from Ebola, MERS and potential new outbreaks warrant significant investment, which should be directed not just to vaccines, but also development of molecular diagnostics and other POC tests.

A worldwide research and development fund for POC diagnostics should be set up, as recommended by the Harvard Global Health Institute-London School of Tropical Medicine and Hygiene Independent Panel (Moon *et al.* 2015).

3. Waiting for patients to present symptomatic, sick and scared at treatment centres perpetuates outbreaks, unnecessary mortality, and collateral deaths in those not infected. Alternative care facilities and diagnostic centres with integrated logistics for community SWNs will allow communities to respond efficiently and effectively.
4. Ultrahigh sensitive and specific assays that detect high-risk diseases quickly can stop outbreaks from escalating into devastating epidemics. Companion diagnostics, such as coagulopathy clusters (PT/INR, D-dimer, fibrinogen and platelets), viral load assays and digital PCR will help predict outcomes (Faye *et al.* 2015), streamline therapeutic monitoring, identify and detect relapses and allow social workers to counsel patients regarding sexual transmission.
5. Diagnosis should occur upstream in SCPs™ in homes, primary care and ERs using FAST•POC™ and POCT•PODs™ before patients disseminate disease throughout the community. SCPs™ consolidate process steps to stop spread of outbreaks, while diagnostic centres with controlled environments placed along SCPs™ consolidate community efforts on a cost-effective scale.
6. Public health practitioners must work in the field closer to points of need and use new strategies, such as SCPs™, ACFs, diagnostic centres, POCT•PODs™ and geospatially optimised FAST•POC™. SCPs™ can facilitate contact tracing, counteract community resistance and denial, protect health workers, ease overburdened treatment centres and reduce patient loss to follow-up. Based on modelling predictions (Nouvellet *et al.* 2015), rapid POCT with confirmatory nucleic acid testing will reduce the scale of epidemics >33%, if implemented using the optimised strategies presented here.
7. Epidemiologists should build and publish knowledge bases of POC test sensitivity, specificity and predictive values. These data will facilitate diagnostic device maturation, refine evidence-based medicine for targeted diseases and prepare first responders for future outbreaks.
8. POC diagnostics should be available for immigration screening, on cruise ships, in industrial sites abroad, within airline terminals and at other points of first encounter worldwide. Adaptations in hospitals have not generated isolation bed capacity adequate to deal with potentially large numbers of cases, so new outbreaks will require ACFs.
9. Individual communities should engage ACF planning, matrix education, PPE rehearsals and community POC training to ameliorate civil rights issues through equitable care during military lockdowns, quarantines and forced confinements. Social scientists should educate response teams about cultural factors relevant to outbreak control, and specifically, about POC culture, investigated with objective surveys (Kost and Curtis 2015).
10. POC experts, professionally certified POC coordinators and geospatial scientists should design SCPs™ in the context of cohesive national strategies. The recent outbreaks motivate national policies and guidelines for POCT, in order to assure appropriate infrastructure can be designed, funded and distributed evenly.

## ACKNOWLEDGEMENTS

This work was supported by the POCT•CTR and Dr Kost, Founding Director. Spatial Care Path™ (SCP™) is a trademark by Gerald Kost and William Ferguson. FAST•POC™ and POCT•POD™ are trademarks of Gerald Kost. Angela Kost created Fig. 24.4. Figures and tables are provided courtesy and permission of Knowledge Optimization®, Davis, California.

## REFERENCES

Broadhurst MJ, Kelly JD, Miller A, Semper A, Bailey D, Gropelli E, *et al.* (2015) ReEBOV antigen rapid test kit for point-of-care and laboratory-based testing for Ebola virus disease: a field evaluation study. *Lancet* **386**, 867–874. doi:10.1016/S0140-6736(15)61042-X

Chua AC, Cunningham J, Moussy F, Perkins MD, Formenty P (2015) The case for improved diagnostic tools to control Ebola virus disease in West Africa and how to get there. *PLoS Neglected Tropical Diseases* **9**, e0003734. doi:10.1371/journal.pntd.0003734

Faye O, Ansdronico A, Faye O, Saije H, Boelle P-Y, Magassouba N'F *et al.* (2015) Use of viremia to evaluate the baseline care fatality ratio of Ebola virus disease and inform treatment studies: a retrospective cohort study. *PLoS Medicine* **12**, e1001908. doi:10.1371/journal.pmed.1001908

Hongoltz-Hetling M (2015) Ebola is now killing people who aren't even infected. *Foreign Policy* Online 7 December 2015, <http://foreignpolicy.com/2015/12/07/ebola-is-now-killing-people-who-arent-even-infected-sierra-leone/>.

Kost GJ (2015) Using small-world networks to optimise preparedness, response, and resilience. In *Global Point of Care: Strategies for Disasters, Emergencies, and Public Health Resilience.* (Eds GJ Kost and CM Curtis) pp. 539–568. AACC Press, Washington DC, USA.

Kost GJ, Curtis CM (Eds) (2015) *Global Point of Care: Strategies for Disasters, Emergencies, and Public Health Resilience.* AACC Press, Washington DC, USA.

Kost GJ, Zhou Y, Katip P (2015a) Understanding point of care culture improves resiliency and standards of care in resource-limited countries. In *Global Point of Care: Strategies for Disasters, Emergencies, and Public Health Resilience.* (Eds GJ Kost and CM Curtis) pp. 471–490. AACC Press, Washington DC, USA.

Kost GJ, Ferguson WJ, Hoe J, Truong A-T, Banpavichit A, Kongpila S (2015b) The Ebola Spatial Care Path™: accelerating point-of-care diagnosis, decision making, and community resilience in outbreaks. *American Journal of Disaster Medicine* **10**, 121–143. doi:10.5055/ajdm.2015.0196

Kost GJ, Ferguson WJ, Troung A-T, Hoe J, Prom D, Banpavachit A, *et al.* (2015c) Molecular detection and point-of-care testing in Ebola virus disease and other threats: a new global public health framework to stop outbreaks. *Expert Review of Molecular Diagnostics* **15**, 1245–1259. doi:10.1586/14737159.2015.1079776

Liu X, Kost GJ, Liu J, Liu X (2016) *The Origin and Definition of Point of Careology.* International Collaborative Document [English-Chinese].

Moon S, Sridhar D, Pate MA, Jha AK, Clinton C, Delaunay S, *et al.* (2015) Will Ebola change the game? Ten essential reforms before the next pandemic. The report of the Harvard-LSHTM Independent Panel on the global response to Ebola. *Lancet* **386**, 2204–2221. doi:10.1016/S0140-6736(15)00946-0

Nouvellet P, Garske T, Mills HL, Nediati-Gilani G, Hinsley W, Blake IM, *et al.* (2015) The role of rapid diagnostics in managing Ebola epidemics. *Nature* **3**, 5109–5116.

Okeke N, Manning RS, Peiffer T (2014) Diagnostic schemes for reducing epidemic size of African viral hemorrhagic fever. *Journal of Infection in Developing Countries* **8**, 1148–1159. doi:10.3855/jidc.4636

Oleś K, Gudowska-Nowak E, Kleczkowski A (2012) Understanding disease control: influence of epidemiological and economic factors. *PLoS One* **7**, e36026. doi:10.1371/journal.pone.0036026

Strecker T, Palyi B, Ellerbrok H, Jonckeere S, deClerck H, Bore JA, *et al.* (2015) Field evaluation of capillary blood samples as a collection specimen for the rapid diagnosis of Ebola virus infection during an outbreak emergency. *Clinical Infectious Diseases* **61**(Supplement 1), 669–675. doi:10.1093/cid/civ397

# 25 Point-of-care testing for C-reactive protein

*Rogier Hopstaken and Lara Harmans*

**Summary**

C-reactive protein (CRP) is a rapid and sensitive inflammation marker for diagnosis of disease. CRP point-of-care testing (POCT) is currently used by general practitioners (GPs) in a selective number of countries, mainly in Europe. Aided by similar guidelines, CRP is mostly used for diagnosis and antibiotic stewardship in adults with lower respiratory tract infections, but is also suggested for upper respiratory tract infections, diverticulitis, appendicitis and chronic obstructive pulmonary disease (COPD) exacerbations. Even though CRP correlates well with the severity of illness, it cannot determine aetiology nor can it accurately discriminate between bacterial and viral infections in general practice. So far, cost-effectiveness is mostly in the longer term: reduced antibiotic prescribing and quality-adjusted life years (QALYs) gained. There are currently several POC devices available for CRP (or even high sensitivity CRP) of acceptable quality for use in general practice.

## INTRODUCTION

This chapter introduces the C-reactive protein (CRP) test and its clinical use in respiratory infections (notably its use in reducing antibiotic prescription rates), with some commentary on the extent of its use in the general practice/primary care sector, particularly in Europe but also in other regions of the world.

## BACKGROUND

C-reactive protein (CRP) is an acute-phase biomarker released by the liver during the systemic response to inflammation (Pepys 1981; Volanakis 2001). Circulating levels are low in healthy individuals. The levels rise quickly (within 4–6 h) and remain high during active inflammation/infection, with maximal concentrations after 36–50 h, and with a rapid decline upon recovery (Becker *et al.* 2004; Volanakis 2001). Serial measurements can be useful to monitor the course of illness and response to (antibiotic) therapy. A 1000-fold rise of the normal value (generally <10 mg/L) is possible. CRP is therefore a very rapid and sensitive inflammation marker, but non-specific for a particular acute illness when used without clinical context. CRP has been used routinely in hospital settings for all types of inflammations and infections in many countries all over the world, and for many years now. It is an acknowledged and useful biomarker in diagnosis of disease. CRP is also often requested by primary care physicians in many countries as a regular laboratory test. POCT for CRP is, however, only used in a selective number of countries. It was introduced in Scandinavian general practice in the late 1980s. At that time, evidence on the added value of CRP was limited to a Norwegian study on lower respiratory tract infections (LRTI) in general practice (Melbye *et al.* 1988). Since then, it is routinely performed in the Scandinavian countries and Switzerland. Other European countries have recently shown interest in introducing CRP POCT. This follows publications showing convincing evidence of the rather poor clinical diagnosis of pneumonia in general practice, and the added value of CRP POCT in these cases. Moreover, introduction of CRP POCT in general practices resulted in better antibiotic stewardship in lower respiratory tract infections, with broad satisfaction of GPs and patients in general practice (Cals *et al.* 2009; Hopstaken *et al.* 2003; Little *et al.* 2013; van Vugt *et al.* 2013). In 2011, CRP POCT was introduced in the Dutch guideline on lower respiratory tract infections ('acute cough'). This has resulted in a rapidly increasing uptake of CRP POCT by, currently, ~50% of GPs in the Netherlands. The use of CRP (POCT) has recently been recommended by the British guideline on community- and hospital-acquired pneumonia in adults by the National Institute for Health and Care Excellence (NICE) (Eccles *et al.* 2014).

## EVIDENCE

The contribution of CRP POCT in patients with a possible inflammation process or infection needs to be assessed on top of the available clinical information from medical history and physical examination. Most evidence is available for adults with acute cough due to a LRTI.

### Diagnosis of pneumonia

After Laennec had described the added value of indirect auscultation (using a stethoscope) compared with direct auscultation (ear on the chest) in 1819 (Laennec 1819), it took until the mid-1980s before formal diagnostic studies on the predictive value of symptoms and signs for the diagnosis of pneumonia were performed in emergency departments and general practice settings (Metlay *et al.* 1997). Classical symptoms and signs, derived from observations in hospital settings, turned out to have rather poor predictive value for the diagnosis of pneumonia in general practice, due to the lower incidence and (generally) less severe extent of the disease found in a primary care setting. Overall, the clinical diagnosis of pneumonia was poor compared with the (non-perfect) reference standard: judgment of pneumonia by (a panel of) radiologists based on chest radiographs. The overall contribution of the clinical judgement for pneumonia, summarised as area under the curve (AUC) in ROC curves, was 70%, both in a Dutch study, as well as in the large GRACE study in 12 European countries (Hopstaken *et al.* 2003; van Vugt *et al.* 2013). Addition of CRP to the GP's clinical judgment raised this to 90% and 79%, respectively. In particular, exclusion of pneumonia with low CRP test results (<20 mg/L), present in most of all adult acute cough patients, is of importance to reassure both the GP and the patient of the presence of the non-severe illness. Other (less formal) diagnostic studies performed in primary care and emergency departments have all pointed to the same direction of this significant added value of CRP for the diagnosis (and exclusion) of pneumonia.

### Antibiotic stewardship

CRP POCT has the potential to reduce many unnecessary antibiotic prescriptions in the combat of emerging bacterial resistance worldwide. Cough is the most common acute reason for consulting a general practitioner. In a 13-country study, the prescription rates in primary care of antibiotics for acute cough varied from 28 to 92% (Butler *et al.* 2009). Cough due to LRTIs accounts for 28 million GP consultations per year in the USA and Europe (Macfarlane *et al.* 2001; Schappert and Burt 2006). Up to 90% of oral antibiotics are prescribed in primary care, mostly for respiratory tract infections (Goossens *et al.* 2005). Differentiating severe LRTI (mostly pneumonia, 5–20% of LRTI patients consulting a GP) from non-severe LRTI (mostly acute bronchitis; 80–95% of LRTI patients) is important, because antibiotics are not helpful for most patients with acute bronchitis (Little *et al.* 2013; Smith *et al.* 2014), but considered necessary for pneumonia.

The challenge for primary care doctors is the risk of not treating a potentially life-threatening pneumonia on the one hand, and prescribing unnecessary antibiotics in the generally self-limiting acute bronchitis on the other hand (André *et al.* 2004; Hopstaken *et al.* 2003). Diagnostic uncertainty, (perceived) patient pressure, cultural habits and the common belief that bacterial resistance is caused by others are important reasons for huge antibiotic overprescribing in most countries in the world (Coenen *et al.* 2013; McCullough *et al.* 2015). The first two factors can be influenced by CRP POCT. In the two available, high-quality cluster-randomised controlled trials, CRP POCT indeed reduced antibiotic prescribing without compromising recovery and satisfaction with

**Table 25.1.** Guidelines for antibiotic prescription in primary care based on CRP test result (Sources: Eccles *et al.* 2014; Verlee *et al.* 2012)

| **CRP levels <20 mg/L**<br>**Self-limiting RTI** | **CRP 20–100 mg/L**<br>**Consider a delayed antibiotic prescription** | **CRP >100 mg/L**<br>**Severe infection** |
|---|---|---|
| Pneumonia unlikely | Clinical presentation decisive | High risk of pneumonia |
| Do not routinely offer antibiotic therapy; give education | Prescribe antibiotics only in patients with a high risk of complications | Offer antibiotic therapy |

care (Cals *et al.* 2009; Little *et al.* 2013). Enhanced general consultation skills enlarged this effect. Regarding CRP POCT, participating GPs were advised to prescribe according to the guidelines in Table 25.1. Similar guidelines with algorithms using CRP thresholds for antibiotic prescribing in primary care are implemented in the Netherlands and the UK. These guidelines state that a (POC) CRP test should be considered if a patient presents with a suspected LRTI if it is not clear after clinical examination whether antibiotics should be prescribed.

A Cochrane review on biomarkers as POC tests to guide prescription of antibiotics in patients with both upper and lower acute respiratory infections in primary care judged six CRP POCT randomised controlled trials, involving 3284 mostly adult patients (Aabenhus *et al.* 2014). Antibiotic use was 22% lower in the group of patients with CRP POCT, giving a risk ratio of 0.78 (95% CI 0.66 to 0.92; I2 = 68%; Fig. 25.1). Reported reductions were 36.2% in patients presenting with acute cough/lower respiratory tract infection.

Medicalisation effects of introducing CRP POCT may be possible, but CRP POCT used by GPs did not affect office visit rates related to LRTI, shown in the only study evaluating this possible effect (Cals *et al.* 2013).

Fig. 25.2 shows a flowchart for management of respiratory tract infections that was used in the guideline on acute cough of the Dutch College of GPs (Verheij *et al.* 2011). It is primarily based on the results of a Dutch diagnostic study on LRTI (Hopstaken *et al.* 2003) and the Dutch cluster-randomised controlled trial (Cals *et al.* 2009).

Comparable conclusions derived from the European GRACE studies were the basis for the recent introduction of CRP POCT in the British NICE guideline on diagnosis and management of community- and hospital-acquired pneumonia in adults. It is advised to 'consider a point-of-care C-reactive protein test if after clinical assessment a diagnosis of pneumonia has not been made and it is not clear whether antibiotics should be prescribed.' Cut-off points of 20 and 100 mg/L were used in a comparable way

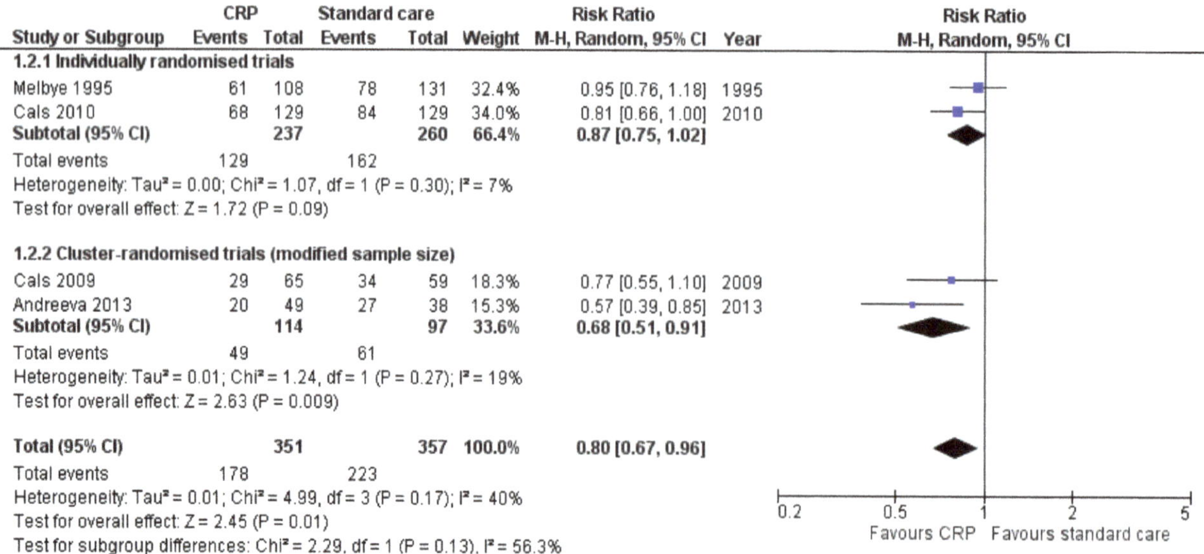


**Fig. 25.1.** Forest plots for randomised and cluster randomised controlled trials. (Source: Reproduced from Aabenhus *et al.* (2014) with permission of John Wiley & Sons)

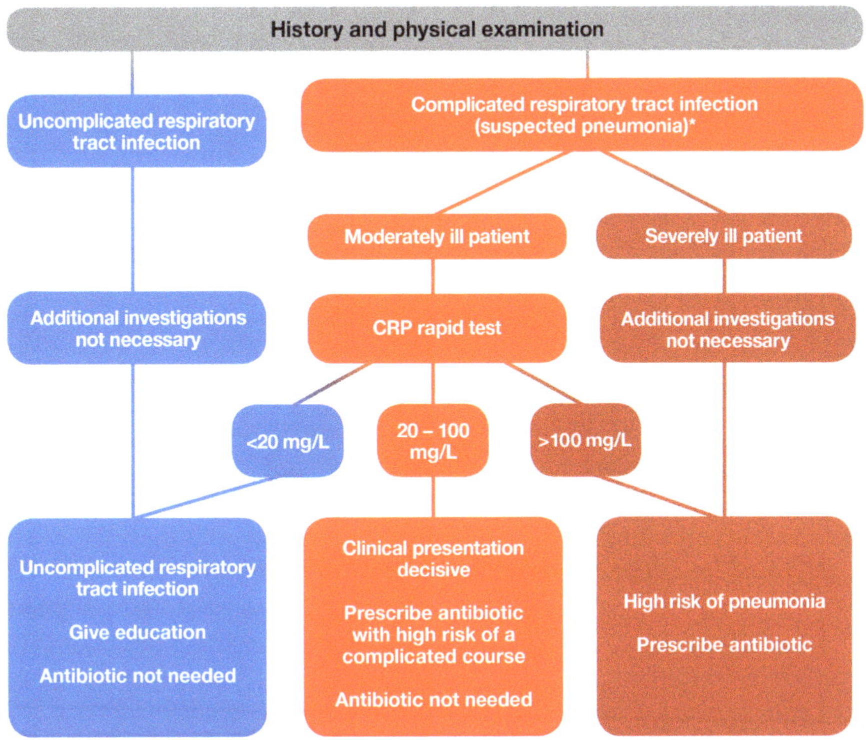


**Fig. 25.2.** Management of respiratory functions. (Source: Modified from Verlee *et al.* 2012)

as described in Table 25.1. The guideline for the management of adult LRTI by the European Respiratory Society uses the same approach, although does not specifically comment on CRP test results between 20 and 99 mg/L (Woodhead *et al.* 2011).

Because resistant pneumonia bacteria can cause infections that result in increased mortality, prolonged hospital stays, and increased costs (Feikin *et al.* 2000), the most predominant outcome measure is reduction in antibiotic prescriptions (Joshi *et al.* 2013). Another study demonstrated that the introduction of CRP POCT could reduce antibiotic prescription rates and radiology referrals, most likely without negative effects on patient recovery rates (Andreeva and Melbye 2014). When comparing GP communication skills training with use of CRP POCT, similar potential to reduce antibiotic use was shown: a combination of the interventions showed an additive effect (Little *et al.* 2013).

## Cost-effectiveness

Cost-effectiveness of introducing CRP POCT in primary care for LRTIs was shown in the three studies performed so far (Cals *et al.* 2011; Hunter 2015; Oppong *et al.* 2013).

Hunter (2015) presented three models of CRP POCT use in patients with RTI symptoms in a 3-year study in England: a group of GPs performing CRP POCT; a group of practice nurses performing CRP POCT; and a group of GPs performing CRP POCT that have been trained in specific communication skills. All three models showed favourable results over the groups not using CRP POCT at all: the additional cost per patient of the test is outweighed by the cost savings and QALYs gained of reduced infections in the long run.

Cals *et al.* (2011) performed an observational study on the effects of CRP POCT use on antibiotic prescription rates in patients presenting with acute cough in the Netherlands. The patients who received usual care had a mean cost of €35.96 (with 68% prescribed antibiotics), patients managed by GPs using CRP POCT €37.58 (with 39% prescribed antibiotics), patients managed by GPs trained in enhanced communication skills €25.61 (with 33% prescribed antibiotics), and patients managed by GPs with both interventions €37.78 (with 23% prescribed antibiotics). At very low or no willingness-to-pay, the interventions were cost-effective to reduce antibiotic prescribing in any combination.

In a study in Norway and Sweden, Oppong *et al.* (2013) found a non-significant reduction in antibiotic prescribing ($P$ = 0.078) and increased cost of GPs using CRP POCT ($P$ = 0.092). A cost-effectiveness analysis showed, however, that the increased short-term costs of CRP POCT (€11.27 per patient) were followed by a long-term cost reduction of €112.70 per antibiotic prescription avoided. The use of CRP POCT was also associated with an improved quality of life: a cost per QALY gain of €9391 was calculated.

### Conditions other than LRTI

The value of CRP POCT has mostly been studied in LRTI, but could also be beneficial in the diagnostic process of other respiratory tract infections, diverticulitis, appendicitis, COPD and other complaints resulting from a possible inflammation. Evidence from primary care is, however, scarce.

#### Upper respiratory tract infections (URTI)

Antibiotic prescribing may be reduced when GPs use CRP POCT for rhinosinusitis (Bjerrum *et al.* 2004; Cals *et al.* 2010) but the results are conflicting (Diederichsen *et al.* 2000) and relatively weak in countries where overall antibiotic prescribing is already low. It seems that antibiotics are withheld when a low CRP test result is obtained, but frequently started when CRP test results are only moderately elevated (>25 mg/L). The risk of overuse of CRP POCT is not neglectable (André *et al.* 2004).

#### Diverticulitis

CRP POCT may be advised as an additional test to support the diagnosis of diverticulitis (CRP >20 mg/L), as well as for differentiating uncomplicated from possibly complicated (>100 mg/L) diverticulitis (de Wit *et al.* 2012). A CRP test result above 50 mg/L was one of three strong predictors of diverticulitis in a hospital study (Andeweg *et al.* 2011), but primary care studies are lacking.

#### COPD

CRP POCT can be helpful to discriminate infectious from non-infectious exacerbations of COPD in line with (other) LRTI (Geijer *et al.* 2015). A Norwegian guideline on COPD uses a cut-off point of CRP >50 mg/L for antibiotic treatment (Helsedirektoratet 2012). CRP has also shown to be of prognostic value for clinical outcome in exacerbations of mild to moderate COPD (Llor *et al.* 2012).

#### Appendicitis

A CRP POC test is often used in patients with a suspected appendicitis in hospitals. Sensitivity, particularly in the early stages of disease, is not high enough to safely rule out appendicitis with a low CRP test result. The positive likelihood ratio was good enough in a recent systematic review to advise CRP POCT when appendicitis is suspected. Accuracy of CRP as a single test for appendicitis was 75% (Yu *et al.* 2013).

## CURRENT ISSUES/LIMITATIONS

CRP correlates well with severity of an illness, but cannot determine aetiology (Aabenhus *et al.* 2014). CRP levels are typically lower in patients with viral infections than in patients with bacterial infections (Cooke *et al.* 2015), but it cannot be confirmed that CRP can differentiate between bacterial and viral infections accurately in general practice (Hopstaken *et al.* 2005; Melbye *et al.* 2004).

Even though children are often subject to LRTIs and antibiotic prescription rates are very high, studies on CRP POCT in children are lacking in general practice. The diagnostic value of CRP POCT for pneumonia in adults cannot be automatically extrapolated to children, due to differences in immunity, causal agents, anatomy and physiology, particularly in the very young (Chang 2010). CRP levels correlate with chances of having pneumonia, but pneumonia cannot be safely ruled-out with low levels (Koster *et al.* 2013; Oostenbrink *et al.* 2013). Pneumonia was present in 28% of children with CRP levels below 20 mg/L in a hospital study. High values increase the likelihood of the diagnosis: CRP raised the pre-test probability of 52 to 63%. The measurement of CRP may be more beneficial in a primary care setting, where pre-test probabilities are much lower (Koster *et al.* 2013).

Above all, CRP POCT is a diagnostic tool that may have added value after clinical work-up and in selected cases. GPs are the experts who can turn this non-specific test into a specific one, when combined with other available diagnostic information.

## OTHER MARKERS OF INFECTION

### Procalcitonin (PCT)

PCT may be an effective and safe tool for guiding antibiotic stewardship in patients with acute respiratory infections. In secondary care settings, PCT has shown to have

Table 25.2. Selected specifications of the five CRP devices used in the study of Minnaard *et al.* (2013)

| Device | Afinion™ AS 100 | Nycocard™ Reader II | Eurolyser Smart 700/340 CRP | QuickRead go | QuickRead 101 |
|---|---|---|---|---|---|
| Manufacturer | Alere/Axis Shield, Norway | Alere/Axis Shield, Norway | Eurolyser, Austria | Orion Diagnostica, Finland | Orion Diagnostica, Finland |
| Method | Solid phase, sandwich immunometric | Solid phase, sandwich immunometric | Solid phase immunologic | Immunoturbidimetric | Immunoturbidimetric |
| Size (cm) | 17 × 32 × 17 | 17 × 20 × 10 | 14 × 14.5 × 26 | 28 × 16 × 16 | 14 × 22 × 8 |
| Weight (kg) | 5 | 0.5 | 3.4 | 1.5 | 1.0 |
| Connectivity | Yes | No | Yes | Yes | No |
| Analysis time | 3 min 45 s | 3 min 20 s | 4 min 20 s | 3 min 30 s | 1 min |
| Measuring range (mg/L) | 5–160 | 5–120 | 1–120 | 5–120 | 8–160 |
| Other tests | HbA1c, UACR, lipids | HbA1c, UAlb, D-dimer | HbA1c, UAlb, D-dimer, hsCRP, INR, ferritin, homocysteine, lipoprotein | No | Strep A, UAlb, faecal occult blood |

greater sensitivity and specificity in distinguishing bacterial and viral infections than CRP (Simon *et al.* 2004), but CRP seems to do better when ruling out pneumonia in primary care (van Vugt *et al.* 2013).

In general practice, PCT does not add sufficient value for decision making (Schuetz *et al.* 2012). Moreover, PCT POCT currently yields test results in 18 min, which usually does not fit neatly with most busy general practices. Addition of PCT to clinical judgment raised the accuracy for pneumonia from 70 to 71%, which was lower than addition of CRP (79%) (van Vugt *et al.* 2013).

### Hs-CRP

A specific CRP test that measures low grades of inflammation (0–10 mg/L) is called high-sensitive CRP (hs-CRP). Some CRP devices have the option to test for hs-CRP. Hs-CRP is an independent predictor of increased cardiovascular risks. It may also have predictive abilities for cardiovascular events. Hs-CRP consistently predicts new coronary events in patients with unstable angina and acute myocardial infarction (Pearson *et al.* 2003). Hs-CRP could also be used to identify patients who may be at higher absolute risk for developing cardiovascular disease than estimated by traditional, major risk factors, including biochemical risk markers (Rifai and Ridker 2001). However, the benefits of this strategy, or any treatment based on this strategy, is still not determined.

## SYNOPSIS OF CRP POCT DEVICES CURRENTLY AVAILABLE

Various POCT devices for CRP are on the market, offering both quantitative and semiquantitative tests, and venous and capillary sampling. Most devices provide test results within 3–5 min. Generally a single cut-off value in qualitative tests is not informative enough, because there is a strong correlation between the CRP value and the severity of infection/inflammation. Hence, this section is limited to a description of quantitative capillary CRP POCT, because these are most suitable for and most widely used in primary care.

Analytical performance, agreement and user-friendliness of five quantitative CRP POC devices (Afinion™, Eurolyser Smart, NycoCard™ Reader II, QuikRead 101 and QuikRead Go) was studied at an accredited laboratory, using a central laboratory analyser as the reference method (Minnaard *et al.* 2013). Selected specifications for these devices are provided in Table 25.2. Between-day imprecisions of <10% were reported with four of the POC devices (Afinion, NycoCard Reader II, QuikRead 101 and QuikRead Go) using two plasma pools with CRP concentrations of ~20 mg/L and 100 mg/L, respectively. Using eight serum pools with varying concentrations, mean differences (as assessed by Bland Altman plots) were <2 mg/L (at CRP concentrations <20 mg/L) and <6 mg/L at CRPs (between 20 and 100 mg/L) for all five devices. For CRP levels above 100 mg/L, agreement with the laboratory results systematically decreased for all POCT devices. The same research group performed a second study to determine the added diagnostic value of the five CRP POC tests in detecting pneumonia in primary care (Minnaard *et al.* 2015). They used venous samples from adult patients with acute cough from the European GRACE study with a proportion of 50% having radiographically proven pneumonia. All five CRP test devices and the laboratory analyser performed with similar accuracy in detecting pneumonia both as single test, and when used in addition to clinical findings. The authors conclude that 'variability in results obtained from standard CRP laboratory and POC test devices do not translate into clinically relevant differences when used for prediction of pneumonia in patients with acute cough in primary care.'

A third study was also a systematic multi-device evaluation for CRP POCT on adult venous blood samples, to determine the accuracy of the POCT results compared with a laboratory analyser. The conclusion from this study was that the general agreement between the POC tests (Afinion, Eurolyser Smart, iChroma, Microsemi and QuikRead Go) and the laboratory analyser was not very good, but acceptable for use in general practice (Brouwer and van Pelt 2015).

## CONCLUSION

CRP by POCT is a highly sensitive test, and can only be a specific test when integrated with the patient's clinical context. The value of CRP POCT is mostly studied and proven for the diagnosis and management of adult patients with lower respiratory tract infections (LRTIs), but may also have added value in children and in patients with abdominal complaints (acute diverticulitis and acute appendicitis), exacerbations of COPD, and other generalised inflammations or infections. In addition to the clinical work-up, CRP cut-off values of 20 mg/L and 100 mg/L are generally used for management decisions. CRP POCT can result in a reduction of unnecessary antibiotic prescriptions and a better selection of the right patients with LRTI to prescribe antibiotics to. High-quality CRP POCT is currently only routinely used in Scandinavian countries, Switzerland and the Netherlands.

## CASE STUDY 1.1: MR PETERS IS ILL

The 52-year old Mr Peters has not been feeling well for 5 days, and has a nasty cough. A combination of cough syrup and plenty of sleep did not help. He decides to consult his GP, Dr Laven. Mr Peters feels generally unwell, has a dry cough, and he feels tired all day long. He is not short of breath. Mr Peters is overall healthy, a non-smoker, does not use any medicines, and does not experience any problems at home or at work. The GP records: patient looks tired, moderately ill, not dyspneic; rectal temperature 38.4°C, heart rate 90 bpm, lymph nodes not enlarged, percussion normal. Auscultation reveals some crackles and rhonchi in both lower lung fields, left more than right.

Dr Laven explains to Mr Peters that he might suffer from acute bronchitis, a mostly mild and self-limiting illness, or pneumonia, which requires antibiotic treatment. To exclude the latter she asks Mr Peters to go to the practice nurse for a finger-prick test to measure CRP with a drop of blood. Dr Laven asks Mr Peters to return to his consultation room, when the test result is available – in just a few minutes. The CRP POC test result is 18 mg/L. Dr Laven explains that this value is low, which indicates that a pneumonia is very unlikely. She advises him to get plenty of rest and drink lots of fluids, and to come back if the symptoms get worse or the fever persists for 3 more days. Dr Laven reminds Mr Peters that the bothersome cough and fatigue usually diminish rapidly, but may last, less severely, for up to 3–4 weeks. After a week, Mr Peters phones cheerfully and tells the practice assistant to record that he is feeling a lot better, except for some coughing, especially at night.

## CASE STUDY 1.2: DR LAVEN AND HIGH-QUALITY CRP POCT

Dr Laven is happy that her patient Mr Peters feels much better now. She looks back on a good consultation and is happy that she had decided, earlier that month, to follow the Dutch guideline on POCT in general practice. She had started a collaboration with a primary care laboratory to jointly set up CRP POCT in her office. She admits, at first, she had to get used to the idea that she had to be certified by completing an online training on CRP POCT before she could start. She even had to sign a POCT contract with the laboratory on 'rights and obligations'. The primary care laboratory had selected the best available device for routine use in general practice after evaluating test quality, user-friendliness and robustness of various CRP POCT systems. When the device was placed, her practice nurse received hands-on training on how to perform the test, as well as on general issues of quality assurance, logistics and communication of the test results and controls. A dedicated IT system was installed that automatically connected patient information with the test device, via the cloud, with the laboratory system, and back to the electronic patient record to minimise human errors. It also allowed for device controls and user controls with a central server. The laboratory's POCT team checks the quality of the POCT system 24/7 and acts instantly on problems from a distance and by visiting the practice site. Dr Laven has learned that CRP POCT is not 'just a rapid test', but a process in which all elements need to be taken into account to improve patient care with maximal patient safety.

## REFERENCES


Aabenhus R, Jensen JU, Jørgensen KJ, Hróbjartsson A, Bjerrum L (2014) Biomarkers as point-of-care tests to guide prescription of antibiotics in patients with acute respiratory infections in primary care. *Cochrane Database of Systematic Reviews* **11**, CD010130. doi:10.1002/14651858.CD010130.pub2

Andeweg CS, Knobben L, Hendriks JC, Bleichrodt RP, van Goor H (2011) How to diagnose acute left-sided colonic diverticulitis: proposal for a clinical scoring system. *Annals of Surgery* **253**, 940–946. doi:10.1097/SLA.0b013e3182113614

André M, Schwan A, Odenholt I (2004) The use of CRP tests in patients with respiratory tract infections in primary care in Sweden can be questioned. *Scandinavian Journal of Infectious Diseases* **36**, 192–197. doi:10.1080/00365540410019372

Andreeva E, Melbye H (2014) Usefulness of C-reactive protein testing in acute cough/respiratory tract infection: an open cluster-randomized clinical trial with C-reactive protein testing in the intervention group. *BMC Family Practice* **15**, 80. doi:10.1186/1471-2296-15-80

Becker KL, Nylen ES, White JC, Muller B, Snider RH Jr (2004) Clinical review 167: Procalcitonin and the calcitonin gene family of peptides in inflammation, infection, and sepsis: a journey from calcitonin back to its precursors. *The Journal of Clinical Endocrinology and Metabolism* **89**, 1512–1525. doi:10.1210/jc.2002-021444

Bjerrum L, Gahrn-Hansen B, Munck AP (2004) C-reactive protein measurement in general practice may lead to lower antibiotic prescribing for sinusitis. *The British Journal of General Practice* **54**, 659–662.

Brouwer N, van Pelt J (2015) Validation and evaluation of eight commercially available point of care CRP methods. *Clinica Chimica Acta* **439**, 195–201. doi:10.1016/j.cca.2014.10.028

Butler CC, Hood K, Verheij T, Little P, Melbye H, Nuttall J, *et al.* (2009) Variation in antibiotic prescribing and its impact on recovery in patients with acute cough in primary care: prospective study in 13 countries. *British Medical Journal* **338**, b2242. doi:10.1136/bmj.b2242

Cals JWL, Butler CC, Hopstaken RM, Hood K, Dinant GJ (2009) Effect of point of care testing for C-reactive protein and training in communication skills on antibiotic use in lower respiratory tract infections: cluster randomised trial. *British Medical Journal* **338**, b1374. doi:10.1136/bmj.b1374

Cals JWL, Schot MJC, de Jong SAM, Dinant G-J, Hopstaken RM (2010) Point-of-care C-reactive protein testing and antibiotic prescribing for respiratory tract infections: a randomized controlled trial. *Annals of Family Medicine* **8**, 124–133. doi:10.1370/afm.1090

Cals JW, Ament AJ, Hood K, Butler CC, Hopstaken RM, Wassink GF, *et al.* (2011) C-reactive protein point of care testing and physician communication skills training for lower respiratory tract infections in general practice: economic evaluation of a cluster randomized trial. *Journal of Evaluation in Clinical Practice* **17**, 1059–1069. doi:10.1111/j.1365-2753.2010.01472.x

Cals JWL, de Bock L, Beckers PHW, Francis NA, Hopstaken RM, Hood K, *et al.* (2013) Enhanced communication skills and C-reactive protein point-of-care testing for respiratory tract infection: 3.5-year follow-up of a cluster randomized trial. *Annals of Family Medicine* **11**, 157–164. doi:10.1370/afm.1477

Chang AB (2010) Pediatric cough: children are not miniature adults. *Lung* **188**(Supplement 1), 33–40. doi:10.1007/s00408-009-9166-2

Coenen S, Francis N, Kelly M, Hood K, Nuttall J, Little P, *et al.* (2013) Are patient views about antibiotics related to clinician perceptions, management and outcome? A multi-country study in outpatients with acute cough. *PLoS One* **8**, e76691. doi:10.1371/journal.pone.0076691

Cooke J, Butler C, Hopstaken R, Dryden MS, McNulty C, Hurding S, *et al.* (2015) Narrative review of primary care point-of-care testing (POCT) and antibacterial use in respiratory tract infection (RTI). *BMJ Open Respiratory Research* **2**, e000086. doi:10.1136/bmjresp-2015-000086

de Wit NJ, Berger MY, Vogelenzang R, Wetzels RV, van Rijn-van Kortenhof NM, Opstelten W, *et al.* (2012) Summary of the Dutch College of General Practitioners (NHG) practice guideline on diverticulitis. *Nederlands Tijdschrift voor Geneeskunde* **156**, A4140.

Diederichsen HZ, Skamling M, Diederichsen A, Grinsted P, Antonsen S, Petersen PH, *et al.* (2000) Randomised controlled trial of CRP rapid test as a guide to treatment of respiratory infections in general practice. *Scandinavian Journal of Primary Health Care* **18**, 39–43. doi:10.1080/02813430050202541

Eccles S, Pincus C, Higgins B, Woodhead M on behalf of the Guideline Development Group (2014) Diagnosis and management of community and hospital acquired pneumonia in adults: summary of NICE guidance. *British Medical Journal* **349**, g6722. doi:10.1136/bmj.g6722

Feikin DR, Schuchat A, Kolczak M, Barrett NL, Harrison LH, Lefkowitz L, *et al.* (2000) Mortality from invasive pneumococcal pneumonia in the era of antibiotic resistance, 1995–1997. *American Journal of Public Health* **90**, 223–229. doi:10.2105/AJPH.90.2.223

Geijer RM, Tuut MK, in't Veen JC, Broekhuizen BD, Chavannes NH, Smeele IJ (2015) The NHG guidelines 'Adult asthma' and 'COPD'. *Nederlands Tijdschrift voor Geneeskunde* **159**, A9076.

Goossens H, Ferench M, Vander SR, Elseviers M (2005) Outpatient antibiotics use in Europe and association with resistance: a cross-national database study. *Lancet* **365**, 579–587. doi:10.1016/S0140-6736(05)70799-6

Helsedirektoratet (2012) *KOLS-Nasjonal Faglig Retningslinje og Veileder for Forebygging, Diagnostisering og Oppfølging av Personer med kols.* Helsedirektoratet, Oslo, Norway.

Hopstaken RM, Muris JW, Knottnerus JA, Kester AD, Rinkens PE, Dinant GJ (2003) Contributions of symptoms, signs, erythrocyte sedimentation rate, and C-reactive protein to a diagnosis of pneumonia in acute lower respiratory tract infection. *The British Journal of General Practice* **53**, 358–364.

Hopstaken RM, Stobberingh EE, Knottnerus JA, Muris JW, Nelemans P, Rinkens PE, *et al.* (2005) Clinical items not helpful in differentiating viral from bacterial lower respiratory tract infections in general practice. *Journal of Clinical Epidemiology* **58**, 175–183. doi:10.1016/j.jclinepi.2004.08.004

Hunter R (2015) Cost-effectiveness of point-of-care C-reactive protein tests for respiratory tract infection in primary care in England. *Advances in Therapy* **32**, 69–85. doi:10.1007/s12325-015-0180-x

Joshi A, Perin DP, Gehle A, Nsiah-Kumi PA (2013) Feasibility of using C-reactive protein for point-of-care testing. *Technology and Health Care* **21**, 233–240.

Koster MJ, Broekhuizen BD, Minnaard MC, Balemans WA, Hopstaken RM, de Jong PA, *et al.* (2013) Diagnostic properties of C-reactive protein for detecting pneumonia in children. *Respiratory Medicine* **107**, 1087–1093. doi:10.1016/j.rmed.2013.04.012

Laennec RTH (1819) De *L'auscultation Mediate ou Traite du Diagnostic des Maladies des Poumons et du Coeur (On Mediate Auscultation or Treatise on the Diagnosis of the Diseases of the Lungs And Heart).* Brosson & Chaude. Paris, France.

Little P, Stuart B, Francis N, Douglas E, Tonkin-Crine S, Anthierens S, *et al.* on behalf of the GRACE consortium (2013) Effects of internet-based training on antibiotic prescribing rates for acute respiratory-tract infections: a multinational, cluster, randomised, factorial, controlled trial. *Lancet* **382**, 1175–1182. doi:10.1016/S0140-6736(13)60994-0

Llor C, Moragas A, Hernández S, Bayona C, Miravitlles M (2012) Efficacy of antibiotic therapy for acute exacerbations of mild to moderate chronic obstructive pulmonary disease. *American Journal of Respiratory and Critical Care Medicine* **186**, 716–723. doi:10.1164/rccm.201206-0996OC

Macfarlane J, Holmes W, Gard P, Macfarlane R, Rose D, Weston V, *et al.* (2001) Prospective study of the incidence, aetiology and outcome of adult lower respiratory tract illness in the community. *Thorax* **56**, 109–114. doi:10.1136/thorax.56.2.109

McCullough AR, Rathbone J, Parekh S, Hoffmann TC, Del Mar CB (2015) Not in my backyard: a systematic review of clinicians' knowledge and beliefs about antibiotic resistance. *The Journal of Antimicrobial Chemotherapy* **70**, 2465–2473. doi:10.1093/jac/dkv164

Melbye H, Straume B, Aasebo U, Brox J (1988) The diagnosis of adult pneumonia in general practice. The diagnostic value of history, physical examination and some blood tests. *Scandinavian Journal of Primary Health Care* **6**, 111–117. doi:10.3109/02813438809009300

Melbye H, Hvidsten D, Holm A, Nordbø SA, Brox J (2004) The course of C-reactive protein response in untreated upper respiratory tract infection. *The British Journal of General Practice* **54**, 653–658.

Metlay JP, Kapoor WN, Fine MJ (1997) Does this patient have community-acquired pneumonia? Diagnosing pneumonia by history and physical examination. *Journal of the American Medical Association* **278**, 1440–1445. doi:10.1001/jama.1997.03550170070035

Minnaard MC, van de Pol AC, Broekhuizen BD, Verheij TJ, Hopstaken RM, van Delft S, *et al.* (2013) Analytical performance, agreement and user-friendliness of five C-reactive protein point-of-care tests. *Scandinavian Journal of Clinical and Laboratory Investigation* **73**, 627–634. doi:10.3109/00365513.2013.841985

Minnaard MC, van de Pol AC, de Groot JA, De Wit NJ, Hopstaken RM, van Delft S, *et al.* (2015) The added diagnostic value of five different C-reactive protein point-of-care test devices in detecting pneumonia in primary care: a nested case-control study. *Scandinavian Journal of Clinical and Laboratory Investigation* **75**, 291–295. doi:10.3109/00365513.2015.1006136

Oostenbrink R, Thompson M, Lakhanpaul M, Steyerberg EW, Coad N, Moll HA (2013) Children with fever and cough at emergency care: diagnostic accuracy of a clinical model to identify children at low risk of pneumonia. *European Journal of Emergency Medicine* **20**, 273–280. doi:10.1097/MEJ.0b013e32835771fd

Oppong R, Jit M, Smith RD, Butler CC, Melbye H, Mölstad S, Coast J (2013) Cost-effectiveness of point-of-care C-reactive protein testing to inform antibiotic prescribing decisions. *The British Journal of General Practice* **63**, e465–e471. doi:10.3399/bjgp13X669185

Pearson TA, Mensah GA, Alexander RW, Anderson JL, Cannon RO 3rd, Criqui M, *et al.* (2003) Markers of inflammation and cardiovascular disease: application to clinical and public health practice: a statement for healthcare professionals from the Centers for Disease Control and Prevention and the American Heart Association. *Circulation* **107**, 499–511. doi:10.1161/01.CIR.0000052939.59093.45

Pepys MB (1981) C-reactive protein fifty years on. *Lancet* **317**, 653–657. doi:10.1016/S0140-6736(81)91565-8

Rifai N, Ridker PM (2001) High-sensitivity C-reactive protein: a novel and promising marker of coronary heart disease. *Clinical Chemistry* **47**, 403–411.

Schappert SM, Burt CW (2006) Ambulatory care visits to physician offices, hospital outpatient departments, and emergency departments: United States, 2001–02. *Vital and Health Statistics. Series 13, Data from the National Health Survey* **13**, 1–66.

Schuetz P, Müller B, Christ-Crain M, Stolz D, Tamm M, Bouadma L, *et al.* (2012) Procalcitonin to initiate or discontinue antibiotics in acute respiratory tract infections. *Cochrane Database of Systematic Reviews* **12**, CD007498.

Simon L, Gauvin F, Amre DK, Saint-Louis P, Lacroix J (2004) Serum procalcitonin and C-reactive protein levels as markers of bacterial infection: a systematic review and meta-analysis. *Clinical Infectious Diseases* **39**, 206–217. doi:10.1086/421997

Smith SM, Fahey T, Smucny J, Becker LA (2014) Antibiotics for acute bronchitis. *Cochrane Database of Systematic Reviews* **4**, CD000245.

van Vugt SF, Broekhuizen BD, Lammens C, Zuithoff NP, de Jong PA, Coenen S, *et al.* on behalf of the GRACE consortium (2013) Use of serum C reactive protein and procalcitonin concentrations in addition to symptoms and signs to predict pneumonia in patients presenting to primary care with acute cough: diagnostic study. *British Medical Journal* **346**, f2450. doi:10.1136/bmj.f2450

Verheij ThJM, Hopstaken RM, Prins JM, Salomé PhL, Bindels PJ, Ponsioen BP, *et al.* (2011) *M78 NHG Guideline Acute Cough.* Dutch College of General Practitioners, The Netherlands. <www.nhg.org>.

Verlee L, Verheij TJM, Hopstaken RM, Prins JM, Salome PL, Bindels PJE (2012) Samenvatting van de NHG-standaard 'Acuut hoesten'. *Nederlands Tijdschrift voor Geneeskunde* **156**, A4188, <https://www.ntvg.nl/artikelen/samenvatting-van-de-nhg-standaard-%E2%80%98acuut-hoesten%E2%80%99>.

Volanakis JE (2001) Human C-reactive protein: expression, structure, and function. *Molecular Immunology* **38**, 189–197. doi:10.1016/S0161-5890(01)00042-6

Woodhead M, Blasi F, Ewig S, Garau J, Huchon G, Ieven M, *et al.* (2011) Joint Taskforce of the European Respiratory Society and European Society for Clinical Microbiology and Infectious Diseases. Guidelines for the management of adult lower respiratory tract infections–full version. *Clinical Microbiology and Infection* **17**(Supplement 6), E1–E59. doi:10.1111/j.1469-0691.2011.03672.x

Yu CW, Juan LI, Wu MH, Shen CJ, Wu JY, Lee CC (2013) Systematic review and meta-analysis of the diagnostic accuracy of procalcitonin, C-reactive protein and white blood cell count for suspected acute appendicitis. *British Journal of Surgery* **100**, 322–329. doi:10.1002/bjs.9008

# 26 Point-of-care testing for drugs of abuse

*Santiago Vazquez and Brooke Spaeth*

**Summary**

The United Nations Office on Drug and Crime (UNODC) estimated that 246 million people between the ages of 15 and 64 years used an illicit drug in 2013. The advantages of point-of-care testing (POCT) for drugs of abuse are the ability to have results without delay and reduced cost of testing. Urine and oral fluid (saliva) are the preferred matrix analysed by POCT drugs of abuse devices, which use immuno-chromatography to detect the drug or drug metabolite. A range of devices is available for POC drug testing, from simple dipsticks, to cups with incorporated test strips, to instrument-based readers. POCT for drugs of abuse can be used in roadside drugs testing, workplace testing, judicial drug testing and rehabilitation clinics. The limitation of POCT for drugs of abuse is that a positive result needs confirmatory testing by a laboratory.

## GLOBAL DRUG USE TRENDS

According to the *World Drug Report* (UNODC 2015), 246 million people between the ages of 15 and 64 years are estimated to have used an illicit drug in 2013. This equates to 1 in 20 people globally. Of these drug users, more than 1 in 10 is considered a problem drug user, suffering from drug use disorders or drug dependence. General USA workforce urine drug test data released by Quest Diagnostics® showed that the percentage of American workers testing positive for illicit drugs including marijuana, cocaine and methamphetamine has increased for the second consecutive year. These are the first increases observed since 2003 (McKetin *et al.* 2014).

Cannabis is the most commonly used illicit drug and its use continues to rise. Improvements in cannabis plant cultivation techniques and the use of genetically selected strains have produced increases in yield and potency of cannabis. This has led to a growing concern that cannabis may be becoming more harmful, with increasing numbers of users seeking treatment for cannabis use disorders (UNODC 2015).

Opiate use remains the most problematic form of drug use globally due to the relationship between opiates and injecting drug use, blood-borne viruses (BBV) and overdose deaths. In 2014, opium poppy cultivation reached the highest level since the late 1930s. The effects of these record crops are yet to be seen on the global opiate market (UNODC 2015).

Cocaine use continues to decline in Western and Central Europe and North America although it remains the primary drug of concern in Latin America and the Caribbean. Supply reduction measures may have contributed to the decline in coca bush cultivation in coca-producing countries, now with the lowest levels of cultivation since the mid-1980s, leading to a reduction in the availability of cocaine and the reduction of some of the principal cocaine markets (UNODC 2015).

Methamphetamine continues to dominate the global market for amphetamine type substances (ATS). In North America, Europe and Australia there are increasing trends towards the use of methamphetamine in its purest form known as crystal methamphetamine or 'ice' rather than methamphetamine in its powdered form known as 'speed' (AIHW 2014; UNODC 2015). The 'high' experienced from ice is much more intense than other drugs and has a greater potential for the user to develop dependence (addiction) and psychosis, as well as long-term physical and mental health problems.

New psychoactive substances (NPS) are recent additions to the recreational drug market and are marketed as alternatives to traditional drugs. NPS often have chemical structures similar to 'traditional' illicit drugs and are purported to mimic their mind-altering effects; however, they are generally not detectable by conventional drug screening tests. Marketing as legal or herbal highs has yielded market acceptance. NPS continue to proliferate; by the end of 2014 a total of 541 NPS had been reported in the global marketplace. Information and research on the potential harm caused by NPS is limited; however, worrying developments such as the injecting use of NPS and poly-drug use involving NPS have the potential to pose serious risks to public health and safety (UNODC 2015).

Prescription drug misuse is higher globally in the female population compared with males (UNODC 2015). Women are twice as likely as men to use tranquillisers, but both have roughly equal levels of use of prescription opioids. Data from the National Drug Strategy Household Survey 2013 found that pain-killers/analgesics (e.g. over-the-counter and prescription codeine combination products) were the most commonly misused pharmaceutical drugs, followed by tranquillisers/sleeping pills (e.g. benzodiazepines) as the second most commonly misused pharmaceutical drug (AIHW 2014).

## THE HEALTH BURDEN OF DRUG USE

Globally, drug use accounted for an estimated 187 100 drug-related deaths in 2013 (UNODC 2015). Illicit drug use is an increasingly significant contributor to the global burden of disease/illness, rising from 25th to 19th ranking between 1990 and 2010 (Degenhardt *et al.* 2013; Lim *et al.* 2012). Drug abuse is associated with numerous health impacts ranging from the mild, such as headaches and altered mental states, to life-threatening situations such as suicide, coma, seizures and violence towards others. The health risks of drug use increase with the frequency, quantity and number of drugs used. Intravenous drug use amplifies the potential for deleterious health effects through the potential transmission of BBV, including HIV, hepatitis C and hepatitis B, as well as bacterial infections including bacterial endocarditis, osteomyelitis and abscesses (Karch 2007). In fact, the level of mortality among injecting drug users is nearly 15 times higher than would be normally expected among people of comparable age and gender in the general population. There is no 'quick fix' for drug dependence: it is a chronic health condition. Affected persons may remain vulnerable for a lifetime and require long-term and continued treatment.

## HISTORICAL MILESTONES OF DRUG TESTING

Workplace drug testing has developed steadily through a series of events and technological developments. The most significant milestones are detailed in Table 26.1.

## THE DRUG TESTING PROCESS

Drug testing is generally a two-step process: an initial drug screen and, if required, a confirmatory test. The drug screen is a qualitative analysis that does not measure the quantity of a drug group, drug or its metabolites, but quickly establishes the presence or absence of a drug/drug group and/or its metabolites in a particular specimen. This is usually an immunoassay, performed either on an automated instrument in the laboratory or by a POCT device. Immunoassays are calibrated at the cut-off concentrations, and a specimen that yields a response greater or equal to this calibration point is positive, and negative if the response is less. Initial immunoassay positive results should be referred to as 'presumptive positive' until confirmatory testing is performed. This is necessary because screening assays do not have a high degree of specificity and substances chemically similar to the drug/s being tested can cross-react yielding false positive results. For example, the consumption of poppy seeds can yield a false positive result for opiates.

**Table 26.1.** Major historical events in the development of drug testing

| Year | Event | Comments |
|---|---|---|
| Pre 1960s | Limited ability to drug test | Capacity to chemically identify the use of common drugs has been available for approximately a century; however, the ability to engage in mass drug screening was limited primarily by inefficient and non-specific techniques (Lewis 2001). |
| 1966 | Drug testing for methadone substitution therapy | Drug testing was introduced in the USA as a means of monitoring patients who were undergoing methadone substitution therapy for heroin addiction. Testing was carried out primarily by performing thin layer chromatography (Dole *et al.* 1966). |
| 1971 | Nixon declares war on drugs | US President Nixon names drug abuse as 'public enemy number one in the United States.' During the Nixon era, for the only time in the history of the war on drugs, the majority of funding goes towards treatment, rather than law enforcement (Kuzmarov 2009). |
| | Operation Golden Flow | In June 1971, following the public relations fallout surrounding drug addicted army personnel in Vietnam, President Nixon enacted a urine drug testing program on USA military personnel known as Operation Golden Flow (Kuzmarov 2009). |
| 1972 | First immunoassay drug screening assay released | Originally developed to be used in the methadone maintenance treatment programs the enzyme multiplied immunoassay technique (EMIT®) assay, developed by Syva®, was automated, didn't require separation and used easily available spectrophotometers (Schneider *et al.* 1973). |
| 1986 | President Reagan signs The Anti-Drug Abuse Act 1986 | US President Reagan's Executive Order 12564 required all federal agencies to develop programs and policies to achieve a drug-free federal workplace (Normand *et al.* 1994). |
| 1988 | Micro-particle based drug screening devices FDA approved | The first wave of practical, micro-particle-based, POCT drug screening devices received FDA approval. These devices, using latex agglutination-inhibition, allowed results to be visually read in 4 min, rather than after 2 h of incubation (Karch 2007). |
| | The first mandatory guidelines for workplace drug testing published | The USA Department of Health and Human Services drug testing standards 'Mandatory Guidelines for Federal Workplace Drug Testing Programs' were published. |
| Mid-1990s | Proliferation of membrane based lateral flow drug screening devices | By the mid-1990s, as many as twelve membrane-based lateral flow devices for screening drugs of abuse in urine were available. These devices have further evolved and have become the primary technique for POC drug testing (Karch 2007). |
| 1995 | Australian standard for urine drug testing published | Standards Australia published AS 4308 'Procedures for specimen collection and the detection and quantitation of drugs of abuse in urine' (Standards Australia 1995). |
| Late 1990s | First lateral-flow POCT oral fluid (OF) device available | The first on-site screening devices for drug testing in oral fluids were developed in the late 1990s. By 1999, three on-site oral fluid devices were available (Verstraete 2005). |
| 2001 | ROSITA study released | The 21-month Roadside Testing Assessment (ROSITA) project included the on-site immunoassay detection of drugs in urine, oral fluid and/or sweat in 2968 subjects in European Union countries. |
| 2002 | European guidelines released | European guidelines for legally defensible workplace drug testing prepared by the European Workplace Drug Testing Society were released. |
| 2006 | Australian standard for oral fluid drug testing published | Standards Australia published AS 4760 'Procedures for specimen collection and the detection and quantitation of drugs in oral fluid' (Standards Australia 2006). |

The purpose of the confirmatory test is to unequivocally verify or negate the drug screen result. If present, the specific drug and/or its metabolite are identified and quantified. Confirmatory tests are performed in a laboratory setting and employ analytical techniques that have a higher degree of specificity and sensitivity than the initial screen. The use of mass spectrometric techniques coupled with chromatographic techniques such as liquid chromatography (LC) or gas chromatography (GC) are required to achieve the near absolute specificity essential for confirmatory work. These tests involve higher costs due to the high degree of skill and effort required, as well as higher cost of instrumentation. Confirmation is essential where punitive consequences may follow a positive result such as in workplace or judicial settings.

## DRUGS OF ABUSE TESTING STANDARDS AND GUIDELINES

Every form of drugs of abuse testing is contingent on the use of a cut-off. Functionally, it is an administrative decision point. If a specimen contains a target drug above this threshold concentration value the specimen is reported as positive. Below this concentration, a specimen is reported as negative. Prior to 1988, when the US government published 'Mandatory Guidelines for Federal Workplace Drug Testing Programs', guidelines and standards for drugs of abuse testing did not exist. Standardised cut-offs did not exist. Screening cut-offs were established by individual manufacturers of POCT devices while confirmatory cut-offs were determined by the laboratory performing confirmatory analysis. Confirmatory cut-offs varied from laboratory to laboratory and depended upon the sensitivity of the laboratory's equipment.

Setting standardised cut-offs aimed to minimise the risk of a positive result from incidental exposure to a target drug, such as passive marijuana smoke, and ensure uniformity of testing and reporting across laboratories. Initially, guidelines were developed only for urine drug testing, with guidelines for oral fluid testing preceding the advent of oral fluid POCT devices.

Screening and confirmation cut-offs for urine and oral fluid guidelines and standards used in the USA and Australia are listed in Tables 26.2–26.5. Similar guidelines are also available for Europe (European Workplace Drug Testing Society 2015a,b). Confirmatory cut-off concentrations are generally lower than screening cut-offs because confirmation targets a particular drug, while a screening cut-off accommodates immunoassay testing in which the total response is the sum of the response by the target drug as well as any cross reacting drugs and/or metabolites. Cut-offs are largely quite closely aligned across all regions where testing is performed; however, differences do exist. The most significant differences exist between US guidelines for urine screening cut-offs for amphetamines and opiates, where they are significantly greater than those used in other countries such as

**Table 26.2.** Screening and confirmation cut-off concentrations, in urine, as stated in the US Mandatory Guidelines for Federal Workplace Drug Testing Programs. Cut-offs are subject to change as revision of mandatory guidelines is currently under consideration (Sources: SAMHSA 2015a,b, 2008).

| Screening test analyte/s | Screening cut-off concentration (ng/mL) | Confirmatory test analyte | Confirmatory cut-off concentration (ng/mL) |
|---|---|---|---|
| Marijuana (THC-COOH) | 50 | THC-COOH[a] | 15 |
| Benzoylecgonine | 150 | Benzoylecgonine | 100 |
| Codeine/morphine | 2000 | Codeine | 2000 |
| | | Morphine | 2000 |
| Hydrocodone/hydromorphone | 300 | Hydrocodone | 100 |
| | | Hydromorphone | 100 |
| Oxycodone/oxymorphone | 100 | Oxycodone | 50 |
| | | Oxymorphone | 50 |
| 6-MAM | 10 | 6-MAM | 10 |
| Phencyclidine | 25 | Phencyclidine | 25 |
| Amphetamine/methamphetamine | 500 | Amphetamine | 250 |
| | | Methamphetamine | 250 |
| MDMA/MDA/MDEA | 500 | MDMA | 250 |
| | | MDA | 250 |
| | | MDEA | 250 |

[a]Delta-9-tetrahydrocannabinol-9-carboxylic acid

**Table 26.3.** Screening and confirmation cut-off concentrations, in oral fluid, as stated in the US Mandatory Guidelines for Federal Workplace Drug Testing Programs. Cut-offs subject to change as revision of mandatory guidelines is currently under consideration.

| Screening test analyte/s | Screening cut-off concentration (ng/mL) | Confirmatory test analyte | Confirmatory cut-off concentration (ng/mL) |
|---|---|---|---|
| Marijuana (THC) | 4 | THC | 2 |
| Cocaine/benzoylecgonine | 15 | Cocaine | 8 |
| | | Benzoylecgonine | 8 |
| Codeine/morphine | 30 | Codeine | 15 |
| | | Morphine | 15 |
| Hydrocodone/hydromorphone | 30 | Hydrocodone | 15 |
| | | Hydromorphone | 15 |
| Oxycodone/oxymorphone | 30 | Oxycodone | 15 |
| | | Oxymorphone | 15 |
| 6-MAM | 3 | 6-MAM | 2 |
| Phencyclidine | 3 | Phencyclidine | 2 |
| Amphetamine/methamphetamine | 25 | Amphetamine | 15 |
| | | Methamphetamine | 15 |
| MDMA/MDA/MDEA | 25 | MDMA | 15 |
| | | MDA | 15 |
| | | MDEA | 15 |

in Europe and Australia. These differences may become an issue when POCT devices are purchased from uninformed device suppliers who source product intended for markets in foreign countries where different cut-offs are used. For example, kits developed for the US market, if used in Australia, may cause false negative screening results for opiates and amphetamines because of the higher cut-offs for these target drugs.

Currently, with the exception of the AS/NZS 4308:2008, all standards and guidelines mentioned in this chapter are under review or open for public comment. With the increasing concern that drug abuse is not limited to illicit substances, guidelines and standards are including additional substances particularly pharmaceutical drugs.

## SPECIMENS FOR DRUGS OF ABUSE TESTING

Almost any biological matrix can be used for testing for the presence of drugs or their metabolites; however, matrix selection is essential in evaluating an individual's likelihood of impairment or historical drug use. The more common matrices include blood, urine, oral fluid and hair. Other matrices that are not widely used include sweat, meconium, breast milk, vernix caseosa (a waxy cheese-like substance found coating the skin of newborn babies), semen and nails. Only urine and oral fluid are commonly analysed using POCT devices.

### Blood

Blood is widely regarded as the specimen offering the best correlation with the degree of impairment. However, not all drugs of abuse have been subjected to controlled studies to define this relationship. Drugs are present in blood most commonly as the parent compound and not the respective metabolites, which may be present at low concentrations and are relatively short-lived. The analysis of drugs in blood is complex and time-consuming. Collection of specimen is invasive and the possibility of transmission of infectious disease is greater than with other matrices.

### Urine

Urine is the biological matrix of choice when it comes to the detection of drug use in an individual. It offers numerous distinct advantages including:

- large specimen volumes
- drugs/metabolites bio-concentrate into urine (up to 100-fold)

**Table 26.4.** Urine screening and confirmation cut-off concentrations as stated in the Australian and New Zealand standard AS/NZS 4308:2008 (Source: Standards Australia and Standards New Zealand 2008)

| Screening test analyte/s | Screening cut-off concentration (ng/mL) | Confirmatory test analyte | Confirmatory cut-off concentration (ng/mL) |
|---|---|---|---|
| Amphetamine-type substances | 300 | Amphetamine | 150 |
| | | Methamphetamine | 150 |
| | | MDA | 150 |
| | | MDMA | 150 |
| | | Benzylpiperazine[a] | 500 |
| | | Phentermine[a] | 500 |
| | | Ephedrine[a] | 500 |
| | | Pseudoephedrine[a] | 500 |
| Benzodiazepines | 200 | Diazepam | 200 |
| | | Nordiazepam | 200 |
| | | Oxazepam | 200 |
| | | Temazepam | 200 |
| | | $\alpha$-Hydroxyl-alprazolam | 100 |
| | | 7-Amino-clonazepam | 100 |
| | | 7-Amino-flunitrazepam | 100 |
| | | 7-Amino-nitrazepam | 100 |
| Cocaine metabolites | 300 | Benzoylecgonine | 150 |
| | | Ecgonine methyl ester | 150 |
| Opiates | 300 | Codeine | 300 |
| | | Morphine | 300 |
| | | 6-MAM[a] | 10 |
| Cannabis metabolites | 50 | 11-nor-delta-9-tetrahydrocannabinol-9-carboxylic acid | 15 |

[a]These drugs may be optionally tested within each class

**Table 26.5.** Oral fluid screening and confirmation cut-off concentrations as stated in the Australian standard AS 4760–2004 oral fluid (Source: Standards Australia 2006)

| Screening test analyte/s | Screening cut-off concentration (ng/mL) | Confirmatory test analyte | Confirmatory cut-off concentration (ng/mL) |
|---|---|---|---|
| Amphetamine-type stimulants | 50 | Amphetamine | 25 |
| | | Methamphetamine | 25 |
| | | MDA | 25 |
| | | MDMA | 25 |
| Cocaine and metabolites | 50 | Benzoylecgonine | 150 |
| | | Ecgonine methyl ester | 150 |
| Opiates | 50 | Codeine | 25 |
| | | Morphine | 25 |
| | | 6-MAM | 10 |
| Δ9-tetrahydrocannabinol (THC) | 25 | Δ9-tetrahydrocannabinol | 10 |

- variety of POCT devices available
- extensive literature regarding analytical methods
- long history of case law regarding workplace use.

Drugs are generally present in the urine as phase I and phase II metabolites of the respective parent compound.

Some of the challenges include:

- invasion of privacy
- potential for adulteration
- potential for physiological dilution
- also correlation between urine drug/metabolite levels and the likelihood of impairment is difficult.

### Oral fluid

Oral fluid is a mixture of various fluids, including saliva, from the oral cavity and is effectively an ultra-filtrate of blood and consequently the drug in circulation, usually the parent drug, is found in oral fluid. The major factors affecting drug entry into oral fluid are a drug's lipophilicity and ionisability at typical oral fluid pH (normal pH is ~6.7). Oral fluid is increasingly becoming the drug testing matrix of choice spurred on by: the global experience with roadside drug testing programs; availability of POCT devices; collection process that minimises privacy and gender related issues; and specimens present fewer opportunities for adulteration or substitution and the perception that results are more closely correlated with impairment.

Some of the challenges include:

- volume of oral fluid collected is limited
- drug concentrations are low
- some medications, illegal drugs and medical conditions cause dry mouth syndrome (or xerostomia) making specimen collection difficult (Drummer 2006).

Additionally, detection of cannabis use can be challenging because cannabinoids are not secreted from blood into oral fluid and detection is generally considered to be the result of relatively short-lived contamination of the oral cavity following smoking or ingestion. Anecdotally, this may be beneficial where the goal of drug testing is the demonstration of possible impairment. Analysis of benzodiazepines can also be challenging for analysis due to their low therapeutic concentrations in blood.

### Hair

Hair testing appears to be best suited for detecting prior frequent heavy use rather than for detection of very recent or occasional drug use (Dolan *et al.* 2004). Drugs and/or metabolites are assumed to be incorporated into the hair shaft during growth, by direct transfer from the bloodstream through hair follicles and secretions of the sebaceous and sweat glands in the scalp (Musshoff and Madea 2006). Drugs can be detected in the hair shaft ~7–10 days after drug ingestion.

Specimen collection is relatively easy and non-invasive and hair has the longest window of detection compared with other matrices. Furthermore, it may give an indication of the chronology of drug use or abstinence if segmental analysis along the length of the hair shaft is performed.

Challenges of hair based drug testing include:

- analysis is very costly and labour intensive
- few laboratories are capable of performing analysis
- POCT devices are unavailable
- specimen can be removed by shaving
- significantly, results can be difficult to interpret because drugs may also be incorporated into hair through environmental drug exposure (Wong and Tse 2005).

Additional controversies exist about the effect of biophysical attributes on the concentrations of drugs in hair. Studies have shown that hair structure, growth rate, melanin content, hygiene and cosmetic hair treatments, such as bleaching, have an effect (Dasgupta 2008).

## POCT DEVICES – LATERAL FLOW METHODS

A range of devices is now available for POC drug testing, from simple dipsticks, to cups with incorporated test strips, to instrument-based readers. The appeal of modern lateral flow devices for drugs of abuse testing lies in the specificity and rapidity of result delivery – anywhere from a few to 15 min. Devices are available in single assay or multi-assay formats with adulterant and creatinine testing. Devices use well-established immunoassay technologies, which involve antigen–antibody reactions in chromatographic strips, with this form of immunoassay testing referred to as immunochromatography. Antibodies are directed to the specific drug and/or metabolites to be detected and are labelled with either colloidal gold or coloured latex spheres as a means of visualisation.

A POC drug testing device consists of three regions: sample introduction, test and waste areas as shown in Fig. 26.1.

The sample introduction area consists of a sample pad, which overlaps the conjugate pad, which in turn

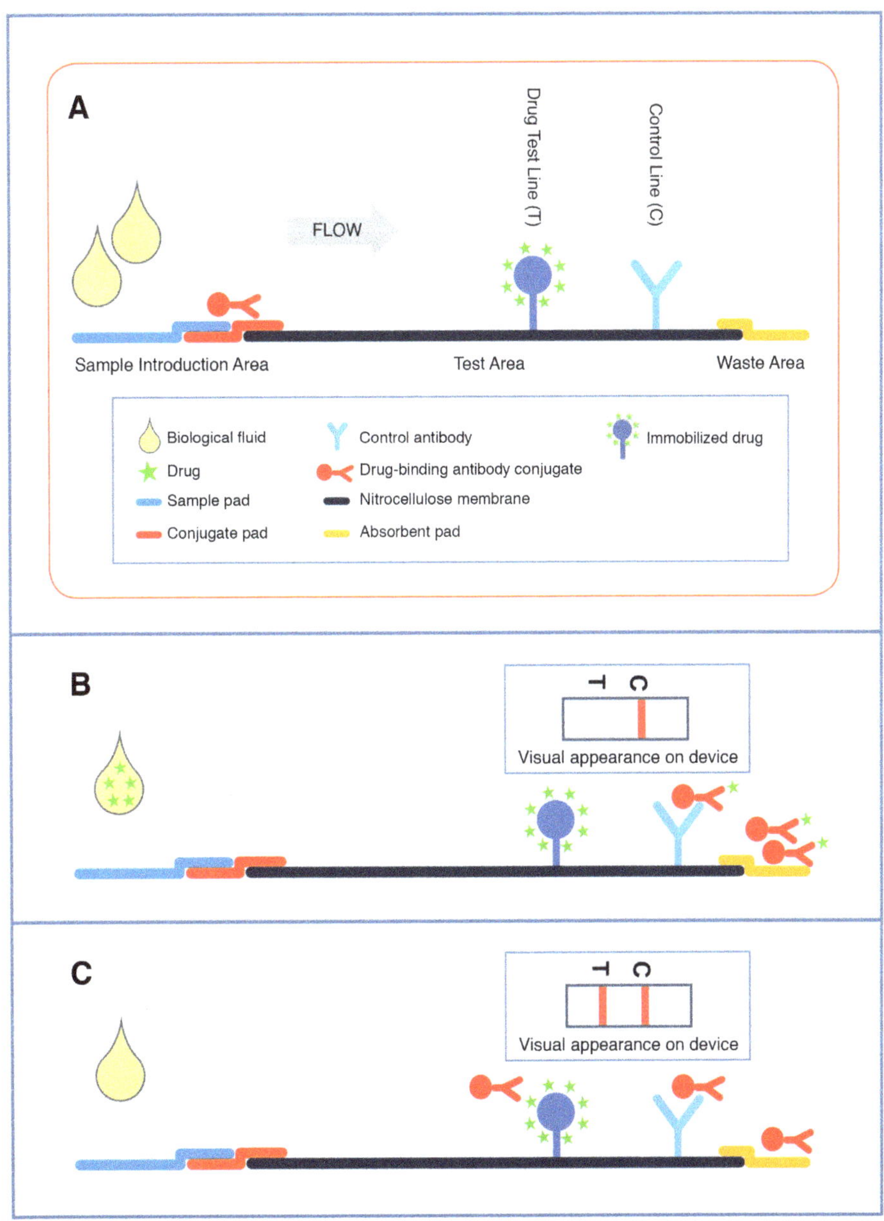


**Fig. 26.1.** (A) Layout of a point-of-care drug testing device; (B) addition of a specimen containing drug at a concentration at or above the cut-off producing a single line result; (C) addition of a specimen free of drug or containing drug at a concentration below the cut-off concentration produces a two line result.

overlaps the nitrocellulose membrane. This membrane acts as the separation and reaction medium. The sample pad is impregnated with a buffer and surfactant matrix, to ensure optimal immunoreactions, and the conjugate pad is impregnated with the drug-binding labelled-antibody. The test area is situated on the nitrocellulose membrane and comprises a drug test line and a control line. The drug test line consists of a drug covalently bound to a large molecular weight carrier protein (drug conjugate) immobilised on the nitrocellulose membrane. The control line is a single line of immobilised antibodies specifically directed to bind to the labelled antibody. This control line is a functional control and only determines serviceability of the device. It is not a drug-based quality control test of assay performance. The waste area consists of a final porous pad, which overlaps the nitrocellulose membrane and acts as a waste capture container.

**Table 26.6.** The POCT drug testing market can be divided into two major categories: those supplied by prominent companies and those supplied by manufacturers in China (these are too numerous to list)

| Company | Qualitative urine POCT | Quantitative urine POCT | Qualitative oral fluid POCT | Quantitative oral fluid POCT |
|---|---|---|---|---|
| Branan Medical Corporation™+ | Fastect®II, ToxCup®, QuickTox®, Monitect® | | Oratect®, OratectPlus®, Oratect® III | |
| Alere™ | SureStep™ Drug Screen Cassette, SureStep™ Drug Screen Cup | Alere Triage® MeterPro | Alere iScreen® OFD Test | Alere™ DDS®2 |
| Bio-Rad™ | TOX/See Rapid Urine Drug Screen Test+ | | | |
| US Diagnostics Inc.[a] | ProScreen® Cup, ProScreen® Dip, ProScreen® Cassette, UScreen Cup, UScreen Dip, E-Z Cup | | UScreen Oral, USD Oral | |
| Clonal Technologies | | | Clonal Oral Fluid DoA | |
| Dräger | | | | Dräger DrugTest® 5000 |
| Thermo Fisher Scientific | MicroScreen™ Drug testing Cup+, MicroTox 6 Panel Drug Test Cassette+ | | | |
| Securetec AG | | | DrugWipe 5S, DrugWipe 6S | |

[a]An Alere subsidiary
+Manufactured by Alere or Alere subsidiary

When sample is introduced to the sample pad, it rehydrates the buffer and surfactant compounds. The sample then migrates to the conjugate pad where it rehydrates and mixes with the labelled antibody. The mixture then migrates along the nitrocellulose membrane through the test area by capillary action to the waste area. Once the test has been performed, the test result is evaluated visually by the presence or absence of a coloured line at the drug test and/or control line.

When a drug is present in the test sample above the cut-off concentration, the drug populates all possible binding sites on the labelled antibody and prohibits it from binding to the drug conjugate. The labelled antibody is still able to bind to the control line giving the single line at the control line, as shown in Fig. 26.1B, indicative of a non-negative result. In contrast, when no drug is present in the specimen or is present below the cut-off concentration, binding sites on the labelled antibody are available to bind to the immobilised drug conjugate on the membrane as well as with the control line giving rise to two lines, which corresponds to a negative result, as depicted in Fig. 26.1C, which is why results are often referred to as 'negative read'. The absence of any line is indicative of a failed test possibly due to incorrect application of the test, poor storage of the device or manufacturing issues. In such cases, testing of the specimen should be repeated (Ropero-Miller *et al.* 2009).

A limitation of these devices is the necessity for the operator to visually interpret the result, which is subjective and can be influenced by the individual's visual acuity, level of training and adherence to the device manufacturer's operating instructions. Increasingly, vendors are developing instruments and readers of POC devices to provide objective interpretation of results.

Table 26.6 lists representative examples of some qualitative and quantitative drugs of abuse devices that are available on the global market.

## LIMITATIONS OF POCT

The utility and ease-of-use of POCT devices has enabled access to drug of abuse testing across all sections of society. Consequently, non-technically trained or inexperienced operators have the confidence to apply testing. However, deficiencies in the understanding of POCT device limitations, performance and troubleshooting of problematic specimens can compromise the accuracy of the results reported.

Result reading from POCT devices, in the main, is quite facile because the test line will be intense when drug is not present in the specimen, or not visible when the concentration of drug is well above the cut-off. In situations, however, where the drug concentration in the specimen is present at a concentration near its respective cut-off, either above or below, the test line may appear very faint and difficult to determine if present or absent. This situation is often referred to as a 'near cut-off' concentration reading. Factors such as the visual acuity of the reader, lighting conditions and colour vision deficiency, such as protanopia (inability to perceive red light) could all have an impact on the ability of the user to read a result and thus give rise to the subjective nature of result reading. This is a concern for test accuracy. In a study by Kadehjian, the near cut-off performance of five POCT devices was evaluated. Sixty clinical specimens for each of the five SAMHSA-specified drug categories (cocaine, THC-COOH, amphetamines, opiates and phencyclidine) were selected with drug concentration near the POCT device screening cut-offs. POCT device results were read independently by both a scientist and a non-scientist and compared with results from an immunoassay analyser (Emit reagents) and gas chromatography-mass spectrometry (GC-MS). An overall accuracy of only 70% (66–74%), compared with GC-MS, was found (Kadehjian 2001).

Adulterants can affect immunoassay testing by affecting drug–antibody interactions. Most POCT device manufactures offer the option to manufacture devices with on-board adulterant testing strips; for example, the detection of dilution and oxidants. In addition to chemical adulterants (including glutaraldehyde, nitrites, chromium VI compounds or bleach), to which instrumental based immunoassays systems are susceptible, POCT devices are also at risk from adulterants that can impede flow, such as particulate matter. Such adulterants prevent the development of a control line and thus invalidate testing. Oral fluid, as a matrix, is susceptible to poor flow of matrix through POCT membranes due to viscosity issues and debris in the oral cavity without attempts at adulteration. In situations where possible adulteration is detected or suspected, operating procedures should allow for re-collection of a specimen and referral of both to the laboratory for analysis.

A significant challenge for oral fluid-based POCT devices is the non-specific binding of drug to device surfaces limiting drug recovery from the device and therefore the usability of some devices. Numerous devices demonstrate poor THC recoveries (Drummer 2006).

## WINDOW OF DETECTION

The length of time that a drug or its metabolites can be detected in a biological specimen, or matrix, is referred to as the detection time or the window of detection. Many factors influence the window of detection for a drug and, as such, only an estimate of this length of time can be given. Factors that influence the window of detection include:

- drug half-life
- frequency of drug use
- quantity of the drug ingested
- individual metabolism rates and excretion routes
- route of administration
- sensitivity and specificity of the test
- cut-off concentration used
- the individual's health, diet, weight, amount of body fat, gender, fluid intake, and pharmacogenomic profile
- matrix tested.

Fig. 26.2 shows a comparison of the detection times in various matrices.

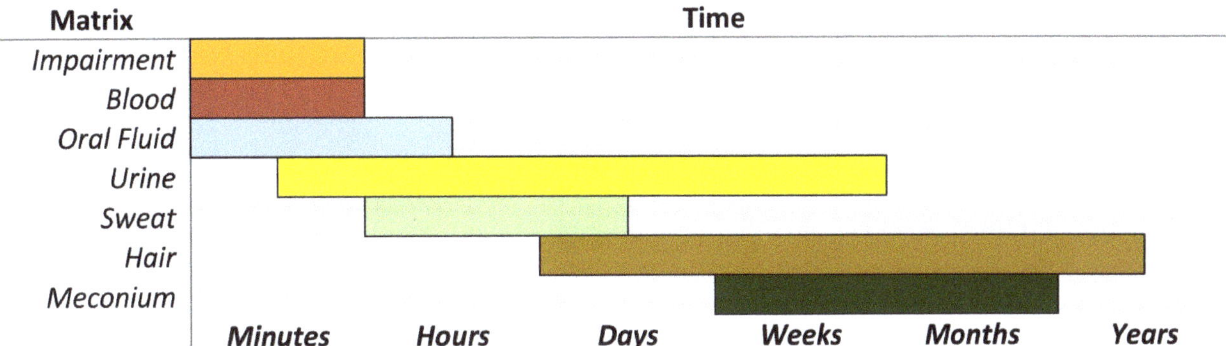


**Fig. 26.2.** Windows of detection of drugs in various matrices. Time ranges are very broad and are dependent on numerous factors including drug taken, frequency of use, drug half-life and the individual. (Source: Dasgupta 2008)

## PHARMACOLOGY AND METABOLISM OF MAJOR CLASSES OF DRUGS MEASURED BY POCT

### Amphetamines

Amphetamines refers to the group of substances that primarily include methamphetamine, amphetamine, methylenedioxyamphetamine (MDA) and methylenedioxymethamphetamine (MDMA). These low-molecular weight drugs are abused for their central nervous system (CNS) and cardiovascular stimulant activity. These effects are mediated by increasing synaptic concentrations of noradrenalin and dopamine either by stimulating neurotransmitter release or inhibiting uptake or both. The effects are longer lasting than cocaine and may prevent fatigue and suppress appetite. Heavy users of the drug may consume up to 2000 mg per day.

Amphetamine is metabolised by deamination, oxidation and hydroxylation as shown in Fig. 26.3. Methamphetamine in humans primarily undergoes N-demethylation to yield amphetamine, the major metabolite of methamphetamine. Methamphetamine may also undergo hydroxylation to give *p*-hydroxymethamphetamine. Under normal conditions ~40% of a D-methamphetamine dose is excreted in urine in the first 24 h and <10% is present as amphetamine. MDMA is metabolised to MDA with ~70% of the dose excreted as the parent drug within 3 days. Both MDMA and MDA are hydroxylated to mono and di-hydroxy derivatives before conjugation and elimination (Karch 2007).

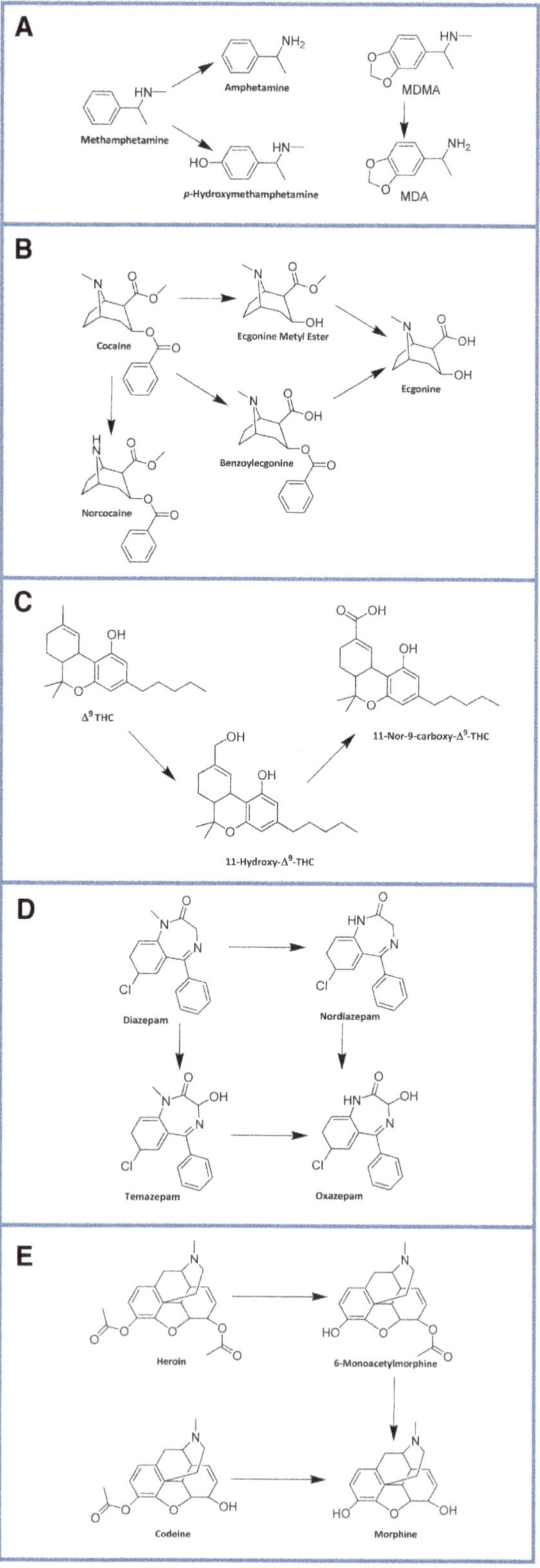


**Fig. 26.3.** The major metabolic pathways of (A) methamphetamine and MDMA, (B) cocaine, (C) THC, (D) benzodiazepines and (E) opiates.

### Cocaine

Cocaine is a naturally occurring alkaloid obtained from the plant *Erythroxylon coca*. Cocaine inhibits the presynaptic re-uptake of the neurotransmitters noradrenalin, serotonin and dopamine at synaptic junctions, resulting in stimulation of the sympathetic nervous system. This drug is abused for its euphoria, increased alertness and energy, heightened sexual excitement and self-confidence. The physiological effects of this stimulation include tachycardia, hypertension, vasoconstriction, mydriasis (prolonged dilation of the pupil) and hyperthermia. Cocaine also acts as a local anaesthetic through its ability to block sodium channels in neuronal cells.

In humans, the primary route of metabolism of cocaine is through hydrolysis of the ester linkages to give benzoylecgonine (BE) and ecgonine methyl ester (EME). Further metabolism of these metabolites produces ecgonine. Cocaine can also be *N*-demethylated to give norcocaine. It is estimated that up to 90% of cocaine dose is excreted in the urine in 24 h. Parent, un-metabolised, drug accounts for <10% while the amount of BE and EME can each account for ~30–50% of the dose depending upon urine pH (Karch 2007).

### Marijuana

Marijuana refers to all parts of the plant *Cannabis sativa* – the leaf, seed and resin – the primary active constituent being tetrahydrocannabinol (THC). The pharmacological effects of marijuana include sedation, euphoria, hallucinations and temporal distortion. THC binds to the cannabinoid receptors in the brain and in immune tissues such as the spleen, tonsils and thymus. In addition THC possesses activity at benzodiazepine and opioid receptors. THC may act as a direct or indirect dopamine agonist to stimulate the brain's reward circuits (Shaw *et al.* 2001). Over 20 metabolites of THC have been identified in human urine and faeces.

More than 60% of the drug is excreted in faeces, while ~20% of the drug is excreted in urine. Following a single dose, 80–90% of the drug is excreted within 5 days – mostly as the hydroxylated and carboxylated metabolites (Shaw *et al.* 2001). However, clearance times may extend to weeks or months with chronic users.

### Benzodiazepines

Benzodiazepines are the most commonly prescribed medications encountered in drug screening. Abuse of these drugs usually occurs either through long-term use, longer than recommended use or illicit use. Long-term prescription use typically involves use at low doses, while illicit use involves high doses and clear indications of intoxication. The effects of benzodiazepine intoxication are similar to those of alcohol intoxication. Benzodiazepines have central nervous system (CNS) depressant effects and they are used as muscle relaxants, anticonvulsants, sedative-hypnotics and anti-anxiety medications.

Metabolism of benzodiazepines produces numerous metabolites. Metabolism typically involves hydroxylation, demethylation and glucuronidation. Diazepam undergoes N-demethylation to nordiazepam, both of which can undergo hydroxylation to yield temazepam and oxazepam, respectively. In urine, only small amounts of diazepam or nordiazepam are detected. From a single diazepam dose typically both temazepam and oxazepam and sometimes nordiazepam are observed, and occasionally diazepam (Karch 2007).

Diazepam, nordiazepam and oxazepam are long-acting benzodiazepines and are typically prescribed at high doses. Following chronic use, they can be detected in urine for weeks or months. Short-acting benzodiazepines such as in urine can be detected for only a few days (Karch 2007).

### Opiates

Opiates produce their pharmacological effects by binding to opiate receptors in the body. Three types of opiate receptors are recognised, with the μ receptor considered to be the most important. Opiates act as μ-receptor agonists and exert a direct effect on brain stem respiratory centres, reducing their responsiveness to carbon dioxide causing respiratory depression. μ receptors are responsible for euphoria, supraspinal analgesia, respiratory depression, reduced gastrointestinal motility and physical tolerance and dependence.

Heroin is very rapidly metabolised by deacetylation to 6-monoacetylmorphine (6-MAM), which is further metabolised to morphine. The presence of 6-MAM in urine is definitive evidence of recent heroin use. Codeine is metabolised by *O*-demethylation to morphine and *N*-demethylation to norcodeine. Codeine concentration in urine is usually highest in the initial phase of elimination, but morphine conjugates are the major products found in urine over the 20–40 h period. Morphine is metabolised by conjugation to its glucuronide and by sulfation. It can also undergo *N*-demethylation and *N*-oxide formation. Approximately 90% of a morphine dose is excreted within 72 h (Shaw *et al.* 2001). The presence of morphine in urine can be attributed to morphine use itself or the metabolism of codeine or heroin to morphine. Therefore, it can be difficult to determine the source of morphine without further information. This can be further complicated, because the consumption of poppy seed can also produce codeine and morphine concentrations in urine above screening cut-offs.

## POCT DRUG TESTING IN DIFFERENT SETTINGS

### Clinical

In the clinical setting, urine is the preferred biological matrix for testing. Clinical situations where drug POCT can be useful include:

- emergency medicine
- mental health management and identifying substance use disorders
- prevention of dangerous medication interactions
- identifying/refuting maternal drug use
- monitoring patient compliance (SAMHSA 2012).

However, controversy exists regarding the value of drug testing in clinical settings. Reasons include methods used, targeted analytes and the level of understanding of the physician using the data (Hammett-Stabler *et al.* 2002). Additionally, testing is often limited to screening without the benefit of confirmatory testing and tests are commonly optimised for workplace testing where cut-offs are set high enough to be indicative of drug abuse. Therefore, therapeutic concentrations of medications may not be detected. Nevertheless, the rapidity of result production together with the cost of laboratory-centric drug screening has made POCT a valuable option, particularly in emergency medicine and mental health settings. Clinicians should be guided on the range of detectable analytes and cut-off concentrations used in drug testing of their patients.

## Workplace

Worldwide, workplace drug testing is not legislatively mandated, except in the USA where workplace drug testing is mandated for all government sector workers. Due to the liabilities associated with unsafe workplaces, many private sector corporations, particularly those involved in safety-sensitive areas, have drug testing policies. These policies are generally directed towards pre-employment screening, random screening as a workplace deterrent, reasonable suspicion, post incident investigation and return to duty following detection. The immediacy and timely delivery of results is of concern because workers are often stood down on full pay until results are confirmed by a laboratory. As such, POCT is almost exclusively used in these settings. Although urine is the biological matrix commonly selected for testing, increasingly, negotiations between unions and individual corporations are favouring oral fluid as the testing matrix, due to the belief that detection of drugs in oral fluid may be a better indication of possible impairment. The move towards drug screening in oral fluid has been facilitated by increasing numbers of laboratories gaining accreditation for the provision of confirmation services in oral fluid. The menu of target analytes is directed towards the detection of illicit substances and pharmaceutical drugs such as benzodiazepines, opiates and opioids. Due to the medico-legal implications and potential impact of non-negative results, confirmatory testing should follow.

## Judicial

The criminal justice setting encompasses drug courts, probation and parole and correctional facilities. Carried out under supervision of the courts or parole boards, sample collection and testing is scheduled and directed by the relevant judicial authority. Financial resources for testing are limited because funding is provided by the federal, state or local governments. Depending on the country or state, the drug testing of individuals in the criminal justice setting is often covered by specific legislation. Cut-offs used are often aligned with recommended workplace cut-offs in the respective country. Due to time and budgetary constraints, there is an increasing shift towards POCT for drugs of abuse in these settings.

Urine is the biological matrix of choice; however, there is movement towards the testing of oral fluid, particularly in the community setting where corrections officers may randomly turn up at an offender's residential address for testing. Depending on the severity of the offence, the rigour of testing may vary; for example, with lower level offenders, judicial monitoring is focussed on rehabilitation of the individual, non-negative results may not be confirmed and are treated as positives. In monitoring high-risk offenders, where judicial intervention may be required, non-negative results are confirmed and certificates of analysis are provided to the requesting organisation by the issuing laboratory.

In judicial settings, the range of illicit substances abused reflects patterns of abuse in the general population. However, in the custodial environment where access to illicit substances is limited, abuse of pharmaceutical substances is equally if not more prevalent. Depending on the class of drug, the detection of abused pharmaceutical substances using POCT can be limited due to the availability of a test for that particular pharmaceutical.

## Roadside

Although roadside alcohol breath testing has, undeniably, reduced the number of alcohol-associated fatalities, the same cannot be said about driving while under the influence of drugs. Increasingly, governments are establishing roadside drug testing programs and these programs are yielding surprisingly high drug detection rates. For example, the New South Wales Police Force in Australia started testing for cannabis, methamphetamine and ecstasy by the roadside in 2007 (Centre for Road Safety 2015). During 2013, roadside drug tests detected the presence of illicit drugs in oral fluid in about one in 40 light vehicle drivers. Since 2013, roadside drug testing has become more targeted and, during 2014, as many as one in 10 drivers were detected with the presence of one of the three targeted drugs. Comparatively, only one in every 236 drivers randomly tested for alcohol returned a positive reading in the period from 2010 to 2013 (Centre for Road Safety 2015).

Screening is performed by the roadside generally using POCT devices and specimens are sent to the laboratory for confirmatory analysis when necessary. Although numerous matrices have been investigated, oral fluid is the preferred matrix in this setting because it offers the advantages of ready availability, less invasive collection and results are more likely to be reflective of impairment.

## QUALITY PRACTICES

Good quality practices are necessary throughout the entire drug testing process from the point of collection through to the issuing of results. Manufacturers of POCT devices that follow good manufacturing practices typically employ lot-based quality controls (QC) throughout each stage of the manufacturing process, from test strip production to the device assembly stage. Nevertheless, lot-to-lot variations in performance can be seen from time-to-time at the end-user stage. In addition, poor storage or use of devices in temperature extremes, and new or poorly trained users, can also cause variations in performance. End-users should be aware of these factors and at a minimum use QC material to monitor the ongoing performance of POCT devices and testing programs regularly. This is one of the many quality management practices necessary to maintain an effective drug testing program. There is often resistance to QC procedures due to the additional cost. If, however, the potential costs and impacts of failed testing are considered, the additional cost of QC is only a minor concern. Furthermore, standards and guidelines mandate the use of quality management processes in testing; and participation in nationally or internationally recognised proficiency testing (PT) programs. Participation in PT programs provides independent assessment of an end-users performance and comparison of performance with other end-users. PT programs are readily available for urine, as are QC materials. On the other hand, PT programs and QC materials to support oral fluid testing are difficult to find and the range of target drugs offered may be limited. The end-user's QA processes should allow for evaluation of QC and PT program results and detail acceptance criteria and the course of action to be taken should performance fail to meet the acceptance criteria.

## REFERENCES

AIHW (Australian Institute of Health and Welfare) (2014) 'National Drug Strategy Household Survey detailed report: 2013'. Drug statistics series no. 28. Cat. no. PHE 183. Canberra, Australia.

Centre for Road Safety (2015) 'Drug driving Fact sheet'. NSW Government Department of Transport, Sydney, Australia.

Dasgupta A (2008) *Handbook of Drug Monitoring Methods - Therapeutics and Drugs of Abuse*. Humana Press, Totowa NJ, USA.

Degenhardt L, Whiteford HA, Ferrari AJ, Baxter AJ, Charlson FJ, Hall WD, *et al.* (2013) Global burden of disease attributable to illicit drug use and dependence: findings from the Global Burden of Disease Study 2010. *Lancet* **382**, 1564–1574. doi:10.1016/S0140-6736(13)61530-5

Dolan K, Rouen D, Kimber J (2004) An overview of the use of urine, hair, sweat and saliva to detect drug use. *Drug and Alcohol Review* **23**, 213–217. doi:10.1080/0959523041000170 4208

Dole VP, Kim WK, Eglitis I (1966) Detection of narcotic drugs, tranquilizers, amphetamines and barbiturates in urine. *Journal of the American Medical Association* **198**, 349–352. doi:10.1001/jama.1966.03110170061017

Drummer OH (2006) Drug testing in oral fluid. *The Clinical Biochemist Reviews* **27**, 147–159.

European Workplace Drug Testing Society (2015a) *European Guidelines for Workplace Drug Testing in Urine*. <http://www.ewdts.org/ewdts-guidelines.html>.

European Workplace Drug Testing Society (2015b) *European Guidelines for Workplace Drug Testing in Oral Fluid*. <http://www.ewdts.org/ewdts-guidelines.html>.

Hammett-Stabler CA, Pesce AJ, Cannon DJ (2002) Urine drug screening in the medical setting. *Clinica Chimica Acta* **315**, 125–135. doi:10.1016/S0009-8981(01)00714-8

Kadehjian LJ (2001) Performance of five non-instrumented urine drug-testing devices with challenging near-cut-off specimens. *Journal of Analytical Toxicology* **25**, 670–679. doi:10.1093/jat/25.8.670

Karch SB (2007) *Drug Abuse Handbook*. 2nd edn. CRC Press, Boca Raton FL, USA.

Kuzmarov J (2009) *The Myth of the Addicted Army: Vietnam and the Modern War on Drugs*. University of Massachusetts Press, Boston MA, USA.

Lewis JH (2001) *No. 205 Drug Detection and its Role in Law Enforcement*. Australian Institute of Criminology, Canberra.

Lim SS, Vos T, Flaxman AD, Danaei G, Shibuya K, Adair-Rohani H, *et al.* (2012) A comparative risk assessment of burden of disease and injury attributable to 67 risk factors and risk factor clusters in 21 regions, 1990–2010: a systematic analysis for the Global Burden of Disease Study. *Lancet* **380**, 2224–2260. doi:10.1016/S0140-6736(12)61766-8

McKetin R, Black E, Shakeshaft A, Newton N, Teesson M, Farrell M, *et al.* (2014) *Methamphetamine – What You Need to Know About Speed, Ice, Crystal, Base and Meth.* National Drug and Alcohol Research Centre, Canberra.

Musshoff F, Madea B (2006) Review of biologic matrices (urine, blood, hair) as indicators of recent or ongoing cannabis use. *Therapeutic Drug Monitoring* **28**, 155–163. doi:10.1097/01.ftd.0000197091.07807.22

Normand J, Lempert RO, O'Brien CP (1994) *Under the Influence? Drugs and the American Workforce.* National Academy Press, Washington DC, USA.

Ropero-Miller JD, Goldberger BA, Liu RH (2009) *Handbook of Workplace Drug Testing.* AACC Press, Washington DC, USA.

SAMHSA (Substance Abuse and Mental Health Services Administration) (2008) *Mandatory Guidelines for Federal Workplace Drug Testing Programs.* Department of Health and Human Services, Rockville MD USA.

SAMHSA (2012) *Clinical Drug Testing in Primary Care.* Technical Assistance Publication (TAP) 32. Department of Health and Human Services, Rockville MD, USA.

SAMHSA (2015a) *Mandatory Guidelines for Federal Workplace Drug Testing Programs – Urine.* Department of Health and Human Services, Rockville MD, USA.

SAMHSA (2015b) *Mandatory Guidelines for Federal Workplace Drug Testing Programs – Oral Fluid.* Department of Health and Human Services, Rockville MD, USA.

Schneider RS, Lindquist P, Wong ET, Ruebenstein KE, Ullman EF (1973) Homogeneous enzyme immunoassay for opiates in urine. *Clinical Chemistry* **19**, 821–825.

Shaw ML, Kwong TC, Rosano TG, Orsulak PJ, Wolf BA, Magnani B (2001) *The Clinical Toxicology Laboratory: Contemporary Practice of Poisoning Evaluation.* AACC Press, Washington DC, USA.

Standards Australia (1995) *Recommended Practice for the Collection, Detection and Quantitation of Drugs of Abuse in Urine – AS/NZS 4308:1995.* Standards Australia, Sydney.

Standards Australia (2006) *Procedures for Specimen Collection and the Detection and Quantitation of Drugs of Abuse in Oral Fluid – AS 4760:2006.* Standards Australia, Sydney.

Standards Australia and Standards New Zealand (2008) *Procedures for Specimen Collection and the Detection and Quantitation of Drugs of Abuse in urine - AS/NZS 4308:2008.* Standards Australia, Sydney.

UNODC (United Nations Office on Drugs and Crime) (2015) *World Drug Report 2015.* UN Office on Drugs and Crime, Vienna, Austria.

Verstraete AG (2005) Oral fluid testing for driving under the influence of drugs: history, recent progress and remaining challenges. *Forensic Science International* **150**, 143–150. doi:10.1016/j.forsciint.2004.11.023

Wong RC, Tse HY (2005) *Drugs of Abuse: Body Fluid Testing.* Humana Press, Totowa NJ, USA.

# THEME 3

# POINT-OF-CARE TESTING FOR SPECIFIC CLINICAL SETTINGS

# 27 Point-of-care testing in general practice

*Mark Shephard and Michael Kidd*

**Summary**

General practice, its practice teams and their primary health care relationships comprise the foundations of an effective health-care system. The current focus of general practice runs in parallel with the changing social context of health and with advances in technology and telehealth. Point-of-care testing (POCT) is an example of a rapidly evolving technology that has many advantages for general practice. The Point-of-Care Testing in General Practice Trial conducted in Australia (2005–2007) demonstrated the safety, clinical efficacy and acceptability of POCT in general practice for chronic diseases. Although the needs, utility and limitations of POCT in general practice are well characterised in developed countries, much work is needed to meet needs and overcome barriers for POCT in general practices in developing countries.

## AN INTRODUCTION TO GENERAL PRACTICE

### What is general practice?

General practice and family medicine are terms used interchangeably in different countries to describe the speciality of medicine that provides person-centred, continuing, comprehensive and coordinated medical care at the primary care level for individuals, families and communities (Kidd 2013; Murtagh and Rosenblatt 2011).

The general practitioner (GP) – also known as the family doctor or family physician in different parts of the world – is a medical practitioner trained in the speciality of general practice, who is primarily responsible for providing first contact and delivering comprehensive health care to every individual seeking medical care and advice, and for arranging other health personnel to provide services when necessary (Villanueva *et al.* 2013).

As a sector, general practice, its practice teams and their primary health care relationships comprise the foundations of an effective health-care system in many nations (RACGP 2015). The core attributes of general practice are summarised in Table 27.1.

### WONCA – representing the profession of general practice globally

Globally, the profession of general practice is represented by the World Organization of Family Doctors (abbreviated WONCA, an acronym comprising the first five initials of the World Organization of National Colleges, Academies and Academic Associations of General Practitioners/Family Physicians). WONCA is a not-for-profit organisation and was founded in 1972 by member organisations in 18 countries. WONCA now has 118 member organisations in 131 countries and territories with

**Table 27.1.** Core values and key principles that underpin general practice as a profession (Source: adapted with permission from Kidd 2013 Chapter 3 and RACGP 2015)

| Attribute | Commentary |
|---|---|
| General | General practice deals with the unselected health problems of the whole population; it does not exclude certain categories of the population because of age, sex, social class, race or religion, or any category of complaint or health-related problem; access to it is not limited by geographical, cultural, administrative or financial barriers. |
| Person-centred care | GPs understand that health, illness and disease are ultimately personal experiences, and that their principal role is to relieve personal disease in all its forms, in the manner best suited to each individual. The patient's needs, values and desired health outcomes always remain central to the GP's evaluation and management processes. |
| Continuous | Based on a long-standing personal relationship built on mutual knowledge, trust and respect between the patient and the doctor, GPs seek to build health, wellbeing and resilience by covering individuals' health care longitudinally over substantial periods of their lives and not being limited to one particular episode of an illness. |
| Comprehensive | The scope of general practice is challenging: spanning prevention, health promotion, early intervention for those at risk, and the management of acute, chronic and complex conditions within the practice population whether in the home, practice, health service, outreach clinic, hospital or community. |
| Coordinated | General practice deals with many of the health problems presented by individuals at their first contact with their family physician but, whenever necessary, the GP should ensure appropriate and timely referral of the patient to specialist services or to another health professional. GPs contribute to, and actively participate in, a well-functioning multidisciplinary care team and must be prepared to exercise leadership of the team. The GP is increasingly the custodian of, and conduit for, key patient clinical information. |
| Whole-of-person health care ('holism') | An appreciation of the interplay between biomedical, behavioural and socio-economic contributors to health leads to a deep understanding of the whole person, and the ability to manage complex conditions and circumstances. The GP functions as a physician, counsellor, advocate and agent of change for individuals, families and their communities. |
| Diagnostic and therapeutic skills | GPs are skilled in managing uncertainty, undifferentiated illness and complexity, able to use best-practice evidence in the light of individual circumstances, and engage patients and families in understanding, planning and managing their health according to individual capacities. |
| Continuing quality improvement | GPs are able to assess their professional capabilities, expand existing skills and acquire new skills over a professional lifetime in response to changing clinical and community contexts. |
| Leadership, advocacy and equity | GPs understand the socio-economic and environmental determinants of health and the contribution made by other health professionals, sectors and community groups, resulting in collaboration, advocacy and leadership, influencing local environments to the benefit of individuals, families and communities, especially those most marginalised and at risk. |

membership of ~500 000 family doctors (http://www.globalfamilydoctor.com/AboutWonca).

WONCA represents and acts as an advocate for its members at an international level where it interacts with world bodies such as the World Health Organization (WHO), with which it has official relations as a non-governmental organisation and is engaged in several collaborative projects. WONCA's mission is to improve the quality of life of people of the world by fostering high standards of care in general practice/family medicine. WONCA also represents the educational, research and service provision activities of general practice/family medicine globally.

## THE EVOLVING ROLE AND SCOPE OF GENERAL PRACTICE

For most people in many countries, their general practice represents the first and most commonly used point of access to health care. Consultation with the GP remains at the core of general practice, regardless of whether the purpose of the consultation is to actively manage a pre-existing condition or to make an effective diagnosis of a presenting condition.

Today, general practices can be: (i) small in size and run by a single GP (the 'solo' practice); (ii) large multi-partner ('group') practices employing a variety of clinical staff; (iii) include speciality clinics within a general practice; or (iv) part of 'polyclinics', where GPs co-locate with other specialists and a range of allied health services (e.g. podiatry, physiotherapy, nutrition, pharmacy and/or phlebotomy centres). General practice teams are tending to become larger, multidisciplinary and multi-skilled and may comprise a range of health professional staff that, as well as the GP, include, in different nations in different settings, nurses, nurse practitioners, physician assistants, health-care assistants, practice managers, IT support staff and receptionists (Goodwin *et al.* 2011).

Today, GPs must possess the skills, knowledge and clinical judgement to deal with a wide range of problems/presentations seen in the general practice setting; these may range from a variety of targeted procedural activities (e.g. skin biopsies, suturing lacerations and obstetric deliveries), to managing and co-coordinating care of many complicated or specialised disorders (such as acute emergencies, stabilisation of trauma, serious infections, and a range of chronic diseases and mental health concerns).

In this context, the current focus of general practice now tends to run in parallel with the changing social context of health (Goodwin *et al.* 2011). Most developed countries now have an ageing population where people are living longer but the additional years of life are likely to be compromised by long-term chronic illnesses (such as diabetes, renal or heart diseases) that require continuing management. Therefore, rather than treating episodic periods of illness, the GP is increasingly working in partnership with patients who have various co-morbidities to help them maintain stability in their lifestyles. Further, 'more informed' patients now have greater access to health-related information through the internet and, as a result, are become more demanding in their expectations of the family doctor and have a stronger desire to take more responsibility for managing their own health and health care.

Advances in technology and telehealth more generally mean that patients can now self-monitor their own conditions, download and send test results to their GP, as well as access disease-related or health promotion information through mobile phone applications.

POCT is an example of a rapidly evolving technology that has many potential advantages for the general practice setting. Intuitively, POCT conducted in general practices provides a convenient and accessible service for patients; with pathology testing performed, tests results available, treatment adjusted and medication prescribed during a single consultation with the GP. For the GP, the availability of immediate pathology results can support clinical judgement and decision making. Murtagh and Rosenblatt (2011) provided an historical list of the 20 most frequently managed disorders/diagnoses seen in Australian and USA family practices; they include hypertension, diabetes, lipid metabolism disorders, urinary tract infections, respiratory tract infections and viral diseases. Cooke *et al.* (2013) recently listed the top 10 and top 30 most frequently managed problems encountered in Australian general practices; they include (with rank order in parentheses) hypertension (1), upper respiratory tract infection (3), diabetes (5), lipid disorders (6), urinary tract infection (17), atrial fibrillation (26) and ischaemic heart disease (29). These top 30 problems accounted for ~48% of GP problems managed. There are 'matching' POC tests for each of these diseases/conditions (Table 27.2), which represent the 'tip of the iceberg' in realising the full potential of POCT in this setting, particularly

**Table 27.2.** Examples of common clinical presentations in Australian and US family practices and matched POC tests currently available

| Presentations | Examples of matched POC tests available |
|---|---|
| Hypertension | Blood pressure |
| Respiratory tract infections (bacterial and viral) | C-reactive protein, procalcitonin, influenza, group A streptococcus (GAS), Streptococcus pneumoniae, respiratory syncytial virus (RSV) |
| Diabetes | Glucose, HbA1c, creatinine, urine albumin:creatinine ratio (ACR), lactate |
| Lipid metabolism disorders | Total, HDL- and LDL-cholesterol, triglycerides |
| Urinary tract infections | Urine dipsticks for nitrite and leucocyte |
| Atrial fibrillation | International normalised ratio (INR) |
| Ischaemic heart disease | Cardiac troponin I and T, electrocardiogram (ECG) |

when considering the prevalence of communicable diseases in many low- and middle-income countries where sexually transmitted infections, malaria, drug-resistant tuberculosis and dengue fever, for example, also contribute significantly to disease burden.

## AN OVERVIEW OF POINT-OF-CARE TESTING IN GENERAL PRACTICE

This section reviews the early and recent literature on POCT in general practice, examines the key findings of the largest randomised controlled trial of POCT in the sector, explores the POC tests most wanted by the profession and describes some of the current limitations and barriers to the uptake of POCT in general practice.

### Reviewing the literature on POCT in general practice over the past 20 years

Hobbs *et al.* (1997) conducted the first detailed systematic review of POCT in primary care for the National Health Services' Health Technology Assessment (HTA) Program in the United Kingdom (UK). This study identified just over 100 published papers covering POC tests used in primary care for diabetes, haematuria, home pregnancy, cardiac enzymes, allergy, anticoagulation, anaemia, deep vein thrombosis, streptococcal throat, chlamydia, HIV and urinary tract infections, as well as markers of general inflammation/infection. However, the quality of these papers was generally poor and no randomised controlled trials were sourced. Only 32 papers passed quality filters for detailed appraisal in this systematic review, with >70% of these studies relating solely to the analytical performance of these tests and <10% of the studies reporting both test performance and an outcome measure. The major findings of this detailed review were summarised 2 years later by Delaney *et al.* (1999) who concluded there was limited evidence to support the general introduction of POCT in general practice; they stated: 'almost no reports were found of unbiased assessment of the effect of near patient tests in primary care on patient outcomes, organisational outcomes [including patient satisfaction], or cost.' Indeed, the lack of quality evidence for the effectiveness of POCT in primary care at this time led to the publishing of criteria required for evaluations to be undertaken in this setting (Delaney *et al.* 2000). They stated: 'there is a need for a formal statement of the criteria by which to judge the quality of evaluations in this field … seven questions need to be addressed. These cover the performance, reliability and acceptability of the test, its impact on decision-making, comparison with existing practice, cost-effectiveness of the test and integration with the practitioner's knowledge base.' The criteria they proposed embodied the following: 'demonstration of the need for POCT, definition of the appropriate reference standard, calculation of sample size based on modelling of the decision problem and defining acceptable limits to the likelihood ratio, avoidance of verification bias, selection bias and treatment paradox, testing for the presence of spectrum bias, reporting the sensitivity of the results to changes in setting or prevalence or disease and calculating cost-effectiveness.'

POCT in general practice in Australia was the subject of an extensive literature review by Guibert *et al.* (2001). This review was commissioned by the Australian Government's Department of Health and Ageing in response to a significant lack of information on POCT in this setting in Australia. The study aimed to examine the role and value of POCT in general practice by reviewing current literature, sourcing the opinions of key stakeholders in this field (e.g. consumers, GPs and pathologists) and providing recommendations to the Government on policy and directions for future research for POCT in this setting. The POCT tests reviewed were glucose, lipids, potassium, haemoglobin, human chorionic gonadotropin (HCG), *H. pylori*, Streptococcus A, micro-urine (dipstick urinalysis and urine microscopy), international normalised ratio (INR), haemoglobin A1c (HbA1c), microalbumin, C-reactive protein (CRP) and substances of abuse (with the latter five being only superficially covered). However, the effectiveness of these tests was not discussed in any detail in this review, other than to note the evidence for the clinical and economic benefits of using POCT in general practice was 'patchy and generally not high level by NHMRC criteria.' Nevertheless, this review documented several key recommendations regarding how POCT should be conducted in general practice in Australia and it highlighted that rural and remote general practices could potentially be the main beneficiaries of POCT but that further work was needed to determine the clinical and economic benefits of POCT in general practice.

Later, a further systematic review of POCT for patients with diabetes, hyperlipidaemia or coagulation disorders in general practice was conducted by Australian authors working on the Point-of-Care Testing in General Practice Trial (Gialamas *et al.* 2010a). Nine papers from six randomised or quasi-randomised trials were included in this review (three related to type 2 diabetes, one to hyperlipidaemia and five to anticoagulation therapy). They found there was no robust evidence that POCT in general practice had comparable analytical quality to laboratory testing nor that is was clinically or operationally effective. The review was limited by the low number of trials sourced, the short period of follow-up of patients and the large between-study heterogeneity.

### The Australian Point-of-Care Testing in General Practice (Randomised Controlled) Trial

In 2005, the Australian Government recommended that a randomised controlled trial of POCT in general practice be conducted in Australia, due in part to address the lack of quality evidence for the efficacy of POCT in this sector identified by the earlier systematic reviews. The objectives of the trial were to investigate the safety, clinical effectiveness, cost effectiveness and acceptability of POCT in general practice. The trial was conducted within a structured quality management framework comprising:

- a set of interim standards for POCT in general practice
- a comprehensive training and competency assessment program for practice nurse device operators
- a quality control (QC) and external proficiency testing (PT) program to monitor the analytical quality of POCT performed during the trial
- an interim accreditation program (Laurence *et al.* 2008a,b). The design for the trial and an evaluation framework were developed before the commencement of the trial.

The 18-month cluster randomised controlled trial (RCT) commenced in September 2005 and was completed in February 2007. The trial was conducted in 53 general practices, with approximately equal numbers of practices recruited from the Adelaide, South Australia (urban), Bendigo, Victoria (rural) and Dubbo, New South Wales (remote) geographic regions. Just under 5000 patients (4968) were recruited for the trial, making this study the largest RCT conducted in the general practice sector globally. A total of 3010 patients from 30 practices were randomised to have pathology testing performed on-site by POCT (intervention group) and 1958 patients from 23 practices had their pathology samples performed by their usual laboratory (control group). All patients were required to have a pre-existing diagnosis of type 2 diabetes or hyperlipidaemia or be on anticoagulation therapy. POC tests measured for the trial included HbA1c and urine ACR (for diabetes management), lipids (for monitoring patients with hyperlipidaemia who were being prescribed lipid lowering drugs) and INR (for measuring clotting time for patients receiving warfarin therapy).

The principal clinical effectiveness outcome measures for the trial are summarised in Table 27.3. They show that POCT was not inferior to (i.e. it was the same or better

**Table 27.3.** Clinical effectiveness of POCT in the Point-of-Care Testing in General Practice Trial (Source: adapted from Bubner *et al.* 2009)

| Proportion of patients with results in target range (%) | | | |
|---|---|---|---|
| **POC test** | **Intervention (POCT)** | **Control** | **Difference** |
| HbA1c | 65.5 | 56.2 | 9.3[a] |
| ACR | 77.4 | 74.2 | 3.2[a] |
| Total cholesterol | 38.7 | 21.6 | 17.0[a] |
| Triglyceride | 70.9 | 68.8 | 2.0[a] |
| HDL cholesterol | 73.5 | 82.7 | –9.2 |
| INR | 57.0 | 61.5 | –4.5 |
| **Proportion of tests with results in target range (%)** | | | |
| **POC test** | **Intervention (POCT)** | **Control** | **Difference** |
| HbA1c | 64.1 | 54.7 | 9.4[a] |
| ACR | 77.0 | 72.6 | 4.4[a] |
| Total cholesterol | 34.9 | 20.9 | 14.0[a] |
| Triglyceride | 67.0 | 65.4 | 1.7[a] |
| HDL cholesterol | 74.9 | 83.5 | –9.1 |
| INR | 55.8 | 57.6 | –1.8[a] |

Note: ACR = urine albumin:creatinine ratio; INR = international normalised ratio
[a]Difference was statistically significant ($P$ <0.05)

than) laboratory testing of patients in terms of (i) the proportion of patients whose tests results were in the target range for all tests except INR and HDL cholesterol and (ii) the proportion of tests within the target range for all tests except HDL cholesterol. For example, for HbA1c, there was a 9.3% improvement in the percentage of patients with results in the target range in the POCT group compared with the control group; while, for total cholesterol, there was a 14% improvement in the percentage of tests with results in the target range in the POCT group compared with the control group.

In relation to the proportion of patients showing an improvement in their test result from baseline, POCT was again non-inferior to pathology testing for HbA1c (57% with POCT *v.* 45% with laboratory testing); total cholesterol (74% *v.* 57%) and triglyceride (55% *v.* 51%) (*P* ≤0.001 in each case), but not for HDL cholesterol.

Clinical effectiveness was also assessed by measuring patients' adherence to medication by a self-administered questionnaire using a five-item medication adherence report scale (MARS-5) and non-inferiority analysis (Gialamas *et al.* 2009). Results showed that having access to POCT was associated with the same or better medication adherence compared with having test results provided by the laboratory (39.3% medication adherence in POCT group compared with 37.0% with control group, difference 2.3%, *P* <0.001). This trend was consistent across all three patients conditions monitored (i.e. diabetes, hyperlipidaemia and anticoagulation disorders).

In summary, in terms of therapeutic control, POCT was found to be the same or better than pathology laboratory testing for most tests, suggesting that POCT could assist GPs in better management of some chronic conditions, while the results also suggested that having an

**Table 27.4.** Between-group comparisons of patient satisfaction with POCT for all chronic conditions assessed in the Trial (Source: modified from figure by Laurence *et al.* 2010a, with permission from the *British Journal of General Practice*, the journal of the Royal College of General Practitioners)

| Areas | Statements | Intervention median satisfaction score (mean transformed satisfaction score) | Control median satisfaction score (mean transformed satisfaction score) | Difference (intervention – control) in mean transformed satisfaction score (95% CI) | *P*-value |
|---|---|---|---|---|---|
| Collection process | I would rather have blood taken by a finger prick than by needle in my arm | 7.8 (0.92) | 5.1 (1.64) | –0.73 (–0.89 to –0.57) | <0.001 |
| Confidence in the process | Laboratories have better hygiene than point-of-care testing | 4.3 (1.65) | 4.6 (2.07) | –0.43 (–0.62 to –0.23) | <0.001 |
| Confidence in the results | I have confidence in the information given by my GP or practice regarding my pathology test result | 9.0 (0.06) | 8.9 (0.18) | –0.12 (–0.21 to –0.03) | 0.010 |
| Convenience | Not having to travel to an outside laboratory would be convenient | 8.9 (0.17) | 8.7 (0.36) | –0.20 (–0.34 to –0.05) | 0.009 |
| Cost | Outside pathology laboratories involves extra time and transport costs | 8.5 (0.44) | 8.6 (0.39) | 0.06 (–0.11 to 0.23) | 0.510 |
| Disease management | Having immediate feedback of the test result for my condition was important as it allowed/would allow me to discuss the management of my condition with my GP | 9.0 (0.12) | 8.7 (0.30) | –0.18 (–0.30 to –0.06) | 0.003 |
| | I am/would be more motivated to look after my condition because of regular point-of-care testing | 8.9 (0.29) | 8.2 (0.64) | –0.36 (–0.49 to –0.22) | <0.001 |
| | Point-of-care-testing strengthened/would strengthen my relationship with my GP | 8.3 (0.52) | 8.1 (0.72) | –0.20 (–0.35 to –0.05) | 0.010 |

**Table 27.5.** Summary of the median within-practice imprecision by geographic region, and comparison with analytical goals for imprecision set for the POCT in General Practice Trial (Source: adapted from Shephard *et al.* 2009)

| | | | Median within-practice imprecision (CV%) | | | | | |
|---|---|---|---|---|---|---|---|---|
| | | Imprecision goal (CV%) set | QC level 1 | | | QC level 2 | | |
| POC test | Lot | for trial | Urban | Rural | Remote | Urban | Rural | Remote |
| HbA1c | 1 | 4 | 3.3 | 2.2 | 2.4 | 3.4 | 3.4 | 2.7 |
| | 2 | 4 | 2.6 | 2.9 | 3.0 | 3.9 | 3.2 | 3.2 |
| Urine ACR | 1 | 12 | 5.0 | 5.1 | 5.0 | 3.4 | 4.0 | 4.1 |
| Total cholesterol | 1 | 5 | 3.4 | 3.1 | 3.2 | 4.1 | 3.0 | 2.7 |
| | 2 | 5 | 2.3 | 2.1 | 2.6 | 2.8 | 2.1 | 3.2 |
| Triglyceride | 1 | 7.5 | 4.3 | 3.3 | 4.5 | 3.7 | 3.2 | 4.0 |
| | 2 | 7.5 | 3.8 | 5.0 | 5.3 | 3.7 | 5.1 | 6.1 |
| HDL cholesterol | 1 | 6 | 6.4 | 4.9 | 5.5 | 4.5 | 3.1 | 4.0 |
| | 2 | 6 | 5.1 | 6.5 | 8.8 | 4.7 | 3.9 | 5.1 |
| INR | 1 | 10 | 7.1 | 6.1 | 7.9 | na | na | na |
| | 2 | 10 | 6.5 | 6.9 | 6.2 | na | na | na |

immediate test result was beneficial for patients in terms of medication compliance.

Patient satisfaction with POCT in general practice was also assessed during the trial by the level of agreement with statements about different aspects of POCT using a visual analogue scale and a mixed model analysis of variance with allowance for clustering at the practice level (Laurence *et al.* 2010a). A total of 4573 questionnaires were distributed, with an 88% response rate (87% intervention and 89% control groups, respectively). Patients accessing POCT had (statistically significantly) higher levels of satisfaction than the control group with the collection process (finger-prick versus venous sampling) and with confidence in the testing process and test results. Patients accessing POCT also reported that POCT motivated them to 'look after their condition' better and strengthened their relationship with their doctor (Table 27.4).

The trial also concluded it was safe to perform POCT in the general practice setting, as assessed by:

- the competency of the 80 device operators trained (Shephard *et al.* 2009a)
- the general analytical standards achieved for QC and PT (Shephard *et al.* 2009b)
- the agreement between POCT and laboratory testing conducted during the trial (with POCT sites being required to send an equivalent sample to the laboratory for each POC test performed) (Gialamas *et al.* 2010b)
- compliance with the standards established for the trial (assessed by the interim accreditation program) (Tirimacco *et al.* 2011)
- an assessment of serious adverse events (SAE) that occurred during the trial – with no SAE being attributable to POCT; the number of SAEs per 10 000 person-years was lower for the intervention group (1320) than for the control group (1446) overall and for all three conditions and, overall, the proportion of patients experiencing one or more SAE was the same for both the intervention (13%) and control (13%) groups (Laurence *et al.* 2008a).

As mentioned, analytical quality of the POCT devices used during the trial (DCA 2000, Cholestech LDX and Coaguchek S) was assessed throughout its duration by both QC and PT. The overall participation rate for QC and PT testing across the trial averaged >90% for all POC tests. Device operators conducted QC testing to an analytical standard that met the imprecision goals set for the trial for all POC tests and all lot numbers tested (except for one level of HDL-cholesterol QC) (Shephard *et al.* 2009b). As shown in Table 27.5, there was also no difference between the imprecision observed for QC testing across the testing that occurred in the urban, rural and remote geographic locations of the practices in the trial (Shephard 2009).

Device operators also conducted PT to an acceptable level of accuracy when compared with pathology

Table 27.6. Comparison of surveys concerning POC tests currently used and those desired by general practitioners (top 5 tests)

| Current POC tests most widely used | | POC tests needed for the future | |
|---|---|---|---|
| **Howick *et al.* (2014)** | **WONCA Survey 2014–2015** | **Howick *et al.* 2014** | **WONCA Survey 2014–2015** |
| Urine pregnancy | Glucose | D-dimer | HbA1c |
| Urinalysis | Urinalysis | Cardiac troponin | Cardiac markers |
| Glucose | Lipids | Chlamydia | Full blood count |
| INR | Haemoglobin | BNP | INR |
| Haemoglobin | Urine pregnancy | CRP and Gonorrhoea (equal) | Electrolytes |

laboratories (84% to 98% acceptable results, depending on the test), although imprecision goals for PT were not met for total and HDL cholesterol.

Finally, cost effectiveness was evaluated by assessing incremental cost-effectiveness of a clinical strategy based on performing POCT in general practice compared with pathology testing through a laboratory (Laurence *et al.* 2010b). Overall findings were varied, with the incremental cost-effective ratio (ICER) for POCT found to be favourable for urine ACR but unfavourable for INR, with uncertainty surrounding the cost efficiency of POCT for HbA1c and lipids.

### What POC tests do general practitioners currently use and what do they want?

A recent international survey of over 2770 GPs and family physicians from Australia, Belgium, the Netherlands, UK and USA was undertaken by Howick *et al.* (2014). The survey sought to gain information on (i) clinical conditions for which a POC test may be useful, (ii) which POC tests are used currently by survey respondents and (iii) which POC tests GPs would like to use in the future. Part of the survey's aim was to raise awareness among GPs of new POC technologies available and also to help industry prioritise tests that are likely to be required in the future GP market.

The two most common clinical conditions for which GPs sought a POC test were urinary tract infections (Australia, UK, USA) and pulmonary embolism/deep vein thrombosis (Belgium and the Netherlands). GPs in all five countries also listed diabetes, acute cardiac disease and anaemia among their top 10 conditions.

The three most common current POC tests used by >80% of responding GPs were urine pregnancy tests, urine leucocytes/nitrites and blood glucose, followed by INR (31%) and haemoglobin (28%). INR POCT was used by almost half of the GPs from Australia, the USA and the UK. Haemoglobin was the most popular POC test among Dutch and the USA GPs. C-reactive protein (CRP) was used widely by GPs from the Netherlands (48%) but by <15% of GPs in the remaining four countries.

In terms of their 'wish list', POC tests for D-dimer, troponin, chlamydia, gonorrhoea, brain natriuretic peptide (BNP), CRP, HbA1c, white cell count and haemoglobin were wanted by more than half of the responding GPs across all countries. Although comprehensive, this survey only sought the views of GPs working in developed countries and therefore the needs of clinicians from developing countries are not represented in this survey.

In 2013, WONCA established a Special Interest Group on Global Point-of-Care Testing. The Special Interest Group provides a forum for family doctors of all countries to meet, discuss, learn about, promote, advocate for and research the clinical utility and effectiveness of POCT (WONCA SIG 2015). This group also conducted a survey of member GPs (albeit on a smaller scale) to ascertain current and future POCT needs, as well as barriers and limitations to the implementation of POCT. The WONCA survey received responses from GPs in each of WONCA's 7 regional sectors ($n$ = 150), but the responses were weighted heavily from the European zone. A comparison of findings between the surveys of Howick *et al.* (2014) and the WONCA Special Interest Group are summarised in Table 27.6.

## FACILITATORS, LIMITATIONS AND BARRIERS TO THE USE OF POINT-OF-CARE TESTING IN GENERAL PRACTICE

Jones *et al.* (2013) conducted a systematic review of the attitudes of GPs towards POCT. They found that GPs believed POCT improved diagnostic certainty, facilitated self-management of chronic conditions, improved the doctor–patient relationship, which in turn enhanced

**Table 27.7.** Ten-point plan for the introduction of POCT into general practice (Source: adapted from Cals and van Weert 2013)

| **Use and quality requirements in a family practice** | |
|---|---|
| Test accuracy | Essential that POCT results are accurate, precise and robust |
| Time to decision | POC test result must be available within the timeframe in which a clinical decision has to be made |
| Usability | The POCT device must be easy to use from an operator perspective |
| Frequency of use | The POC test should be used frequently enough within the practice, ensuring limited wastage of consumables |
| Quality control | Essential that quality testing requirements are feasible within the practice workflow and are not too costly and/or complicated |
| **Indication and efficacy in a family medicine setting** | |
| Indication for testing | The clinical reason for using the test should be clearly defined |
| Test interpretation | Enough information should be available for the correct interpretation of the POC test result, taking into account (and knowing) the test limitations |
| Immediate effect on GP's decision | Will the test have direct consequences for the GP's decision making? |
| Effect on patient outcomes | Does the POC test provide results that will benefit patients with the relevant clinical condition? |
| Cost-effectiveness | Will the POC test be cost-effective in the practice? |

communication and shared decision making, and resulted in fewer re-consultations for the same or future episodes of illness. The WONCA Special Interest Group survey identified the most valuable attributes of POCT in general practice as being its capacity to provide rapid diagnosis and treatment (88%), convenience for the patient (75%), ease of use (60%), improved doctor–patient relationship (57%) and improved patient adherence to medication (55%).

However, like Delaney *et al.* more than a decade earlier, Cals and van Weert (2013) warn that POC tests need to be introduced cautiously in general practice and only after establishing their added value in this setting. They argue that, while POC tests can be helpful in the 'grey area of diagnostic uncertainty', POCT must be part of a 'balanced process in which the test result is an integral part of the way GPs decide on diagnosis and prognosis

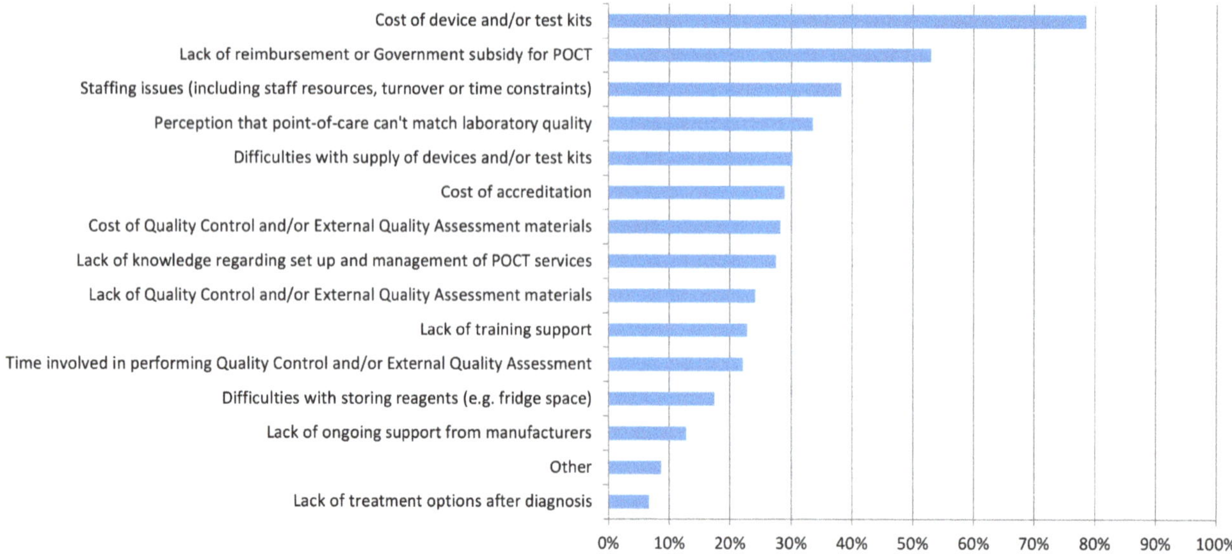


**Fig. 27.1.** Current barriers to the implementation of POCT in general practice, identified by the WONCA Special Interest Group on Global Point-of-Care Testing.

and communicate with their patients.' They also proposed a 10-point framework by which POCT should be introduced into a general practice setting (Table 27.7).

Jones *et al.* (2013) identified the five main barriers to the adoption of POCT in general practice as concerns over test accuracy, an over-reliance on POC tests (potentially undermining clinical skills), the cost of funding POCT and equipment maintenance, and the usefulness of POCT being limited to certain clinical scenarios and patients. The main barriers to POCT identified in the WONCA Special Interest Group survey are shown in Fig. 27.1.

The cost of implementing POCT is clearly a major impediment to its uptake in general practice and, where government reimbursement for POCT is not available, sustainability becomes increasingly difficult and costs are often transferred to the patient – a burden that patients in many developing countries cannot afford. As Howick *et al.* (2014) state: 'the difference in reimbursement and care models across countries for POC tests needs to be explored further to discover whether and how specific POC tests might improve patient outcomes in specified settings.' Staff turnover is a constant issue, particularly for general practices in rural or remote locations (Shephard *et al.* 2009a). The cost and time involved in performing quality testing to ensure analytical quality needs to realistic, practical and affordable within the busy general practice environment.

In conclusion, the potential use and scope of POCT in general practice is ever broadening, but its uptake must be balanced by the local or regional clinical conditions for which POCT is most needed, while more cost effectiveness studies of high quality are required to provide greater justification for reimbursement of POCT to be supported by governments of the world. Although the needs, utility and limitations of POCT in the general practice setting is relatively well characterised in countries of the developed world, much more work needs to be undertaken in terms of the implementation, needs and barriers for POCT in general practices within developing countries, where burdens of communicable and non-communicable diseases are highest.

## REFERENCES


Bubner TK, Laurence CO, Gialamas A, Yelland LN, Ryan P, Willson KJ, *et al.* (2009) Effectiveness of point-of-care testing for therapeutic control of chronic conditions: results from the PoCT in General Practice Trial. *The Medical Journal of Australia* **190**, 624–626.

Cals J, van Weert H (2013) Point-of-care tests in general practice: hope or hype? *The European Journal of General Practice* **19**, 251–256. doi:10.3109/13814788.2013.800041

Cooke G, Valenti L, Glasziou P, Britt H (2013) Common general practice presentations and publication frequency. *Australian Family Physician* **42**, 65–68.

Delaney B, Hyde C, McManus R, Wilson S, Fitzmaurice DA, Jowett S, *et al.* (1999) Systematic review of near patient test evaluations in primary care. *British Medical Journal* **319**, 824–827. doi:10.1136/bmj.319.7213.824

Delaney B, Wilson S, Fitzmaurice DA, Hyde C, Hobbs R (2000) Near patient tests in primary care: setting the standards for evaluation. *Journal of Health Services Research & Policy* **5**, 37–41.

Gialamas A, Yelland LN, Ryan P, Willson K, Laurence CO, Bubner TK, *et al.* (2009) Does point-of-care testing lead to the same or better adherence to medication? A randomised controlled trial: the PoCT in General Practice Trial. *The Medical Journal of Australia* **191**, 487–491.

Gialamas A, St John A, Laurence CO, Bubner TK, members of the PoCT Management Committee (2010a) Point-of-care testing for patients with diabetes, hyperlipidaemia or coagulation disorders in the general practice setting: a systematic review. *Family Practice* **27**, 17–24. doi:10.1093/fampra/cmp084

Gialamas A, Laurence C, Yelland L, Tideman P, Worley P, Shephard M, *et al.* (2010b) Assessing agreement between point of care and laboratory results for lipid testing from a clinical perspective. *Clinical Biochemistry* **43**, 515–518. doi:10.1016/j.clinbiochem.2009.11.014

Goodwin N, Dixon A, Poole T, Raleigh V (2011) 'Improving the quality of care in general practice: Report of an independent inquiry commissioned by The King's Fund'. The King's Fund, London, UK.

Guibert R, Schattner P, Sikaris K, Churilov L, Leibowitz R, Matthews M (2001) 'Review of the role and value of near patient testing in general practice'. Report to the Pathology Section, Diagnostic and Technology Branch, Commonwealth Department of Health and Aged Care, Melbourne.

Hobbs F, Delaney B, Fitzmaurice D, *et al.* (1997) A review of near patient testing in primary care. *Health Technology Assessment* **1**, 1–229.

Howick J, Cals JWL, Jones C, Price CP, Pluddemann A, Heneghan C, *et al.* (2014) Current and future use of point-of-care tests in primary care: an international survey in Australia, Belgium, the Netherlands, the UK and the USA. *British Medical Journal Open* **4**, e005611, <http://bmjopen.bmj.com/content/4/8/e005611.short>.

Jones CHD, Howick J, Roberts NW, Price CP, Heneghan C, Pluddermann A, *et al.* (2013) Primary care clinicians' attitudes towards point-of-care blood testing: a systematic review of qualitative studies. *BMC Family Practice* **14**, 117. doi:10.1186/1471-2296-14-117

Kidd M (Ed.) (2013) *The Contribution of Family Medicine to Improving Health Systems.* Radcliffe Publishing, London, UK.

Laurence C, Gialamas A, Yelland L, Bubner T, Glastonbury B, Beilby J, Members of the Evaluation Working Group (2008a) 'Point of Care Testing in General Practice Trial. Final Report'. Australian Government Department of Health and Ageing, Canberra.

Laurence C, Gialamas A, Yelland L, Bubner T, Ryan P, Wilson K, *et al.* (2008b) A pragmatic cluster, randomised trial to evaluate the safety, clinical effectiveness, cost effectiveness and satisfaction with point of care testing in a general practice setting – rationale, design and baseline characteristics. *Trials* **9**, 50. doi:10.1186/1745-6215-9-50

Laurence CO, Gialamas A, Bubner T, Yelland L, Willson K, Ryan P, *et al.* (2010a) Patient satisfaction with point-of-care testing in general practice. *The British Journal of General Practice* **60**, e98–e104. doi:10.3399/bjgp10X483508

Laurence CO, Moss JR, Briggs NE, Beilby JJ (2010b) The cost-effectiveness of point of care testing in a general practice setting: results from a randomised controlled trial. *BMC Health Services Research* **10**, 165. doi:10.1186/1472-6963-10-165

Murtagh J, Rosenblatt J (2011) *Murtagh's General Practice.* 5th edn. McGraw-Hill, Sydney.

Shephard M (2009) The influence of geography on the performance of quality control testing in the Australian Government's Point of Care Testing in General Practice Trial. *Clinical Biochemistry* **42**, 1325–1327. doi:10.1016/j.clinbiochem.2009.05.008

Shephard M, Mazzachi B, Watkinson L, Shephard A, Laurence A, Gialamas A, *et al.* (2009a) Evaluation of a training program for device operators in the Australian Government's Point of Care Testing in General Practice Trial. *Rural and Remote Health* **9**, 1189, <http://www.rrh.org.au/publishedarticles/article_print_1189.pdf>.

Shephard M, Shephard A, Watkinson L, Mazzachi B, Worley P (2009b) Design, implementation and results of the quality control program for the Australian Government's Point of Care Testing in General Practice Trial. *Annals of Clinical Biochemistry* **46**, 413–419. doi:10.1258/acb.2009.009045

Tirimacco R, Glastonbury B, Laurence C, Bubner T, Shephard M, Beilby J (2011) Development of an accreditation program for Point of Care Testing (PoCT) in general practice. *Australian Health Review* **35**, 230–234. doi:10.1071/AH09792

Villanueva T, Arroll B, Cavadas LF, Gusso G, Gerva J, Griswold K, *et al.* (2013) Family doctors in health systems. In *The Contribution of Family Medicine to Improving Health Systems.* (Ed. M Kidd) pp. 41–73. Radcliffe Publishing, London, UK.

WONCA SIG (WONCA Special Interest Group on Global Point-of-Care Testing) (2015) WONCA website, <http://www.globalfamilydoctor.com/groups/SpecialInterestGroups/Pointofcaretesting.aspx>.

# 28 Point-of-care testing in rural, remote and Indigenous settings

*Mark Shephard, Louise Causer and Rebecca Guy*

**Summary**

Rural and remote communities experience higher mortality rates and poorer health status than metropolitan regions. Nowhere is this health divide more profound than for Indigenous people. Point-of-care testing (POCT) has a particular niche within rural and remote health and its astute and practical application can be an 'inventive solution' for improving health-care delivery in these locations. This chapter showcases three current POCT models working in rural and remote Indigenous Australia that support the detection and/or management of chronic, acute and infectious diseases.

## AN INTRODUCTION TO RURAL, REMOTE AND INDIGENOUS HEALTH

The terms 'rural' and 'remote' generally refer to those towns and populations that exist outside major metropolitan and urban areas, with remote environments being most distant in terms of geographical isolation, space, time and connection (Kelly and Dade Smith 2007).

The International Labour Office (2015) recently concluded there were 'significant if not extreme' differences between rural and urban populations in health coverage and access at global, regional and national levels, with 56% of the global rural population lacking health coverage compared with 22% of the urban population. Some of their key findings are summarised in Table 28.1.

Strasser (2003) notes that, even in countries where the majority of the population lives in rural areas, the resources remain concentrated in the cities. He argues there is a need to focus on health and wellbeing in rural and remote areas where the provision of health services is severely affected by limited funding and resource constraints, due largely to government and urban planners thinking that 'the country is just like the city'. In reality, the characteristics of rural health and the issues driving the delivery of health-care services are very different to those of metropolitan centres. Isolation by geography and the effect this has on access to health services is the defining element of rural health (Kelly and Dade Smith 2007). Differing social, lifestyle and environmental determinants of rural health, including greater degree of cultural diversity, lack of employment opportunities, lower income levels and poorer access to housing, education and transport significantly influence the mode of health-care delivery, health status and patterns of disease. Overall, the rural sector experiences higher mortality rates and poorer health status than metropolitan regions, a trend that increases with increasing degree of remoteness. Prevalence rates for communicable and non-communicable diseases are generally higher in rural than metropolitan environments, and greatest in remote regions (Simmons and Hsu-Hage 2002).

**Table 28.1.** Key messages regarding inequities between rural and urban health (Source: ILO 2015)

| |
|---|
| • The rural/urban divide is a consistent feature across the world, existing in all regions and all countries. |
| • Rural/urban inequalities result in higher rural mortality. |
| • The rural/urban divide is aggravated by extreme health workforce shortages in rural areas (with a global shortfall of ~7 million missing health workers to deliver services in rural areas compared with a lack of 3 million skilled staff in urban areas). |
| • The deficit in per capita health spending is twice as large in rural areas as in urban environments. |
| • Fundamental rights to health and social protection remain largely unfulfilled in rural populations. |
| • While core issues leading to inequality can be identified within the health sector, many of the root causes – poverty, informality, discrimination and lack of voice and power – are found beyond the sector itself. |
| • Looking forward, those living in rural areas should have access to health protection and services that meet the criteria of availability, affordability, accessibility, acceptability and quality. |

The challenge of reducing the health differential between rural and metropolitan environments lies with the development of inventive solutions to specific local health problems. The astute and practical application of POCT can unquestionably be one of those 'inventive solutions' for improving rural health-care delivery – across chronic, acute and infectious diseases.

## Indigenous health

Nowhere is this health differential between remote and urban environments more profound than for Indigenous people. For example, in Australia, Indigenous Australians living in remote areas were nearly twice as likely to have diabetes as those living in non-remote areas (9% *v.* 5%) (Atkinson *et al.* 2008); incidence of end-stage renal disease in certain remote Indigenous regions are 30-times the national incidence (Cass *et al.* 2002), and rates of gonorrhoea are 60-times higher in remote Indigenous communities than in non-Indigenous populations (Kirby Institute 2012). Many countries have endeavoured to close the gap in Indigenous disadvantage related to broad social determinants of health, but Mitrou *et al.* (2014) reported that Indigenous populations in Australia, Canada and New Zealand were just as disadvantaged in 2006 as they were in 1981 in terms of employment and income, and more disadvantaged in the education domain. Difference in life expectancy between Indigenous and non-Indigenous people has closed to ~7 years in Canada and the USA and to 7.5 years in New Zealand, but in Australia remain at 20 years (NACCHO and Oxfam Australia 2007). Decreases in mortality in Canada and USA were attributed to decreases in deaths due to injuries and in Maori people to reductions in deaths due to circulatory conditions. In some Australian states and territories, some gains have been made in slowing death rates due to chronic diseases, while deaths due to infectious disease have significantly declined. These gains have been attributed to improved access to primary health-care programs supported by well-constructed, well-resourced secondary prevention and health-promotion programs (Freemantle *et al.* 2007).

Indeed, it is within the Indigenous rural and remote primary health sector that POCT can potentially have the greatest application and benefit. Having said this, nowhere does the implementation and sustainability of POCT face greater challenges. In working with Indigenous communities, it is crucial the POCT researcher undertakes cultural awareness training before implementing a program and works in a culturally safe manner at all times during the program. The South Australian Health and Medical Research Institute (SAHMRI), through its Wardliparingga Aboriginal Research Unit, released a companion document as part of the 'South Australian Aboriginal Health Research Accord', which concisely elucidated a set of nine key principles for the conduct of Indigenous research; these principles, outlined in Table 28.2, provide a culturally safe framework for POCT researchers both within and outside Australia to follow when implementing programs within an Indigenous community (SAHMRI/Wardliparingga Aboriginal Research Unit 2014).

## The 'fit' between POCT and rural, remote and Indigenous health

The remaining sections of this chapter describe three current POCT models working in rural and remote Indigenous Australia. Each model is founded on the principles outlined in the SAHMRI Accord. The models showcase POCT programs for chronic, acute and infectious disease.

**Table 28.2.** Principles of the South Australian Aboriginal Health Research Accord (SAHMRI/Wardliparingga Aboriginal Research Unit 2014)

| Principle | Descriptor |
|---|---|
| Priorities | Research should be conducted on priorities arising from and endorsed by the Aboriginal community to enhance acceptability, relevance and accountability. |
| Involvement | The involvement of Aboriginal people and organisations is essential in developing, implementing and translating research. |
| Partnership | Research should be based on the establishment of mutual trust, and equivalent partnerships, and the ability to work competently across cultures. |
| Respect | Researchers must demonstrate respect for Aboriginal knowledge systems and custodianship of that knowledge. |
| Communication | Communication must be culturally and community relevant and involve a willingness to listen and learn. |
| Reciprocity | Research should deliver tangible benefits to Aboriginal communities. These benefits should be determined by Aboriginal people themselves and consider outcomes and processes during, and as a result of, the research. |
| Ownership | Researchers should acknowledge, respect, and protect Aboriginal intellectual property rights and transparent negotiation of intellectual property use and benefit sharing should be ensured. |
| Control | Researchers must ensure the respectful and culturally appropriate management of all biological and non-biological research materials. |
| Knowledge translation | Sharing and translation of knowledge generated through research must be integrated into all elements of the research process to maximise impact on policy and practice. |

## THE QAAMS POCT PROGRAM FOR DIABETES MANAGEMENT

### Background

Type 2 diabetes and its principal complication, renal disease, are responsible for a significant burden of morbidity, mortality, social and cultural trauma in Australia's Aboriginal and Torres Strait Islander people. Rates of diabetes in many Indigenous communities are as high as 30–40%, deaths due to diabetes in Indigenous Australians are 12- to 17-times that of non-Indigenous Australians, and 47% of all cases of end-stage renal disease in Indigenous patients are directly attributable to diabetes (Shephard and Gill 2010).

In 1998, Australia's National Diabetes Strategy and Implementation Plan recommended that a trial of POCT for HbA1c on the DCA 2000® (Siemens) be conducted in Australian Aboriginal medical services to assist diabetes management for Indigenous people. The resultant QAAMS (Quality Assurance for Aboriginal and Torres Strait Islander Medical Services) Program commenced as a pilot in 45 Aboriginal medical services in June 1999. Seventeen years on, the QAAMS Program is the largest national POCT field program in Australia and now supports the quality-assured conduct of POCT for HbA1c and urine albumin:creatinine ratio (ACR) in 200 Indigenous sites across Australia, 80% of which are rural or remote (Fig. 28.1). Since 2008, the DCA Vantage® has been used to measure these markers. QAAMS has been continuously funded by the Australian Government Department of Health since 1999 and the program is now embedded in the mainstream practice of diabetes care for Indigenous people.

### Program design

The Program is managed for the Australian Government by the Flinders University International Centre for Point-of-Care Testing and the RCPA Quality Assurance Programs Pty Ltd provides the proficiency testing component.

The long-term sustainability of the QAAMS Program is due to a commitment and adherence to four underlying principles/activities:

- continuing education, training and competency assessment of POCT device operators. Training is available in flexible formats including face-to-face (on-site visits, regional and annual workshops) or e-learning options (videoconferencing and web-streamed videos that are available at any time via the QAAMS website www.qaams.org.au). Competency assessment can be undertaken at face-to-face training sessions or on-line.
- regular surveillance of analytical quality through tailored monthly quality control (QC) and proficiency

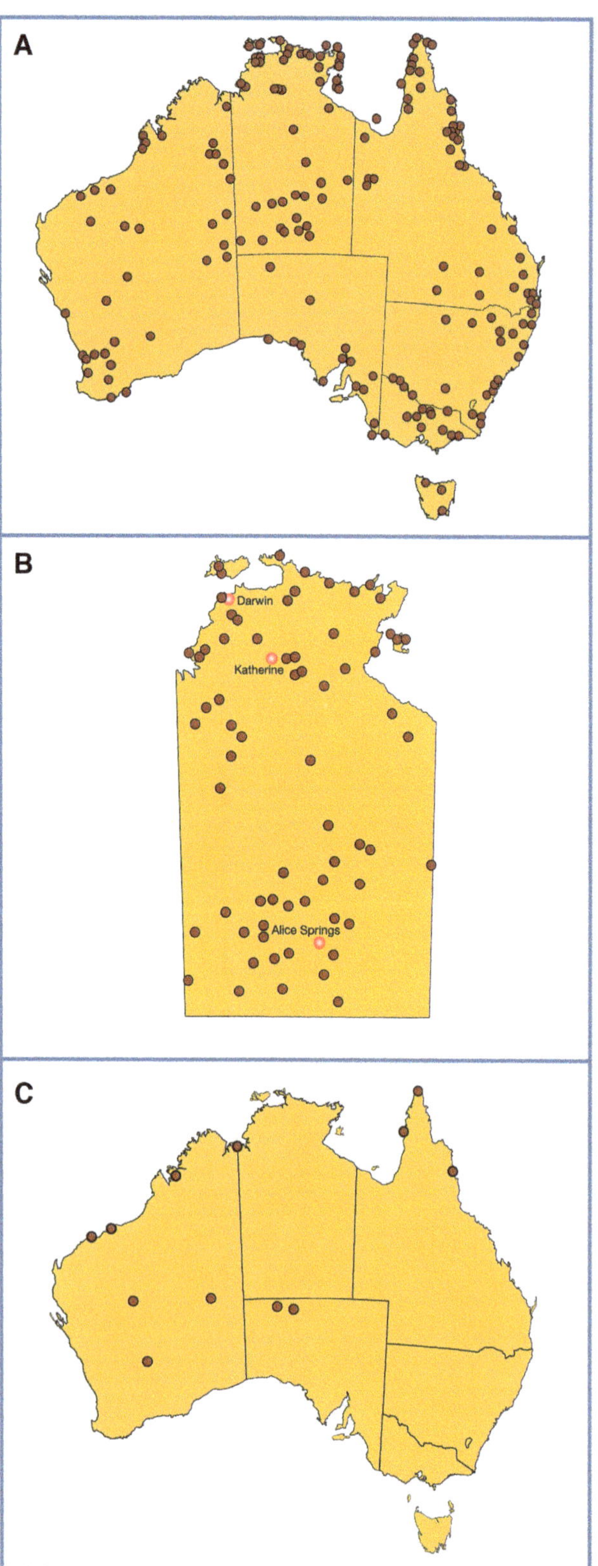


Fig. 28.1. General location of medical services participating in showcase POCT models (A) QAAMS; (B) the Northern Territory POCT Program; and (C) TTANGO.

testing (PT) procedures, with participants being able to electronically submit their results of testing.

- ongoing support services for participating sites (such as regular newsletters, website updates and telephone hotline services).
- continuous research, evaluation and quality improvement of the Program (focussed on evaluation of key performance indicators for the Program – see below) (Shephard and Gill 2010).

The training of Aboriginal Health Workers (Aboriginal people who live and work in the community and have training in primary care) as the principal POCT device operators has provided them with a strong sense of empowerment, responsibility and commitment to the Program: a role that has become highly valued and respected by the Indigenous patients they serve (Shephard 2006; Shephard *et al.* 2015a). This strategy has proven crucial to the overall acceptance of the Program in the Indigenous community setting.

The establishment of a QAAMS Indigenous Leaders Team in 2008 enabled Indigenous participants to provide strong advocacy and have a strong Indigenous voice at the national governance level of the Program (Shephard *et al.* 2015a). The QAAMS Leaders Team comprises an Aboriginal Health Worker from each state and territory who has demonstrated outstanding leadership and commitment to the Program. They meet regularly with the QAAMS Program Management Group and are active participants in regional training sessions and the QAAMS Annual Workshop.

## Results

There is a strong evidence base from continuous quality audits that the QAAMS Program is:

- *clinically effective*; a series of observational studies conducted from 2006 to 2012 show either (i) statistically significant reductions in absolute HbA1c concentration or (ii) improvements in the percentage of patients achieving glycaemic targets (HbA1c <7% [53 mmol/mol]) and a decrease in the percentage of patients with poor glycaemic control (HbA1c >10% [86 mmol/mol]) post the introduction of POCT in groups of diabetes patients both within and between different communities (Shephard *et al.* 2015b).
- *operationally effective*; an audit of 40 diabetes patients from remote Northern Territory (Spaeth *et al.* 2014) showed that, before POCT when the laboratory was used

for testing HbA1c, patients had an average of 2.7 (±1.7) HbA1c tests performed over a 15-month period and the mean turnaround time for clinical follow-up and consultation was 24 (±15) days. Post the introduction of POCT, testing frequency over the equivalent time period was 4.2 (±0.8) tests, while turnaround for follow-up and consultation was <15 min.

- *culturally effective*; the results of community-based qualitative surveys undertaken among key stakeholders, including doctors, device operators and patients with diabetes, show high levels of satisfaction with POCT (Table 28.3) (Shephard 2006; Shephard *et al.* 2015a). Doctors were confident with the accuracy and reliability of POCT results and felt that POCT contributed positively to patient care and enhanced their relationship with their patients. Operators felt being responsible for conducting POCT was culturally empowering, while POCT was effective in improving clinical outcomes and raising awareness of diabetes more broadly in the community. Patients indicated that receiving an immediate POCT result was more convenient than having to come back for a follow-up visit and that their doctor was better able to manage their diabetes by having rapid access to their results.
- *analytically sound*; the DCA 2000/Vantage devices have consistently met national laboratory and profession-derived benchmarks for analytical quality. Since 2010, there has been no statistically significant difference between the imprecision achieved by QAAMS and Australian laboratories for HbA1c, with the median imprecision for PT testing on the DCA Vantage averaging 2.45% ±0.16 for QAAMS sites and 2.34% ±0.14 for Australian laboratories (all methods) ($P = 0.08$). For quality control testing across the same 6 year period, the median imprecision for HbA1c testing has averaged 2.59% (±0.49) for the level 1 QC and 3.04% (±0.46) for the level 2 QC used in the Program. The desired imprecision goal for HbA1c testing in Australia (for both laboratory and POCT methods) is a CV% ≤3%.
- *cost-effective and sustainable*; the provision of government rebates for POCT HbA1c and urine ACR, which reimburse for the cost of testing cartridges for participating services, has ensured the Program is cost neutral for services. In October 2015, the Australian Government approved a rebate for the use of HbA1c for diagnosis of diabetes in QAAMS. These three POCT rebates are only available through the QAAMS Program.

Table 28.3 summarises the satisfaction with pathology services before and after POCT was introduced to the services in QAAMS (and the Northern Territory POCT programs). There was a statistically significant increase in satisfaction levels post POCT for both programs ($P < 0.05$, Fischers exact chi-square test).

The Australian Government has commissioned two independent evaluations of the QAAMS Program. Their most recent evaluation concluded 'All sources of evidence suggest the QAAMS Program is meeting best practice standards in the areas of Indigenous healthcare, diabetes management and point of care testing' and 'QAAMS is one of the few programs to successfully navigate the cultural complexities and potential pitfalls of chronic disease management in Indigenous communities' (Campbell

**Table 28.3.** Satisfaction with pathology services before (when the laboratory was used) and after the introduction of POCT

| Program | Stakeholder | POC test | Satisfaction | Unsatisfied (%) | Unsure (%) | Satisfied (%) | n |
|---|---|---|---|---|---|---|---|
| QAAMS | Operators | HbA1c | Before POCT | 30 | 28 | 42 | 57 |
| | | | After POCT | 4 | 7 | 90 | |
| | Patients | HbA1c | Before POCT | 11 | 28 | 61 | 159 |
| | | | After POCT | 3 | 6 | 91 | |
| NT POCT | Operators | Electrolytes | Before POCT | 34 | 13 | 54 | 24 |
| | | | After POCT | 0 | 4 | 96 | |
| | Operators | Troponin | Before POCT | 52 | 18 | 31 | 23 |
| | | | After POCT | 0 | 4 | 96 | |
| | Operators | INR | Before POCT | 42 | 12 | 46 | 24 |
| | | | After POCT | 0 | 0 | 100 | |

Research and Consulting 2008). In 2013, the QAAMS Program was the recipient of an international award called 'Projects that Work'. The award recognised sustained excellence in regional and community-based health care and was presented by the Foundation for the Advancement of International Medical Education and Research (FAIMER).

### Transferability

Since 2011, the foundation elements of QAAMS have been translated to an international POCT model for diabetes management called ACE ('Analytical and Clinical Excellence'). The ACE Program has commenced in 35 rural and remote primary care services in Canada, South Africa, East Timor, Papua New Guinea, Western Samoa, Solomon Islands and Thailand (Motta and Shephard 2015). Like QAAMS, ACE has a strong emphasis on community engagement and empowerment. High levels of poor glycaemic control were initially identified across all countries, with between 25 and 38% of patients tested having an HbA1c ≥10.5% (91 mmol/mol). In countries where this test was not available before POCT being introduced, such as East Timor, HbA1c testing has also been used for prevalence estimates and for diagnosis of patients with diabetes. Of 283 patients being assessed for cataract surgery at the National Eye Centre in Dili, Timor-Leste, 27 (10%) were newly diagnosed with diabetes and had a mean HbA1c of 9.7% (83 mmol/mol) (Dawkins *et al.* 2015).

## THE NORTHERN TERRITORY POCT PROGRAM FOR ACUTE CARE

### Background

The Northern Territory of Australia is a land of spectacular ancient landscapes and remarkable cultural and biological diversity, but it is a very remote and harsh environment. Government health services in the Territory are provided through remote health centres, which service local communities comprising mainly Indigenous people and which are located between 100 and 700 km from the nearest tertiary hospital. Aboriginal people may also access health services in the Territory through Aboriginal Community Controlled Health Services (ACCHS), which are managed by boards comprising local Indigenous community members. ACCHS provide leadership in exercising self-determination, taking active responsibility for improving Aboriginal and Torres Strait Islander health, and setting the frameworks to underpin the shift to healthy or well communities (Panaretto *et al.* 2014).

In 2007, a review of pathology services in the Territory showed that, in the Top End (the Territory's tropical north), only 10 out of 28 remote health centres had daily access to pathology, while in Central Australia (a mainly desert environment), almost no remote health centres had daily access to pathology services. This led the Northern Territory Government to investigate POCT as a potential solution to tackle poor access to pathology services. The Northern Territory POCT Program commenced in 2008 and initially involved 33 remote health centres (Shephard *et al.* 2012) allowing POCT for acute and chronic conditions to be conducted safely for patient care. All centres were equipped with an Abbott i-STAT® POCT device, which measured electrolytes, urea, creatinine, glucose and haemoglobin (the last calculated from the haematocrit) (on the Chem 8+ cartridge type), blood gases and lactate (CG4+), cardiac troponin I and international normalised ratio, according to defined clinical protocols. In mid-2015, the Program was expanded Territory-wide to include 72 remote health centres and ACCHS (Fig. 28.1B).

### Program design

The Program is overseen by a POCT Management Committee comprising representatives from the Flinders University International Centre for Point-of-Care Testing (Chair and POCT Coordinator), the NT Government's Remote Health Branch (District Medical Officer, Regional POCT Supervisors from Central Australia and the Top End, representatives from the Remote Health Quality and Safety Team and Regional District Managers) and a medical officer from Aboriginal Medical Services Alliance NT (AMSANT), the peak body representing the ACCHS sector in the Territory.

Flexible training options have been developed to deal with issues associated with the high level of staff turnover and the remote location of health service staff. These include: face-to-face onsite training sessions; centrally/regionally located training workshops; weekly training sessions via GoToMeeting teleconferencing; and self-directed learning using a variety of targeted training resources, including a training manual, DVD and step-by-step poster guides. GoToMeeting (www.gotomeeting.com.au) allows the POCT Coordinator and participants to dial in to a training session and for participants to view a PowerPoint presentation of training over the internet,

**Table 28.4.** Between-site imprecision for quality control testing on the i-STAT in the Northern Territory POCT Program during 2015

| Analyte | Number of analyses | Analyte concentration | Unit | Imprecision (CV%) observed | Goal (CV%) by laboratories[a] |
|---|---|---|---|---|---|
| Sodium | 129 | 122 | mmol/L | 0.5 | 0.6 |
| Potassium | 111 | 6.1 | mmol/L | 1.1 | 1.3 |
| Urea | 129 | 19.9 | mmol/L | 1.8 | 3.4 |
| Creatinine | 129 | 350 | µmol/L | 2.4 | 4.8 |
| Glucose | 126 | 15.2 | mmol/L | 0.9 | 2.5 |
| pH | 121 | 7.07 | n/a | 0.18 | 1.6 |
| Lactate | 121 | 7.1 | mmol/L | 1.6 | 5.0 |
| Troponin I | 48 | 0.5 | ng/mL | 6.6 | 6.4[b] |

[a]Median imprecision achieved by laboratories in the RCPA Blood gas and Co-oximetry Quality Assurance Program, cycle 56, 2015
[b]Median imprecision achieved by sites in the RCPA POCT Troponin I Quality Assurance Program, cycle 14, 2015

listen to the Coordinator deliver the presentation and ask questions during the session. This training format has proven popular among participants, with multiple sites being able to link in to a single training session.

In addition to quality testing procedures, all sites are required to perform weekly electronic QC (simulator) checks on the i-STAT device.

POCT feedback reports to health centre managers were introduced in 2010 to provide a monthly overview of i-STAT testing performed at each service in the Program. The feedback reports highlight the following statistics across the previous month: cartridge usage, individual operator usage of the i-STAT, common errors and participation rates in quality testing. This information assists managers in ordering stock, identifying additional staff training requirements and ensuring quality testing is completed on time.

A set of agreed research outcomes have been developed to assess and validate the operational and clinical effectiveness, as well as the analytical safety, of POCT in remote NT health centres.

## Results

The volume of i-STAT patient testing has continued to rise steadily across each year of the program, from 1754 tests in year 1 to 10 181 tests in year 7. Almost 50 000 tests have been performed since the Program commenced. INR testing has been the most commonly performed patient test (42% of total testing), followed by Chem8+ tests (29%), Troponin I (20%) and CG4+ tests (9%).

Since the Program commenced, 917 remote health staff (Aboriginal health practitioners, remote area nurses and doctors) have been trained as POCT operators (including 142 new operators during 2015).

Analytical quality for i-STAT POCT has consistently met profession-based analytical goals and/or state-of-the art laboratory performance (Shephard *et al.* 2014, 2015b). Between-site imprecision observed during 2015 for selected analytes and lot numbers of quality control material with the highest number of repeated analyses are shown in Table 28.4.

Satisfaction with POCT in the Northern Territory Program was validated using qualitative surveys of device operators in the Program's first year. The percentage of respondents ($n$ = 39) who were satisfied with their pathology service increased (depending on the test concerned) from between 29% and 54% when the laboratory was used to between 84% and 100% after the i-STAT was introduced ($P$ <0.001, Fishers exact chi-square test). When asked in what ways POCT had improved pathology service delivery at their remote health centre, 95% of respondents stated that it was more convenient than the laboratory service and 84% believed it had assisted in the stabilisation of acutely ill patients (Shephard *et al.* 2012).

In terms of clinical effectiveness, the ability to make an informed on-site clinical decision on acutely ill patients as to whether they could be stabilised *in situ* or required a medical evacuation to a tertiary hospital has been crucial in improving both clinical (and operational) outcomes. An illustrative case study is presented below.

## Case study

A young mother presented to a remote health clinic with a 22-month-old child who had a 24-h history of vomiting and diarrhoea and a fever of 38.5°C. Another family member of her household had recently been treated for rotavirus. A stool sample was sent to the nearest microbiology laboratory (900 km away) for investigation of the presence of rotavirus. The child was treated initially with paracetamol and his temperature fell to 37.3°C. The treating clinician advised the mother to return with the child the next day for review or earlier if the patient's condition deteriorated. The mother returned to the clinic several hours later because the child had a temperature of 40.1°C. The District Medical Officer was consulted by phone and he recommended that further paracetamol be given and the patient's electrolytes be measured on the i-STAT; a normal sodium but a low potassium of 2.4 mmol/L (paediatric reference interval 3.5–5.0 mmol/L) was recorded. The patient then experienced a further two episodes of diarrhoea, after which the child was prescribed oral rehydration solution (ORS). Over the next day, the child was given oral potassium and potassium levels were measured regularly on the i-STAT and titrated back to normal. The patient regained muscle turgor, resumed eating and drinking well, and the fever resolved. The microbiology results were received at the clinic 2 days later and were negative for rotavirus, highlighting the long turnaround time for results from the central laboratory to this remote centre. This case highlights the ability of the i-STAT to assist in the stabilisation of an acutely ill paediatric patient on-site and an evacuation from a remote region was avoided, allowing the patient and the family to remain in the community.

### Cost-effectiveness

An initial assessment of the cost effectiveness of the NT POCT Program was undertaken from July 2011 to June 2012; this preliminary study found that the evacuations of 80 patients were prevented specifically due to the availability of the on-site i-STAT results (equating to a cost saving of A$640 000, based on an average evacuation cost of A$8000). A detailed cost-effectiveness study is currently being undertaken across 2015/16 at six remote health centres through an Emergency Medicine Foundation grant.

### Summary

The NT POCT Program has demonstrated that POCT has been operationally and clinically effective and well accepted by remote health service staff. Immediate pathology results by POCT deliver significant real-time benefits that include optimising patient safety and quality of care when stabilising a patient (either before an evacuation or allowing the patient to remain and be treated in the community), reducing the number of unnecessary medical retrievals and contributing to significant cost savings.

## THE TTANGO TRIAL FOR POC CHLAMYDIA AND GONORRHOEA TESTING

### Background

At any given time, just under half of young people aged 16–19 years in many remote Aboriginal communities have a curable sexually transmissible infection (STI) (Guy *et al.* 2015), with infection rates being considerably higher than those among non-Indigenous young people (Kirby Institute 2015). As described in Chapter 17, due to the distance from laboratories, many people are lost to follow-up before receiving treatment or treatment is considerably delayed. The Test Treat And Go (TTANGO) trial (Guy *et al.* 2013) was designed to comprehensively evaluate the clinical effectiveness, cost-effectiveness, feasibility and acceptability of the GeneXpert® (Cepheid, USA) for POCT of chlamydia (CT) and gonorrhoea (NG) in primary health services. The TTANGO trial itself represents the first use globally of the GeneXpert in the hands of clinical staff in the primary health-care setting for routine STI management. The TTANGO trial results will provide evidence to support the programmatic implementation of this technology in settings in Australia where STI infection rates are highest.

### Study design

TTANGO was a crossover cluster-randomised controlled trial, led by the Kirby Institute (UNSW Australia) and conducted in collaboration with Aboriginal community controlled and government-run health services seeing predominantly Aboriginal people in remote Australia. In consultation with government and ACCHSs, 12 primary care health services were invited to participate and enrolled in the TTANGO trial, with eight classified as being located in very remote areas, two in remote and two in outer regional areas. The health services are from five geographical regions across Australia (Fig. 28.1C).

During the trial, participating services conducted clinical management of CT and NG infections under two alternative modalities/phases sequentially – 'Standard Practice phase' or 'POC phase'. Health services were randomised to commence with one of these phases then shift to the alternate phase after 12 months.

During the Standard Practice phase, health services maintained routine STI testing and management practices involving syndromic management, and sending off specimens (swabs and/or urine) to laboratories for routine nucleic acid amplification tests (NAATs), with treatment and management of asymptomatic infections based on the results that were received from the laboratory. The NAATs commonly used at the laboratories were the Roche Cobas and the Gen Probe Aptima.

During the POC phase, health services continued routine STI testing and management practices (syndromic management, and sending off specimens to laboratories for routine NAATs) but supplemented their activity with CT and NG POCT using the GeneXpert and using the POC test result to guide treatment and management at the time of initial consultation. GeneXpert testing was conducted by health service staff according to manufacturer recommendations using either 1 mL of urine or a swab specimen (the same specimen as sent to the laboratory).

GeneXpert devices, test cartridges and specimen collection kits were supplied to the participating health services free of charge for the duration of the TTANGO trial. The GeneXpert test is a molecular-based test platform suited for use at the point of care (see Chapter 17 for further details). Results generated by the GeneXpert at the conclusion of testing for each specimen (taking ~90 min) are reported separately for CT and NG and also include information relating to test cycle thresholds, sample adequacy and test running time. Any specimen generating an error result was re-tested where sufficient specimen volume remained. Errors were investigated by study coordinators to identify possible causes.

Study coordinators delivered standardised training to nominated clinical staff (Aboriginal health workers/practitioners, nurses, doctors) at each participating health service. Training was conducted in-person over 1 or 2 days on-site and included: instruction on the TTANGO protocol, trial and results documentation and data collection; performing the GeneXpert test, maintenance of the device and quality testing processes; and concluded with an assessment of competency for those staff designated to be responsible to perform the test at the service ('operators'). Staff received a competency certificate valid for 2 years if successful. Health services were provided with a training manual and briefer wall charts that covered the key procedural steps. On-line refresher training was also available. Study coordinators monitored POCT remotely (test numbers and results, including errors) and made regular visits to services (approximately every 6 months) to discuss STI testing reports generated from data collected during TTANGO and encourage best practice STI management at the service.

As part of TTANGO, all participating services were enrolled in an external PT program supported by the National Serology Reference Laboratory (NRL) Australia. QC was monitored monthly with services performing the GeneXpert test using positive CT and NG specimens supplied by The University of Queensland.

The TTANGO study protocol was approved by five ethics committees from participating jurisdictions.

## Preliminary results

The TTANGO trial implementation was completed at the end of 2015, with available preliminary results described below.

*Stakeholder acceptability:* The potential impact on clinical practices was explored through in-depth qualitative interviews with stakeholders in the early stages of TTANGO (see Table 17.5).

- Participants believed that: POCT could reduce the time to treatment and infectious period and expedite partner notification, improve testing coverage and result in more targeted prescribing, thereby minimising the risk of antibiotic resistance.
- Participants highlighted the need for systems to be developed to: maintain the completeness of communicable disease surveillance data given the current dependence on reporting from pathology laboratories; maintain and improve the flow of NG antibiotic sensitivity data, already compromised by the shift to nucleic acid-based testing; provide flexible training models; and ensure the quality of testing.
- Financing of POCT emerged as an important theme, with the cost of POCT equipment, consumables, quality assurance and servicing all important considerations (Natoli *et al.* 2015a).

*Staff acceptability*: This was explored with in-depth interviews and self-administered questionnaires. Most staff reported:

- The GeneXpert was both easy to use and useful in their setting.

| | | NAAT Result | | |
|---|---|---|---|---|
| | | Positive | Negative | Total |
| GeneXpert Result | Positive | 209 | 11 | 220 |
| | Negative | 3 | 2263 | 2266 |
| | Total | 212 | 2274 | 2486 |
| | **%Concordant (95%CI)** | **98.6 (95.9-99.7)** | **99.5 (99.1-99.8)** | **99.4 (99.1-99.8)** |

**Fig. 28.2.** Concordance between GeneXpert and conventional laboratory NAAT results for *Chlamydia trachomatis* (CT)

- POCT had improved STI management, resulting in more timely and targeted treatment, earlier commencement of partner notification, and reduced time and effort associated with client recall (Natoli *et al.* 2015b).

For some, challenges included the manual documentation processes and managing positive test results in a shorter time frame.

*Patient acceptability*: Surveys of patients indicated that the GeneXpert CT/NG test platform was highly acceptable to patients; 88% of patients indicated that getting their results today was the thing they liked most about the GeneXpert CT/NG test, followed by getting their medicine today, if needed (74%). Despite the result being available in 90 min, only 19% of patients disliked having to wait around for their results.

*Operational performance:* Analyses of test data to evaluate the operational performance of the GeneXpert demonstrated that the GeneXpert was highly concordant with the best alternative tests available (laboratory-based NAATs) (Figs 28.2 and 28.3). Overall concordance for CT was 99.4% (95% CI: 99.1–99.8) and for NG was 99.9% (95% CI: 99.1–100.0) (Causer *et al.* 2015). The majority of the discordant results (0.6%) identified were for CT tests ($n$ = 14), with 11 positive on GeneXpert and negative on laboratory NAAT and three negative on GeneXpert but positive on laboratory NAAT (Causer *et al.* 2015). Both discordant NG results were positive on GeneXpert but negative on the laboratory NAAT. These discordant results appeared to occur more frequently when specimens had lower organism loads at the threshold of test detection. Around 3% of the GeneXpert tests led to an error result when first run, but most returned a valid result when repeated.

*Time to treatment*: Preliminary time to treatment data suggests most patients with a positive POC test result were treated on the same day compared with previous reports in a similar setting that indicate 20% of those diagnosed with an STI do not receive treatment, and for those treated, the average time to initiation is around 3 weeks (Guy *et al.* 2012; Guy and Swan 2015; Huang *et al.* 2015).

*Clinical impact*: Analyses to evaluate infection averted, reduction in re-infection rates and cost-effectiveness will be determined during 2016.

## Next steps

In 2015, the NHMRC and Australian Government Department of Health provided funding to expand the use of the GeneXpert to a wider network of remote health

| | | NAAT Result | | |
|---|---|---|---|---|
| | | Positive | Negative | Total |
| GeneXpert Result | Positive | 145 | 2 | 147 |
| | Negative | 0 | 2339 | 2339 |
| | Total | 145 | 2341 | 2486 |
| | **%Concordant (95%CI)** | **100 (97.5-100.0)** | **99.9 (99.7-100.0)** | **99.9 (99.7-100.0)** |

**Fig. 28.3.** Concordance between GeneXpert and conventional laboratory NAAT results for *Neisseria gonorrhea* (NG)

services where rates of STI infections are high, including those already participating in TTANGO. Key partners involved in this expanded program are government, community health organisations, the commercial developer of the technology, laboratories and other research organisations. This expanded program, known as 'TTANGO2', commenced in 2015 and is funded for 5 years. TTANGO2 is designed to support and evaluate the programmatic implementation of POCT for STI using the GeneXpert and strategies to increase STI testing across a network of ~33 primary health services in regional and remote areas over a 5-year period. A new assay for detection of *Trichomonas vaginalis* (TV) using the same GeneXpert platform will also be included, once approved by the Therapeutic Goods Administration (TGA). A formal, comprehensive evaluation of TTANGO2 will be conducted to determine the long-term uptake, sustainability and impact of STI POCT in these services and the communities they serve.

## ACKNOWLEDGEMENTS

The TTANGO Program is funded by a grant from the National Health and Medical Research Council (NHMRC). In addition to the authors of this chapter, TTANGO Investigators include: David Anderson, Steven Badman, Basil Donovan, Christopher Fairley, Belinda Hengel, John Kaldor, Lisa Natoli, David Regan, Sepehr Tabrizi, Annie Tangey, Handan Wand, James Ward, David Whiley and David Wilson.

The QAAMS Program is funded by the Australian Government's Department of Health.

## REFERENCES

Atkinson D, Murray R, Couzos S (2008) Diabetes. In *Aboriginal Primary Health Care. An Evidence-based Approach.* 3rd edn. (Eds S Couzos and R Murray) pp. 521–574. Oxford University Press, Melbourne.

Campbell Research and Consulting (2008) 'Mid-term evaluation of the Quality Assurance for Aboriginal Medical Services Program. Final report'. Department of Health and Ageing, Canberra.

Cass A, Cunningham J, Wang Z, Hoy W (2002) Regional variation in the incidence of end-stage renal disease in indigenous Australians. *The Medical Journal of Australia* **175**, 24–27.

Causer LM, Tangey A, Badman SG, Hengel B, Natoli L, Speers D, *et al.* (2015) Operational performance of a new molecular-based point-of-care test for diagnosis of *Chlamydia trachomatis* and *Neisseria gonorrhoeae* infection: concordance with conventional laboratory testing. *World STI and HIV Congress.* 13–16 September, Brisbane.

Dawkins RCH, Oliver GF, Sharma M, Pinto BM, Jeronimo B, Pereira B, *et al.* (2015) An estimation of the prevalence of diabetes mellitus and diabetic nephropathy in adults in Timor-Leste. *BMC Research Notes* **8**, 249. doi:10.1186/s13104-015-1171-3

Freemantle J, Officer K, McAullay D, Anderson I (2007) *Australian Indigenous Health – Within an International Context.* Telethon Institute for Child Health Research and Centre for Child Health, University of Western Australia, Perth, <https://www.lowitja.org.au/sites/default/files/docs/AustIndigneousHealthReport.pdf>.

Guy RJ, Swan C (2015) TTANGO (Test, Treat and Go); use of molecular point-of-care tests to detect and treat sexually transmissible infections in young Aboriginal people in remote communities. *World STI and HIV Congress.* 13–16 September, Brisbane.

Guy R, Ward JS, Smith KS, Su JY, Huang RL, Tangey A, *et al.* (2012) The impact of sexually transmissible infection programs in remote Aboriginal communities in Australia: a systematic review. *Sexual Health* **9**, 205–212. doi:10.1071/SH11074

Guy RJ, Natoli L, Ward J, Causer L, Hengel B, Whiley D, *et al.* (2013) A randomised trial of point-of-care tests for chlamydia and gonorrhoea infections in remote Aboriginal communities: Test, Treat ANd GO- the "TTANGO" trial protocol. *BMC Infectious Diseases* **13**, 485. doi:10.1186/1471-2334-13-485

Guy R, Ward J, Wand H, Rumbold A, Garton L, Hengel B, *et al.* (2015) Coinfection with *Chlamydia trachomatis, Neisseria gonorrhoeae* and *Trichomonas vaginalis*: a cross-sectional analysis of positivity and risk factors in remote Australian Aboriginal communities. *Sexually Transmitted Infections* **91**, 201–206. doi:10.1136/sextrans-2014-051535

Huang R, Ward J, Tangey A, Causer L, Guy R and on behalf of the TTANGO investigators (2015) New molecular point-of-care test improves timeliness of treatment for *Chlamydia trachomatis* (CT) and *Neisseria gonorrhoea* (NG) in a remote Aboriginal health clinic. *World STI and HIV Congress.* 13–16 September, Brisbane.

International Labour Office (2015) *Global Evidence on Inequalities for Rural Health Protection. New Data on Rural Deficits in Health Coverage for 174 Countries.* International Labour Office, Social Protection Department, Geneva, Switzerland.

Kelly K, Dade Smith J (2007) What and where is rural and remote Australia? In *Australia's Rural and Remote Health: A Social Justice Perspective.* 2nd edn. (Ed. J Dade Smith) pp. 86–106. Tertiary Press, Melbourne.

Kirby Institute (2012) 'Bloodborne viral and sexually transmitted infections in Aboriginal and Torres Strait Islander People. Surveillance and Evaluation Report 2012'. Kirby Institute, Sydney.

Kirby Institute (2015) 'Bloodborne viral and sexually transmissible infections in Aboriginal and Torres Strait Islander people: Annual Surveillance Report 2015'. Kirby Institute, Sydney.

Mitrou F, Cooke M, Lawrence D, Povah D, Mobilia E, Guimond E (2014) Gaps in Indigenous disadvantage not closing: a census cohort study of social determinants of health in Australia, Canada and New Zealand from 1981–2006. *BMC Public Health* **14**, 201. doi:10.1186/1471-2458-14-201

Motta L, Shephard M (2015) The international ACE Program – Point-of-care testing for diabetes management. *Point of Care* **14**, 76–80. doi:10.1097/POC.0000000000000053

NACCHO (National Aboriginal Community Controlled Health Organisation) and Oxfam Australia (2007) *Closing the Gap. Solutions to the Indigenous Health Crisis Facing Australia*. NACCHO, Melbourne.

Natoli L, Guy RJ, Shephard M, Whiley D, Tabrizi SN, Ward J, *et al.* (2015a) Public health implications of molecular point-of-care testing for chlamydia and gonorrhoea in remote primary care services in Australia: a qualitative study. *BMJ Open* **5**, e006922. doi:10.1136/bmjopen-2014-006922

Natoli L, Guy RJ, Shephard M, Causer L, Badman SG, Hengel B, *et al.* (2015b) "I Do Feel Like a Scientist at Times": a qualitative study of the acceptability of molecular point-of-care testing for Chlamydia and Gonorrhoea to primary care professionals in a remote high STI burden setting. *PLoS One* **10**, e0145993. doi:10.1371/journal.pone.0145993

Panaretto KS, Wenitong M, Button S, Ring IT (2014) Aboriginal community controlled health services: leading the way in primary care. *The Medical Journal of Australia* **200**, 649–652. doi:10.5694/mja13.00005

SAHMRI (South Australian Health and Medical Research Institute)/Wardliparingga Aboriginal Research Unit (2014) *South Australian Aboriginal Health Research Accord Companion Document*. SAHMRI, Adelaide.

Shephard MD (2006) Cultural and clinical effectiveness of the 'QAAMS' point-of-care testing model for diabetes management in Australian Aboriginal medical services. *The Clinical Biochemist Reviews* **27**, 161–170.

Shephard MDS, Gill JP (2010) The National QAAMS program. *The Clinical Biochemist Reviews* **31**, 95–99.

Shephard M, Spaeth B, Mazzachi B, Auld M, Schatz S, Loudon J, *et al.* (2012) Design, implementation and initial assessment of the Northern Territory Point-of-Care Testing Program. *The Australian Journal of Rural Health* **20**, 16–21. doi:10.1111/j.1440-1584.2011.01243.x

Shephard M, Spaeth B, Auld M, Schatz M, Lingwood A, Loudon J, *et al.* (2014) Towards sustainable point-of-care testing in remote Australia – the Northern Territory i-STAT point-of-care testing program. *Point of Care* **13**, 6–11. doi:10.1097/POC.0000000000000009

Shephard M, O'Brien C, Burgoyne A, Croft J, Garlett T, Barancek K, *et al.* (2015a) A review of the cultural safety of a national indigenous point-of-care testing program for diabetes management. *Australian Journal of Primary Health* **9**, (September). doi:10.1071.PY15050

Shephard M, Spaeth B, Motta L, Shephard A (2015b) Point-of-care testing in Australia: practical advantages and benefits of community resiliency for improving outcomes. In *Global Point-of-Care – Strategies for Disasters, Emergencies, and Public Health Resilience*. (Eds G Kost and C Curtis) pp. 527-535. AACC Press, Washington DC, USA.

Simmons D, Hsu-Hage B (2002) Determinants of health, disease and disability: differences between country and city. In *The New Rural Health*. (Eds D Wilkinson D and I Blue) pp. 79–93. Oxford University Press, South Melbourne.

Spaeth BA, Shephard MDS, Schatz S (2014) Point-of-care testing for haemoglobin A1c in remote Australian Indigenous communities improves timeliness of diabetes care. *Rural and Remote Health* **14**, 2849, <http://www.rrh.org.au/articles/subviewnew.asp?ArticleID=2849>.

Strasser R (2003) Rural health around the world: challenges and solutions. *Family Practice* **20**, 457–463. doi:10.1093/fampra/cmg422

# 29 Point-of-care testing in the hospital setting

*Geoff Herd and Samarina MA Musaad*

**Summary**

Point-of-care testing (POCT) is an essential component of laboratory testing in modern hospitals. It is not only surviving but flourishing in an era when patient-centred care is a focal point for health-care delivery and more care is devolved to the community. POCT is capable of reducing emergency department (ED) overcrowding, accelerating management, reducing hospital admissions, supporting appropriate treatment plans, and assisting and extending laboratory testing within the hospital. For successful implementation there needs to be a culture within hospitals that prioritises quality, an attitude that spotlights the patient, education on intricacies of POCT and managerial support.

## INTRODUCTION

### An overview of point-of-care testing in the hospital setting from a global perspective

POCT is now widespread throughout hospitals where testing sites include intensive care units (ICUs), coronary care units (CCUs), emergency departments (EDs), high dependency units, special care baby units, maternity assessment units (MAUs), operating theatres (ORs), speciality clinics and wards such as haematology or burns units, and even hospitals' central laboratories. Different settings have different needs and accordingly tailored processes. Advances in information technology (IT) have revolutionised POCT. Wireless technology means wherever the patient is in a hospital, a POC test can be performed. POCT in hospitals was historically siloed (typically involving a patient–doctor encounter with basic documentation and not part of a standard management plan), whereas now it is integrated into clinical pathways. Furthermore, although POC tests in the hospital environment were previously performed mainly by hospital laboratory scientists, they are now ubiquitous with many health professionals being primary users.

As patient-centred care and safety become even more at the forefront, POCT has assumed vital importance in hospitals. Examples include, but are not limited to, rule-in or rule-out conditions in EDs, such as natriuretic polypeptides and cardiac troponins (cTn) for heart failure and acute coronary syndromes (ACS), respectively, assessment of renal dysfunction by measuring creatinine before using radio-contrast media and prediction of foetal distress in delivery suites by measuring foetal scalp lactate. This trend has been paralleled by commercial growth of the available POCT devices in the last decade (Huckle 2006; Nichols 2005; Price and Kricka 2007).

All POCT services in hospitals should ideally be under laboratory supervision and be governed and supported by a POCT committee with representation and accountability from all stakeholders. Quality should be comparable to that of an accredited laboratory in context of the POC test being fit for clinical purpose.

A global trend towards a reduction in health-care budgets means that there should be a strong evidence-base for introducing new testing modalities and economic benefit aligned with improved patient outcomes. Management styles have evolved to parallel the above trends and health funders and managers have become more accepting of the role POCT can potentially play in achieving goals, key performance indicators and clinical targets.

In developed nations, POCT in hospitals supports clinical pathways for both acute and chronic conditions, is used to reduce overcrowding in EDs, to reduce length of stay (LOS) in the hospital or ICU, to reduce operating time in ORs and to support maternity services. It rarely replaces traditional laboratory testing because the latter can meet most relevant turnaround times (TAT) and is done in a rigorously quality controlled environment with expert oversight; in this context POCT becomes an extension of laboratory medicine. In contrast in remote, under resourced and/or underdeveloped populations POCT can be the sole provider for laboratory testing. Reasons include lack of infrastructure, inadequate water supply, unreliable electrical supply, and building facilities that are inadequate to house large analysers.

Globalisation has resulted in faster and easier movement of large numbers of humans and pathogens across geographical and political boundaries. This can lead to rapid spread of diseases in rapidly developing pandemics. The recent Ebola outbreak, for example, has seen major hospitals in many countries, including New Zealand, use POCT as a tool to manage potential cases (MoH 2015). Hospitals were prepared with isolation wards, equipped with POCT devices for diagnosis and management of people with or suspected to have the disease.

Changes to health-care delivery internationally have led to increased centralisation of services and consolidation of laboratories in developed countries, mainly to manage health budgets and resources better. At the same time, there is a focus on patient-centric care and a seemingly paradoxical trend towards decreased hospital-based care, which is a critical driver for hospital POCT. POCT is expanding in scope and scale in countries such as Germany and the Netherlands. In Italy, POCT is mostly administered in hospitals. Driven by geographical barriers and the remoteness of some populations, community POCT is on the rise in Australia and Canada.

With the current global trends, it is not possible to foresee a future without well-established POCT systems in hospitals all around the world.

## THE MAIN CLINICAL NEEDS/ PRESENTATIONS SEEN IN THE HOSPITAL SETTING AND NEEDS FOR POINT-OF-CARE TESTING

Table 29.1 and Fig. 29.1 show a snapshot of POC tests used in hospitals, the clinical condition/s for which the tests are requested, common sites in hospitals and types of hospitals that usually provide the service. This list of POC tests is not exhaustive, but is designed to illustrate the routine scope and scale of POC testing in multi-speciality metropolitan and remote or rural hospitals.

The range of POC technologies used within different types of hospitals encompasses many devices and common laboratory tests such as blood gases, electrolytes, urinalysis and glucose. However, some POC tests, such as toxicology and cardiac markers, are more likely to be available in a remote hospital ED because of lack of on-site laboratory services and to inform patient transfers to tertiary hospitals. In both metropolitan and rural hospitals, POC devices may also be used as back-up devices to provide a limited range of tests when a laboratory analyser is unavailable or being serviced. Hospitals can also be responsible for administering, supervising and providing oversight to POCT community programs; for example, the Community Pharmacy Anticoagulant Management Service (CPAMS) in New Zealand (described in Chapters 13 and 34).

## BENEFITS AND RISKS OF IMPLEMENTING POINT-OF-CARE TESTING IN HOSPITALS

POCT in hospitals is underpinned by the speed of result availability. When embedded within a clear process or clinical pathway and well governed, POCT can shorten the patient's journey, from presentation to discharge, and render it more clinically and cost-effective.

However, as shown in Fig. 29.2, there are risks and benefits with POCT in hospitals and the clinical and operational factors and advantages overlap, such as a shortened decision cycle time in turn reduces LOS, which ultimately benefits the patient.

From the patient's and the hospital's perspective, the goal is to assess patients in a timely fashion in ED (or any other ward/department that receives acute patients) and to facilitate discharging the patient to the relevant department, ward or home. The sheer number of

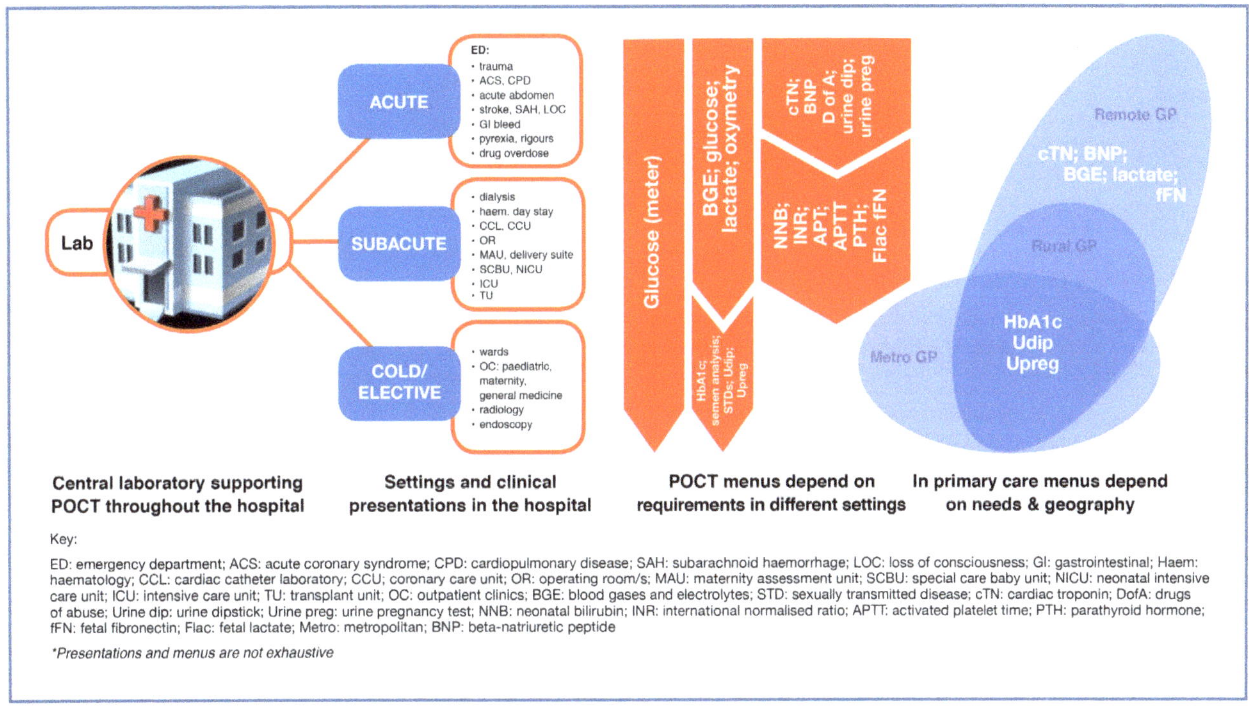


**Fig. 29.1.** The scope and scale of POCT in today's hospitals.

inpatients and patients presenting to ED in a hospital can be substantial. Testing samples from all these patients can overwhelm the central laboratory in terms of meeting turnaround times, staffing and testing capacity. By providing POCT that is supervised by the laboratory in relevant departments and wards, POC testing can support the central laboratory and help mitigate delays in testing that ultimately advantage the patient.

Rural or remote hospitals have limited services and are a long distance from tertiary care centres and speciality units. By providing the result for a critical analyte such as cTn at the POC, a decision to transport the patient for specialised treatment can be made with confidence. This prevents unnecessary transfers, which can inconvenience the patient, and reduces associated costs. (A description of the successful implementation of

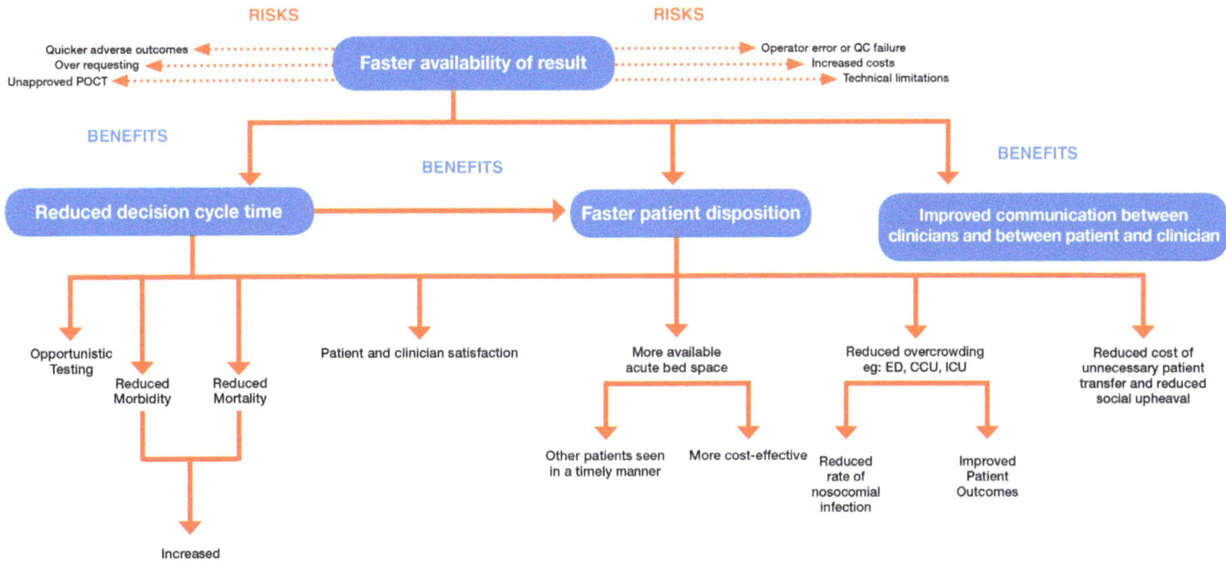


**Fig. 29.2.** Risks and benefits with POCT in hospitals.

**Table 29.1.** The scope and scale of POCT in the modern-day hospital setting

| Tests/assays[a] | Clinical use/presentation[b] | Hospital site/s[c] | Type of hospital[d] |
|---|---|---|---|
| **General** | | | |
| cTn | Rule in ACS, baseline in dialysis patients | ED, CCU, DU, CCL | M/R |
| BNP | Rule in heart failure | ED, cardiology OPC | M |
| | Rule in cardio-embolic stroke | ED | |
| Electrolytes | Shock, LOC, delirium | ED, ICU, DU, NICU, SCBU, TU, BCU/IW | M/R |
| Ionised calcium | Seizures, tetanus | ED, OR, DU | M |
| Full blood count | Shock, sepsis, blood loss, all patient requests when main analyser is being serviced (back-up) | ED, OR, haematology day stay, CCL, NICU, SCBU, CL, BCU/IW, mental health units for patients on clozapine | M/R |
| Co-oximetry | Blood loss, anaemia, polycythaemia, cyanosis, carbon-monoxide (CO) poisoning | ED, OR, ICU | M/R |
| Lactate-adult/ paediatric | Sepsis, shock, trauma, metabolic acidosis | ED, OR | M/R |
| $sO_2$ | Monitoring oxygen therapy | ED, OR, ICU | M/R |
| Pro-calcitonin | Sepsis | ED (especially paediatric) | M |
| CRP | Sepsis | ED (especially paediatric) | M/R |
| Creatinine | Renal impairment, CKD, back-up, prevention of contrast induced nephropathy | OR, radiology, ED, DU, CL, BCU/IW | M/R |
| Faecal occult blood | GI bleeding | ED, wards, colonoscopy and OPCs | M/R |
| Urine dipstick | UTI, sepsis, PIH | ED, obstetric OPC, wards | M/R |
| Urine and whole blood pregnancy | Exclude pregnancy (intrauterine/ectopic) | ED, radiology, wards | M/R |
| Urine specific gravity | Paediatric: metabolic /endocrine disorders | Wards, OPCs | M |
| **Obstetrics and neonatal** | | | |
| fFN | Symptomatic of PTL | MAU, ED, obstetric ward | M/R |
| Lactate-neonate | Foetal distress | DS | M/R |
| Total bilirubin (transcutaneous-spectrophotometric) | Neonatal hyperbilirubinaemia | NICU, post-natal ward | M/R |
| pH (strips) | NG feeding | SCBU | M |
| Glucose | Neonatal hypoglycaemia | NICU, SCBU, post-natal ward | M/R |
| **Coagulation** | | | |
| PT/INR | Monitoring warfarin therapy | ED, haematology day stay, haematology anticoagulation clinic, endoscopy unit, BCU/IW | M/R |
| | Used pre-operatively to check that patients have stopped warfarin before surgery | | M |
| APTT | Possibility of bleeding | OR, DU, TU | M |
| | Stroke | ED, radiology | |
| D-dimer | VTE, PE | ED, OR | M/R |
| TEG | Haemorrhage, coagulopathy, cardiac and hepatic surgery | ED, OR | M |
| ACT | Heparinisation | OR (cardiac surgery) | M |
| Platelet function PFA | Patients on aspirin and clopidogrel (Personalised antiplatelet therapy) | OR (cardiac surgery) | M |

| Tests/assays[a] | Clinical use/presentation[b] | Hospital site/s[c] | Type of hospital[d] |
|---|---|---|---|
| **Metabolic** | | | |
| Glucose | LOC, delirium, DKA, GDM | ED, OPC, DU, TU, BCU/IW, MAU | M/R |
| Urine ketones | DKA | ED | M/R |
| Beta-hydroxy butyrate | DKA | ED | M/R |
| Urea | Shock, LOC, delirium, pyrexia, acute abdomen, acute GI bleeding | ED, DU, BCU/IW | M/R |
| Amylase/lipase | Acute abdomen, back-up | ED | R |
| Liver function (e.g. enzymes, protein, albumin, bilirubin) | Shock, LOC, delirium, pyrexia, acute abdomen, back-up | ED, TU, CL, BCU/IW | M/R |
| Total $CO_2$ | Metabolic acidosis/alkalosis | ED | M |
| Blood gases and pH | Shock, LOC, delirium, pyrexia, RTA, trauma, ACS, CPD, back-up | ED, OR, ICU, CCU, CCL, CL, BCU/IW | M/R |
| Drugs of abuse | Drug overdose, LOC, addict | ED, detoxification units | M |
| Parathyroid hormone | Parathyroid surgery | OR | M |
| **Infection** | | | |
| Sexually transmitted diseases | High risk, symptomatic | OPC and Sexual Health Clinic | M/R |
| HIV and HCV | Suspected infection | ED, wards, AAW, OPC | High prevalence population, high-risk individual |
| Malaria | Symptomatic | ED, OPC | Endemic areas |
| Influenza | Symptomatic | ED, AAW | M: High-risk individuals |
| Pneumococcal | Symptomatic | ED, AAW | M: High-risk individuals |
| RSV | Symptomatic | ED, AAW | M: High-risk individuals |
| Urease | Gastric ulcer/gastritis (gastric biopsy to test for *Helicobacter pylori)* | Endoscopy units | M |
| **Other** | | | |
| Semen analysis | Fertility assessment | Fertility clinics | M |
| HbA1c | Diabetic patients or diabetes in pregnancy | Diabetes OPCs | M/R |
| Urine protein or albumin:creatinine ratio | Diabetic patients or diabetes in pregnancy | Diabetes OPCs | |
| Blood grouping | 'Bedside' blood grouping is performed before transfusion in France and Germany | | |

[a]Tests/assays: HIV: human immunodeficiency virus; HCV: hepatitis C virus; RSV: respiratory syncytial virus; BNP: b-type natriuretic peptide; TEG: thromboelastography; fFN: foetal fibronectin; $sO_2$: oxygen saturation

[b]Clinical use/presentation: ACS: acute coronary syndrome; DKA: diabetic ketoacidosis; LOC: loss of consciousness; PTL: preterm labour; VTE: venous thromboembolism; PE: pulmonary embolism; GDM: gestational diabetes mellitus; RTA: road traffic accident; CPD: cardiopulmonary disease; PIH: pregnancy-induced hypertension

[c]Hospital site/s: ED: emergency department; OR: operating theatre; CL: central laboratory; DU: dialysis unit; AAW: acute admission ward; NG: nasogastric; CCU: coronary care unit; CCL: cardiac catheterisation laboratory; OPC: outpatient clinic; ICU: intensive care unit; NICU: neonatal intensive care unit; SCBU: special care baby unit; TU: transplant unit; OR: operating theatre; MAU: maternity assessment unit; DU: delivery unit; BCU/IW: bio-containment units/isolation wards

[d]Type of hospital: M: metropolitan; R: remote or rural

POCT in a small remote hospital in New Zealand is provided later in this chapter.) Concomitantly, resources will be devoted to patients in true need who will be transferred and receive adequate management. Furthermore, in the absence of a 24/7 laboratory service, POCT provided after hours for acute admissions for essential analytes, such as cTn, BNP, electrolytes, full blood count, international normalised ratio (INR), bilirubin and CRP, can fill a gap in the service. Patients presenting outside laboratory working hours will not be disadvantaged or clinically compromised.

Opportunistic testing, long distance transfers from remote hospitals and provision of laboratory testing 24 h a day in a rural or remote area are all measures that can mitigate inequity (the unjustified and unequal provision of health care).

There are risks associated with pathology testing, and POCT is no exception. It bears the additional burden of distinctive risks purely because of its one characteristic: speed. An incorrect result available quickly can be acted upon quickly (e.g. patient discharged inappropriately or unnecessary medication administered, with adverse consequences). Recognition of risk is the first step towards mitigating it, which, in turn, is pivotal to a POCT service reaching its full potential. Continuous education and audits can help mitigate these risks. Governance using best practice guidelines and accreditation for POCT against ISO 22870:2006 is a key quality assurance element to reduce the risks associated with POCT in hospitals.

Table 29.2 summarises common barriers and limitations to implementing a successful POCT service in a hospital and recommendations for overcoming them. The key to mitigation of these issues and the hospital 'silo mentality' is *governance* and recognition of the complementary expertise of physicians, nurses, scientists, pathologists and managers to meet analytical, clinical, operational, fiscal and patient requirements.

## OVERVIEW OF THE EVIDENCE BASE FOR POINT-OF-CARE TESTING IN HOSPITALS

Availability of good clinical evidence is disproportionate to the scale, scope and rate of expansion of POCT. Barriers for conducting statistically powered randomised controlled trials (RCT), the second best source of evidence after meta-analyses in evidence-based laboratory medicine (Price 2012), include:

- limited funds.
- the need for multidisciplinary cooperation between different departments and/or health sectors and long-term follow up. Most commonly clinical outcomes for POCT are demonstrable in faster patient recovery, fewer admissions and readmissions, lower morbidity or mortality rates or reduced transmission of infectious diseases. POCT clinical outcome studies therefore need time, a large number of participants considering the varied endpoints, as well as a requirement for blinded randomisation to minimise bias.
- outcome myopia. Faster turnaround time (TAT), which is an *operational* outcome, is assumed to improve *clinical* outcome and generate savings. In the short term a faster result may, for instance, lead to less crowded EDs. However, an operational advantage at one phase of the patient's journey does not imply the same for other phases, nor does it guarantee improved clinical and fiscal outcomes.
- POCT can be viewed as 'simple' testing with no analytical limitations or caveats and minimal need for training, so why conduct potentially demanding studies?

These limitations also have an impact on cost-effectiveness studies. Operational and analytical outcome studies are therefore more common.

In the review below, we draw on selected evidence to evaluate the significance of POCT in hospitals. Some of the data has been critiqued in order to emphasise that there is no perfect study and findings always need to be taken in context of strengths and limitations of individual investigations.

Rooney and Schilling (2014) conducted a literature review on the impact of POCT on the rapidity of assessment and diagnosis of patients admitted to the ED; their premise being POCT may reduce overcrowding compared with laboratory testing. Overcrowding is associated with higher mortality rates, delays in management and reduced ED effectiveness. The authors focussed on common clinical problems, namely ACS, venous thromboembolism (VTE), severe sepsis and stroke. The POC test menus used for assessment included cTn, D-dimer, lactate, INR and activated partial thromboplastin time (APTT).

They concluded that with use of POCT:

- Fewer patients needed admission (e.g. 14% drop by introducing rapid D-dimer testing).
- Faster result TATs allowed more efficient triage and reduced delays to start treatment; for example, cTn

**Table 29.2.** Barriers, limitations and recommendations for implementing POCT in hospitals (Source: Herd and Musaad 2015)

| Barriers, challenges and limitations | Recommendations to remove or mitigate barriers and limitations |
|---|---|
| Lack of governance | Getting all stakeholders involved and setting up a POCT committee at a hospital level |
| Introduction of unapproved POCT into hospitals | All POCT needs to be approved by a governance group to avoid clinical and financial risk |
| Lack of accreditation and the use of guidelines | Providers should seek laboratory support for ISO 22870:2006 accreditation for POCT |
| Lack of connectivity (ability of devices to transmit information to other information systems) | Procurement specifications for devices need to state that devices are POCT1-A2 compliant for quality assurance where practicable |
| Staff variety and numbers | Establishing a well-defined training program allowing for continuous re-training and re-certification |
| Large scope of tests and large scale of testing | Recognition by executive teams that the scale of POCT is large and expanding and that it needs adequate support in the form of clinical and management expertise |
| | Governance and oversight by a POC Manager or Coordinator, acknowledging POCT is performed in many locations, some of which may be physically remote from the hospital |
| Overuse of POC tests | Staff education and training programs, connectivity of devices to the hospital information system, and regular audits |
| Laboratory staff perspectives: deskilling and erosion of workplace | Educating, training and job retention |
| Attitudes towards quality control and certification | Educating on risk management and presenting case studies |
| Prevalence of silo mentality and budget | Cooperating with stakeholders and underscoring the importance of including the entire patient journey |
| | Management decisions need to be taken with full appreciation of the clinical needs |
| False perception that POCT is too expensive | Promoting a cost-effective approach. Note: Some tests can be less expensive compared with laboratory assays (e.g. BNP) |
| Lack of appreciation of technical and analytical nuances of POCT and that devices are deceptively simple to use | Educating |
| | Promoting a culture of quality |
| | Establishing relations with stakeholders |
| Tests must be analytically 'fit-for-purpose'; that is, appropriate for the clinical setting in context of the population to be tested and the clinical condition/s to be considered | Careful selection of devices |
| | Ensure there is good correlation between POC and laboratory test results for a given test |
| | Seek advice from pathologists and scientists in accredited laboratories |
| Limitations of individual test methods (e.g. antibiotic interference with POC glucose, and timing for strip tests). | Careful laboratory validation of POC tests |
| | Seek advice from pathologists and scientists in accredited laboratories on performance and analytical interference with assays |
| Paucity of evidence base | Maximise benefit from available evidence |
| | Base implementation on sound defensible scientific rationale |
| | Develop systematic protocols for the clinical evaluation of devices |
| Lack of an adverse event management system (AEMS) (Musaad *et al.* 2015) | Robust training and quality management systems |
| | Early warning system for anomalous results and trends |
| | Involve stakeholders in feedback and resolution after implementation |
| | Escalation of incidents for review at clinical governance level where appropriate |

results were viewed 42 min sooner by physicians compared with results from the central laboratory; D-dimer results available 101 min earlier; lactate results 151 min sooner; and there was earlier percutaneous intervention (PCI) and earlier thrombolysis.

The authors concluded that 'POCT, when used effectively, may alleviate the negative impacts of overcrowding on the safety, effectiveness, and person-centeredness care in ED.'

The RATPAC (Randomised Assessment of Treatment using Panel Assay of Cardiac markers) trial, a multi-centre RCT with economic evaluation, was conducted in six EDs in the United Kingdom (Goodacre *et al.* 2011). The objective was to assess the effectiveness of using a POCT cardiac marker panel in patients with suspected acute myocardial infarction (AMI). The panel consisted of creatine kinase (CK-mass), myoglobin and cTnI. A total of 2243 patients were included. Thirty two per cent of patients in the POCT group were successfully discharged within 4 h of presentation, as opposed to 13% in the control group with an odds ratio (OR) adjusted for age, gender and history of coronary heart disease of 3.81 (95% CI 3.01 to 4.82, $P < 0.001$). Although the difference in mean length of initial hospital stay was not significant, 54% of the intervention (POCT) group were not admitted during follow up compared with 40% of the control group. The rate of major adverse events was not different at 3% and 2%, respectively. Cost analysis demonstrated a higher cost for the POCT group at £1217 per patient with the control group costing £1006 per patient. Mean quality-adjusted life-years (QALYs) were comparable at 0.158 and 0.161, respectively (Fitzgerald *et al.* 2011; Goodacre *et al.* 2011). POCT was deemed not cost-effective even though it supported successful and safe discharge of more patients and reduced the median, but not mean, length of hospital stay.

In an RCT in West Africa, a treat-test package including a rapid diagnostic test for all *Plasmodium* (malaria) species and a urine dipstick was used to investigate the resolution of febrile illnesses on day 7 after presentation and management at a hospital outpatient clinic (Ameyaw *et al.* 2014). Other parameters in the package were clinical examination of the ear, nose, throat and chest, and treatment with antipyretics with or without antimalarials and/or antibiotics. The study included a total of 240 children between the ages of 6 months and 12 years presenting with pyrexia.

Results of POCT were compared with central laboratory findings. All children in the control group were diagnosed with malaria or malaria plus a bacterial infection (roughly 50% each). In the intervention (POCT) group, however, 33% and 16% were diagnosed with viral and bacterial infection, respectively, 37% having been diagnosed with malaria and 14% with malaria and bacterial infection.

At initial diagnosis, none of the control group received only antibiotics or antipyretics, 51% received antimalarials only and 48.7% antimalarials and antibiotics as opposed to 16%, 33%, 37% and 14%, respectively, in the intervention group. At day 2 review, 14 children in the control group needed a change of medication, whereas only one child needed that in the intervention group. Ten per cent (12 children) from the control group remained febrile at the end of the study as opposed to 0.8% (one child) from the intervention group.

In the context of over-diagnosis of malaria, frequently encountered antibiotic and antimalarial resistance, and in an environment with limited resources, this study demonstrated how POCT can be part of a successful 'package deal' to improve clinical outcomes and tackle inappropriate prescribing in a heavily under-resourced hospital setting by modern standards.

The National Institute for Health Research (NIHR) investigated the impact of POCT and/or rapid molecular tests (RMT) on diagnosing and managing acute respiratory tract infection admissions caused by three pathogens in the elderly and high-risk individuals (Nicholson *et al.* 2014). The study was conducted in acute medical admissions units and medical wards of two teaching hospitals in the UK. A total of 1172 participants with either acute exacerbation of chronic cardiopulmonary disease or an acute cardiopulmonary illness were included and randomised to either conventional laboratory testing, POCT for influenza and pneumococcal infection, or RMT for influenza and respiratory syncytial virus (RSV). Conventional laboratory methods were viral culture, sputum culture and polymerase chain reaction (PCR). Objectives included: to compare clinical and prescribing outcomes and QALYs for the POCT patients, RMT patients and patients randomised to conventional laboratory testing; to conduct a systematic review on diagnostic accuracy of POCT for influenza; and to compare the diagnostic accuracy of PCR and POCT with culture methods.

Findings are summarised as follows:

- There was no difference in prescribing or clinical outcomes between the groups.
- PCR and POCT were not better than culture methods.
- Difference in cost-effectiveness and QALY analysis did not reach statistical significance. POCT had higher cost that was not offset by a higher gain in terms of QALYs.
- Systematic review and meta-analysis of 70 similar studies showed overall sensitivity of POCT for influenza to be 74% with a specificity of 99%. Further analysis demonstrated sensitivity for children of 86%, compared with 67% for mixed age populations.

Findings therefore did not support routine POCT or RMT for influenza, RSV or pneumococcal infection in this particular study. However, this raises the question: can these devices prove useful where laboratory culture is not an option? POCT and RMT were more expensive but simpler to use and did not cause a drop in QALYs, so the answer is probably yes.

Results from POCT are by definition available much sooner than results from conventional laboratory testing, usually within minutes. However, when conventional laboratory results take weeks to be available, 48 h result availability can indeed be considered a POCT application. Such an application of 'simulated POCT' was found to have positive clinical outcomes for HIV positive children in paediatric wards in a Malawi hospital in Africa (McCollum *et al.* 2014).

The POC test used was a rapid HIV RNA PCR test. Three hundred children with a history of exposure to HIV, all less than 12 months of age, were randomised to receive standard care using World Health Organization (WHO) algorithms and HIV DNA laboratory tests with results available in weeks (control) or rapid PCR with results available in 48 h and antiretroviral therapy (ART) initiated accordingly. All children were followed up 1 month after discharge or initiation of ART at a hospital clinic.

The rate of HIV diagnosis was similar in both groups. The difference in days for receipt of molecular test results was 30 days (32.5 for the control group versus 2.5 days for the intervention group). None of the children who tested negative with rapid PCR received ART, whereas 27% of the control group did. Seventy-two per cent of HIV positive children in the intervention group received in-hospital ART compared with 47% in the control group.

This study shows HIV rapid PCR helped access ART when needed, while preventing unnecessary exposure to ART in patients testing negative.

A Health Technology and Assessment Report described results from a series of RCTs and diagnostic accuracy studies designed to assess the clinical and analytical effectiveness and incremental cost of using rapid foetal fibronectin (fFN) on predicting preterm delivery (PTD) in patients presenting to hospitals with relevant symptoms and <37 weeks of gestation, compared with standard care when the test was not used (Deshpande *et al.* 2013). Twenty studies were included in total.

Foetal fibronectin is a matrix glycoprotein needed to 'glue' cells together. It is found in the placental decidua. When it leaks into cervicovaginal secretions in relatively large quantities, it predicts imminent delivery. The ability to predict (or exclude) imminent delivery in patients presenting to hospital with symptoms of preterm labour is valuable because it allows appropriate and timely management to mitigate foetal and maternal complications.

The study found no evidence for improved clinical outcomes and the accuracy of the fFN test was reported to be moderate, with the highest reported sensitivity of 77% for predicting PTD within 7–10 days and specificity of 85% for predicting PTD at <37 weeks. One RCT reported a reduction of 40% in length of hospital stay for patients found to be fFN negative. The ability of the test to impart savings was uncertain.

POCT for fFN was integrated in clinical pathways but failed to deliver the expected outcomes. The ability to predict PTD accurately is the holy grail of obstetric practice. When the POC fFN test first appeared in the market, there was much optimism and obstetric departments were very eager to acquire it. The reality that multiple studies, albeit across many different study designs and locations, have failed to prove significant clinical and fiscal benefit has bewildered some health professionals, yet most will not part with it. The strength of the test lies in its negative predictive value (NPV) because there are many factors that can give a false positive result (e.g. lubricants and inadequate sampling).

It is safe, however, to conclude that in most cases unless a negative fFN result secures early discharge there will be no fiscal gains. It is most likely that fFN would be very useful at reasonably excluding the possibility of PTD within a certain timeframe in remote areas, avoiding the need for costly and distant transfers to health centres and the social upheaval of an expectant mother being away from her family.

In a 76 000 patient a year ED in a tertiary teaching hospital in Foshan, China, the clinical efficacy of POCT brain natriuretic peptide (BNP) for distinguishing patients with cardio-embolic stroke (CE) from patients with stroke of a different aetiology was investigated (Wu *et al.* 2015). BNP is a protein released by cardiac muscle when it is stretched and/or damaged and, in the case of CE, stroke is associated with abnormal heart rhythm and size of the brain infarct. The rationale of this study was that, compared with other causes of stroke, BNP in CE stroke is elevated and this characteristic would help in early identification of afflicted patients, who have a higher recurrence rate for stroke and worse outcomes compared with victims of other ischaemic stroke subtypes. Early detection may lead to a critical attempt at risk modification with anticoagulation.

The study was conducted in a high prevalence population; there are nearly 2 million new stroke victims annually in China. Prospective consecutive adults with clinical acute ischaemic stroke were enrolled. Clinicians were blinded to the BNP level taken on admission and routine care was administered in accordance with the American Heart Association and American Stroke Association (AHA/ASA) Guidelines. Stratification of patients was based on the five TOAST (Trial of ORG 10172 in Acute Stroke Treatment) stroke aetiological subtypes. Based on the authors' prior work and that of others, a BNP of 66.5 pg/mL (7.8 pmol/L) correlated with CE stroke (sensitivity 75%, specificity 89%).

A total of 172 stroke patients were included of whom 45 (26.2%) were classified as having CE stroke on discharge based on standard care (clinical and neuro-radiological imaging). Based on BNP, CE was suspected in 50 (29%) patients of whom 16 were subsequently found to be false positives based on standard care. Of the 122 ruled out by BNP, 11 were reclassified as CE upon discharge (false negatives). Sensitivity and specificity of the test were 76% (95% CI: 69.13–81.99) and 87% (95% CI: 82.44–92.36), respectively. Importantly, the positive predictive value (PPV) was 68% (95% CI: 65.33–70.67) and negative predictive value (NPV) was 91% (95% CI: 86.71–92.25). Mean BNP concentration was found to be significantly higher in patients with CE stroke (176.9 ±87.1 *v.* 114.1 ±90.8 pg/mL [21 pmol/L ±10 versus 13 pmol/L ±11] for the whole cohort). Similarly, BNP was higher in the CE group compared with other stroke subtypes (176.9 *v.* 46.4, 48.1, 45.8 pg/mL in the three other subtypes, $P < 0.01$).

The significant burden that stroke poses on a health system means that a mechanism that helps focus on a critical subtype makes sense both from a patient-centred perspective and an operational perspective. This particular study demonstrated an important NPV of POC BNP testing, ruling out CE stroke with a proposed clinically viable cut-off value. Arguably, stroke would not be ruled out without appropriate clinical assessment and radiological imaging, but excluding the possibility of CE stroke with reasonable certainty would be useful in facilitating patient flow through busy ED departments and streamlining management protocols. Because predictive values are factors of population prevalence, POCT BNP used to help identify stroke of CE aetiology would be most valuable in populations with a high disease burden.

Lee-Lewandrowski *et al.* (2009) investigated the impact of introducing D-dimer POCT to the busy ED (84 000 visits a year) at Massachusetts General Hospital. They attempted to test the hypothesis 'the availability of a rapid whole blood D-dimer test would decrease the time needed to evaluate patients suspected of having venous thromboembolism (VTE) and thus permit more rapid decisions concerning appropriate disposition' and to evaluate the impact the new POCT would have on radiological studies and the rate of admission whether to the observation unit or medical beds.

A D-dimer POC test was introduced in the ED satellite laboratory. The total number of patients included was 463; 252 before implementation and 211 afterwards. The latter group had paired samples taken for simultaneous POCT and laboratory testing of D-dimer. Total test TAT (TTTAT) was defined as time from blood draw to availability of result.

TTTAT dropped by 79% after implementation of POCT, from 2 hours to 25 min and ED LOS fell by 1.3 h and 30 min in mean and median LOS, respectively. There was a significant drop of 14% in patients admitted to hospital, and an increase of 7% and 6% in patients discharged from ED and admitted for observation only, respectively. There was no difference observed in utilisation of follow-up radiological studies. Both laboratory testing and POCT showed a sensitivity of 100% and a NPV of 100%.

This study demonstrated that a POC D-dimer test used to exclude VTE in low-risk individuals in a busy ED can help reduce ED LOS and efficiently reduce the number of admissions without increasing the number of relevant radiological studies and without increasing patient morbidity. Indeed POCT for D-dimer was permanently introduced in this ED without the need for confirmatory laboratory testing. This is an example of a benefit of POCT in ED: namely, reduced rates of admission, which is realised outside of ED, in the hospital ward.

When a myocardial infarction (MI) is associated with typical electrocardiographic (ECG) changes it is termed S-T segment elevation MI (STEMI). It is easy to diagnose because of the these changes; however, when there are no ECG changes, as with non-STEMI (NSTEMI), biochemical confirmation by elevation of cTn becomes paramount and speed of availability of cTn level assumes critical importance. The impact of introducing cTnI POCT in ED for NSTEMI patients was investigated in a non-blinded RCT in an ED of a 900-bed tertiary care hospital in Paris (Renaud *et al.* 2008). Patients were stratified into two groups based on risk factors.

From a total of 833 patients enrolled, 419 were allocated to POCT and 414 to central laboratory testing. The median time from blood collection to physician notification of the first cTnI result dropped by 71 min (from 109 to 38 min) in the POCT cohort but most importantly this translated to a decrease in time from presentation to treatment of 47 min (198 to 151 min). Furthermore there was no significant difference in either 30-day or 90-day mortality between the groups. LOS was not different between the groups.

When a result for the POC cTnI test was available, nurses did not deliver it to the caring physician until it was requested in order to mimic physician behaviour when results were released from the central laboratory and mitigate potential bias that may be introduced by a change in behaviour caused by the nurses' and doctors' awareness of results (Hawthorne effect). Furthermore, testing time for both POCT and laboratory-generated results was comparable (15 min versus 17 min, respectively). In spite of these factors, the clinical outcomes were encouraging: ~45 min in the context of MI management is a significant improvement.

This study underscores the supportive role POCT can play when targeted to a particular patient group. The lack of improvement in LOS highlights the multiplicity of factors involved in patient care apart from speed of result availability: a fact well demonstrated in a study by Ryan *et al.* (2009). This study included 2000 patients in a four-centre ED RCT in the USA. It was a complex trial run over 2 years involving many ED physicians and at least two different clinical pathways used throughout the different centres. Patients were randomised to receive cTnI testing by POCT (with simultaneous laboratory testing) or by laboratory testing alone. They attempted to test the hypothesis 'point-care-testing decreases time to discharge compared with a central laboratory testing strategy in patients presenting to the ED with possible acute coronary syndrome (ACS).' The primary outcome measure was time from presentation to disposition and secondary outcome was time from presentation to departure from ED.

There was a definite reduction in test TAT from 58 min for laboratory testing to 15 min with POCT. There was a general trend towards a decrease in the median time to disposition by approximately half-an-hour with a fall in median time to discharge by 12 min only. When analysing individual centres, only one demonstrated a significant reduction in time to disposition by 22 min and time to departure by 45 min for patients being admitted with no improvement in either parameter for patients discharged. On the other hand, another centre showed an actual increase of 90 min for both parameters in discharged patients.

Thus, sooner decision making did not necessarily translate to sooner action (discharge) and outcomes in various centres were quite different. This study emphasises the importance of other operational factors involved in patient disposition. The authors claim that, if four patients are evaluated for ACS daily and discharged from ED saving 30 min of ED bed-time, an extra 60 h of ED bed space would be available monthly. With this expectation in mind, the study confirms the potential POCT for cTn can have on bed space savings, a critical factor in EDs.

As opposed to targeting POCT to a single test or condition, Jang *et al.* (2013) investigated the impact a comprehensive metabolic POCT panel would have on ED patient flow. The study was a non-blinded single-centre RCT conducted in a teaching hospital in Korea with ~54 000 visits annually. A total of 10 244 patients, who were aged 15 years and above and whose ED physician had requested a comprehensive metabolic panel within an 8 month timeframe, were included in the study. The POCT panel included liver function tests, electrolytes, urea, creatinine, glucose, calcium and total carbon dioxide. Testing was conducted by trained emergency medicine technicians (EMT) who, after drawing blood samples, randomised the patients to either central laboratory testing (5090) or POCT (5154).

Median ED LOS for patients assigned to POCT was 350 min, as opposed to 372 min for patients assigned to central laboratory testing (i.e. a median drop of 22 min). When sub-categorising patients, it was found that the median LOS for those discharged fell by 12 min; for emergency index level 3 patients, the commonest index severity classification of participants in the study (87%), the median LOS decreased by 22 min. Of those who received a computerised tomography (CT) scan, median time to CT scan in the POCT group fell by 11 min and median LOS fell by 58 min (not statistically significant).

The clinical utility of POC lactate measurement in the stratification of patients at risk for sepsis was the subject of a brief report by Singer *et al.* (2014). Sepsis, a systemic response to inflammation, has a mortality of 20–50%. Early knowledge of lactate levels helps identify patients at highest risk for adverse outcomes and enables early institution of supportive measures such as intravenous (IV) fluids and IV antibiotics. Investigators aimed to test the hypothesis 'compared with central laboratory testing, bedside POC lactate testing would reduce the time to intravenous fluid and antibiotic administration in ED patients with sepsis.'

This 'before and after' study was conducted in a tertiary care hospital with 90 000 annual ED visits. Patients had at least two systemic inflammatory response syndrome (SIRS) criteria, a blood lactate of at least 2 mmol/L and had not received IV antibiotics in the preceding 24 h. SIRS criteria are a list of findings that help identify patients with sepsis; they include a temperature of 38°C or more, a temperature of 35°C or less, heart rate ≥90 beats/min, respiratory rate ≥20 breaths/min, a systolic blood pressure <90 mmHg or an acute change in mental status. Eighty consecutive patients before, and 80 after, implementation of POC lactate testing were included. All clinical decisions were based on POCT results for the latter group. POC lactate results were simultaneously compared with central laboratory lactate levels to determine relative accuracy. All POCT results were immediately communicated to the caring physician. The primary outcome for the study was time from ED triage to IV antibiotics and fluids administration.

Although time to result availability was significantly less in the 'after' group versus the 'before' group (median 34 and 122 min, respectively), there was no change in time to ordering of IV fluids or antibiotics. There was a reduction in the median time to *initiation* of IV fluids of 16 min in the 'after' group but no change in the time to initiation of IV antibiotics. In-hospital mortality decreased from 19 to 6% and the percentage of patients admitted to ICU fell from 51 to 33% after implementation of POC lactate testing. Only two patients had discrepant lactate levels (with POC lactate ≥2 mmol/L and laboratory lactate <2 mmol/L).

The authors judged that a reduction of 30 min in time to initiation of IV fluids and antibiotics would be clinically relevant. This limited study failed to deliver this outcome. They argued that the physical proximity of IV fluids to the patient and ease of administration compared with IV antibiotics may have played a role. Nevertheless, other findings were significant and associated with the introduction of faster (bedside) lactate measurement, a measure recommended by guidelines that deal with management of patients with suspected sepsis.

Thromboelastography (TEG®) and rotational thromboelastometry (ROTEM®) are tests used to measure the visco-elastic properties of whole blood clot formation under low shear stress. These two haemostatic assays, which are now available in POC platforms, help assess bleeding and thrombotic risks; they are widely used in patients undergoing cardiac surgery or liver transplantation and can achieve savings related to reductions in blood products transfused for cardiac surgery and liver transplantation. From a patient's perspective, the main benefit of having these tests performed is reduction or avoidance of inappropriate blood transfusions.

Spalding *et al.* (2007) described a retrospective study of 1422 patients undergoing cardiac surgery. This study compared the costs of blood products and coagulation factors before (729 patients) and after (693 patients) the implementation of bedside ROTEM testing. It resulted in a reduction in the use of blood products – from €125 828 to €55 925: a cost saving of 44%, which exceeded the cost of the ROTEM testing.

A clinical and cost-effectiveness economic model by National Health Service Quality Improvement Scotland Health Technology Assessment (HTA) was reported in 2008 (NHSQIS 2008). The model showed that, for 200 tests on cardiac surgery patients, intra-operative and post-operative TEG was less expensive than the use of standard laboratory coagulation tests (SLTs) such as prothrombin time/INR, activated partial thromboplastin time (APTT) and clinical discretion alone. The cost at 1 month per cohort of 1000 patients was £1 058 770 with TE versus £1 184 390 with SLTs and £1 662 060 with clinical discretion. At 1 year, these trends in cost savings were repeated. The model showed that fewer patients would need transfusion with TEG and there was a small increase in QALYs gained at 1 month after transfusion. For liver transplantation patients, TEG was also less expensive than SLTs and clinical discretion alone at both 1 month and 1 year. This HTA report also recommended that, from an operational perspective, TEG should be implemented with appropriate clinical governance and quality assurance.

A systematic review of the clinical effectiveness of viscoelastometry (VE) by Whiting *et al.* (2015) comprised 31 studies. The review included 11 RCTs involving 1089 cardiac surgery patients, six assessed TEG and five ROTEM. There was a significant reduction in red blood cell transfusion (relative risk (RR) 0.88, 95% CI 0.80–0.96; six studies), platelet transfusion (RR 0.72, 95% CI 0.58–0.89; six studies) and fresh frozen plasma transfusion (RR 0.47, 95% CI 0.35–0.65; five studies) in VE testing groups compared with control. VE testing was more cost-effective than SLTs for cardiac surgery; the cost saving was £43 for ROTEM, £79 for TEG and £132 for Sonoclot.

In summary, POCT will not be the magic bullet to fix all challenges faced by modern day hospitals, be they in developed or underdeveloped regions, but POCT certainly has a significant role and potential to have a positive impact. Faster result availability is one piece of the operational jigsaw that needs to marry up to achieve full potential. Use of POCT in hospitals may reduce ED overcrowding, streamline pathways, treat patients faster and reduce morbidity, as well as bolster community efforts and public health initiatives beyond hospital systems.

## CASE STUDY OF A CURRENT AND SUCCESSFUL HOSPITAL POCT SERVICE – IMPLEMENTATION OF POCT IN RAWENE HOSPITAL IN NEW ZEALAND

The Hokianga district in Northland, New Zealand covers a geographical area of 1520 km$^2$ and serves a population of 6350 people, of whom 70% are Maori. The area has a high deprivation rating and receives many visitors and tourists all year. Access to health services is challenged at times by flooding, rough terrain, unsealed roads and a ferry crossing across the Hokianga Harbour. Rawene Hospital provides an accident and emergency service, maternity and acute patient treatment locally but is located 2 hours by road from Whangarei Hospital, the only major hospital in Northland.

Rawene Hospital does not have an on-site laboratory service and therefore specimens for non-urgent investigations are sent by road to Northland Pathology Laboratory in Whangarei. These specimens are dispatched Monday to Friday at 10:00 a.m. and the test results transmitted in late afternoon: a delay of at least 8 h. There is no laboratory service after 10:00 a.m. on Friday or at weekends and on public holidays.

In 2008, an Abbott i-STAT analyser was installed to provide the following POC tests: blood gases and lactate, electrolytes, urea, creatinine, glucose, cTnI and BNP. The POCT service was implemented using the Northland District Health Board POCT quality management system, which includes a staff training and certification program, and internal and external quality control tests with oversight from the NDHB POC coordinator.

The POCT service was evaluated by Blattner *et al.* (2010) and showed that it improved diagnostic certainty from 2.5 diagnoses pre-test to 1.3 diagnoses post-test ($P$ <0.001) and changed patient disposition for 43% of patients ($P$ <0.001) by reducing transfers to the base hospital by 62% (52 pre-test and 20 post-test) and increasing discharges by 480% (7 pre-test and 34 post-test). Substantial treatment changes occurred in 75% of cases, with some change in 22% and no change in 3% of cases. The overall cost to Rawene Hospital was NZ$90 222 during the first year of operation but this cost also included treatment costs, and more and longer bed stays for patients who, before the POCT service was implemented, would have required transfer to Whangarei Hospital for treatment, which entails a 2-hour journey by road ambulance transport. As a result, the net savings in reduced transfers and costs to Whangarei Hospital was NZ$362 138. The additional benefits include better continuity of care and patients not being separated from whanau or family.

## REFERENCES

Ameyaw E, Nguah SB, Ansong D, Page I, Guillerm M, Bates I (2014) The outcome of a test-treat package versus routine outpatient care for Ghanaian children with fever: a pragmatic randomized control trial. *Malaria Journal* **13**, 461. doi:10.1186/1475-2875-13-461

Blattner K, Nixon G, Dovey S, Jaye C, Wigglesworth J (2010) Changes in clinical practice and patient disposition following the introduction of point-of-care testing in a rural hospital. *Health Policy* **96**, 7–12. doi:10.1016/j.healthpol.2009.12.002

Deshpande SN, van Asselt ADI, Tomini F, Armstrong N, Allen A, Noake C, *et al.* (2013) Rapid fetal fibronectin testing to predict preterm birth in women with symptoms of premature labour: a systematic review and cost analysis. *Health Technology Assessment* **17**, 1–138. doi:10.3310/hta17400

Fitzgerald P, Goodacre SW, Cross E, Dixon S, on behalf of the RATPAC Research Team (2011) Cost-effectiveness of point-of-care biomarker assessment for suspected myocardial infarction: the Randomized Assessment of Treatment Using Panel Assay of Cardiac Markers (RATPAC) Trial. *Academic Emergency Medicine* **18**, 488–495. doi:10.1111/j.1553-2712.2011.01068.x

Goodacre S, Bradburn M, Fitzgerald P, Cross E, Collinson P, Gray A, *et al.* (2011) The RATPAC (Randomised Assessment of Treatment using Panel Assay of Cardiac markers) trial: a randomised controlled trial of point-of-care cardiac markers in the emergency department. *Health Technology Assessment* **15**(23). doi.org/10.3310/hta15230

Herd G, Musaad SMA (2015) Clinical governance and point-of-care testing at health provider level. *The New Zealand Medical Journal* **128**, 41–46.

Huckle D (2006) Point-of-care diagnostics: will the hurdles be overcome this time? *Expert Review of Medical Devices* **3**, 421–426. doi:10.1586/17434440.3.4.421

Jang JY, Shin SD, Lee EJ, Park CB, Song KJ, Singer AJ (2013) Use of a comprehensive metabolic panel point-of-care test to reduce length of stay in the emergency department: a randomized controlled trial. *Annals of Emergency Medicine* **61**, 145–151. doi:10.1016/j.annemergmed.2012.07.021

Lee-Lewandrowski E, Nichols J, Van Cott E, Grisson R, Louissaint A, Benzer T, *et al.* (2009) Implementation of a rapid whole blood D-Dimer test in the emergency department of an urban academic medical center. Impact on ED length of stay and ancillary test utilization. *American Journal of Clinical Pathology* **132**, 326–331. doi:10.1309/AJCP6US3ILGEAREE

McCollum ED, Preidis GA, Maliwichi M, Olson D, McCrary M, Kazembe PN, *et al.* (2014) Clinical versus rapid molecular HIV diagnosis in hospitalized African infants: a randomized controlled trial simulating point of-care infant testing. *Journal of Acquired Immune Deficiency Syndromes* **66**, e23–e30. doi:10.1097/QAI.0000000000000080

MoH (Ministry of Health) (2015) *Ebola Information for Health Professionals*. New Zealand, <www.health.govt.nz>.

Musaad SMA, Khan SA, Herd G (2015) Point-of-care testing: high time for a dedicated national adverse event monitoring system. *The Clinical Biochemist Reviews* **36**, 3–6.

NHS QIS (National Health Service Quality Improvement Scotland) (2008) 'The clinical and cost effectiveness of thromboelastography/thromboelastometry.' Health Technology Assessment Report. Glasgow, UK, <www.nhshealthquality.org>.

Nichols JH (2005) Point-of-care testing. In *The Immunoassay Handbook*. 2nd edn. (Ed. D Wild) Nature Publishing Group, London, UK.

Nicholson KG, Abrams KR, Batham S, Medina MJ, Warren FC, Barer M, *et al.* (2014) Randomised controlled trial and health economic evaluation of the impact of diagnostic testing for influenza, respiratory syncytial virus and Streptococcus pneumoniae infection on the management of acute admissions in the elderly and high-risk 18- to 64-year-olds. *Health Technology Assessment* **18**, 1–274, vii–viii. doi:10.3310/hta8360

Price CP (2012) Evidence-based laboratory medicine: is it working in practice? *The Clinical Biochemist Reviews* **33**, 13–19.

Price CP, Kricka LJ (2007) Improving healthcare accessibility through point-of-care technologies. *Clinical Chemistry* **53**, 1665–1675. doi:10.1373/clinchem.2006.084707

Renaud B, Maison P, Ngako A, Cunin P, Santin A, Hervé J, *et al.* (2008) Impact of point-of-care testing in the emergency department evaluation and treatment of patients with suspected acute coronary syndromes. *Academic Emergency Medicine* **15**, 216–224. doi:10.1111/j.1553-2712.2008.00069.x

Rooney KD, Schilling UM (2014) Point-of-care testing in the overcrowded emergency department – can it make a difference? *Critical Care* **18**, 692. doi:10.1186/s13054-014-0692-9

Ryan R, Lindsell CJ, Hollander JE, O'Neil B, Jackson R, Shreiber D, *et al.* (2009) A multicenter randomized controlled trial comparing central laboratory and point-of-care cardiac marker testing strategies: the disposition impacted by serial point of care markers in acute coronary syndromes (DISPO-ACS) Trial. *Annals of Emergency Medicine* **53**, 321–328. doi:10.1016/j.annemergmed.2008.06.464

Singer AJ, Taylor M, LeBlanc D, Williams J, Thode HC Jr (2014) ED bedside point-of-care lactate in patients with suspected sepsis is associated with reduced time to iv fluids and mortality. *The American Journal of Emergency Medicine* **32**, 1120–1124. doi:10.1016/j.ajem.2014.06.027

Spalding GJ, Hartrumpf M, Sierig T, Oesberg N, Kirschke CG, Albes JM (2007) Cost reduction of perioperative coagulation management in cardiac surgery: value of "bedside" thromboelastography (ROTEM). *European Journal of Cardio-Thoracic Surgery* **31**, 1052–1057. doi:10.1016/j.ejcts.2007.02.022

Whiting P, Al M, Westwood M, Ramos IC, Ryder S, Armstrong N, *et al.* (2015) Viscoelastic point-of-care testing to assist with the diagnosis, management and monitoring of haemostasis: a systematic review and cost-effectiveness analysis. *Health Technology Assessment* **19**, 1–228. doi:10.3310/hta19580

Wu Z, Zhao M, He M, Zeng H, Tan F, Li K, *et al.* (2015) Validation of the use of B-type natriuretic peptide point-of-care test platform in preliminary recognition of cardioembolic stroke in patients in the ED. *The American Journal of Emergency Medicine* **33**, 521–526. doi:10.1016/j.ajem.2015.01.013

# 30 Point-of-care testing for paramedic services

*Hugh Grantham and Timothy Pointon*

**Summary**

Point-of-care testing (POCT) for paramedic services has evolved from the simplest POCT of blood glucose and ECG monitoring to a sophisticated and integrated use of POCT in assessment and monitoring of prehospital patients. This evolution has been rapid, as has the evolution of the professional paramedic. This chapter describes the role of POCT in the paramedic environment and discusses the issues associated with providing POCT in this diverse and challenging environment.

## CLINICAL EXAMPLE OF PARAMEDIC USE OF POINT-OF-CARE TESTING

An elderly lady with dementia in a residential care facility has clear anticipatory directions that decline hospital management, but have a focus on comfort care, while not declining all treatment. This is a typical anticipatory care direction expressed by a large percentage of the residential care population (Silvester *et al.* 2013). When she developed confusion and a change in behaviour, the need for a clinical assessment was identified. Even if an emergency department (ED) assessment and evaluation was deemed appropriate, it is not consistent with the wishes expressed in the anticipatory directions. Consequently, a clinical assessment by extended care paramedics was performed as an appropriate alternative. This assessment noted the history of type 2 diabetes and a point-of-care (POC) test for glucose returned a value of 15.5 mmol/L. The exact value is not critical to clinical assessment but the fact that it is raised to the point where it would be causing osmotic diuresis is noted. Furthermore, as her medication has not changed and her blood glucose levels had been previously well controlled, an underlying infection can be suspected.

Clinical evaluation reveals a low blood pressure (BP) of 90/60 mmHg with a relatively normal pulse of 88 beats per minute in a patient with a pacemaker. Abdominal discomfort, a mildly raised temperature and cloudy urine from a catheter specimen raises the possibility of urosepsis. POC dipstick testing confirms the presence of blood, nitrites, leucocytes and protein in her urine.

The clinical decision in this case becomes less dependent on the diagnosis and more focussed on how to respect her wishes and not be too invasive. In this case, an intravenous cannula for blood sampling and fluid or drug administration is acceptable to her daughter who is her substitute decision maker. POCT of a venous blood sample reveals acutely raised urea, relatively low sodium and potassium, associated with diuresis, and a lactate of 4.5 mmol/L (reference interval <1.7 mmol/L). There is evidence of dehydration associated with the osmotic diuresis and lactic acidosis associated with poor perfusion and sepsis.

A clinical treatment plan involving the patient's daughter, as substitute decision maker, and the patient's general practitioner (GP) is devised, which includes intravenous antibiotics and intravenous fluid resuscitation with normal saline supported, oral potassium supplements and a small dose of rapid acting insulin. All of this can be achieved with minimal distress to the patient and without moving her to the ED. Her GP can assess her within 24 h to evaluate the response to treatment and discuss with her daughter the next steps in treatment, which might include a course of oral antibiotics if she is recovering or a decision not to escalate care because she is not responding.

In this case, patient-focussed care has been delivered that respected the patient's wishes and accurately took into account the clinical problem. POCT assisted in this process by measuring and monitoring the glucose, assessing the renal function and electrolytes levels, thus allowing correction and assessing the degree of lactic acidosis, providing guidance for the fluid resuscitation. If the patient had been transferred to the hospital situation, a non-response to simple treatment would result in escalation of care, such as the use of inotropes and probably transfer to the intensive care unit. POCT in this example allowed this patient the opportunity to recover.

## OVERVIEW OF THE PARAMEDIC SETTING FROM AN AUSTRALIAN, REGIONAL AND/OR GLOBAL PERSPECTIVE

As one of the newest professions, paramedics have undergone a significant evolution in a very short space of time. Prior to the 1960s, very little had changed from the original concept of mobile stretcher-bearers that were attributed to Napoléon Bonaparte's chief of surgery, Baron von Larrey, among others (Pruitt 2006). The origins of modern paramedics started with combat medics in the military translating their skills to the civilian environment in the 1960s. The first portable cardiac care with cardiopulmonary resuscitation as we now know it, and the first portable defibrillators in the field, belong to this era (Eisenberg *et al.* 1996).

The early paramedics made the first significant step in their professional evolution by carrying out treatment in the field and in transit. The treatment that was carried out was governed by protocols and by medical control and allowed early assessment and management of acute conditions such as cardiac dysrhythmia and hypovolaemia. The transition from a purely transport to hospital role to implementing assessment and management to the patient in the field marks the first utilisation of POC assessment.

If we take an inclusive view of POCT, we certainly have to include the first electrocardiogram (ECG) rhythms recorded in the field, which provided information upon which treatment was based. One of the earliest monitor/defibrillators was the LIFEPAK® 5, which had the advantage of simplicity and robustness. This device allowed the paramedic to improve resuscitation outcomes by the early identification of life-threatening arrhythmias and the application of defibrillation. The LIFEPAK® 5 retains a very important position in the history of POC assessment and monitoring as a benchmark for portability, reliability and robustness. The 1980s saw a rapid expansion of paramedic treatments in both Australia and America. To facilitate this increased scope of practice, paramedics were being equipped with more assessment tools and were now able to assess a variety of physiological parameters, such as blood glucose (Holstein *et al.* 2000; Jones *et al.* 1992), pulse oximetry (Aughey *et al.* 1991; Brown *et al.* 1996; Cydulka *et al.* 1992) and non-invasive blood pressure monitoring. A similar evolution occurred in Europe, notably in France and Germany, where physician-staffed ambulances used the same assessment tools. The early pulse oximeters were bulky and a little temperamental (Sinex 1999), but for the first time gave real-time feedback on oxygenation. In Australia, the first pulse oximeters appeared on ambulances in the late 1980s and had become almost universal by the mid-1990s. This rapid and extensive uptake was appropriate for a device that provided useful information that could not be obtained in another way in a timely fashion with minimum effort on the part of the clinician. The characteristics valued by prehospital clinicians, be they paramedics or doctors, were beginning to emerge as reliability, simplicity and portability. By the end of the 1990s, the range of physiological parameter measures available to paramedics included blood glucose, electrocardiograms (ECG) (including 12 lead ECG), blood pressure monitoring (invasive and non-invasive), oximetry and end-tidal $CO_2$. The advances in professional practice and education allowed the next step of the expansion of the paramedic role – the extended care paramedic.

The next decade from 2000 to 2010 saw the expansion of the extended care paramedic role into an autonomous practice that permitted assessment and treatment of more complex and chronic conditions (Evans *et al.* 2014).

Extended care paramedics have evolved in Canada, the United Kingdom, Australia and New Zealand. Although a significant variation in extent of practice exists between different models, they all relied on high-quality assessment of patients using POCT. The possibility of basing complex clinical decisions upon POCT blood results has become a reality. Paramedics whose treatment will be influenced by the results can now carry out POCT in the patient's home, in a disaster setting and in the field. The values of reliability, simplicity and portability are still the yardstick for assessing POCT equipment for use in a paramedic environment.

## THE CLINICAL ROLE OF POCT IN A PARAMEDIC SETTING

Considering POCT in the more usually accepted sense of blood tests carried out in the field, the greatest amount of experience in this area has been obtained by the extended care paramedics. These paramedics manage patients in their own home environments using POCT to guide clinical management in specific conditions (Fig. 30.1). Assessing and managing patients in their own home, as opposed to an already overcrowded hospital system, has some advantages: not only does this approach meet the needs and wishes of the patient but also offers savings in both fiscal terms and logistics for the health system. Patients who may benefit from this care provided in their own home include: those with simple problems amenable to a standardised simple management pathway; those with complex problems but who do not chose to be managed in hospital; and those with a specific subset of the complex problems in palliative care.

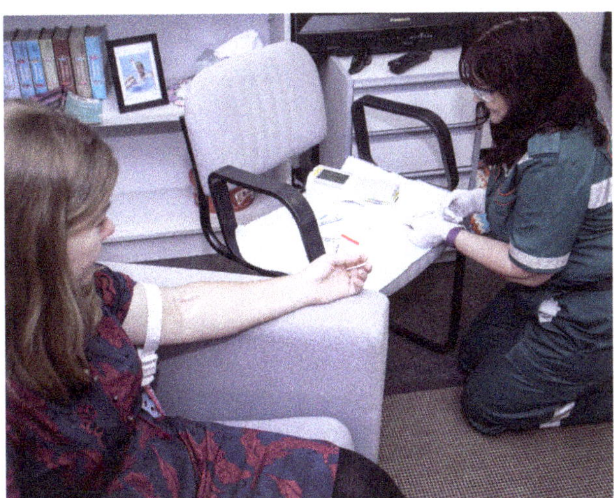

**Fig. 30.1.** Paramedic conducting POCT in a patient's home.

The simplest blood-based POCT device widely used in ambulance services is the blood glucose meter. Knowing the patient's blood glucose allows a paramedic to quickly identify hypoglycaemia as the cause of a decreased consciousness level and to manage that effectively in the field (Strote *et al.* 2005). It also allows the paramedic to initiate a care pathway, which will generally involve hospital stabilisation. Blood glucose monitoring is also used to evaluate the out-of-hospital management strategy, such as glucagon or glucose (administered orally or intravenously). A common presentation for a paramedic is the patient who has their hypoglycaemic event fully reversed by the paramedic intervention in the field. Accurate identification of normal blood glucose levels allows for safe non-transport decisions to be made, without the risk of recurrent hypoglycaemia (Cain *et al.* 2003).

The requirement for absolute accuracy of blood glucose measurement in the prehospital setting is not as important as the clear identification of hypo, hyper or normoglycaemia, which is used as a basis for providing treatment. The values of reliability, simplicity and portability coupled with low cost are going to determine paramedic preferences between POCT blood glucose systems.

Tortella *et al.* (1996) introduced the benefit of using handheld whole blood analysers in the prehospital setting to help field treatment and triage of patients. Obtaining a routine set of electrolytes, urea and creatinine in the field influences the decision-making capacity of extended care paramedics when considering the disposition (hospital or alternative management) of a patient in the out-of-hospital setting. Knowledge of the urea and electrolytes is an important component in assessing the status of a patient with dehydration associated with gastroenteritis and an unremarkable test result will contribute to a decision as to whether it is safe and appropriate to leave the patient at home with simple treatment.

Many of the patients attended by extended care paramedics are elderly with a degree of renal impairment. Being able to assess renal function in the field allows comparison with previous results, stored on the health system computer, and therefore supports an assessment of trends, which is invaluable in making decisions on both hospital disposition and treatment choices. Primary health-care screening for chronic renal failure in Australia has been shown to be beneficial for the early identification and referral of patients (Mathew *et al.* 2010).

Renal impairment often presents with effects from increasing therapeutic levels of drugs, which may be responsible for a variety of symptoms (Bell *et al.* 2013). Among those patients who have complex problems, but may not wish to go the hospital, are the elderly patients with urosepsis. An accurate assessment of renal function is useful in considering dosage and ongoing administration of antibiotics, in particular gentamicin, which is particularly useful for urosepsis. The extended care paramedic, armed with a current assessment of renal function and the ability to compare this with previous records, can make better and more profound decisions, which can be shared with the patient's usual clinician in a culture of team work and joint management.

Haemoglobin evaluation is a useful discriminator between acute and chronic blood loss and, when considered in conjunction with previous results, influences decisions on hospital admission versus home treatment. Blood transfusion delivered in the patient's home is being considered in some settings and offers an attractive alternative to a hospital admission for a group of elderly frail patients who receive frequent transfusions (Ademokun *et al.* 2005). Decisions on transfusion have to be based upon blood results and POCT allows this to occur rapidly at the time of presentation.

The role of POCT in coagulation monitoring in the primary health-care setting has progressed significantly over the last decade, particularly with the monitoring of international normalised ratio (INR) in patients using warfarin. Self-monitoring and self-management has been proposed as a viable model for long-term management (Bussey *et al.* 2013; Heneghan *et al.* 2012; Sharma *et al.* 2015). Several studies have shown improved time within therapeutic range and less time at extreme INR values. However, not all patients are capable of self-management, thus the management may be conducted by the extended care paramedic in collaboration with the GP. The value of elderly frail patients being assessed in their own environment by an extended care paramedic, rather than having to be transported to an ED for assessment of an abnormal coagulation result, is clear when considering the cost and impact to the patient.

The use of POCT for INR monitoring has provoked some debate, with close attention paid to precision and accuracy when compared with laboratory based testing (Hobbs *et al.* 1999; Kitchen *et al.* 2015; Perry *et al.* 2010; Tripodi *et al.* 2003). It should be noted that there is a variation between INR results obtained using different reagents in different laboratories, which can present a challenge in patient's management. However, with suitable training, quality management systems and attention to instrument calibration, POCT for INR appears to be safe, reliable and provides timely and beneficial oral anticoagulant dosing adjustments (Beynon *et al.* 2015; Christensen and Larsen 2012; St John *et al.* 2015). Close collaboration between the extended care paramedic and the medical officer has the potential to more effectively manage the patient's INR levels in a timely fashion.

Out-of-hospital POC troponin testing offers useful evidence to consider when assessing ischaemic heart disease (Sørensen *et al.* 2011; Stengaard *et al.* 2013). In reality, those patients at high risk of myocardial infarction should be assessed within the hospital system, regardless of troponin levels, on the presumption they will need rapid access to reperfusion therapy. The value of early troponin measurements has been questioned on the basis of the reported accuracy of prehospital diagnosis based on troponin levels and the length of time taken for troponin levels to rise after a myocardial infarction (Schuchert *et al.* 1999; van der Laarse *et al.* 2013). Those patients who would not accept reperfusion therapy for reasons of patient choice do not require troponin testing. The remaining role for POC troponin testing is to reassure both patient and clinician in cases where acute coronary syndrome is considered unlikely and the chest pain has been present for >4 h. It should be noted that troponin levels can rise with a variety of non-cardiac conditions, making a change in level in a series of tests far more useful than a single result.

Venous blood gas testing is practical in the field and can provide limited information about the acutely ill patient (Kelly *et al.* 2014). In the physician staffed prehospital setting, arterial blood gas monitoring is beginning to appear, allowing the practitioner to tailor management appropriately (Jousi *et al.* 2010; Mikkelsen *et al.* 2015). Apart from assessment of chronic respiratory disease and $CO_2$ retention, the other particularly useful area is assessment of the metabolic acidosis and lactic acid levels associated with poor perfusion and sepsis (Guyette *et al.* 2011; Seymour *et al.* 2012). In terms of influencing management decisions, a normal pH and normal lactate are very reassuring when considering out-of-hospital management.

Thus far we have considered POCT in the environment of a patient's own home or residential care facility, where the clinical decision is about hospital or out-of-hospital management of the condition. Paramedics also work in hostile environments where patient assessments occur in the field. These hostile environments can include vehicle trauma at the roadside, remote bush environments, military operations and disaster settings. As the logistical separation from hospital assessment and management increases, the potential benefits of POC assessment also increase.

POC assessment in a wilderness or distant environment, where extrication is likely to take many hours, allows initial stabilisation to be guided and monitored for its effectiveness during that time. A high lactate level, for instance, may provide evidence of the primary lactic acidosis associated with poor perfusion and serial measurements may indicate the effectiveness of the ongoing management during the period of extrication. In the combat setting, POCT used by surgeons and medics allows for close monitoring of coagulopathies associated with severe trauma (Cotte *et al.* 2013). When paramedics manage the patient who is remote from care because of logistical issues, they can be responsible for assessment and management over an extended period of hours.

The remote environment provides some drivers that influence the design and functionality of purpose-built POCT equipment. Robustness and weight become key elements, because every piece of equipment has to be carried in to the scene and then work flawlessly once there. These issues are also part of the disaster scenario and influence the choice of equipment used in disasters (Kost *et al.* 2012). The equipment also needs to be able to function at extremes of temperature and tolerate exposure to the elements. Readout screens need to be clear when viewed in bright sunlight. Although these elements are also important for POC equipment design used in hospitals and clinics, they become much more important in this setting.

Remote industrial sites are particularly suited to the use of POCT for assessment of patients and monitoring of chronic conditions (Acker *et al.* 2014). Larger industrial sites should be staffed by nursing or paramedic health professionals and should have a dedicated medical centre. Unfortunately, not all regulations dictate this standard of care, creating the possibility of the clinical decision being made by individuals lacking a tertiary qualification or equivalent experience. The paramedic or nurse in this setting uses POCT in patient assessment, allowing more detailed clinical assessment to occur and more detailed clinical information to be shared with remote specialists. The value of POCT in this setting is that it allows a greater confidence in decision making regarding evacuation versus treatment on site.

Large industrial settings, typically remote mine sites, rely on a fit and competent workforce to maintain production 24 h a day. An avoidable loss of a productive worker, coupled with the logistical expense of evacuating them, can present a significant burden. The clinician managing these cases is required to make challenging decisions that meet the needs of both the worker and the employer, so accurate assessment information is vital to support the decision. The economic pressures on the clinical environment place the industrial paramedic or nurse in a potentially difficult situation, which can be assisted by access to accurate data from POCT.

Clinicians working in the community setting, the industrial setting or in disaster relief teams will have different needs from their POCT equipment. Each setting will present a slightly different set of patient presentations and test requirements. However, each setting will require robust, reliable POCT that has a high degree of accuracy and reproducibility, which allows the clinician to make complex decisions related to the patient's ongoing care.

## BENEFITS, LIMITATIONS AND BARRIERS IN DELIVERING POCT IN PARAMEDIC SETTINGS

POCT in a paramedic environment offers the benefits of improved patient assessment in the field, which can be translated to more discerning decisions as to which patients are going to benefit from hospital management and which patients can be managed in the community. The greatest benefits are to be found in managing those patients with multiple co-morbidities at the end of life where good decision making can save them a great deal of discomfort and unnecessary disruption associated with hospital attendance. This application of POCT to guide treatment can potentially increase the number of cases in which out-of-hospital management can be offered, thus providing significant economic advantage to the healthcare system.

Other areas of benefit from POCT in the paramedic setting are anticipated to include innovative tests that provide more information for the clinician when managing the acute emergency. Lactate results in predicting cases that are likely to develop septic shock (Seymour *et al.* 2012) and the use of ultrasound to identify internal haemorrhage in the trauma case (Chin *et al.* 2013;

Heegaard *et al.* 2010; Kim *et al.* 2012; Song *et al.* 2013) are examples of new applications of POCT. These tests may provide further information to manage critical cases that are often difficult to identify in the field. Remote industrial sites where paramedics are required to support workers in challenging environments and screen for drug and alcohol use is another positive application of POCT, which is becoming established, but not yet well reported in the literature.

However, POCT must be implemented with caution to ensure that there is a true benefit in terms of patient outcomes and cost of health-care delivery. As the range of POCT options increases, each new test needs to be assessed for potential benefits and appropriateness for paramedic use in the out-of-hospital setting. An appropriate POC test will add clinical value to the decision that can be weighed against the cost of the test. In the paramedic environment, the cost of the test is not merely financial but includes many other factors, such as consequences of misleading results or the time taken to perform the tests.

Test results from POCT in the field may be interpreted incorrectly in the absence of a full clinical picture provided by a more comprehensive hospital-based assessment. Such misinterpretations can have a very significant risk if they lead to inappropriate treatment. Consequently, testing that can produce subtle or misleading results should always be strictly regulated and clinicians working in the field should discuss complex or grossly abnormal results with a physician.

Performing the POC test can be time consuming. Unlike the hospital process, where the main goal is to reach the diagnosis, paramedic practice is often a balance between the quality detailed assessment and keeping the process of moving and minimising the time to definitive treatment. A patient with a suspected myocardial infarction or stroke is a good example of a situation where every action that uses time has to be justified in terms of the value delivered versus the delay in reperfusion. If the patient has a clear clinical indication to warrant urgent transfer to the catheter laboratory for angioplasty and stenting, then there is no value in using time obtaining a POC troponin result. Troponin testing takes ~10 min to perform and can distract the paramedic from patient care during this time. The clinical risk therefore exists that the test may be performed without any tangible benefit to the patient, and possibly with some detriment due to the time delay.

One of the subtle problems of POCT by paramedics is that testing may reassure the clinician to discharge the patient without more exhaustive testing. While beneficial for many cases, it is possible that further testing would have produced the key information necessary to manage a patient. For example, a patient who receives routine biochemical blood tests in the hospital ED is likely to be subjected to imaging and more detailed testing as a routine action. The patient who is reassured by normal POCT results in the field may not have the opportunity to benefit from follow-up assessments.

POCT can also come at a logistical cost if the equipment itself is fragile, heavy or sensitive to environmental stressors. The ideal POCT equipment should be light and robust, and be able to run on multiple different power sources with simple changeable batteries. For paramedics, POCT may be performed in a variety of settings, including outdoors, roadside and industrial sites with the associated varying environmental conditions. Reagents should ideally not require refrigeration and special packaging, although this can be difficult to achieve. Maintaining a stable environment for storage of the reagent cartridges also becomes a problem in a mobile environment; for example, where a refrigerator in a vehicle is required to maintain a constant temperature even when the vehicle is not running. Instrument displays should be easily readable in bright sunlight and results should be stored for later downloading to a permanent written record or an electronic patient management system. Finally, the cost of POCT equipment is an important consideration for any large ambulance service.

There is a further barrier to the use of POCT in the paramedic environment once the clinical risk, financial and logistical issues have been considered. This barrier relates to the perceived role of the paramedic and the clinical culture of the system in which they work. Paramedics have only recently appeared in this space in response to an unmet need. This recent arrival creates a potential for conflict when other clinicians do not see this as an appropriate paramedic role. This cultural constraint is likely to have a far greater influence on the use of POCT by paramedics than any of the logistical or clinical considerations. It is important that paramedic POCT should be seen as part of an integrated health-care system, with an emphasis on teamwork for the benefit of the patient. In practical terms, this means a great deal of attention needs to be devoted to communication and consultation with those members of the clinical team responsible for the patient's ongoing management. This cultural communication focus is a key element of the successful extended paramedic program.

As previously described, POCT is becoming standard in paramedic practice. It is hoped that the prehospital care drivers will influence the design and provision of POC equipment for the field. This equipment will differ from equipment designed for use in the hospital or clinic, with more emphasis placed on the prehospital values of reliability, simplicity and portability, with the ability to perform consistently in the hostile environments of out-of-hospital care, remote industrial sites, disaster relief activities and the military combat setting.

## CURRENT CLINICAL USE OF POCT BY PARAMEDICS

The extended care paramedic system in South Australia represents an example of an early adopter of POCT in a paramedic environment. POCT has been integrated within the clinical assessment of patients by extended care paramedics and is used regularly to guide clinical practice. The most commonly used modalities include assessing electrolytes, urea and creatinine for renal function, as well as haemoglobin and the INR of patients on warfarin. Lactate is measured, but whether this influences clinical decision making is the subject of ongoing analysis. Troponin is occasionally measured but does not often influence clinical decision making.

Associated costs of training and the logistical support including maintaining a working environment are borne within the extended care paramedic budget. Although an individual cost–benefit analysis of the POCT element of the system has not been conducted, extended care paramedics deliver significant savings to the health system when budget lines are considered globally. Global evaluation of budget lines implies considering the costs to ambulance services and hospitals together, rather than in individual organisations.

The use of POCT by paramedics allows for high levels of clinical discretion management of the patient in the community. This discretion promotes better patient outcomes in both supporting decisions not to transport patients and identifying patients who benefit from hospital management.

## REFERENCES


Acker JJ, Johnston TM, Lazarsfeld-Jensen A (2014) Industrial paramedics, out on site but not out of mind. *Rural and Remote Health* **14**, 2856, <http://www.rrh.org.au/articles/subviewnew.asp?ArticleID=2856>.

Ademokun A, Kaznica S, Deas S (2005) Home blood transfusion: a necessary service development. *Transfusion Medicine (Oxford, England)* **15**, 219–222. doi:10.1111/j.1365-3148.2005.00574.x

Aughey K, Hess D, Eitel D, Bleecher K, Cooley M, Ogden C, *et al.* (1991) An evaluation of pulse oximetry in prehospital care. *Annals of Emergency Medicine* **20**, 887–891. doi:10.1016/S0196-0644(05)81432-5

Bell JS, Blacker N, Leblanc VT, Alderman CP, Phillips A, Rowett D, *et al.* (2013) Prescribing for older people with chronic renal impairment. *Australian Family Physician* **42**, 24–28.

Beynon C, Erk AG, Potzy A, Mohr S, Popp E (2015) Point of care coagulometry in prehospital emergency care: an observational study. *Scandinavian Journal of Trauma, Resuscitation and Emergency Medicine* **23**, 58. doi:10.1186/s13049-015-0139-6

Brown LH, Manring EA, Kornegay HB, Prasad NH (1996) Can prehospital personnel detect hypoxemia without the aid of pulse oximeters? *The American Journal of Emergency Medicine* **14**, 43–44. doi:10.1016/S0735-6757(96)90012-1

Bussey HI, Bussey M, Bussey-Smith KL, Frei CR (2013) Evaluation of warfarin management with international normalized ratio self-testing and online remote monitoring and management plus low-dose vitamin K with genomic considerations: a pilot study. *Pharmacotherapy* **33**, 1136–1146. doi:10.1002/phar.1343

Cain E, Ackroyd-Stolarz S, Alexiadis P, Murray D (2003) Prehospital hypoglycemia: the safety of not transporting treated patients. *Prehospital Emergency Care* **7**, 458–465. doi:10.1080/312703002193

Chin EJ, Chan CH, Mortazavi R, Anderson CL, Kahn CA, Summers S, *et al.* (2013) A pilot study examining the viability of a Prehospital Assessment with UltraSound for Emergencies (PAUSE) protocol. *The Journal of Emergency Medicine* **44**, 142–149. doi:10.1016/j.jemermed.2012.02.032

Christensen TD, Larsen TB (2012) Precision and accuracy of point-of-care testing coagulometers used for self-testing and self-management of oral anticoagulation therapy. *Journal of Thrombosis and Haemostasis* **10**, 251–260. doi:10.1111/j.1538-7836.2011.04568.x

Cotte J, D'Aanda E, Chauvin V, Kaiser E, Meaudre E (2013) Point-of-care coagulation testing for trauma patients in a military setting: a prospective study. *Journal of Special Operations Medicine* **13**, 59–62.

Cydulka RK, Shade B, Emerman CL, Gershman H, Kubincanek J (1992) Prehospital pulse oximetry: useful or misused? *Annals of Emergency Medicine* **21**, 675–679. doi:10.1016/S0196-0644(05)82778-7

Eisenberg MS, Pantridge J, Cobb LA, Geddes JS (1996) The revolution and evolution of prehospital cardiac care. *Archives of Internal Medicine* **156**, 1611–1619. doi:10.1001/archinte.1996.00440140021002

Evans R, McGovern R, Birch J, Newbury-Birch D (2014) Which extended paramedic skills are making an impact in emergency care and can be related to the UK paramedic system? A systematic review of the literature. *Emergency Medicine Journal* **31**, 594–603. doi:10.1136/emermed-2012-202129

Guyette F, Suffoletto B, Castillo JL, Quintero J, Callaway C, Puyana JC (2011) Prehospital serum lactate as a predictor of outcomes in trauma patients: a retrospective observational study. *The Journal of Trauma* **70**, 782–786. doi:10.1097/TA.0b013e318210f5c9

Heegaard W, Hildebrandt D, Spear D, Chason K, Nelson B, Ho J (2010) Prehospital ultrasound by paramedics: results of field trial. *Academic Emergency Medicine* **17**, 624–630. doi:10.1111/j.1553-2712.2010.00755.x

Heneghan C, Ward A, Perera R, Bankhead C, Fuller A, Stevens R, *et al.* (2012) Self-monitoring of oral anticoagulation: systematic review and meta-analysis of individual patient data. *Lancet* **379**, 322–334. doi:10.1016/S0140-6736(11)61294-4

Hobbs FD, Fitzmaurice DA, Murray ET, Holder R, Rose PE, Roper JL (1999) Is the international normalised ratio (INR) reliable? A trial of comparative measurements in hospital laboratory and primary care settings. *Journal of Clinical Pathology* **52**, 494–497. doi:10.1136/jcp.52.7.494

Holstein A, Kuhne D, Elsing HG, Thiessen E, Plaschke A, Widjaja A, *et al.* (2000) Practicality and accuracy of prehospital rapid venous blood glucose determination. *The American Journal of Emergency Medicine* **18**, 690–694. doi:10.1053/ajem.2000.7324

Jones JL, Ray VG, Gough JE, Garrison HG, Whitley TW (1992) Determination of prehospital blood glucose: a prospective, controlled study. *The Journal of Emergency Medicine* **10**, 679–682. doi:10.1016/0736-4679(92)90524-W

Jousi M, Reitala J, Lund V, Katila A, Leppaniemi A (2010) The role of pre-hospital blood gas analysis in trauma resuscitation. *World Journal of Emergency Surgery* **5**, 10. doi:10.1186/1749-7922-5-10

Kelly AM, Klim S, Rees SE (2014) Agreement between mathematically arterialised venous versus arterial blood gas values in patients undergoing non-invasive ventilation: a cohort study. *Emergency Medicine Journal* **31**, e46–e49. doi:10.1136/emermed-2013-202879

Kim CH, Shin SD, Song KJ, Park CB (2012) Diagnostic accuracy of focused assessment with sonography for trauma (FAST) examinations performed by emergency medical technicians. *Prehospital Emergency Care* **16**, 400–406. doi:10.3109/10903127.2012.664242

Kitchen DP, Jennings I, Kitchen S, Woods TA, Walker ID (2015) Bridging the gap between point-of-care testing and laboratory testing in hemostasis. *Seminars in Thrombosis and Hemostasis* **41**, 272–278. doi:10.1055/s-0035-1544197

Kost GJ, Katip P, Curtis CM (2012) Strategic point-of-care requirements of hospitals and public health for preparedness in regions at risk. *Point of Care* **11**, 114–118. doi:10.1097/POC.0b013e31825a2442

Mathew TH, Corso O, Ludlow M, Boyle A, Cass A, Chadban SJ, *et al.* (2010) Screening for chronic kidney disease in Australia: a pilot study in the community and workplace. *Kidney International* **77**(Supplement 116), S9–S16. doi:10. 1038/ki.2009.538

Mikkelsen S, Wolsing-Hansen J, Nybo M, Maegaard CU, Jepsen S (2015) Implementation of the ABL-90 blood gas analyzer in a ground-based mobile emergency care unit. *Scandinavian Journal of Trauma, Resuscitation and Emergency Medicine* **23**, 54. doi:10.1186/s13049-015-0134-y

Perry DJ, Fitzmaurice DA, Kitchen S, Mackie IJ, Mallett S (2010) Point-of-care testing in haemostasis. *British Journal of Haematology* **150**, 501–514. doi:10.1111/j.1365-2141.2010.08223.x

Pruitt BA Jr (2006) Combat casualty care and surgical progress. *Annals of Surgery* **243**, 715–729. doi:10.1097/01.sla.0000220038.66466.b5

Schuchert A, Hamm C, Scholz J, Klimmeck S, Goldmann B, Meinertz T (1999) Prehospital testing for troponin T in patients with suspected acute myocardial infarction. *American Heart Journal* **138**, 45–48. doi:10.1016/S0002-8703(99)70244-9

Seymour CW, Rea TD, Kahn JM, Walkey AJ, Yealy DM, Angus DC (2012) Severe sepsis in pre-hospital emergency care: analysis of incidence, care, and outcome. *American Journal of Respiratory and Critical Care Medicine* **186**, 1264–1271. doi:10.1164/rccm.201204-0713OC

Sharma P, Scotland G, Cruickshank M, Tassie E, Fraser C, Burton C, *et al.* (2015) The clinical effectiveness and cost-effectiveness of point-of-care tests (CoaguChek system, INRatio2 PT/INR monitor and ProTime Microcoagulation system) for the self-monitoring of the coagulation status of people receiving long-term vitamin K antagonist therapy, compared with standard UK practice: systematic review and economic evaluation. *Health Technology Assessment* **19**, 1–172.

Silvester W, Parslow RA, Lewis VJ, Fullam RS, Sjanta R, Jackson L, *et al.* (2013) Development and evaluation of an aged care specific advance care plan. *BMJ Supportive & Palliative Care* **3**, 188–195. doi:10.1136/bmjspcare-2012-000392

Sinex JE (1999) Pulse oximetry: principles and limitations. *The American Journal of Emergency Medicine* **17**, 59–66. doi:10.1016/S0735-6757(99)90019-0

Song KJ, Shin SD, Hong KJ, Cheon KW, Shin I, Song SW, *et al.* (2013) Clinical applicability of real-time, prehospital image transmission for FAST (focused assessment with sonography for trauma). *Journal of Telemedicine and Telecare* **19**, 450–455. doi:10.1177/1357633X13512068

Sørensen JT, Terkelsen CJ, Steengaard C, Lassen JF, Trautner S, Christensen EF, *et al.* (2011) Prehospital troponin T testing in the diagnosis and triage of patients with suspected acute myocardial infarction. *The American Journal of Cardiology* **107**, 1436–1440. doi:10.1016/j.amjcard.2011.01.014

St John A, Tirimacco R, Badrick T, Siew L, Simpson P, Cowley P, *et al.* (2015) Internet support for point-of-care testing in primary care. *Australian Family Physician* **44**, 10–11.

Stengaard C, Sørensen JT, Ladefoged SA, Christensen EF, Lassen JF, Bøtker HE, *et al.* (2013) Quantitative point-of-care troponin T measurement for diagnosis and prognosis in patients with a suspected acute myocardial infarction. *The American Journal of Cardiology* **112**, 1361–1366. doi:10.1016/j.amjcard.2013.06.026

Strote J, Cloyd D, Rea T, Eisenberg M (2005) The influence of emergency medical technician glucometry on paramedic involvement. *Prehospital Emergency Care* **9**, 318–321. doi:10.1080/10903120590961987

Tortella BJ, Lavery RF, Doran JV, Siegel JH (1996) Precision, accuracy, and managed care implications of a hand-held whole blood analyzer in the prehospital setting. *American Journal of Clinical Pathology* **106**, 124–127.

Tripodi A, Breukink-Engbers WG, van den Besselaar AM (2003) Oral anticoagulant monitoring by laboratory or near-patient testing: what a clinician should be aware of. *Seminars in Vascular Medicine* **3**, 243–254. doi:10.1055/s-2003-44460

van der Laarse A, Cobbaert CM, Gorgels AP, Swenne CA (2013) Will future troponin measurement overrule the ECG as the primary diagnostic tool in patients with acute coronary syndrome? *Journal of Electrocardiology* **46**, 312–317. doi:10.1016/j.jelectrocard.2013.02.007

# 31 Point-of-care testing for disaster management

*Mark Shephard, Paul Arbon and Gerald J Kost*

**Summary**

The number and severity of disasters, natural and human-initiated, has increased significantly during the past 25 years because of: increases in population, density and mobility; global interconnectedness; climate change and environmental degradation; emergence of old and new infectious diseases; and social and economic inequities.

Disaster management involves preparedness for, response to and recovery from, a disaster. Disaster management requires collaboration and coordination between health professionals, government and non-government agencies and communities. The capacity to use quality-assured, state-of the art, disaster-specific rapid point-of-care testing (POCT) within an integrated plan for clinical care facilitates evidence-based clinical decision making for rapid screening, diagnosis, triage, treatment and follow-up of acutely traumatised patients. However, environmental extremes encountered during or after a disaster can compromise the capacity of POCT devices to perform reliably.

## INTRODUCTION

### Understanding disaster impact

Disasters threaten the safety and health of communities and overwhelm their ability to respond without external assistance. Some occur suddenly with catastrophic impact, while others build more slowly and their effects on health are less immediately evident. The provision of appropriate health-care interventions during disasters is therefore a very broad topic.

Many people associate the health response to disaster with immediate response, emergency care, surgery, and the urgent treatment of life-threatening injury. For most of us, our experience of disaster, and disaster health care, is limited to the images and stories that we see in the mainstream media – especially as international or regional teams respond to these dramatic events – and the television footage is usually focussed on the work of surgical teams and at the site of temporary field hospitals. However, the immediate surgical and emergency care response to disaster has relatively limited impact on the health and recovery of those affected, except at the level of those fortunate to receive life-saving treatment in a timely way. Medical teams generally arrive a little too late to save life and cease to have much impact on survival and longer term recovery a few days or weeks after the disaster event. The real work in preparing for, and recovering from, a disaster is done by community members and embedded health practitioners who have an important role in developing the capacity and resilience of communities so that they are well prepared and, when disaster strikes, able to play their part in re-establishing 'normal' health-care services and providing the rehabilitation and ongoing care that is required by survivors. These inputs have the greatest impact on the survival and recovery of affected populations. As a result, the role of health-care professionals across a broad range of specialties and during all phases of disaster should not be underestimated and the impact of strategies that build improved health and therefore more disaster-resilient communities should be emphasised.

There is no widely accepted definition of disaster. Mayner and Arbon (2015) found over 197 definitions in general use. Their review identified common features of these many definitions and presented the following 'consensus' definition: a disaster is 'an event causing widespread disruption and damage exceeding the local ability to cope and overwhelming resources'.

All disasters are related to specific hazards and are generally categorised as: natural; mixed (natural plus man made); and man-made.

Natural disasters may result from seismic causes and include earthquake, volcanic eruption and tsunami, or arise from climatic causes including high winds, high rainfall, erosion and drought. Mixed disasters arise from a combination of human activity and environmental impacts, and include floods, landslides and fire. Man-made disasters arise from technological causes such as the catastrophic release of harmful chemicals, transport or structural failure, explosion, or from conflict. Human conflict is a complex cause of disaster, and includes war, civil conflict, terrorism and the negative impacts of sanctions and embargoes.

## Quantifying the human and financial toll of disasters

Over the short term, it is difficult to identify trends for the occurrence or severity of natural disasters (Fig. 31.1). The Indian Drought of 2002 was the disaster that affected the most people over the past 25 years.

Regarding fatalities over the longer term (since 1900), there is a decline in the total number of deaths from natural disasters, despite an increase in the number of disasters being reported (due to better reporting and climate change). Catastrophic floods and epidemics as seen in the first half of the 20th century have not resulted in as high a death toll in the last 50 years.

Recent data categorising the types of natural disasters in the last 15 years shows earthquake (including tsunami) as the leading cause of death worldwide since 2000. Two

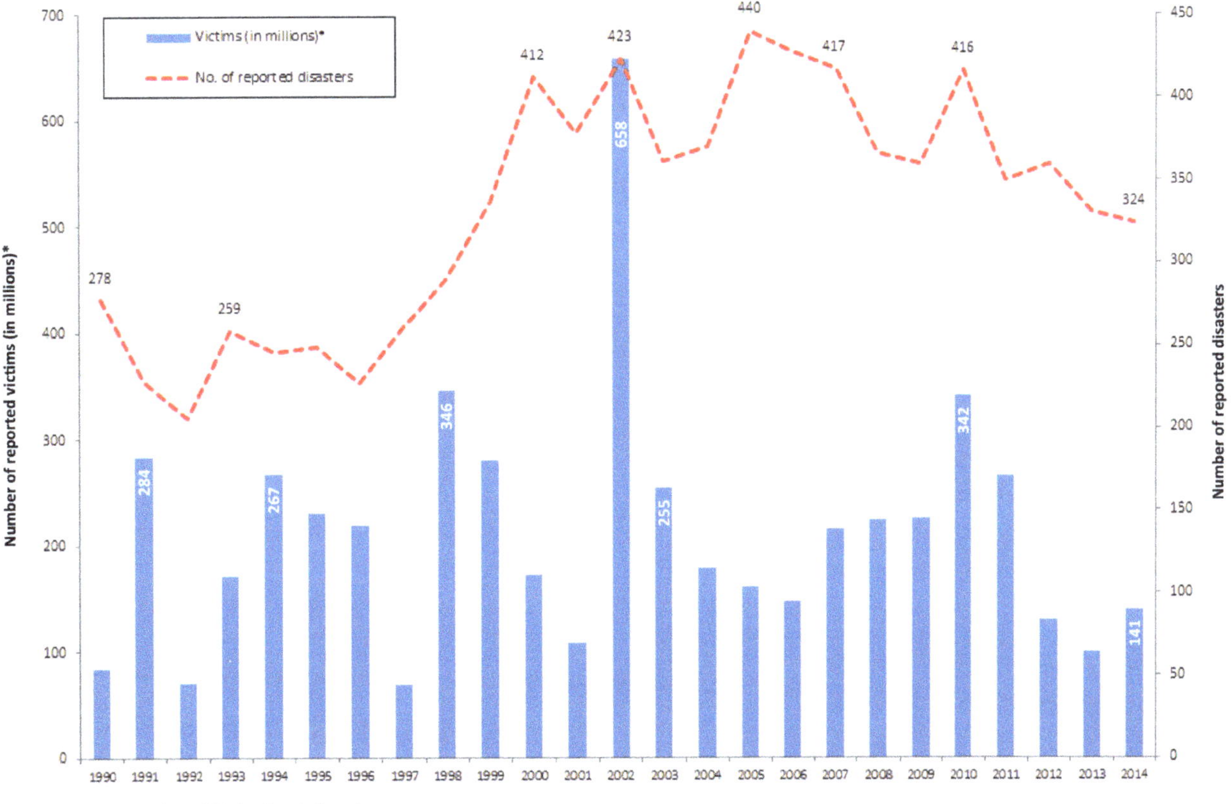


**Fig. 31.1.** Natural disaster occurrence and fatalities per year (since 1990). (Source: Guha-Sapir *et al.* (2015a,b); ©Prof Debarati Guha)

significant events – the Boxing Day Tsunami in 2004 and the Haiti Earthquake in 2010 – dominate the figures for the last 15 years.

Technological disasters are grouped into transport, industrial and miscellaneous. Fortunately, the trend in the deaths from technological disasters has been downwards since 2000. Transport-related disasters, primarily road related disasters, are the leading cause of death for this category, followed by mass explosions and fire.

Comparing economic impact with the death toll from natural disasters tells an interesting story of vulnerability. The most expensive natural disaster was the Tōhoku Earthquake and Tsunami in 2011; however, this resulted in a relatively low death toll when compared with the earthquake events of 2010 (Haiti) and 2004 (Boxing Day Tsunami).

A comparison of fatalities and economic loss for significant comparable events in 2005 (Hurricane Katrina: greater than US$100 billion, 1836 killed) and 2008 (Cyclone Nargis: US$10 billion, 141 000 fatalities) tells a common story of poorer countries' relative vulnerability to natural disasters. Investment in disaster resilience, more commonly seen in developed countries, saves lives, but the damage to infrastructure often has a far higher economic loss. A similar story can be told when comparing localised economic versus human impacts from the Boxing Day Asia Tsunami, with the impact of the Tōhoku Earthquake and Tsunami.

From 1980 to 2012, according to the World Bank, disasters have cost US$3800 billion and show a trend in increasing economic cost of natural disasters; factors including climate change, development and population growth are drivers for this upward trend (World Bank 2013).

A comparison of developing to developed countries shows higher vulnerability of developing countries to natural disasters. Since the 1960s, ~99% of the world population affected by disasters has lived in developing countries and 97% of all deaths have occurred in developing countries.

### Stages of the disaster cycle

The strategic planning for, and management of, disaster events, with particular emphasis on health, encompasses preparedness for, response to and recovery from, a disaster and it is informed by evidence-based disaster research.

Preparedness is the aggregate of all measures and policies adopted before a disaster event that promote mitigation of the damage caused by that event, and minimise the dysfunction that could result from the damage. Planning at all levels of governance is vital and certainly true in the health sphere, where health professionals play a significant role in each stage of the health response to disaster, as well as being required to sustain care services for current clients of the service. A simple, properly disseminated, regularly tested and revised plan for managing a major disaster event is essential (Andress 2010).

Many people associate the health response to disaster with emergency care, surgery, and the urgent treatment of life-threatening injury. Certainly, important early considerations in responding to disaster include establishment of effective triage and managing the initial surge of patients. However, the real work in preparing for, and recovering from, a disaster is done by community members and health practitioners who have an important role to play: (i) in developing the capacity and resilience of communities so that they are well prepared and (ii) when disaster strikes, in re-establishing health-care services and providing the rehabilitation and ongoing care required by survivors. These inputs have the greatest impact on the survival and recovery of affected populations.

The recovery phase of a disaster is the coordinated process of supporting affected communities in the reconstruction of the built environment and the restoration of emotional, social, economic and natural environment wellbeing. Recovery from a disaster can be considered as the bottom of the iceberg. It is in many respects the most complex and difficult phase of disaster management. Communities take on average 10 years to recover from the impact of disaster. The term 'recover' is a misnomer, because communities do not return to their previous state. Rather, they readjust and assimilate the lessons of their recent experience into community and society (Arbon 2010).

There is no distinct point at which immediate response activities change into recovery and then into long-term sustainable development. Progress in some areas is quicker than in others. Physical rehabilitation and reconstruction can sometimes happen more quickly than social or psychological rehabilitation. Recovery from a disaster will only be successful if the community is able to exert a high degree of self-determination in recovery efforts (FitzGerald *et al.* 2010).

## THE ROLE OF POINT-OF-CARE TESTING IN DISASTER MANAGEMENT

POCT has an important, often understated, role in each and every phase of disaster management – preparedness, response and recovery.

## Planning and preparedness for using POCT in a disaster event

Planning for how and when to use POCT optimally in a disaster is a crucial component of preparedness. POCT needs to be integrated within the context of risk analysis, roles and responsibilities of disaster personnel, identification of resources and services needed to combat a disaster, and documentation (and practice readiness) of a disaster plan. How well that planning is undertaken will have a significant bearing on the clinical usefulness and efficiency of POCT in the field following a disaster event.

Despite the well-defined clinical need and potential benefits for rapid POCT in disaster management, regional, national and international policy documents on disaster management developed by governments and professional organisations are currently bereft on information concerning POCT (Kost *et al.* 2011).

The challenge for POCT proponents is to ensure that: (i) policy makers and professional organisations involved in disaster management are aware of the strategic benefits POCT can have; (ii) evidence-based protocols for POCT are embedded within policy documents; and (iii) health professionals and first responders actively involved in mounting disaster responses are well informed, well trained and competent in the quality-assured practice of POCT.

The Clinical and Laboratory Standards Institute (an international interdisciplinary organisation that develops and promotes consensus standards and guidelines within the health-care community) is finalising a Guideline for Emergency and Disaster Point-of-Care Testing POCT-16; this will become an invaluable document. In 2015, Kost and Curtis published a book entitled *Global Point of Care: Strategies for Disasters, Emergencies and Public Health Resilience.* This definitive text adds significantly to the current knowledge on POCT for disaster care. The Flinders University International Centre for Point-of-Care Testing offers postgraduate topics on POCT and disaster management in the Graduate Certificate in Global Point-of-Care Testing (Shephard *et al.* 2015a) and in the Masters in Disaster Health (the latter commencing in the second half of 2016); these two topics prepare health professionals for the role of a POCT Coordinator in a disaster event.

## The role of the POCT Coordinator in providing leadership for POCT in disaster care

The POCT Coordinator (at local, regional, national and international levels) should have a pivotal leadership role in the organisation of POCT preparedness (and, where appropriate or feasible, in on-ground response and recovery) (Mann 2015). A POCT Coordinator is usually a qualified medical scientist or nurse practitioner with advanced knowledge of the principles and practice of POCT and personal experience in coordinating and managing a network of POCT sites. Examples of the responsibilities of a POCT Coordinator in disaster preparedness include: regular review and updating of POCT policy, selection of POCT devices and test clusters, management of reagent stocks and consumables, training and competency assessment and quality assurance/management (Table 31.1).

Two key questions for policy makers (including the POCT Coordinator) regarding analytical quality of POCT field devices used in disaster management are:

- 1. How does one balance the need for speed versus quality of result? In assessing an unconscious patient's glucose levels at a disaster scene, does the responder need to know that the result is 10.1 or 10.2 mmol/L or whether the result is 5, 10 or 20 mmol/L?
- 2. How does one balance the level of quality control (QC) and proficiency testing (PT) testing versus reliance on in-built quality checks to assure a valid test result in a disaster event? There is no 'one-size fits all' answer to this question. As a general rule, the higher number of in-built quality checks, the less the requirement for 'wet' quality testing processes. Wet quality checks can be regularly performed as part of preparedness and practice drill (or 'readiness') activities, but the requirement to perform these checks during a disaster response needs further informed debate.

For US Disaster Medical Assistance Teams (DMATs), QC must be performed by the disaster responder in the field before first use of any POC device. Quality checks should also be performed where devices are exposed to extreme environmental conditions and accurate results are needed for urgent diagnosis and triage of patients.

## Preparedness and location of POCT services at a network level

POCT should be blended synergistically into routine use in health services participating in local or regional POCT networks in areas where there is a high risk of a disaster event occurring (Fig. 31.2). Kost (2006, 2012) uses the term 'small-world networks' to describe these linkages. Device operators in these networks become familiar with and competent in using POCT technology (and associated quality testing procedures) and are therefore able to rapidly 'step up' as front-line responders when/if a

**Table 31.1.** Role and responsibilities for the POCT Coordinator in disaster preparedness

| Role | Responsibilities and general principles |
|---|---|
| Regular policy review | Write, maintain and annually review a master POCT policy document that is linked with overarching disaster planning processes and response systems. |
| | The POCT Policy document should contain information of the specific suite of devices, reagents, tests and quality assurance/management processes required to support a disaster response. |
| | Review of the policy document should include undertaking a needs or 'gap' analysis to rectify any deficiencies identified in the preparedness planning. |
| Selection of POCT device and test clusters | Standardisation of specific devices and test clusters (for use across local, national and international networks) maximises the efficiency of a coordinated POCT response, and enables training to be tailored to, and focussed on, a select suite of devices. |
| | The selection of test clusters should reflect perceived disaster threats (identified as most likely to occur in the hazard vulnerability assessment). |
| | Selected devices and test clusters should streamline seamlessly into established clinical management pathways for triage and treatment. |
| | POCT devices should have environmentally robust connectivity capability to facilitate and maximise the flow of knowledge and information about patient care during a disaster response (Yu *et al.* 2010). The importance of positive patient identification (including the use of bar-coding and other 'new horizon' identification technologies, number of identifiers and how to deal with patients who are unable to be identified) is a critical consideration for patient safety and mitigation of medical errors, and should be built into POCT preparedness plans. |
| Management of reagent stocks and consumables | Planning needs to occur in relation to: |
| | Establishing and maintaining relationships with the industry suppliers of POCT devices, reagents, consumables and quality testing products (including processes for ordering, considerations for stock-piling of reagents, support for device breakdown/repair and links to 24-h hotline support services) |
| | Maintenance of supply chain (including transportation and storage requirements) to ensure reagents are maintained under the environmental controlled conditions recommended by the manufacturer, with consideration being given to use of thermo-modulated transport/storage containers (Rust *et al.* 2012) |
| | Requirements for refrigeration and power supplies (including generators/solar panels). Ideally, devices [of appropriate analytical quality] that are battery operated and reagents that do not require refrigeration are most suited to a disaster scenario. |
| Training and competency assessment | POCT preparedness plans need to allow for pre-disaster training and competency assessment programs for first response medical teams, and staff from primary care units and hospitals in a network or region who have been identified as being likely to participate in a disaster response. |
| | Pre-disaster training programs should be as comprehensive as possible, be available in flexible formats including face-to-face or e-learning options, foster an understanding of the importance of quality testing procedures and incorporate a strong practical component. Resource development should include simple, visual step-by-step guides (posters) on how to conduct POCT to support *in situ* field testing. Following training, all health professional staff should undergo both a written and practical assessment to confirm their competency as a POCT operator and receive a competency certificate. |
| | There also needs to be a documented plan for 'just in time' training (e.g. using e-learning or videoconferencing) with an (online or video/teleconference) certification process, where additional health professional staff can be mobilised rapidly. |
| | POCT training should also be incorporated into broader disaster practice drills. |
| Quality management | POCT should always be undertaken within a documented and systematic quality assurance framework. |
| | In the context of disaster management, POCT quality management procedures are best embedded into preparedness activities in advance of a potential disaster event. |

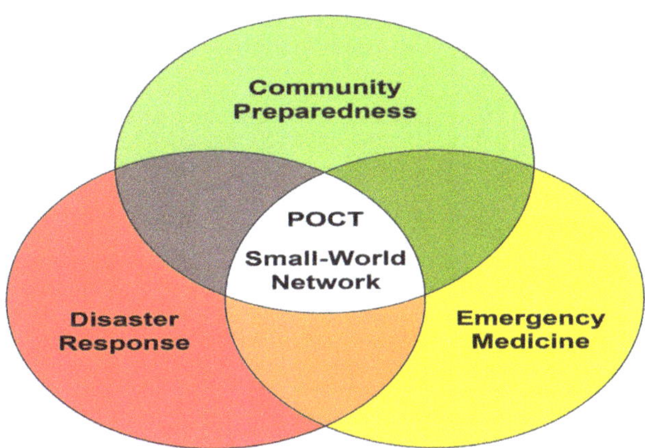


**Fig. 31.2.** The interconnectedness between POCT and community preparedness, emergency medicine and disaster response. (Source: Kost GJ *et al.* (2011). Reproduced with permission from Professor Gerald Kost)

disaster scenario occurs. In essence, device operators have become streamlined for disaster 'readiness' (Shephard *et al.* 2015b).

The strategic location of POCT devices within a local or regional disaster-preparedness network needs to be carefully planned and prioritised, taking into account the likelihood of a disaster occurring. The local topography and population demographics should be considered in this planning; for example, within the geographic confines of the network, where are the pockets of population that are most likely to be affected by a disaster? What transport options will be available following a disaster? Will the area be accessible by road, air or sea? Will ambulances, helicopters, planes, mobile medical units or other alternative testing facilities be accessible or be established in the disaster scene? Answering these questions will assist in the judicious and flexible siting of POCT in the networks in preparedness for a disaster.

## POCT in the response and recovery phases of a disaster event

The capacity to use quality-assured, state-of the art, disaster-specific POCT within an integrated plan for clinical care can have significant benefits. The rapid POCT result at the point of clinical need has high medical impact because it facilitates evidence-based clinical decision making for rapid screening and diagnosis and for efficient triage, treatment and follow-up of acutely traumatised patients. Once the immediate impact of the disaster has passed, and during (but not limited to) times when normal services remain compromised, POCT can be efficiently used in the long-term follow-up of patients, particularly those with chronic diseases.

## How POCT has been used in recent disaster events and what lessons we have learned from these events?

A description of the POCT services available during the Boxing Day Tsunami in 2004 (Kost *et al* 2004), Hurricane Katrina in 2006 (Cefalu *et al.* 2006; Kost *et al.* 2006; Greenough *et al.* 2008) and the Haiti Earthquake in 2010 (Brown and Andrews 2013) is summarised in Table 31.2, together with the lessons learnt from these disasters.

In the Great Bangkok flood of 2011 in Thailand, significant problems occurred with infectious disease outbreaks as a result of major weather disasters. Kost *et al.* (2012a) reviewed the major pathogens (including pandemics) that have been detected following a range of weather-related (and other natural) disasters. Hazards included outbreaks of water- and food-borne infectious diseases and other vector-borne threats such as cholera, malaria, dengue haemorrhagic fever, diarrhoea, skin fungal infections and leptospirosis. There are POC tests available for some of these diseases, but multiplex POCT platforms to detect these disease panels in a disaster scenario do not currently exist. As Louie *et al.* (2008) state: the 'grand challenge' for POCT is for research and development leaders to 'respond with the kind of creative enterprise that is characteristic of past progress in POCT and now revolutionise the fields of emergency and disaster medicine by producing suitably robust POCT that will substantially improve public health preparedness worldwide.'

## What POC tests are most clinically needed in a disaster event?

Table 31.3 broadly summarises the POC tests and test clusters that can support the many clinical presentations encountered in disasters (Kost *et al.* 2011).

Different test clusters may be more applicable/clinically relevant to different types of disasters. Table 31.4 compares and contrasts some of the main clinical presentations seen and the most urgently needed 'first response' POC tests in a bushfire, earthquake, flood, tsunami or infectious disease outbreak.

A recent survey by Brock *et al.* (2010) asked respondents were to rank the importance of POCT pathogen detection in different disaster scenarios; their results can be summarised as follows:

**Table 31.2.** Examples of POCT used in recent disaster events and lessons learned

| Disaster event | Description of POCT services available at the time | Lessons learned |
|---|---|---|
| Boxing Day Tsunami, SE Asia, 2004 | 14 health-care facilities (4 primary care units and 10 hospitals) in Thailand provinces affected by the tsunami. | Medical facilities needed to be located on higher ground 'above elevations attained by future tsunamis'. |
| | POCT was in short supply and poorly organised. POCT available in primary care units was limited to glucose meters, urine dipsticks, urine pregnancy testing, some blood group typing and spun haematocrit. In hospitals, the only available devices were glucose meters and the occasional pulse oximeter. | Community hospitals needed access to whole-blood POCT devices to rapidly perform basic chemistry analyses (such as blood gases, electrolytes, glucose, lactate, haemoglobin and ionised calcium). |
| | One clinical staff member was quoted as saying that he 'decried the lack of electrolyte testing as a critical deficiency' and stated 'cardiac troponin testing was badly needed because patients with chest pain could not be triaged quickly or efficiently, resulting in excess mortality.' | POCT devices needed to be capable of performing: cardiac markers; basic haematology, haemostasis and blood transfusion tests; and infectious disease tests including dengue fever, malaria and tuberculosis. |
| | | The use of POCT must be supported by defined clinical pathways, particularly for acute coronary syndrome and tight glycaemic control. |
| Hurricane Katrina, USA, 2006 | US military services (by sea, land and air) that were engaged to assist with the disaster response were reasonably well equipped with POCT devices, but the flooding that occurred severely limited their capacity to provide on-ground POCT support. | Helicopter, fixed-wing and mobile land units equipped with POCT should be considered as options to help circumvent obstacles in different geographic and topographic settings (where disaster victims are difficult to reach). |
| | 12 hospitals were closed by the Hurricane, while remaining (open) local hospitals, evacuation sites and agencies were underprepared in terms of their POCT resources, being limited to just glucose meters and two i-STATs with a very small number of tests for infectious disease, pregnancy and prothrombin time. | The establishment of 'small world' networks in disaster prone regions is critical in building POCT capacity for disaster response and these networks should have prepositioned POCT, including broad test clusters (notably for cardiac biomarkers and relevant infectious disease), adequately stockpiled disease-specific supplies, and uninterrupted power supplies with adequate fuel for energy production, to optimise performance and 'fast track' emergency patient care during future disasters. |
| | The available POCT provided some capacity for diagnostic testing, but reagents (particularly those for diabetes care) were quickly depleted. | Relating to diabetes specifically, Cefalu *et al.* (2006) stated 'in the future, a stockpile of diabetes-related supplies, pre-packaged as diabetes care kits for shelters and individuals, should be created for rapid deployment after a disaster/evacuation'. |
| | There were as many as 100 000 patients with diabetes who were left stranded in the wake of Hurricane Katrina. Cefalu *et al.* (2006) stated: 'the pressing need for diabetes supplies in shelters, not in hospitals, combined with the size and scope of Katrina, caught the logistics chain 'off guard' and 'the abrupt change in dietary intake and/or composition with a lack of diabetes medication led to significant disruption in glycaemic control, putting patients at risk for both severe hyperglycaemia and hypoglycaemia'. | |

| Disaster event | Description of POCT services available at the time | Lessons learned |
|---|---|---|
| Hurricane Katrina, USA, 2006 (continued) | The health issues that were seen among people displaced by Hurricane Katrina to shelters were reviewed by Greenough *et al.* (2008). They found that 56% of the nearly 500 evacuees taking refuge in Red Cross Shelters in the two weeks after Katrina hit presented with a chronic disease (35% had hypertension, 17% had high cholesterol and 14% had diabetes). In addition, 35% of people arrived with symptoms requiring immediate medical intervention, including dehydration 12%, dyspnoea 12%, injury 9% and chest pain 9.7%. Another 15% arrived with symptoms of communicable disease potential (fever, diarrhoea). Clearly access to POCT would have been most useful in this setting. | |
| Earthquake in Port-au-Prince, in Haiti, 2010. | POCT played a significant role in patient care in the immediate aftermath of the earthquake. The earthquake severely damaged or destroyed more than 60% of Haiti's secondary and tertiary hospitals. Several field hospitals were established in the disaster response phase (with many using the i-STAT POCT device) but almost half of them had left the country 2 weeks after the event.<br><br>The University of Miami/Project Medishare (UMPS) established one of the largest field hospitals during the disaster response phase, and they had a suite of POCT devices including:<br>The Chempaq Diagnostics complete blood count device<br>The HemoCue Hb and WBC analysers for basic haematology measurements<br>The i-STAT, which was used to measure electrolytes, blood gases and lactate<br>Their POCT suite also contained the ability to perform basic urinalysis but their capacity to perform infectious disease testing was limited to rapid salivary HIV testing. | Although the i-STAT was in high demand during the disaster response, its use was compromised by the high temperatures experienced in the field. This limitation is not restricted to the i-STAT and pervades many other disaster POCT platforms. There is a critical need to develop POCT devices that are environmentally robust. |

**Table 31.3.** Examples of common clinical presentations in disaster events and POC test clusters to support these conditions

| Clinical presentation/condition | Examples of POC test clusters |
|---|---|
| Conduction and hydration | Electrolytes, ionised calcium |
| Acid base | Blood gases and related parameters |
| Cardiac injury/assessment | Electrocardiogram (ECG), troponin, CK-MB, myoglobin, BNP, lipids (Tran *et al.* 2012) |
| Sepsis | Lactate, procalcitonin, C-reactive protein, interleukins |
| Crush injury | Creatine kinase, myoglobin |
| Acute kidney injury | Urea, creatinine, NGAL (Tran *et al.* 2012) |
| Haemostasis and coagulation | Complete blood picture (CBP), haemoglobin, total white cell and differential count, platelets, APTT, INR, D-dimer |
| Infectious diseases/pathogen detection | HIV, dengue fever, malaria, cholera, tuberculosis (Tran *et al.* 2012) |
| Blood donor screening | HIV, hepatitis B and C |
| Chronic disease | Glucose, HbA1c, urea, creatinine, urine ACR, urinalysis, lipids |
| Acute abdominal injury | Ultrasound |
| Non-invasive tests for vital signs | $SO_2$ (pulse oximetry), $pCO_2$ (capnography), blood pressure, heart rate, respiratory rate, temperature |

- top 3 disaster pathogen priorities: methicillin-resistant *Staphylococcus aureus* (MRSA), *Vibrio cholera*, *Salmonella typhi*
- top blood stream pathogen priority: MRSA
- top 3 blood donor screening priorities: HIV1/2; hepatitis B and C
- top pandemic screening priorities: influenza A/B; H1N1, avian H5N1, SARS, Ebola, MERS-CoV and Zika.

## What might the 'perfect prototype' for a disaster POCT cache look like?

Kost and colleagues conducted a rigorous series of web-based surveys to identify the most desirable characteristics/specifications for a POC test system for use in urgent, emergency and disaster care (Brock *et al.* 2010; Kost *et al.* 2009, 2010, 2012b,c; Mecozzi *et al.* 2010). The surveys involved different stakeholder groups (disaster experts, subscribers to the journal *Point of Care* and members of the American Association of Clinical Chemistry; $n = 339$) and used visual logistics (graphics and pictorial images) to facilitate ease of response.

Table 31.5 summarises findings from the survey, as well as from other related literature, on the 'ideal' POCT device for use in disasters.

## Which POCT devices currently fill the niche for use in disasters and what gaps still remain?

Many countries are developing POCT 'caches', 'laboratory-in-a-backpack', 'mobile POCT packs' or 'mobile POCT laboratories' (Fig. 31.3) for tailored use in disaster

**Table 31.4.** POC tests and test profiles most needed in specific disaster events (Source: Table prepared by Dr Ian Marr, Royal Darwin Hospital)

| Specific disaster event | Main clinical presentations seen | POC tests/clusters most needed for first response |
|---|---|---|
| Bushfire | Smoke inhalation, CO poisoning, burns, cyanide poisoning | Blood gases, lactate, CO testing (carboxy-hemoglobin level), electrolytes |
| Earthquake | Crush injuries, rhabdomyolysis, skin and soft tissue infections (MRO), haemorrhage | Troponin, CK-MB, myoglobin, C-reactive protein, lactate, procalcitonin, haemoglobin |
| Flood | Diarrhoeal illness (cholera, salmonella, pathogenic E. coli); leptospirosis; skin and soft tissue injuries (MRO); arboviral illness (dengue, RRV, malaria); melioidosis (SE Asia) | Electrolytes, blood gases, lactate, leptospirosis, dengue, malaria, blood glucose |
| Tsunami | Aspiration/near drowning; Skin and soft tissue infections – high rates of MRO (MRSA, *Acinetobacter* spp., *Aeromonas* spp., *Burkholderia* spp. [melioidosis]) plus invasive fungal infection; Trauma/contusion/blood loss | Blood gases, haemoglobin, platelets, INR, APTT, white cell count and differential, electrolytes, C-reactive protein |

Note: MRO = multidrug resistant organisms; MRSA = methicillin-resistant *Staphylococcus aureus*

Table 31.5. Design features for the 'perfect' POCT device prototype

| Parameter | 'Ideal' features |
|---|---|
| Size and weight | Handheld (highest preference), lightweight, highly portable, and simple to use (with a minimum number of manual steps). |
| Power | Minimal power requirements; ideally battery operation with backup. |
| Format | Flexible modular formats capable of performing multiple test profiles across the clinical chemistry, haematology, infectious disease and drugs of abuse suites of tests; to enable modules to be assembled according to the clinical needs for specific types of disaster. |
| Sample matrix | Whole blood should be the preferred testing matrix for chemistry and haematology tests. |
| Sample collection | Direct drawing of blood into a disposable test cassette is preferable to the use of a vacutainer tube for sample collection. |
| Reagents | Reagents need to be usable in environmental extremes; and ideally be inexpensive, able to be stored at room temperature (rather than refrigerated), self-contained and readily disposable. |
| Quality testing | Device should feature as many in-built quality checks as possible (to reduce the need for wet QC and PT quality testing processes). |
| Robustness | Environmentally robust; able to withstand the extremes of temperature, humidity and altitude often encountered in a field disaster. |
| Connectivity | Device should have connectivity capability (including wireless) to facilitate and maximise the flow of knowledge and information about patient care during a disaster response (Yu *et al.* 2010). |
| Waste disposal | Device should store all the biohazard waste in a disposable test cassette. |

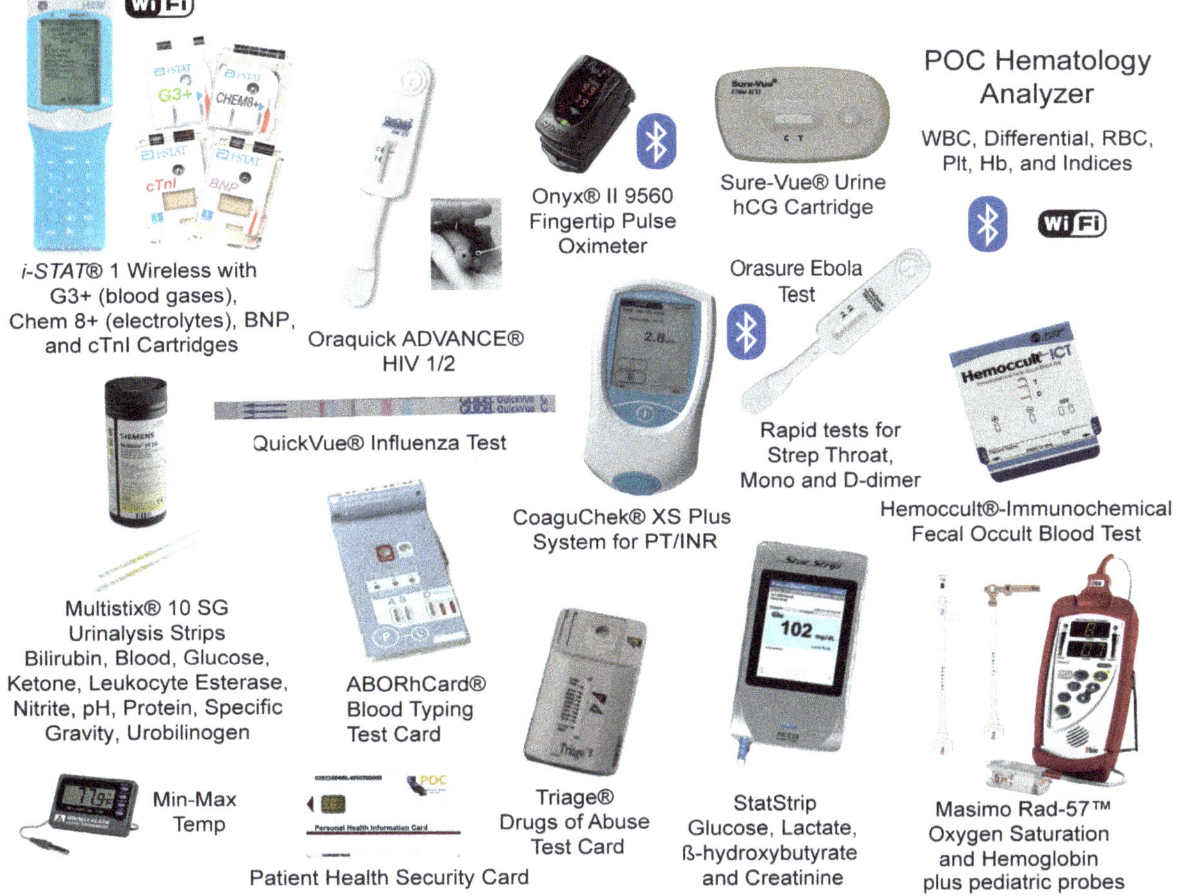


**Fig. 31.3.** POC tests currently recommended for the cache used by US Disaster Medical Assistance Teams (DMATs) and other response teams. (Source: Kost and Curtis (2015), page 423. Modified and reproduced with permission from Professor Gerald Kost)

**Table 31.6.** Selected findings of the effects of temperature and humidity stresses on POC test performance (Source: modified and updated with permission from Kost and Curtis 2015, pp. 298–300)

| Author | Analyte (and system) tested | Environmental stress | Duration of stress | Experimental design | Main findings |
|---|---|---|---|---|---|
| Louie *et al.* 2009 | Glucose test strips, blood gas cartridges (devices were not specified) | Static stress at temperatures of –21°C and +40°C | Up to 4 weeks for glucose strips and up to 72 h for blood gas cartridges | Glucose test strips were heat-stressed on a 40°C water bath and cold-stressed in a –21°C freezer. Frozen glucose strips were also tested after thawing to RT. Blood gas cartridges were heat- and cold-stressed in static conditions. | Heated glucose test strips and blood gas cartridges yielded elevated results. Frozen glucose test strips gave depressed results. Frozen glucose test strips that were thawed recovered partial performance in 2 of 3 blood glucose meters used. Frozen blood gas cartridges failed. |
| Ferguson *et al.* 2012 | Blood gas, electrolytes, glucose and haematocrit (on epoc test cards) | Cards stressed with temperature profile (from –5°C to +20°C) | Repeated for a total of 4 weeks | Test cards were placed in an environmental testing chamber simulating dynamic environmental conditions following the 2011 Great East Japan Earthquake. Thermally stressed test cards and control test cards were evaluated in pairs using three levels of QC material at stress durations of 24, 72, 168 (1 week) and 672 h (4 weeks). | Epoc test cards were largely unaffected by the simulated dynamic cold conditions. Temperature and humidity stresses on epoc test cards produced no statistically significant differences between stress and control analyte measurement for each QC (apart from sodium, potassium and $PO_2$ for the level 3 QC). |
| Tang *et al.* 2012 | QC solutions for blood glucose (measured by two glucose-oxidase blood glucose meter systems – StatStrip and Accuchek) | Temperature: 20°C to 45°C. Humidity: 31–96% | Up to 4 weeks | QC solutions were placed in an environmental chamber simulating conditions during Hurricane Katrina. Solutions stressed for durations of 24, 72, 168 (1 week), 336 (2 weeks), and 672 h (4 weeks) were evaluated at a temperature of 23°C and humidity of 90.6%. Those stressed for durations of 8, 32, 80, 172, 344, and 680 h were evaluated at a temperature of 45°C and humidity of 31.0%. | Dynamic stresses affected the performance of QC solutions and, consequently, results given by the two glucose meter systems (GMS). For GMS1, glucose median paired differences (stressed v. control) decreased significantly for QC levels 1 and 3 after 8 h and increased for level 1 after 336 and 344 h. For solutions tested on GMS2, median paired differences in QC reagents were decreased for both levels at each time point tested at 45°C. |

| Author | Analyte (and system) tested | Environmental stress | Duration of stress | Experimental design | Main findings |
|---|---|---|---|---|---|
| Louie *et al.* 2013 | CK-MB, myoglobin, cardiac troponin I, BNP, D-dimer (measured by multiplex test cassettes) | Temperature: 20–33.9°C. Humidity: 10–79% | Up to 4 weeks | Cardiac biomarker cards were stressed in an environmental chamber using a temperature and humidity profile simulating dynamic flight and ground environmental conditions during a rescue from Hawaii to the Marshall Islands and back. Paired measurements between stressed v. control cassettes at 7 time points (4 during flight and 3 on ground). | Despite moderate short-term temperature elevations, environmental stress conditions led to false negative cardiac troponin and BNP results. Cardiac troponin results from stressed cassettes differed significantly from control (at three timepoints [one flight and two ground]) at concentrations greater than 90 ng/L. BNP from stressed cassettes differed significantly from control at concentrations greater than 108 pg/mL. |
| Lam *et al.* 2014 | Glucose test strips and meters | Exposed to mean relative humidity of 83% and temperature of 42°C | Up to 60 min | Stressed and unstressed glucose meters and strips were tested with spiked blood samples (40 measurements per time point for each of 4 trials) after 15, 30, 45 and 60 min of exposure. | Stressed meters and test strips produced elevated results, with stressed meter bias up to 18% and stressed test strip bias up to 12%. The aggregate stress effect on meter and strips yielded a positive bias of 30% after 15 min. |
| Truong *et al.* 2014 | Glucose and lactate test strips packaged in foil and vials | Exposed to mean relative humidity of 97% | Up to 168 h | Stressed strips removed at defined time points and tested in pairs with unstressed strips using whole blood samples spiked to three glucose concentrations (n = 20 paired measurements per level). | Stressed glucose and lactate strip results differed significantly from unstressed strips; mean glucose paired difference up to 12.5 mg/dL and mean lactate bias –0.2 mmol/L.<br>Both packaging designs protected glucose and lactate strips for at least 1 week of high humidity stress. |

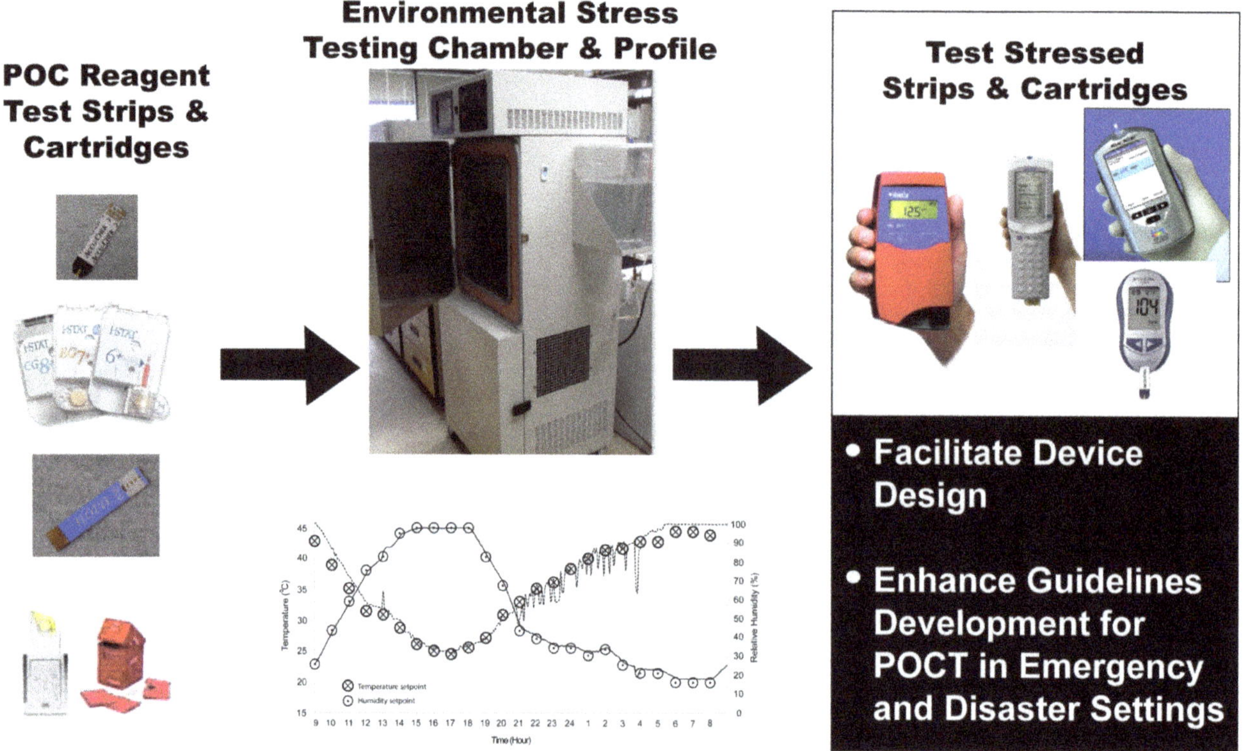


**Fig. 31.4.** The environmental stress testing workflow. (Source: Louie *et al.* (2012). Reproduced with permission from Professor Gerald Kost)

scenarios based on the evidence-based research summarised above.

In the USA, various basic and advanced caches of POCT devices have been developed for use by first responders 'in high crisis' need (Kost *et al.* 2011) and these are been continually refined and customised (Curtis *et al.* 2015; Hoe *et al.* 2015).

### Limitations and barriers to the use of POCT in disaster scenarios

Most POCT devices, reagents and quality materials are designed for use in a controlled laboratory or hospital environment where 'room temperature' conditions (at ~20–23°C) are the norm. Most devices therefore have operating temperature ranges of between 18 and 30°C. Similarly, reagents and quality materials are designed to be transported, stored and used within controlled conditions, generally 'refrigerated' (at around 2–8°C). In a disaster scenario where hospital power sources may be inoperable and extreme environmental conditions (of temperature, humidity and/or altitude) may be experienced in field conditions, POCT devices are often stretched beyond their operable limits and may fail. This is a scenario disaster response teams can ill afford, because they urgently test and triage large numbers of severely injured casualties.

To assure POC test systems (devices, reagents and quality materials) are 'fit for purpose' in a disaster, they need to be rigorously tested under both static and dynamic stress conditions and their limitations need to be well documented and understood by both medical scientists and disaster care workers. Numerous studies conducted over the past decade to examine the ability of POCT devices to withstand the environmental extremes encountered in disaster/emergency scenarios are summarised in Louie *et al.* (2015). Most of this work has been conducted using environmental stress testing chambers (Fig. 31.4) and has focussed on glucose meters, but also includes blood gases and cardiac markers. Table 31.6 summarises selected findings of the effects of temperature and humidity stresses on POC test performance.

As well as devices, innovation in the design of transporting receptacles to minimise vibration and shock and maximise thermoregulation is also required (Rust *et al.* 2012, 2015). The challenge for manufacturers is to improve the durability of POCT devices to withstand a broad range of environmental conditions without compromising the analytical quality of testing.

## CONCLUSIONS

The clinical utility and capability of POCT in disaster medicine will only be maximised if the following principles are adhered to:

- Needs assessment surveys are undertaken to inform the development of new, innovative POCT devices and test systems.
- POC technologies and test clusters specific to the disaster type or pandemic event are developed and, for the latter, molecular diagnostics with flexible choices of bacterial or viral targets of detection are needed.
- POCT devices and reagent systems are clinically validated in field situations and are environmentally robust (confirmed through the use of static and dynamic stress testing).
- POCT is seamlessly integrated within local or regional networks to ensure preparedness and resilience and have a workforce capacity 'at the ready'.

## ACKNOWLEDGEMENT

Dr Ian Marr, Royal Darwin Hospital, is thanked for his input to Table 31.4, while Dr Nick Coatsworth, Executive Director of the National Critical Care and Trauma Response Centre, Darwin, is thanked for his constructive commentary on disaster management.

## REFERENCES

Andress K (2010) Healthcare facility preparedness. In *International Disaster Nursing.* (Eds R Powers and E Daily) pp. 13–28. Cambridge University Press, Washington DC, USA.

Arbon P (2010) Applying lessons learned to the Haiti earthquake response. *Australasian Emergency Nursing Journal* **13**, 4–6. doi:10.1016/j.aenj.2010.02.003

Brock T, Mecozzi D, Sumner S, Kost G (2010) Evidence-based point-of-care tests and device designs for disaster preparedness. *American Journal of Disaster Medicine* **5**, 285–294.

Brown SM, Andrews D (2013) After the disaster. Sustaining quality point-of-care testing in a resource-poor environment. *Point of Care* **12**, 23–26. doi: 10.1097/POC.0b013e318265f773

Cefalu W, Blonde L, Smith S, Fonesca V (2006) The hurricane Katrina aftermath and its impact on diabetes care. *Diabetes Care* **29**, 158–160. doi:10.2337/diacare.29.01.06.dc05-2006

Curtis CM, Louie RF, Kost GJ (2015) The current and future design of point of care in national disaster caches. In *Global Point-of-Care – Strategies for Disasters, Emergencies, and Public Health Resilience.* (Eds G Kost and C Curtis) pp. 413–432. AACC Press, Washington DC, USA.

Ferguson WJ, Vy J, Louie RF, Zhou M, Curtis C, Tang CS, *et al.* (2012) Preliminary evaluation of a point-of-care blood gas-electrolyte analyser potentially robust in cold during emergencies and disasters. *Point of Care* **11**, 152–156. doi:10.1097/POC.0b013e318265f3a3

FitzGerald GJ, Aitken P, Davis ER, Daily E (2010) Disaster recovery. In *International Disaster Nursing.* (Eds R Powers and E Daily) pp. 495–511. Cambridge University Press, New York, USA.

Greenough P, Lappi M, Hsu E, Fink S, Hsieh Y-H, Vu A, *et al.* (2008) Burden of disease and health status among Hurricane Katrina – displaced persons in shelters: a population-based cluster sample. *Annals of Emergency Medicine* **51**, 426–432. doi:10.1016/j.annemergmed.2007.04.004

Guha-Sapir D, Hoyois P, Below R (2015a) *Annual Disaster Statistical Review 2014, the Numbers and Trends.* Centre for Research on the Epidemiology of Disasters, <http://cred.be/download/download.php?file=sites/default/files/ADSR_2014.pdf>.

Guha-Sapir D, Below R, Hoyois P (2015b) *The CRED/OFDA International Disaster Database.* Université Catholique de Louvain, Brussels, <http://www.emdat.be/disaster_trends/index.html>.

Hoe J, Louie R, Truong A-T, Curtis C, Abraham A, Kost G (2015) Enabling mobile medical response with a point-of-care pack. In *Global Point-of-Care – Strategies for Disasters, Emergencies, and Public Health Resilience.* (Eds G Kost and C Curtis) pp. 433–438. AACC Press, Washington DC, USA.

Kost GJ (2006) Newdemics, public health, small-world networks, and point-of-care testing. *Point of Care* **5**, 138–144. doi:10.1097/01.poc.0000232581.36762.21

Kost GJ (2012) Theory, principles, and practice of optimizing point-of-care small-world networks. *Point of Care* **11**, 96–101. doi:10.1097/POC.0b013e31825a25b5

Kost GJ, Curtis CM (Eds) (2015) *Global Point of Care – Strategies for Disasters, Emergencies, and Public Health Resilience.* AACC Press, Washington DC, USA.

Kost GJ, Tran N, Tuntideelert M, Kulrattanamaneeporn S, Peungposop N (2006) Katrina, the tsunami, and point-of-care testing. *American Journal of Clinical Pathology* **126**, 513–520. doi:10.1309/NWU5E6T0L4PFCBD9

Kost GJ, Hale K, Brock T, Louie R, Gentile N, Kitano T, *et al.* (2009) Point-of-care testing for disasters: needs assessment, strategic planning, and future design. *Clinics in Laboratory Medicine* **29**, 583–605. doi:10.1016/j.cll.2009.07.014

Kost GJ, Kost L, Suwanyangyuen A, Cheema S (2010) Emergency cardiac biomarkers and point-of-care testing: optimizing acute coronary syndrome care using small-world networks in rural settings. *Point of Care* **9**, 53–64. doi:10.1097/POC.0b013e3181d9d45c

Kost GJ, Sakaguchi A, Curtis C, Tran N, Katip P, Louie R (2011) Enhancing crisis standards of care using innovative point-of-care testing. *American Journal of Disaster Medicine* **6**, 351–368. doi:10.5055/ajdm.2011.0074

Kost GJ, Katip P, Vinitwatanakhun C (2012a) Diagnostic testing strategies for health care delivery during the Great Bangkok flood and other weather disasters. *Point of Care* **11**, 191–199. doi:10.1097/POC.0b013e318265f255

Kost GJ, Mecozzi D, Brock T, Curtis C (2012b) Assessing point-of-care device specifications and needs for pathogen detection in emergencies and disasters. *Point of Care* **11**, 119–125. doi:10.1097/POC.0b013e31825a25cb

Kost GJ, Katip P, Curtis C (2012c) Strategic point-of-care requirements of hospitals and public health for preparedness in regions at risk. *Point of Care* **11**, 114–118. doi:10.1097/POC.0b013e31825a2442

Lam M, Louie RF, Curtis CM, Ferguson WJ, Vy JH, Truong AT, *et al.* (2014) Short-term thermal-humidity shock affects point-of-care glucose testing: implications for health professionals and patients. *Journal of Diabetes Science and Technology* **8**, 83–88. doi:10.1177/1932296813514325

Louie R, Hindson B, Tran N, Gentile N, Kost G (2008) The grand point-of-care challenge. *Point of Care* **7**, 105–107. doi:10.1097/POC.0b013e318182f9c4

Louie RF, Sumner SL, Belcher S, Mathew R, Tran NK, Kost GJ (2009) Thermal stress and point-of-care testing performance: suitability of glucose test strips and blood gas cartridges for disaster response. *Disaster Medicine and Public Health Preparedness* **3**, 13–17. doi:10.1097/DMP.0b013e3181979a06

Louie RF, Ferguson WJ, Curtis CM, Vy JH, Tang CS, Kost GJ (2013) Effects of environmental conditions on point-of-care cardiac biomarker test performance during a simulated rescue: implications for emergency and disaster response. *American Journal of Disaster Medicine* **8**, 205–212. doi:10.5055/ajdm.2013.0126

Louie RF, Ferguson WJ, Sumner SL, Yu JN, Curtis CM, Kost GJ (2012) Effects of dynamic temperature and humidity stress on point-of-care glucose testing for disaster care. *Disaster Medicine and Public Health Preparedness* **6**, 232–240. doi.org/10.1001/dmp.2012.42

Louie R, Ferguson W, Curtis C, Truong A-H, Lam MH, Kost G (2015) The impact of environmental stress on diagnostic testing and implications for patient care during crisis response. In *Global Point-of-Care – Strategies for Disasters, Emergencies, and Public Health Resilience.* (Eds G Kost and C Curtis) pp. 293–306. AACC Press, Washington DC, USA.

Mann PA (2015) Describing a Point-of-Care Coordinator's potential role in disasters and complex emergencies. In *Global Point-of-Care – Strategies for Disasters, Emergencies, and Public Health Resilience.* (Eds G Kost and C Curtis) pp. 347–356. AACC Press, Washington DC, USA.

Mayner L, Arbon P (2015) Defining disaster: the need for harmonisation of terminology. *Australasian Journal of Disaster and Trauma Studies* **19**, 21–26.

Mecozzi D, Brock T, Tran N, Hale K, Kost G (2010) Evidence-based point-of-care device design for emergency and disaster care. *Point of Care* **9**, 65–69. doi:10.1097/POC.0b013e3181d9d47a

Rust M, Carlson N, Nichols J (2012) A thermo-modulating container for transport and storage of glucose meters in a cold weather environment. *Point of Care* **11**, 157–160. doi:10.1097/POC.0b013e318265f3bb

Rust MJ, Njoroge SW, Nichols J, Louie R (2015) Feasibility of a thermomodulating container to protect devices and reagents from adverse weather conditions. In *Global Point-of-Care – Strategies for Disasters, Emergencies, and Public Health Resilience.* (Eds G Kost and C Curtis) pp. 317–326. AACC Press, Washington DC, USA.

Shephard M, Halls H, Motta L (2015a) Online Point-of-Care Coordinator Graduate Certificate program for global point-of-care testing. In *Global Point-of-Care – Strategies for Disasters, Emergencies, and Public Health Resilience.* (Eds G Kost and C Curtis) pp. 341–346. AACC Press, Washington DC, USA.

Shephard M, Spaeth B, Motta L, Shephard A (2015b) Point-of-care testing in Australia: practical advantages and benefits of community resiliency for improving outcomes. In *Global Point-of-Care – Strategies for Disasters, Emergencies, and Public Health Resilience.* (Eds G Kost and C Curtis) pp. 527–535. AACC Press, Washington DC, USA.

Tang CS, Ferguson WJ, Louie RF, Vy JTH, Sumner SL, Kost G (2012) Ensuring quality control of point-of-care technologies: effects of dynamic temperature and humidity stresses on glucose quality control solutions. *Point of Care* **11**, 147–151. doi:10.1097/POC.0b013e318265f38a

Tran N, Godwin Z, Bockhold J, Kost G (2012) Point-of-care testing at the disaster-emergency-critical care interface. *Point of Care* **11**, 180–183. doi:10.1097/POC.0b013e318265f7d9

Truong AT, Louie RF, Vy JH, Curtis CM, Ferguson WJ, Lam M, *et al.* (2014) Effects of humidity on foil and vial packaging to preserve glucose and lactate test strips for disaster readiness. *Disaster Medicine and Public Health Preparedness* **8**, 51–57. doi:10.1017/dmp.2014.13

World Bank (2013) *Building Resilience: Integrating Climate and Disaster Risk into Development, Lessons from World Bank Group Experience.* The World Bank, Washington DC, USA, <https://www.documentcloud.org/documents/835955-wbg-2013-building-resilience.html>.

Yu J, Brock T, Mecozzi D, Tran N, Kost G (2010) Future connectivity for disaster and emergency point of care. *Point of Care* **9**, 185–192. doi:10.1097/POC.0b013e3181fc95ee

# 32 Point-of-care testing and extreme environments – the Australian Antarctic Division

*Roland Watzl and Jeff Ayton*

**Summary**

Antarctica is one of the most remote places on Earth. Providing medical care, including point-of-care testing (POCT) services in such an extreme environment provides many unique challenges. The fact that each station in Antarctica has to be entirely self-sufficient for the 8 months of complete winter isolation dictates the complexity of the medical support model required. The Australian Antarctic Division (AAD) has nonetheless developed a robust and highly capable POCT diagnostic system to help with medical care in this extreme environment. Our system provides POCT capability on the ground at research stations, in the field, on ships and on aircraft. This POCT system has been field proven and consistently delivers high grade diagnostic information that will influence clinical decision making and decrease diagnostic uncertainty.

## A BRIEF OVERVIEW OF POLAR MEDICINE

There are few places on Earth as remote as Antarctica. There is no permanent population on Earth's southernmost continent. Personnel providing year-round staffing of the numerous international research stations scattered across Antarctica do so only on a temporary basis. During winter, these stations are physically cut off from the rest of the world, owing to extreme weather and pack ice conditions. Access in summer is limited by difficult logistics. Little appears to have changed in this regard in the last 100 years. There have been great advancements with modern technology, yet Antarctica's extreme environment still presents great challenges. Thus humans living and working in Antarctica remain some of the most isolated people on Earth. It is considered easier and quicker to get back to civilisation from the International Space Station than it is to do so from East Antarctica during winter.

Australia has stewardship of 42% of the continent under the Antarctic Treaty system (Fig. 32.1). Australia has had a permanent presence in the deep icy South for 60 years now, ever since Sir Douglas Mawson established the first permanent Australian base at Mawson in 1954. This presence is administered by the AAD, part of the Department of the Environment, based in Hobart, Tasmania.

Providing medical care in such an extreme environment provides many unique challenges. For the last 50 years the AAD has had its own in-house medical support delivered by the Polar Medicine Unit (PMU) or its predecessors, providing holistic medical support to Australia's endeavours in Antarctica and the Southern Ocean. This medical support encompasses medical screening of all expeditioners travelling south, full medical logistic support, as well as recruitment, training and 24/7

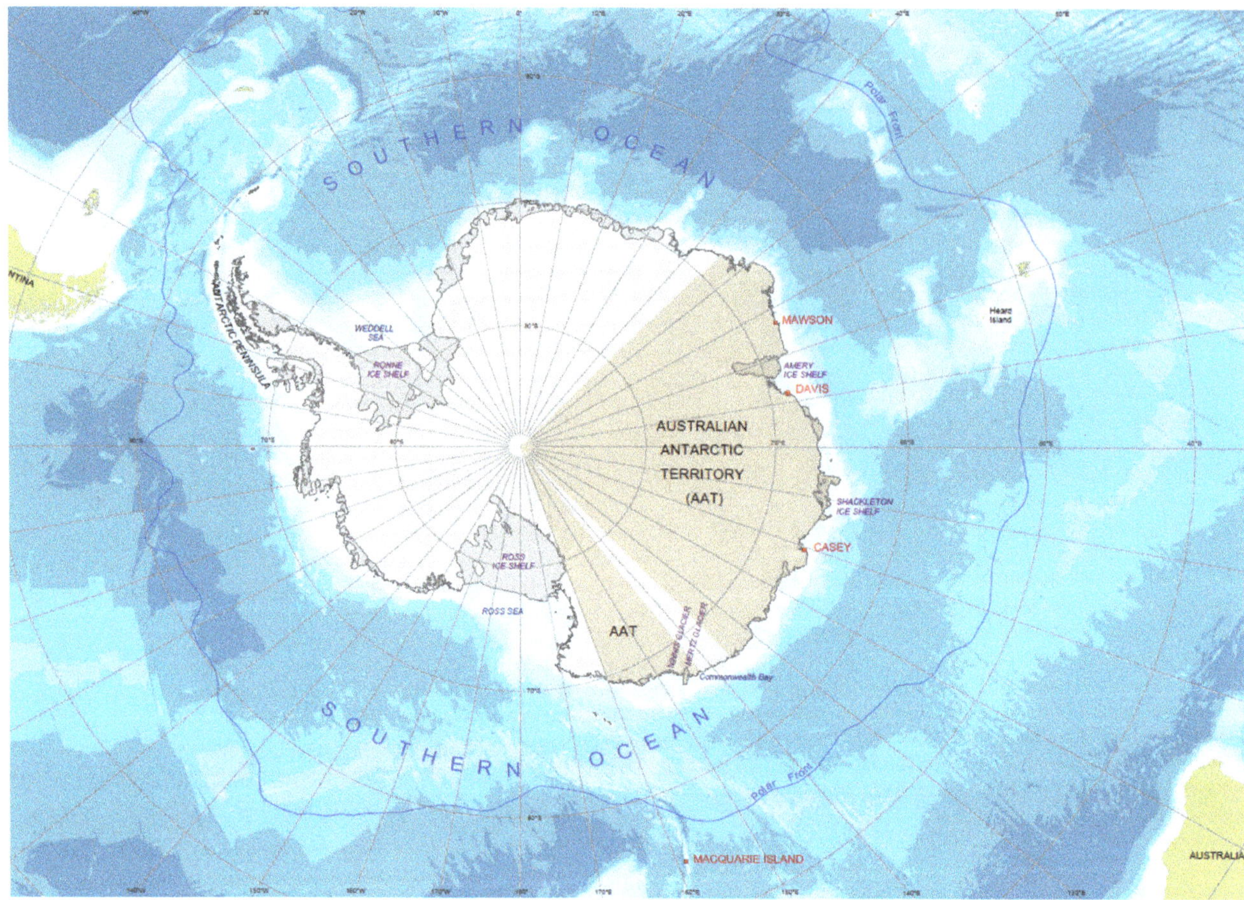


**Fig. 32.1.** Australian Antarctic Territory. (Source: Map courtesy of the Australian Antarctic Division ©Commonwealth of Australia 2015)

telemedicine support for all expedition doctors; these doctors provide the medical support to the expedition at the coalface, be they land or water based or airborne. The expedition doctors are usually generalist practitioners, rather than specialists, and receive critical upskilling before deployment. They are trained and supported to be able to deal with any medical eventuality that might occur. They work in a single doctor model without the on-site support of other trained medical or paramedical staff.

At a time when many Antarctic programs are curtailing their medical capabilities, Australia continues to provide medical support at a high level and within a paradigm where medical evacuation is never first line management. The medical support provided by the PMU is arguable the benchmark against which other support models can be measured. The PMU medical support model has been fine-tuned with the collective Antarctic corporate knowledge and experience gained from providing medical support in the most extreme environment on Earth for 60 years.

This Antarctic medical support model is considered a robust, efficient and effective model from which other extreme environments, for example Space, have sought to learn from and implement similar (e.g. when planning long-term exploratory missions to Mars). Antarctica is considered a valid space analogue with 'real people, under real hazard, undertaking real work, in real isolation without hope of winter evacuation.' (Campbell *et al.* 2004; Lugg and Shepanek 1999; Marchant *et al.* 2002; Nicogossian *et al.* 2006).

## HOW TO DESIGN A POCT SYSTEM FOR AN EXTREME ENVIRONMENT SUCH AS ANTARCTICA

When designing a medical service for any environment, it is always useful to begin by considering what level of service is required and then to determine what level is realistically achievable. This applies to the overall medical

**Table 32.1.** Real-life issues in working in the harsh Antarctic environment

| **Constraints and difficult realities – lessons learned previously** |
|---|
| 1. Limited annual budget |
| 2. Small clinical case load – medical capability provided in case it is needed not because it is needed – low frequency of use – therefore small quantities of supply only – must be able to split consumables for various stations or order in small quantities. |
| 3. Training time for doctors is limited by availability, budget and effectiveness |
| 4. Minimal technical support in Antarctica |
| 5. Extremely restricted supply chain:<br>• environmental extremes, no supply possible for at least 8 months per year<br>• storage and transport difficulties – room temperature storage preferable<br>• servicing issues<br>• need for redundancy |
| 6. Hostile operating environment – constant vibration on ships, highly corrosive maritime environment, potential cold or freeze exposure, high static electricity in Antarctic medical facilities |
| 7. 'Don't put all eggs in one basket' – need back-up systems (critical systems space analogue) – e.g. we provide two different devices to enable haemoglobin and haematocrit measurements, which are critical in determining clinical need for blood transfusion |
| 8. Single doctor model:<br>• solo doctor must perform all tasks required for patient care (generalist 'jack of all trades' but not 'specialist in all')<br>• conflicting priorities in emergency<br>• often minimal technical knowledge |
| 9. Small clinical case load thus:<br>• medical capability provided 'in case' it is needed not because it is needed<br>• low skill retention<br>• POCT devices will spend most of their life in storage – devices requiring daily use/maintenance to ensure ongoing functioning will not reliably work in our environment and will be very difficult to support with a high chance of being unserviceable on the rare occasions where they might be needed urgently (larger wet chemistry analysers are problematic)<br>• only need small quantities of supply for consumables – must be able to split larger units of supply. |

support model, as well as the individual components of that model, including POCT.

For example, the fact that each station group in Antarctica has to be entirely self-sufficient for the 8 months of complete winter isolation dictates the complexity of the medical support model required. However, the actual complexity practically achievable is tempered by the lessons learned previously from the difficult realities inherent in Antarctic operations (Table 32.1). These difficulties include constant annual turn-around of expedition doctors providing medical services (who require training every year), limited budget, difficult logistics and a light clinical workload.

Diagnostic capability is of great importance in providing medical support at any level. The PMU conducted a major review of its laboratory diagnostic capability in 2003/04, which resulted in its current diagnostic system. The (seemingly exponential) proliferation and rapid advancement in POCT technology over the last 20 years has greatly benefitted the Antarctic medical support model. One could of course argue that any diagnostic test done in Antarctica is POCT. All diagnostic tests in Antarctica are essentially performed near the individual at the time of the encounter, with the sole purpose of the result being that it will influence clinical decision making and decrease diagnostic uncertainty. In Antarctica, the operator performing all POCT is usually the doctor.

For the AAD, the overriding principle of diagnostic test selection is 'the right test at the right time for the right condition for the right clinical decision'. This principle is the crux of the ARTS of Remote Medicine (McConnell *et al.* 2007). It is important to note here that in this

A Casey Lab 1973

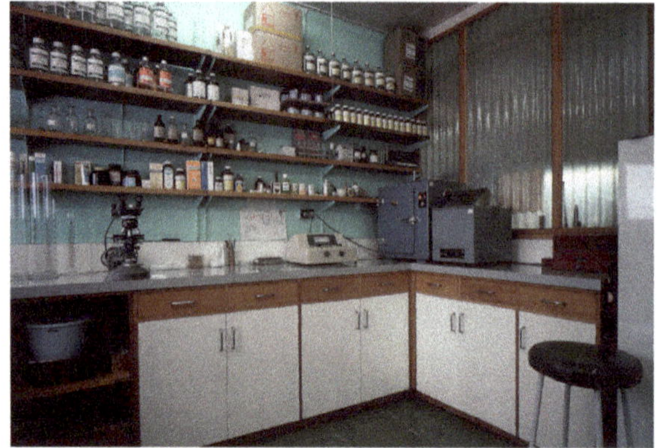

B Casey Lab 2014

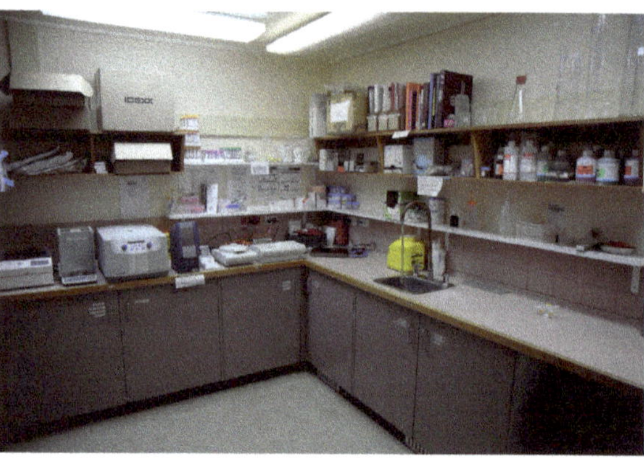

**Fig. 32.2.** Casey station laboratory in 1973 (left) and in 2015 (right). (Source: Photos courtesy of the Australian Antarctic Division ©Commonwealth of Australia 2015).

context a definitive diagnosis in the setting of the extreme environment may never be possible and the results of any diagnostic test are never used in isolation but only ever considered as part of the larger clinical picture, which evolves over time.

Prior to 2003/04, diagnostic capability in Australia's Antarctic program was limited by the paucity of available POC tests and devices (Fig. 32.2). There were very few off-the-shelf POC tests. This at times meant that materials and tests were improvised and based on basic, but robust, third-world medical principles (King 1976). There are anecdotal accounts of improvising a Ziehl-Nielsen stain using battery acid. Some tests were used off-label. There was reliance on product instructions and external protocols that often are written for mainland laboratories. Some diagnostic apparatus in the past, while of superior accuracy, ultimately turned out to be not user friendly in the Antarctic context. Although all capability supplied by the PMU first must undergo critical consideration, inspection and field trial (Kibby and Sullivan 1997), it is important to realise that sometimes only prolonged use will demonstrate shortcomings in an extreme environment, given low patient activity.

The major review undertaken specifically addressed the challenge of designing a revised diagnostic system for Antarctic use with specific reference to known Antarctic constraints and realities, as detailed in Table 32.1, and meeting our unique requirements listed in Table 32.2. Importantly, we accept that while a test may not be perfect, it will nonetheless help to reduce diagnostic uncertainty when applied in appropriate clinical context; for example, a positive qualitative D-dimer test result is not as clinically useful as a negative result and the malaria POC test we use is very good at picking up any type of malaria present (good pan-malarial sensitivity) but is not good at differentiating different types of malaria (sub-optimal specificity for sub-type).

### Reviewing patient population epidemiology and target population specific requirements

In contrast to the Arctic, there is no indigenous population in Antarctica. Visitors to Antarctica come from 20 nations or more via national Antarctic programs (Lugg and Ayton 2009). Additionally, there are visitors via Antarctic tourism, the majority of whom visit areas in the Antarctic Peninsula and the Ross Sea, rather than East Antarctica (where Australian stations are located).

All participants in Australia's Antarctic program are comprehensively medically screened to a high level before deployment. As a general rule, we do not accept anybody whose ongoing wellbeing is dependent on medication. All pre-existing medical conditions are carefully assessed. Being in control of the medical screening process importantly aids in the selection of diagnostic capability, because the medical support system is designed to support essentially fit and well individuals. However, although expeditioners with chronic medical conditions are generally not accepted, chronic medical conditions may develop while on expedition, which then must be diagnosed and monitored.

Table 32.2. Polar Medicine Unit requirements underpinning selection of a diagnostic test for use in Antarctica

| Required characteristics of a POC test used in Antarctica |
|---|
| 1. Aid/influence clinical decision making. The principle of 'the right test at the right time for the right condition for the right clinical decision' (The 'ARTS of Remote Medicine' principles apply) |
| 2. 'Allow sleep at night' – increase the expedition doctor's comfort zone/ avoid unnecessary surgical procedures |
| 3. Be simple to use, reliable and efficient (quick) – 'simplicity of design' |
| 4. Be reproducible and meaningful |
| 5. Be in tune with telemedicine service providers and external specialist networks |
| 6. Allow minimisation of resources/pharmaceutical use |
| 7. Be affordable (small quantities of supply required) |
| 8. Have adequate shelf-life |
| 9. Require only simple room temperature storage |
| 10. Be useful when applied in clinical context (sensitivity *v.* specificity/positive *v.* negative predictive value) |
| 11. Testing can be supported by quality control/proficiency testing wherever possible – we endeavour to meet Australian standards of care wherever possible. If a test has to be used after shelf-life has expired, then we provide 'off-label' quality assurance methods to ascertain that the test is still viable |
| 12. Have minimal environmental foot print |

The AAD has a computerised health register that has been logging data for all health events within Australia's Antarctic program since 1989 (King 1987; Sullivan *et al.* 1991). Analysis of this database, coded using the ICD-9 classification system (WHO 1977), shows that 'injury and poisoning' constitute 38% of the illness and injury burden; 41% of these are musculoskeletal injuries that go hand in hand with working in a high-risk 'slip and fall' environment (Lugg and Ayton 2009). Serious conditions are rare, but have significant implications when they do occur.

The AAD computerised health register also captures all procedures performed since 1989 using the WHO's International Classification of Procedures in Medicine (WHO 1978). This allows analysis of all POCT diagnostic procedures. This was used at the time of a major review of the AAD's diagnostic system in 2004. Fig. 32.3 shows a 10-year analysis of diagnostic tests performed.

It is important to note that the total number of diagnostic investigations was 810, or just 81 across the entire Antarctic program per year. This demonstrates the low

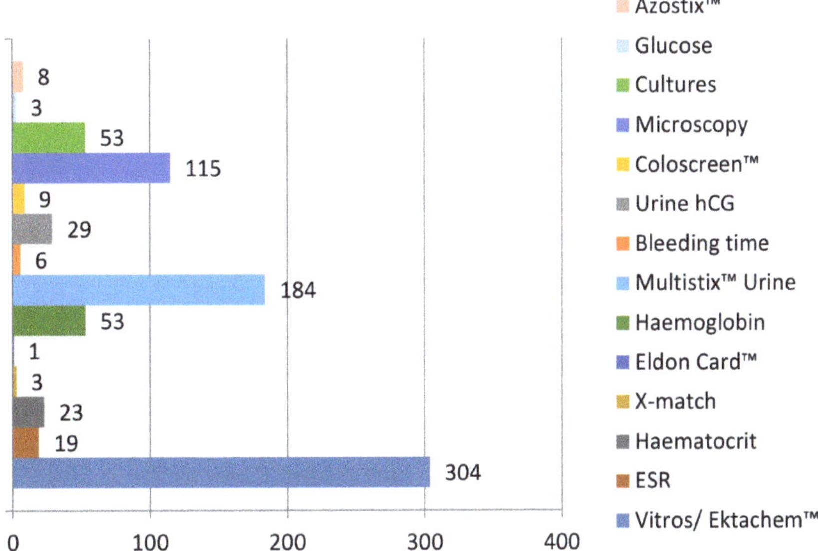


Fig. 32.3. Investigations performed by the Australian Antarctic Division laboratory, by type: 1993–2004 ($n = 810$).

clinical use of diagnostic testing. Little has changed since that time. The humble Multistix™ urine dipstick is probably one of the most useful and most commonly employed diagnostic tools in our setting. The apparent higher number of Ektachem™/Vitros (serum biochemistry) tests is artefactual because the Ektachem™/Vitros analyser is not able to run electrolytes or liver function tests as a single panel, but rather requires the operator to run an individual analysis for each of the constituent analytes (Kibby and Sullivan 1997). Thus a modern POCT device such as the Piccolo™ will analyse 11 analytes in a single test run, whereas this number would be counted as 11 tests when performed on the Ektachem™/Vitros system. Reviewing the above data with this in mind, the urine dipstick clearly holds first place in terms of usage, followed by a revised Ektachem™/Vitros.

## Reviewing basic general diagnostic requirements

Any serious medical condition that may result in shock (cardiogenic, hypovolaemic or septic) may result in multiple organ failure requiring intensive care management. Intensive care management requires monitoring of basic parameters to help deal with intra-venous fluid replacement in the absence of oral intake and organ failure (principally renal and hepatic). Any patient requiring ventilatory support requires blood gas monitoring in addition to basic parameter monitoring. Hence, irrespective of epidemiology or target population considerations, there is the general requirement for monitoring biochemical markers (electrolytes, urea and creatinine), liver function tests, blood gases and haematology parameters (haemoglobin as a minimum, but full differential blood count capability is highly preferable), as well as dipstick urine testing.

Having women of child-bearing age in any patient population also requires basic capacity to diagnose pregnancy (qualitative urine hCG testing) (Ayton 2006) and preferably also to help stage the pregnancy (quantitative serum hCG testing and/or ultrasound examination). In addition, ruling out ectopic pregnancy and assisting in the management of early trimester spontaneous miscarriage is important (using a combination of clinical examination, quantitative serum hCG measurement and ultrasound). Quantitative POCT measurement for hCG only became available in 2014 when Abbott released this test on the i-STAT®. As with all i-STAT® cartridges, a limiting factor is relatively short shelf-life.

## Reviewing the location specific clinical evidence base

Serious medical or surgical conditions in the Antarctic setting are rare, but consequences can be catastrophic. The AAD has extensive experience in managing serious medical conditions in the extremely remote environment where evacuation is not first line treatment (Pardoe 1965; Plowright 2000; Podkolinski and Semmens 1979, 1980; Priddy 1985). This experience critically shapes our selection of POCT.

With significant clinical evidence pertaining to medicine in our extremely remote environment, we have identified specific clinical conditions that have resulted in major clinical problems and sub-optimal clinical outcomes or programmatic impacts in our past experience. These specific conditions include: perforated peptic ulcers, gastrointestinal bleeding, tuberculosis, influenza outbreaks, meningitis and malaria. Consequently, we provide specific POC tests to help deal with diagnosis of these conditions, which also allow rationalisation of pharmaceutical resource use (Goldsmid and Sullivan 1994; Pardoe 1965; Plowright 2000; Podkolinski and Semmens 1979, 1980; Priddy 1985).

For example, using POCT to diagnose an underlying *Helicobacter pylori* infection allows prompt and efficient eradication of the underlying pathogen, optimises pharmaceutical use for symptom control (proton pump inhibitors) and prevents catastrophic complications from perforation of a peptic ulcer, which can cause peritonitis and may require urgent laparotomy and over-sewing of the ulcer with placement of an omental patch (Podkolinski and Semmens 1979, 1980). These potential outcomes, if prevented, can save life and mitigate additional complex medical procedures and therapy.

In the right clinical context, the ability to detect occult gastro-intestinal bleeding is also a critical decision-making tool that allows us to reduce the magnitude of diagnostic uncertainty. A positive test could potentially make the difference between staying in Antarctica and urgent repatriation (if at all possible).

There have been several occurrences in the past where a blood transfusion was required to treat haemorrhagic shock and ongoing internal bleeding. Historically, most of these have been due to gastrointestinal bleeding (Podkolinski and Semmens 1979, 1980; Watzl 2005a). Because there is no access to regular blood banking services in Antarctica, the AAD uses a 'walking' blood bank for this contingency. Although all participants in the Australian program will have a paper cross-match done before departure (i.e. they will have their Landsteiner, Rhesus and Kell groups determined and their blood will be tested for abnormal antibodies), not all potential patients in Antarctica will have a known blood type (e.g. tourists or participants in other international programs). Therefore we offer capability to: (i) rapidly confirm a paper cross match using the Eldon™ card (which allows determination of Landsteiner and Rhesus groups) and (ii) perform a complete forward and reverse cross match using the Bio-rad ID-2™ Gel Card microtyping system. The full cross-match capability is only achievable on Antarctic stations, while ships and field camps have to make do with the Eldon cards. All potential walking blood bank donors are screened before departure and again at the end of summer for the following potentially transmissible infectious agents: hepatitis B, C, HIV1/2, HTLV1/2 and syphilis. Additionally, we are in the process of implementing immunodiagnostic POCT for hepatitis and HIV serology to further help us confirm a safe donor pool contemporaneously with donation.

### Reviewing idiosyncratic medical conditions present in the target population/location

Hobart in Tasmania is Australia's Antarctic gateway. There are several medical conditions that pose specific risks to our patient population, which are the result of local (Australian and Tasmanian) as well as regional (South East Asia) public health considerations. Our diagnostic system is also designed to specifically deal with these risks.

We therefore:

- supplement influenza vaccination with influenza POCT, because Australia's influenza season coincides with early Austral summer activities in Antarctica
- have a specific protocol written for diagnosing and differentiating viral from bacterial meningitis (including off-label use of the urine dipstick test for rapid differentiation) because seasonal meningococcal outbreaks in Tasmania coincide with the Antarctic summer shipping season and with the majority of expeditioners passing through Hobart
- have specific protocols and capability for diagnosing malaria infection because our expeditioners can potentially be exposed and be at risk of infection with malaria while travelling/holidaying in warm South-East Asia before departing for the cold climate in Antarctica. We have had cases of acute malaria while on expedition in Antarctica in the past (Goldsmid and Sullivan 1994).

Given the apparent paradoxical occurrence of malaria, albeit imported, we have implemented latex agglutination POCT to supplement tele-microscopy ability. Blood film analysis can be technically challenging and requires review of micrographs by a trained specialist eye. The rapid immunodiagnostic POC test (BinaxNOW™ Malaria) on the other hand can use finger-prick blood sampling and reliably identifies *P. falciparum* infection; it will also identify the presence of any of the other three sub-types but not differentiate between them. In the extreme remote Antarctic clinical context, this is not a significant shortcoming and again the test is a useful tool that allows us to reduce the magnitude of diagnostic uncertainty, while not entirely removing it.

### Reviewing management of POCT services

There remains the practical reality of operating a POCT service in an extreme environment. There is a multitude of analytical devices on the market but there is little practical information on how they perform in an extreme environment. Larger bench-top analysers require technical support at a level unattainable in the extremely remote setting. Anything that is complex and time consuming to operate takes the single doctor away from patient care in the acute setting, creating a conflict of priority.

The findings following the coroner's inquest into the death of an Australian scientist at the United States Antarctic Program South Pole station in 2000 are instructive (Mervis 2009). The treating doctor's initial diagnosis may have been hampered by the inability to perform specific POCT. This testing would normally have been done on an Ektachem/Vitros™ analyser, but the device at the medical facility had developed a fault that required the treating doctor to re-calibrate the device every time it was turned back on. The fault was due to the failure of a lithium battery responsible for maintaining the device's memory after switching the machine off.

It is important to review likely opportunities to resupply, replenish and/or replace faulty equipment.

Consider the budget and do a cost–benefit analysis reviewing person-days on location, offsetting low patient numbers against the ability and cost of emergency repatriation/evacuation. While all diagnostic testing capability comes at a cost, it is important to put this into proper

Table 32.3. Determining the level of service required for an extreme environment

| Issues for consideration |
|---|
| 1. Review basic general diagnostic requirements (to cater for ubiquitous acute general medical and surgical conditions) |
| 2. Review your patient population's epidemiology and their specific requirements |
| 3. Review idiosyncratic medical conditions present in your target location/population |
| 4. Consider what patients need to be catered for outside of your target patient population |
| 5. Review the location specific medical evidence/database |
| 6. Consider your logistic constraints (ability to repatriate or evacuate patients, opportunities to resupply, replenish or replace faulty equipment); this determines in part the complexity that must or can be supported |
| 7. Consider your budget and do cost–benefit analysis (person-days on location, offsetting low patient numbers against high cost of emergency repatriation/evacuation) |
| 8. Consider operator training and ongoing support requirement |
| 9. Consider ongoing quality testing support for POCT (QC and PT) |

perspective. Averting an emergency medical evacuation also averts significant costs incurred with the retrieval. The immediate cost of a single emergency evacuation by ship from the extreme remoteness of Antarctica can easily exceed A$1 million. Although overall use of POCT may be low, operational cost savings are significant.

Strong consideration should be given to supporting POCT with quality control (QC) and proficiency testing (PT)/quality assurance. Many modern POC devices come with in-built QC. PT is more difficult to achieve in the extremely remote setting of Antarctica. The PMU has participated in PT programs run by the RCPA Quality Assurance Programs Pty Ltd for its benchtop biochemistry analysers for the last 10 years (currently the Piccolo™, previously the Ektachem/Vitros™). This program requires monthly PT specimen preparation and testing. Importantly, this activity ensures monthly use of the devices and confirmation of functionality, flagging technical issues early, and supporting critical evaluation of results obtained in an actual clinical emergency.

Table 32.3 summarises our considerations in designing a POCT system for an extreme environment.

## Limitations and barriers in delivering and implementing POCT in the extreme Antarctic setting

The extreme remoteness of Antarctica means that the accepted model of real world diagnostic support (via NATA accredited specialist laboratories) is a physical impossibility. Mainstream laboratory-grade instrumentation is largely unsupportable in the extreme Antarctic setting, as are frequent servicing requirements.

Software upgrades may need to be delayed to allow use of expired test materials where shelf-life is short and when new supplies cannot be provided because of limited logistic opportunities and during winter isolation. This is particularly true of a device like the i-STAT®. i-STAT® cartridges have relatively short shelf-lives and the device itself requires software updates every 6 months. When this happens during winter in Antarctica, updating the software would immediately render the device inoperable because it will no longer allow use of (recently) expired test cartridges. In our experience, cartridges continue to give reliable results well past their expiry dates if stored correctly.

'Outside the box' approaches are frequently required in an extreme environment, including off-label use of devices in an attempt to reduce diagnostic uncertainty yet never eliminating it.

An example of off-label use of POCT in Antarctica is urine dipstick testing for determining the pH of ocular fluid after chemical eye splash injuries. Urine dipsticks can also be used to help diagnose bacterial peritonitis (Farahmand *et al.* 2013) or the rapid differentiation of viral and bacterial meningitis in CSF fluid (Romanelli *et al.* 2001). For example, the presence of all three of (i) a moderate to major increase in CSF white blood cells (>75 to 500 cells/μL), (ii) a major increase in CSF protein (1–5 g/L) and (iii) a reduced CSF glucose level (a 'normal' result on the Combur 10® reagent strip) is consistent with bacterial meningitis; while the presence of all three of (i) slight or moderate increase in CSF white blood cells, (ii) slight increase in CSF protein and (iii) a normal CSF glucose (50, 100, or 300 mg/dL on a Combur 10® strip) is consistent with viral meningitis. The reliability of the method has been confirmed in other studies (with a sensitivity of 90.7%, specificity 98.1%, positive predictive value 95.1% and negative predictive value 96.4%) (Romanelli *et al.* 2001). Dipsticks for whole blood urea (Azostix™) can be adapted to test peritoneal fluid obtained via diagnostic peritoneal lavage to help determine likelihood of urological tract damage in abdominal trauma (a veterinary medicine concept).

An ESR (erythrocyte sedimentation rate) can be used as a general wellness indicator in an austere environment. It also potentially provides diagnostic information in the setting of metastatic cancer when there is no CT scanning available. It is interesting to note that the ESR was originally invented as a pregnancy test.

Some POCT we use are not in common usage in Australia at the present time, such as procalcitonin testing. Procalcitonin testing is an alternative to C-reactive protein (CRP) and it provides diagnostic (differentiating systemic bacterial infections and sepsis from other systemic inflammatory responses) and prognostic (serial measurements can be used to monitor treatment response) information (Prkno *et al.* 2013; Schuetz *et al.* 2011; Singh and Anand 2014).

Some POCT used in Antarctica is imported from overseas because it is not currently approved for general use in Australia, but in an extreme environment offers benefits. This applies to the ELDON™ card test, which we use to confirm Landsteiner and Rhesus blood groups in the setting of a walking blood bank. This test is a critical component of our blood transfusion capability.

## PATIENT CASE STUDY ILLUSTRATING THE CLINICAL EFFECTIVENESS OF POCT IN THE REMOTE ANTARCTIC SETTING

### Female expeditioner with abdominal pain

A 23-year-old female expeditioner presented to the expedition doctor with a 12-h history of lower abdominal pain, loss of appetite and feeling generally 'out of sorts'. Initial findings were non-specific. A urine sample was obtained and the doctor performed a urine pregnancy test (Clearview hCG II™) and a urine dipstick (Combur 10®). A negative pregnancy test result immediately ruled out pregnancy and thus the important differential diagnosis of an ectopic pregnancy in this clinical setting. The urine dipstick test showed dark urine with a specific gravity of 1.030 and 2+ for ketones, but no other abnormality. These findings were consistent with concentrated urine and dehydration subsequent to poor oral intake. These findings also helped to rule out a urinary tract infection as an underlying cause for the clinical presentation and in the absence of haematuria made a stone in the urinary tract unlikely also. The patient was commenced on simple analgesia and advised to increase their fluid intake and to rest.

Review 6 hours later showed a low grade fever of 38.1°C and more localised tenderness in the right lower abdomen. This was consistent with, but not diagnostic of, early appendicitis. Given the suspicion of appendicitis the following additional tests were performed: full blood count (FBC) (QBC Autoread Plus™), semiquantitative procalcitonin (Brahms PCT-Q™), C-reactive protein (CRP) (Piccolo AmLyte 13™ panel), and electrolytes and renal function (Piccolo Basic Metabolic Plus™ panel).

The FBC showed a white cell count (WCC) of $10.6 \times 10^9$/L (normal range 4.3–10), which was mildly elevated, and a granulocyte count of $6.5 \times 10^9$/L, which was normal and not suggestive of a left shift. Procalcitonin was <0.05 ng/mL (normal) and CRP was 6.5 mg/L (normal), making serious abdominal sepsis unlikely at this stage. Renal function showed urea of 8.5 mmol/L (reference range 2.5–7.9) and a creatinine of 118 µmol/L (reference range 53–106), both mildly elevated and consistent with dehydration.

Active rehydration therapy and a fluid balance chart were started. The patient was put on 2-hourly observation of vital signs.

Review at 12 h showed worsening fever and worsening abdominal pain, now clearly located in the right lower quadrant of the abdomen. The patient looked unwell and, after several initial loose motions, there had been no bowel movement for the last 24 h. Repeat FBC shows an elevated WCC ($16.1 \times 10^9$/L) and a granulocyte count of $8.3 \times 10^9$/L, which was consistent with a left shift. Repeat CRP was now elevated at 25 mg/L, consistent with an acute phase response. Repeat procalcitonin was now <0.5 ng/mL, which is also higher than the previous measurement. Localised infection is possible at this level but bacterial systemic infection is unlikely. These findings in combination were consistent with and highly suggestive of appendicitis (ALVARADO Score = 9) (Wray *et al.* 2013).

The patient was commenced on conservative treatment for appendicitis using intravenous broad spectrum antibiotic cover with ceftriaxone and metronidazole. This treatment is successful in up to 73% of cases of appendicitis, especially if instituted early in the course of the illness (Campbell *et al.* 2004; Svensson *et al.* 2012). Non-responders to this conservative treatment approach will still require emergency appendicectomy.

The patient's clinical condition improved over the next 24 h. Repeat FBC and CRP testing at 24 h showed a fall in WCC to $11.2 \times 10^9$/L and CRP to 12 mg/L. The patient remained afebrile and pain free over the next 24 h and her appetite returned. Repeat testing after 24 h showed a return of the WCC to normal. Urine and renal function results returned to normal and clinically the patient appeared well.

The patient responded to conservative management and the need for an appendectomy was averted. This was welcome news, given it was the middle of winter in Antarctica at the time, being some 5000 km away from the nearest hospital and evacuation not being possible. The patient was switched to oral antibiotics for completion of treatment.

## AUSTRALIAN ANTARCTIC DIVISION'S WORK IN POCT AS AN EXAMPLE OF A SUCCESSFUL MODEL WORKING IN AN EXTREME ENVIRONMENT

Pathology diagnostic techniques available in the Australian Antarctic program, by necessity, continue to be limited.

Given our extensive previous experience in providing medical support in the extreme environment of Antarctica, the sub-Antarctic islands and the Southern Ocean, the AAD has nonetheless developed a robust and highly capable POCT diagnostic system to help with medical care provision in one of the most remote places on Earth. Our system provides capability on the ground at research stations, in the field, on ships and on aircraft. This POCT system has been field proven and consistently delivers high-grade diagnostic information that reduces the diagnostic uncertainty inherent in operating in an extreme environment. It is important to realise that the use of POCT in our extreme environment is not about decision limits, but much more importantly about clinical context and result trends.

This quality system provides the best available diagnostic capability, underpinned by its own *AAD Medical Laboratory Diagnostic Methods Handbook* (an internal AAD document first compiled and published in 2005), which draws together procedures from multiple sources and customises them for the Antarctic context while remaining in tune with real-world telemedicine providers (Watzl 2005b).

The AAD Handbook provides the protocols for the selection, use and application of our POC tests and for the interpretation of the test results. It provides clearly defined instructions covering training retention issues. The POCT system is closely supervised by the AAD Chief Medical Officer and deputies who provide 24/7 guidance to expedition medical officers when they have to use POCT and how to interpret the results obtained.

All expedition medical officers attend a 4-week in-house training course to prepare them for their role. This course includes training in the use of our POCT system and all available POCT devices. This includes specific in-service training for all complex devices and specific refresher training in basic microbiological methods (conducted at the University of Tasmania's medical school). This ensures that all operators are competent to perform our tests and have confidence in the test results obtained. Training records are kept and supplementary training is available as required.

AAD expedition doctors draw on the AAD Handbook to maintain performance standards. Quality assurance, where possible, is achieved by participation in Australian-based PT programs and by selecting high-quality tests that have their own built-in QC and known tolerances.

This approach is in tune with National Pathology Accreditation Advisory Council Guidelines for POCT (NPAAC 2015), which set out best practice guidelines.

Recent connectivity upgrades have also allowed automatic transmission of results from some of our POCT devices directly into our patients' electronic health record, via HL7 data transfer protocols.

The PMU provides its expedition doctors with basic but robust methods in:

- *clinical biochemistry*
- *haematology*
- *microbiology and histopathology* – providing basic capabilities in microbiology limited to the ability to process most clinical specimens to establish whether or not a bacterial infection is present, and to aid in the presumptive diagnosis of some common pathogens. Fine needle aspiration biopsy and urine cytology specimens can be collected for e-medicine if required. This process uses a modified Giemsa stain and digital photo-microscopy. Our methods here were adapted from protocols originally developed in collaboration with the Royal Hobart Hospital.
- *transfusion medicine* – using the concept of a 'walking' blood bank. All expeditioners are screened and grouped before departure. The Biorad™ Gel Card system is used to formally type and cross match blood if required on stations. ELDON™ cards are also provided to confirm ABO and Rhesus groups recorded on expeditioners' medical records. The latter is a useful adjunct on ships where no formal cross-matching capacity exists.
- *potable water testing* – the PMU is also responsible for the monthly testing of drinking water at each

Table 32.4. Current AAD POCT diagnostic capability

| Test | Device/method |
|---|---|
| *Clinical biochemistry* | |
| **General blood/serum biochemistry:** | Piccolo™ Analyser (Abaxis) |
| Alanine aminotransferase, albumin, alkaline phosphatase, amylase, aspartate aminotransferase, calcium, chloride, creatine kinase, creatinine, gamma glutamyl transferase, glucose, lactate dehydrogenase, magnesium, potassium, sodium, total bilirubin, total carbon dioxide, total protein, urea, uric acid, C-reactive protein | |
| **Blood gases/portable biochemistry:** | i-STAT® Handheld Analyser (Abbott) |
| pH, $pCO_2$, base excess (BE), anion gap, sodium, potassium, chloride, urea, (haemoglobin), (haematocrit), quantitative hCG | |
| Dipstick urinalysis | Combur 10® Dipstick (Roche) |
| Faecal occult blood test | bioNexia FOBplus™ (Biomerieux) |
| Blood glucose (digital) | Accu-Check® Performa |
| Blood urea (visual) | Azostix™ |
| Qualitative β-hCG | Clearview™ β-hCG |
| D-dimer | Simplify™ D-Dimer |
| Myoglobin/CK-MB/troponin I | LifeSign MI™ |
| Pro-calcitonin | Brahms PCT-Q™ |
| ***Haematology*** | |
| **General haematology:** | |
| Haemoglobin, haematocrit, platelet count, total white blood cell count, granulocyte count, lymph/monocyte count | QBC Star analyser™ |
| INR | Coaguchek XS Plus® |
| Haemoglobin (stand-alone) | HemoCue® Analyser |
| Haematocrit | Combur™ mini-centrifuge |
| Manual white cell count and differential | Neubauer counting chamber + microscope |
| Erythrocyte sedimentation rate (ESR) | Westergren method |
| Malarial thick and thin films | Giemsa staining and photo-microscopy |
| Malarial latex agglutination test | Binax Now™ test |
| Cell morphology | Leishman Wright stain and photo-microscopy |
| ***Microbiology*** | |
| Basic processing of CSF to differentiate bacterial from viral meningitis | 1. Off-label use of Combur 10® urine dipstick test for rapid determination<br>2. Long method using microscopy, counting chamber and cultures |
| Basic processing of urine to aid in the diagnosis of urinary tract infection | |
| Blood culture | |
| Culture media selected for appropriate use in Antarctic clinical context | Nutrient agar, MacConkey agar, Columbia blood agar base, XLD medium agar, and Sabouraud dextrose agar (Oxoid) |
| Methods for incubation of microbiological cultures | incubators, $CO_2$ enrichment, anaerobic incubation |
| Optochin testing | Optochin discs (Oxoid) |
| Catalase testing | Catalase test strips |

**Table 32.4.** *(continued)*

| Test | Device/method |
|---|---|
| Oxidase testing | Hydrogen peroxide |
| Latex agglutination testing for *S. aureus* | Staphytect Plus™ (Oxoid) |
| Latex agglutination testing for stool antigen of *H. pylori* (equivalent to urea breath testing) | |
| Finger-prick (blood) test for *H. pylori* (equivalent to urea breath testing) | |
| Basic photo-microscopy | Using Gram, Ziehl-Neelsen, Giemsa, India and photo-microscopy, polarised microscopy for crystals |
| Cryogenic storage for transport of microorganisms back to Australia for further study | Protect™ (Oxoid) |
| ***Histopathology*** | |
| Fine needle aspiration biopsy specimens | Giemsa stain and photo-microscopy |
| Urine cytology specimens | Giemsa stain and photo-microscopy |
| ***Transfusion medicine*** | |
| Blood typing | Biorad Gel Card system, ELDON™ cards |
| Forward and reverse cross matching | Biorad Gel Card system |
| ***Potable water testing*** | |
| pH measurement | pH Radiometer |
| Conductivity measurement | Conductivity meter |
| Turbidity measurement | Turbidity meter |
| Coliform testing | Colilert™ test, incubator |
| ***Diagnostic imaging*** | |
| Plain film X-ray radiography | Polymobil Plus mobile X-ray machine and Carestream™ PoC 360 digital processor |
| Dental radiography | Nomad |
| Ultrasonography | General Electric ultrasound |

Australian Antarctic and sub-Antarctic station. This ensures a safe drinking water supply to the Australian Antarctic program. Drinking water testing includes testing and measuring for coliforms, pH, conductivity and turbidity. These methods are described in their own standalone AAD testing manuals.

Table 32.4 summarises current AAD POCT diagnostic capability.

It is critical to point out that all these methods are, of course, further supported by other diagnostic modalities not traditionally thought of as POCT. Thus, in acute coronary syndromes, serial electrocardiograms (ECGs) are performed in addition to troponin testing. Laboratory diagnostic algorithms are interwoven with diagnostic imaging pathways where clinically indicated. Thus, in suspected deep vein thrombosis venous, ultrasonography studies are used in addition to D-dimer testing. Chest radiography is performed in cases of suspected tuberculosis, in addition to sputum analysis and Mantoux testing where indicated. Adding different diagnostic modalities appropriate for clinical context further reduces the diagnostic uncertainty inherent in operating in our extreme environment.

Most importantly, a POCT result is never interpreted in isolation but always used in clinical context, preferably over time to allow analysis of trend, always to support the clinical impression, but never to replace it.

## ACKNOWLEDGEMENTS

Royal Hobart Hospital protocols were originally written by Rob Peterson, Senior Scientist, Microbiology Department, Royal Hobart Hospital and Dr Andrew Parker, Department of Surgical Pathology, Royal Hobart Hospital.

## REFERENCES

Ayton J (2006) Women's health in Antarctica. Antarctic medicine in Australia's Antarctic program. *Obstetrics and Gynaecology Magazine* **8**, 16–18.

Campbell M, Johnston SL, Marshburn T, Kane J, Lugg D (2004) Nonoperative treatment of suspected appendicitis in remote medical care environments: implications for future spaceflight medical care. *Journal of the American College of Surgeons* **198**, 822–830. doi:10.1016/j.jamcollsurg.2004.01.009

Farahmand F, Roze M, Shams S, Ghajarzadeh M, Mohammadi B (2013) Diagnosis of spontaneous bacterial peritonitis in children by reagent strips. *Acta Medica Iranica* **51**, 125–128.

Goldsmid JM, Sullivan P (1994) Malaria in Tasmania 1987–1992. *Journal of Travel Medicine* **1**, 55–56. doi:10.1111/j.1708-8305.1994.tb00557.x

Kibby J, Sullivan P (1997) Evaluation and use of a dry chemistry analyzer in Antarctica. *International Journal of Circumpolar Health* **56**, 142–151.

King M (1976) *A Medical Laboratory for Developing Countries.* Oxford University Press, Oxford, UK.

King H (1987) A new health register for Australian National Antarctic Research Expeditions (ANARE). *The Polar Record* **23**, 719–720. doi:10.1017/S0032247400008445

Lugg D, Ayton J (2009) Polar medicine. In *Expedition and Wilderness Medicine.* (Eds G Bledsoe, M Manyak and D Townes) pp. 197–205. Cambridge University Press, New York NY, USA.

Lugg D, Shepanek M (1999) Space analogue studies in Antarctica. *Acta Astronautica* **44**, 693–699. doi:10.1016/S0094-5765(99)00068-5

Marchant H, Lugg D, Quilty P (Eds) (2002) *Australian Antarctic Science – The first 50 years of ANARE.* Australian Antarctic Division, Kingston, Tasmania.

McConnell F, Pashen D, McLean R (2007) The ARTS of risk management in rural and remote medicine. *Canadian Journal of Rural Medicine* **12**, 231–238.

Mervis J (2009) A death in Antarctica. *Science* **323**, 32–35. doi:10.1126/science.323.5910.32

Nicogossian AE, Lugg DJ, Doarn CR (2006) Civilian telemedicine in remote and extreme environments. In *M-Health: Emerging Mobile Health Systems.* (Eds RSH Istepanian, S Laxminarayan and CS Pattichis) pp. 517–529. Springer Science and Business Media, Inc. New York, USA.

NPAAC (2015) *Guidelines for Point of Care Testing.* National Pathology Accreditation Advisory Council, Commonwealth of Australia, Canberra.

Pardoe R (1965) A ruptured intracranial aneurysm in Antarctica. *The Medical Journal of Australia* **1**, 344–350.

Plowright RK (2000) Crevasse fall in the Antarctic: a patient's perspective. *The Medical Journal of Australia* **173**, 576–578.

Podkolinski MT, Semmens K (1979) Intestinal haemorrhage in Antarctica: a multinational rescue operation. *The Medical Journal of Australia* **2**, 275–277.

Podkolinski MT, Semmens K (1980) Intestinal haemorrhage in Antarctica. *Ambulance World* **4**, 12–15.

Priddy RE (1985) An "acute abdomen" in Antarctica: the problems of diagnosis and management. *The Medical Journal of Australia* **143**, 108–111.

Prkno A, Wacker C, Brunkhorst FM, Schlattmann P (2013) Procalcitonin-guided therapy in intensive care unit patients with severe sepsis and septic shock – a systematic review and meta-analysis. *Critical Care (London, England)* **17**, R291. doi:10.1186/cc13157

Romanelli R, Thome E, Duarte FMC, Gomes RS, Camargo PAM, Freire HBM (2001) Diagnosis of meningitis with reagent strips. *Jornal de Pediatria* **77**, 203–208. doi:10.2223/JPED.207

Schuetz P, Chiappa V, Briel M, Greenwald JL (2011) Procalcitonin algorithms for antibiotic therapy decisions – a systematic review of randomized controlled trials and recommendations for clinical algorithms. *Archives of Internal Medicine* **171**, 1322–1331. doi:10.1001/archinternmed.2011.318

Singh M, Anand L (2014) Bedside procalcitonin and acute care. *International Journal of Critical Illness and Injury Science* **4**, 233–237. doi:10.4103/2229-5151.141437

Sullivan P, Gormly PJ, Lugg DJ, Watts DJ (1991) The Australian National Antarctic Research Expeditions Health Register: three years of operation. In *Circumpolar Health 90. Proceedings of the 8th International Congress on Circumpolar Health.* 20–25 May 1990, Whitehorse, Yukon (Ed. B Postl.) pp. 502–504. University of Manitoba Press, Winnipeg, Canada.

Svensson J, Hall NJ, Eaton S, Pierro A, Wester T (2012) A review of conservative treatment of acute appendicitis. *European Journal of Pediatric Surgery* **22**, 185–194. doi:10.1055/s-0032-1320014

Watzl R (2005a) Transfusion Medicine Management in isolated settings – Antarctica. Presentation at *HSANZ/ANZSBT/ASTH Annual Scientific Meeting.* 15–18 October, Hobart, Tasmania.

Watzl R (2005b) *AAD Medical Laboratory Diagnostic Methods Handbook.* Internal publication, Polar Medicine Unit, Australian Antarctic Division, Kingston, Tasmania.

WHO (World Health Organization) (1977) *International Classification of Diseases, Ninth Revision.* WHO, Geneva, Switzerland.

WHO (1978) *International Classification of Procedures in Medicine, Ninth Revision.* WHO, Geneva, Switzerland.

Wray C, Kao LS, Millas SG, Tsao K, Ko TC (2013) Acute appendicitis: controversies in diagnosis and management. *Current Problems in Surgery* **50**, 54–86. doi:10.1067/j.cpsurg.2012.10.001

# 33 Point-of-care testing in sports science

*Lynda Norton and Kevin Norton*

**Summary**

Professional sports environments involve training programs to maximise physical performance of athletes. This requires conditioning staff prescribing and monitoring training loads as well as medical monitoring to ensure athletes remain healthy. Point-of-care testing (POCT) facilitates rapid decision making and manipulation of training programs, as well as providing important feedback about recovery status and wellbeing. Several biomarkers have been established as reliable indicators of exercise-induced physiological changes in sports science. However, there is still a lack of clarity about the best indicators to measure when monitoring the various phases of training programs. This is a rapidly growing area of scientific research and is a promising area for further developments.

## AN OVERVIEW OF POCT IN SPORTS SCIENCE

Professional athletes undertake extremes of physical training in order to maximise physiological adaptation. During the competition phase, these high levels of exercise are often coupled with limited opportunities for sufficient recovery. The complex interaction of intense physical stress and high training volume, together with the need for time to recover and repair tissues, influence a range of body functions, including health status and performance capacity.

As a consequence, high-performance conditioning and medical staff are increasingly using scientific approaches to prescribe and monitor training loads. For example, there is a range of technologies available to help minimise risks of overtraining and exercise-induced illness and injury, while optimising physical working capacity. Quantifying external training loads has become important in many sports where devices such as power output meters, global positioning devices and accelerometers for g-force-determined body load are often used. Internal load monitoring may involve heart rate patterns in exercise and recovery, perception of effort, sleep quantity and quality, and a range of body fluid biomarkers. Misalignment between external and internal loads often predisposes or reveals potential fatigue-related problems.

Despite an enormous array of biomarkers being routinely measured, there are relatively few definitive markers described in the literature when monitoring athletes' wellbeing. In many ways, this area of research and clinical surveillance is in its infancy but it continues to evolve rapidly (Gleeson 2007; Northoff 2009; Papa *et al.* 2015). The benefits of POCT in sports include an ability to: (i) make training decisions rapidly such as manipulating exercise prescription; (ii) detect biochemical patterns that may relate to interactions of diet, exercise or recovery

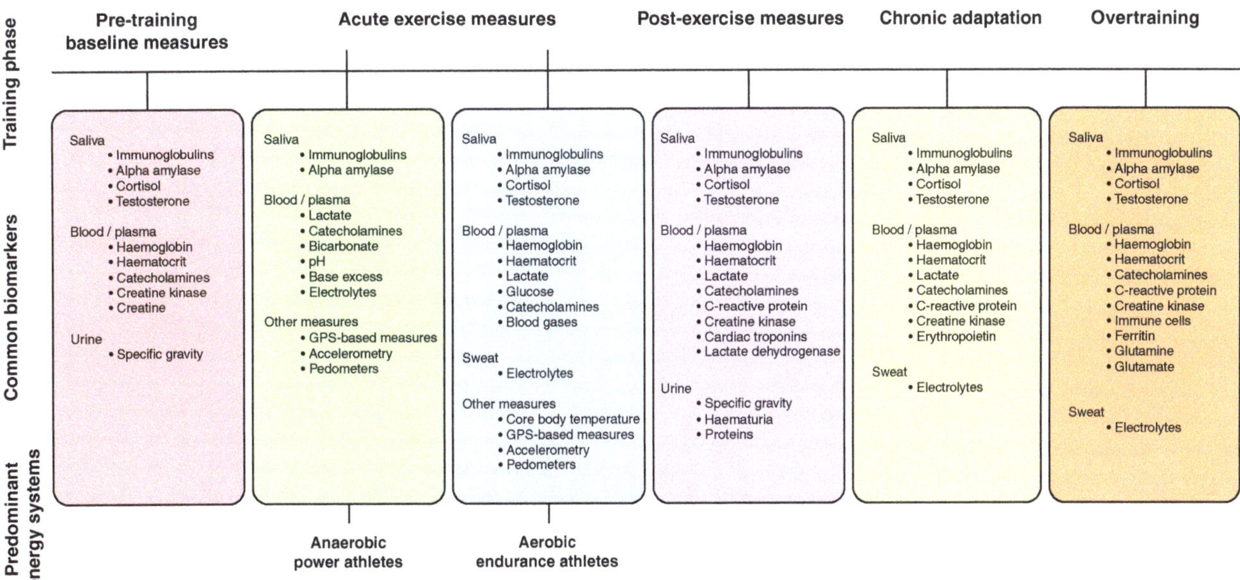


**Fig. 33.1.** Biomarkers and other measures commonly reported in the scientific literature on athlete monitoring. The variables are grouped according to the training phase and energy system of interest, and the medium used for collection.

status; (iii) monitor for overtraining and immune health; (iv) quantify training-induced adaptations; and (v) assess for banned substances.

This chapter on POCT in sports science begins with an overview of common biomarkers within various body fluids used to assess athletes in high-performance sports. These are sub-divided according to the phase of training cycles as well as the predominant energy system under review. The list of variables presented in Fig. 33.1 is not exhaustive, but represents biomarkers and other measures that are often reported in the scientific literature on athlete monitoring.

## TRENDS IN POCT IN SPORT SCIENCE

The very rapid growth of POCT associated with sports performance is illustrated in Fig. 33.2. Two searches were conducted. The first included the terms 'POCT and sport' (among more specific terms) to reflect the 'internal' measures associated with exercise and sport. The second search used the terms 'global positioning and sport' to reflect the rapidly developing use of wearable technologies in sport that assess 'external' measures of human movement. The search results highlight the accelerating outputs within each of the broad pools of research. Furthermore, the searches revealed virtually no overlap in the articles when the terms 'POCT, GPS and sport' were combined, despite the common element that both involve POCT technologies.

Fig. 33.2 shows the results of the database searches for journal articles since 1995. The search was confined to two major databases, although these would capture most of the international journals in the areas.

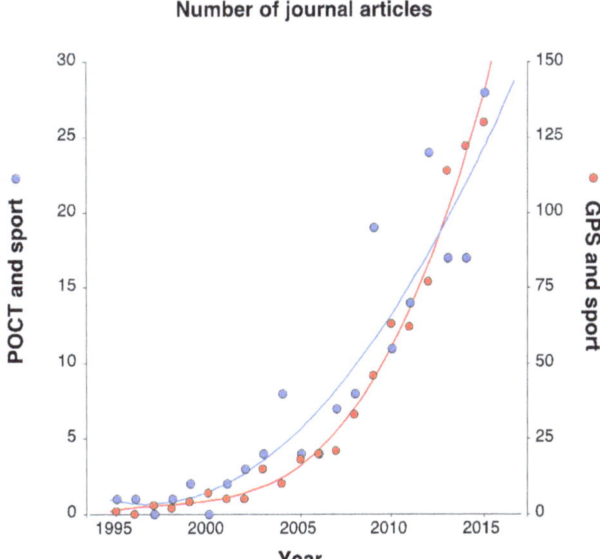


**Fig. 33.2.** The growth in the number of journal articles published since 1995 on both POCT and sport, and GPS and sport. The Internet searches involved Scopus and SportDiscus databases with cross-referencing for duplicates. There was minimal overlap between the articles found in each search indicating the term 'POCT' has rarely been considered to cover wearable technologies such as GPS and accelerometer units. Both areas have grown very rapidly as new technologies and applications have been developed.

## TRAINING PHASE

Exercise science measures are often undertaken according to the periodisation phase of training or specific activity being undertaken. It is useful, for example, to monitor baseline levels of various biochemical markers and then to compare these against changes during or after exercise. Associations are often made between these markers and acute changes in exercise intensity and duration, as well as over the longer term to investigate chronic adaptations. There are five phases of exercise listed in Fig. 33.1 and a range of common biomarkers and other measures that are made within each using POCT are presented. The list shows examples of variables that are regularly measured. However, numerous other markers have been assessed and reported in sport and exercise studies.

### Pre-training/baseline measures

Baseline measures are used to establish within-athlete normative values. These can help to establish typical levels of day-to-day change, and patterns of disruption during and following training. They are also used for an athlete's biological passport, which is a haematological profile based on a series of blood samples, together with a steroid longitudinal profile from urine samples. Only World Anti-Doping Agency (WADA) accredited laboratories can add to the athlete's biological passport and undertake routine doping checks (WADA 2015). These parameters can be tracked consistently to establish an athlete's 'control' levels and, thereby, detect possible outliers (Mørkeberg *et al.* 2009). Notwithstanding, there is a role for POCT. For example, athletes in professional cycling races may have haematocrit measures assessed to prevent starters with levels over 50% and deter the use of recombinant human erythropoietin (rhEPO) (Martin *et al.* 1997).

Baseline measures are important when assessing intervention-induced or time-related changes in biomarkers. Reliable resting or stable measures are most often made at a particular time of the day, typically early morning but this depends on the variable being assessed. It is also important to recognise that pre-competition measures may be very different from resting measures because of the anticipatory effects of the neuroendocrine system and other diurnal influences. Similarly, post-exercise values can also be very different from resting levels. Consequently, if the sample is to be used in connection with the athlete biological passport program to establish baseline measures, the World Anti-Doping Code specifies it shall not be collected within 2 hours following the athlete training or competing (WADA 2013).

### Acute exercise measures

Undertaking an acute bout of exercise induces numerous physiological alterations as the body attempts to cope with the changing demands for fuel supply and energy transfer. There are dramatic disruptions in a range of biomarkers. These often change in an accelerated way in response to linear increases in exercise intensity, and POCT can help to quantify the degree of stress and relative intensity placed on the athlete (Norton *et al.* 2010). The disproportionate changes should be viewed as a stress response whereby high-intensity activity is one of the most potent forms of stressors on the body, even in well-conditioned athletes. A reliable indicator of relative stress can be obtained from blood lactate measures that increase in an accelerated way as exercise intensity rises. This is one of the most common test procedures, both in the laboratory and in the field, to provide evidence of progressively greater anaerobic energy contribution. Table 33.1 lists POCT equipment designed specifically for these measures.

Acute exercise is often categorised according to the predominant energy system used during the activity. Maximal human power is achieved in events of short duration and extreme intensity. Power meters are now an integral part of equipment used by athletes, both in the field and in fitness facilities to provide immediate feedback and assist in exercise prescription. Stored phosphagens and the ability to resynthesise high-energy phosphagens are important in these types of events. Artificially increasing the levels of muscle phosphagens through dietary supplements such as creatine monohydrate and as a normal training response, measuring the rate and capacity of the anaerobic energy system during and after exercise, and assessing the structural damage that can occur as a result of this activity are of most interest. Muscle fibre micro-damage and the consequent release of cellular proteins, enzymes such as lactate dehydrogenase (LDH) and creatine kinase (CK), and other molecules into the blood can yield information about the cyclical nature of exercise-induced damage, repair and performance adaptation.

Aerobic exercise involves continuous activity over a longer period of time. Although the aerobic energy system contributes the majority of the energy transfer in events as short as ~60 s, it generally refers to events of minutes up to hours in duration. Of particular interest is the maximum intensity and duration the exercise can be sustained, and the ability for homeostasis regulation. Endurance training typically shifts the human power curve so that a constant exercise intensity can be sustained for longer, or for a given timeframe at a higher intensity.

Biomarkers of interest often relate to the metabolic activity of long-duration work and oxygen flux from the atmosphere to the mitochondria. This involves many physiological systems and biochemical pathways down to the level of the electron transport chain. The heavy reliance on the capacity to transport sufficient oxygen in the blood means markers such as red cell volume, haemoglobin concentration, oxygen saturation and ferritin levels are important (Chalmers *et al.* 2014; Reinke *et al.* 2012). Moreover, in endurance events there is a need to regulate body temperature, maintain fluid reserves for sweat, regulate electrolyte balance and provide sufficient fuel, among other things (Chalmers *et al.* 2014). These reinforce the importance of markers such as ingestible radio-telemetry temperature sensors (CorTemp, HQ Inc., Palmetto FL, USA), haemoglobin and haematocrit to track plasma volume alterations, electrolyte concentrations in blood (particularly sodium) and sweat, and blood glucose levels, respectively. For example, following several deaths in marathon events, there have been calls to ensure accurate blood sodium measures using POCT before beginning hydration treatment among collapsed runners (Kratz *et al.* 2005).

Wearable tracking devices incorporating a range of microprocessors are increasingly being used for acute activity analysis in sports science (Fig. 33.1). At the novice level, there has been an explosion of wearable heart rate, GPS and accelerometer technologies to monitor training loads, physical activity patterns and energy expenditure, and that are also marketed as fashion accessories. Valid and reliable GPS units have become miniaturised and lightweight over the past decade since they were initially developed for use during professional sports competition in 2003 (Coutts and Duffield 2010). Current systems such as Catapult's 5th generation MinimaxX units contain a 10 Hz GNSS (Global Navigation Satellite System), and a tri-axial accelerometer, gyroscope for rotational velocities and a magnetometer for direction data, all collected at 100 Hz (www.catapultsports.com). These features allow massive datasets in g-force load and movement profiles (such as speed categories and distances, acceleration and deceleration patterns), as well as the number and type of collision impact forces during competition (Wundersitz *et al.* 2015). Numerous validation studies have been undertaken on the use of GPS systems specific to field sports (Cummins *et al.* 2013). Sales in GPS-based professional sports devices grew 64% in 2015 (http://www.fastcompany.com/section/most-innovative-companies-2015). These types of data measurement technologies continue to find applications in everything from footwear and clothing, to sporting equipment such as footballs, golf clubs and tennis racquets.

### Post-exercise measures

Following exercise there are many biomarkers of interest. These may reflect the effects of the acute exercise load on recovery patterns, disruption to anatomical structures, rate of diffusion or resynthesis of molecules affected by the exercise, or acute changes in immune response. The kinetics, degree and capacities of these alterations can also provide information about the training status of the individual, such as the clearance rate of blood lactate. The most common endocrine measures made during the post-competition recovery period among professional athletes are testosterone and cortisol (Cormack *et al.* 2008). Testosterone is a powerful anabolic agent. Depending on the exercise intensity and duration, its concentration in the blood increases following exercise. It is important during recovery due to its role in protein synthesis and to enhance muscle glycogen storage. In overtrained athletes, blood concentrations are generally lower. Cortisol is a stress hormone that acts antagonistically to testosterone to increase protein breakdown and decrease protein synthesis. Because these hormones respond in opposite directions to significant overloads in exercise training, the ratio of these hormones has been used to assess the anabolic: catabolic status of athletes (McLellan *et al.* 2010). Catecholamine levels in urine and plasma reflect the activity of the sympathetic nervous system and are also suppressed in overtrained athletes, as is growth hormone.

Serum CK activity as a measure of muscle damage is popular due to the simplicity of sample collection and analysis. However, variability of this measure by POCT is high, and a poor temporal relationship with muscle recovery has been reported (Twist and Highton 2013).

Both glutamine and glutamate levels rise during exercise but are decreased in plasma following both prolonged

**Table 33.1.** Examples of POCT analysers available for use in sports science for the measurement of lactate and haemoglobin. There are also several devices included that can measure more than one analyte.

| POCT device | Photo | Method principle | Sample volume (µL) | Time for result (min) | Measuring range | Weight (g) | Power source | Long-term reagent storage | Other tests measured |
|---|---|---|---|---|---|---|---|---|---|
| **Lactate** | | | | | | | | | |
| Accutrend® Plus (Roche Diagnostics, Basel, Switzerland) | | Reflectance photometry | 15–50 | Up to 2 depending on analyte | Blood 0.8–21.7 mmol/L; Plasma 0.7–26 mmol/L | 140 | 4 × 1.5V batteries (AAA) | Room temperature | Total cholesterol; triglycerides; glucose |
| Lactate Pro™ (Arkray KDK, Japan) | | Enzymatic-amperometric | 5 | 1 | 0.8–23.3 mmol/L | 50 | 2 × 3 V lithium battery | 2–8°C | |
| Lactate Pro™2 (Arkray KDK, Japan) | | Enzymatic-amperometric | 0.3 | 0.25 | 0.8–23.3 mmol/L | 45 | 1 coin battery CR2032 | Room temperature | |
| Lactate Scout+ (SensLab GmbH, An EKF Diagnostics company, Germany) | | Enzymatic-amperometric | 0.2 | 0.16 | 0.5–25.0 mmol/L | 80 | 2 × 1.5 V batteries (AAA) | Test strips stored at 2–8°C | |
| LAC PRO (BST BioSensor Technology, Germany) | | Enzymatic-amperometric | 6 | 0.10 | 0.5–24.0 mmol/L | 50 | 230 V | Test strips stored at 2–8°C | |

| POCT device | Photo | Method principle | Sample volume (μL) | Time for result (min) | Measuring range | Weight (g) | Power source | Long-term reagent storage | Other tests measured |
|---|---|---|---|---|---|---|---|---|---|
| Lactate Plus (Nova Biomedical, USA) | | Electrochemical lactate oxidase biosensor | 0.7 | 0.25 | 0.5–25.0 mmol/L | 75 | 3 V lithium battery | Test strips stored at room temperature | |
| Nova Statstrip Lactate Express (Nova Biomedical, USA) | | Electrochemical lactate oxidase biosensor | 0.6 | 0.25 | 0.3–20.0 mmol/L | 75 | 3 V lithium battery | Test strips stored at room temperature | Haematocrit |
| YSI 1500 Sport™ analyser (Nova Biomedical, USA) | | Electrochemical lactate oxidase biosensor | 25 | 1 | Lactate to 30 mmol/L Glucose to 50 mmol/L | 4500 | Rechargeable 12 V DC battery with AC adaptor | Room temperature | Glucose |
| **Haemoglobin** | | | | | | | | | |
| HemoCue® Hb201+(Radiometer, Denmark) | | Photometric measurement of azide methaemoglobin | 10 | 1 | 0–256 g/L | 350 | AC adaptor or 4 x AA batteries | 15–30°C | |
| Hemo Control (EKF-diagnostic, Germany) | | Photometric measurement of azide methaemoglobin | 8–10 | 0.5–1 | 0–256 g/L | 700 | Rechargeable batteries | 15–30°C | |

and high intensity exercise. Inadequate recovery between exercise bouts or when athletes suffer from overtraining syndrome are both linked to low levels of these molecules (Newsholme *et al.* 2003). Further, concussive episodes are associated with acute and dramatic elevation of neurotransmitters in the blood and extracellular fluid, including glutamate, and may prove to be a useful diagnostic tool with POCT (Guerriero *et al.* 2015; Hovda 2014).

### Chronic adaptation

Regular and specific overload using exercise training results in physiological and biochemical adaptations. This is referred to as a training response and it generally involves changes that blunt the previous disruption to homeostasis during an absolute level of physical exertion, as well as the capacity to enhance energy transfer and performance. A common test, for example, involves assessing the level of anaerobic energy transfer at a set level of external work by using POCT for metabolites such as blood lactate level. A beneficial exercise response typically reveals a lowered blood lactate level during comparable work after habitual training. Blood lactate transition threshold (speed or workload where lactate rises rapidly) is measured because it is sensitive to training adaptations and correlates well with changes in endurance performance (Demarle *et al.* 2003). Other measures may include concentrations of cellular proteins and hormones, such as CK, cortisol or catecholamines, following a set amount of work, or heart rate at a given intensity that will all show less disruption from baseline following adaptation.

### Overtraining

This refers to the accumulation of both physical training and non-training stressors that result in a decrease in performance or heightened perception of fatigue (Halson *et al.* 2002). It may accumulate over a period of weeks or months and can often be associated with detrimental immune function changes. A relatively large amount of research has been conducted examining a range of biochemical, hormonal and immunological responses to exercise, primarily in a bid to monitor performance and minimise excessive fatigue and illness. A range of POCT systems allow immediacy of results of immune cell profiles, markers of inflammation and tissue damage or stress hormones (Tables 33.1 and 33.2). There are still uncertainties about which biomarkers to measure and several reviews have been published in this area (Meeusen *et al.* 2013; Wyatt *et al.* 2013). Salivary cortisol and testosterone measures have been shown to have an association with performance in the overtrained athlete, as indicated. Other hormonal measures and markers of immune function include salivary immunoglobulin A, natural killer cell activity and neutrophil phagocytic activity (Rietjens *et al.* 2005).

## BIOMARKER SAMPLING MEDIUMS

### Saliva

There are several useful acute and chronic markers that can be obtained using oral-fluid testing (saliva) as a collection medium for POCT. The measurement of physiological biomarkers in saliva offers a valuable tool for assessing the hormonal, immunological and endocrinological status associated with exercise and training (Malon *et al.* 2014; Nater and Rohleder 2009; Papacosta and Nassis 2011). Saliva is easier and safer to collect than urine or blood and generally requires only short disruption to training. However, protein degradation occurs rapidly in saliva at room temperature so it is recommended that samples be frozen immediately after collection to minimise protein breakdown (Esser *et al.* 2008). Despite the low concentration of many of the biomarkers in saliva relative to parallel blood samples, it is becoming increasingly apparent that POCT using saliva sampling and analysis has significant applications in exercise and sport science.

The most common biomarkers assessed in saliva include: (i) α-amylase and cortisol to indicate the stress response to acute and chronic exercise: (ii) testosterone and dehydroepiandrosterone (DHEA) for anabolic adaptations of training; (iii) immunoglobulins and antimicrobial proteins for assessing risk of respiratory infections; and (iv) stimulants such as human growth hormone (hGh), and insulin-like growth factor 1 (IGF-1) that are generally increased following high-intensity exercise.

Alpha amylase is an enzyme associated with starch breakdown and its concentration increases acutely with fear and stress such as exercise under the control of the sympathetic nervous system. It is more often measured in sports science as part of assessment of the hypothalamic-pituitary-adrenal (HPA) axis and impact of chronic physical training. The rapid increase in salivary α-amylase in response to both physical and psychological stress (Nater and Rohleder 2009) is often blunted in the overtrained state (Mckune *et al.* 2014). Studies have shown that acute cortisol responses to exercise are more pronounced in saliva compared with blood, therefore offering a more accurate measure for the assessment of sympathetic nervous system activity (Crewther *et al.* 2010).

Correlations between plasma and salivary testosterone are high (Vittek *et al.* 1985; Yasuda *et al.* 2008) making salivary measurement a simpler option in sports endocrinology. Several researchers have investigated the development of miniaturised, wearable biosensors in mouth guards to enable real-time physiological monitoring (Kim *et al.* 2014; Schabmueller *et al.* 2006). However, issues relating to re-use, hygiene, toxicity and operational stability need to be incorporated in future design and implementation of these biosensors. DHEA, a precursor to testosterone, is also a banned anabolic agent (WADA 2015). It can be measured in saliva to follow the response of this hormone in athletes during competition (Collomp *et al.* 2015). Because the correlation between saliva and serum concentrations is high for steroid hormones, both at rest and during exercise, the initial 'screening' testing can involve saliva analysis but follow-up WADA testing involves sophisticated urinalysis (WADA 2015).

Professional athletes push the limits of physical training loads. As a consequence, higher levels of acute upper respiratory tract infections (URTI) are characteristic among this group (Gleeson 2007; Neville *et al.* 2008; Papacosta and Nassis 2011). Assessment of 'first line of defence' salivary antimicrobial proteins such as salivary IgA (s-IgA), and more recently, salivary lysine (s-lys), α-amylase and lactoferrin may reflect the athlete's tolerance of an exercise training load and the relative risk of respiratory infections (Gleeson 2007; Neville *et al.* 2008; Papacosta and Nassis 2011). For example, reduced s-IgA during periods of heavy training is associated with increased URTI (Walsh *et al.* 2011). Coad and colleagues (2015) recently showed valid and reliable results for s-IgA using the IPRO LFD (IPRO Interactive, Wallingford, UK) immunoassay method.

Stimulants such as hGh and IGF-1 increase both during, and for a short period after, intense exercise, particularly resistance-type activity (Schroeder *et al.* 2013). Exercise influences the salivary concentrations in the same way as serum. However, reports to date indicate the monitoring of these anabolic stimulants has been confined to research studies, although recently there have been calls to broaden the applications (Anizan and Huestis 2014; Gatti and DePalo 2011).

## Blood/plasma

Acute intense exercise is typically associated with significant alterations in lymphocytes. For example, there is a temporary fall in circulating natural killer (NK) cells alongside increases in leukocytes, neutrophils and pro inflammatory cytokines (Brolinson and Elliott 2007; Córdova *et al.* 2010) and these changes may compromise immune function (Gleeson and Walsh 2012). POCT devices that can provide a rapid and complete blood picture for immune-related cells are often used during intense, pre-season training, such as during heat or altitude training camps over days or weeks, and as a monitoring tool across the season.

Many POCT systems use capillary blood samples via finger-tip or ear-lobe puncture. These samples do not need to be centrifuged because measures are made using whole blood. Examples are shown in Tables 33.1 and 33.2.

## Urine

Point-of-care urine analysis is used extensively for patients with various metabolic and kidney disorders. It is being used more widely in sports science to assess for analytes including blood cells and proteins, and metabolites such as creatinine, lactate or glucose. These are typically assessed in endurance or combat athletes who may have suffered, or are susceptible to, acute kidney injury (Coso *et al.* 2012; Hoffman *et al.* 2013).

Urine analysis has also been shown to be a valid and reliable method for determining moderate changes in fluid balance among athletes (Armstrong 2005). Dehydration of only 2–3% can negatively affect performance (Sawka *et al.* 2007). Specific gravity of urine is an indicator of hydration status and is routinely measured using a refractometer in the morning before training and competition (Armstrong 2005). The value is compared with a reference range to help guide hydration management. Other POCT measures such as osmolarity, pH, ketones and bilirubin concentrations, and colour (using strips) are sometimes used (Coso *et al.* 2012). Minimal differences in the accuracy of the related measures of urine specific gravity, osmolarity and colour have been reported (Armstrong *et al.* 1998).

Urine and blood analyses are the only authorised mediums used for WADA drug testing in athletes. Serial urine measures of hormones such as testosterone in accredited laboratories form part of the athlete's biological passport (WADA 2013).

## Sweat

Training-induced adaptations to help maintain adequate hydration levels and core temperature [Tc] regulation

**Table 33.2.** Examples of POCT devices available for use in sports science that can measure a range of test profiles

| POCT device | Photo | Selected examples of test profiles measured | Sample volume (μL) | Time for result (mins) | Weight (kg) | Power source | Long-term reagent storage |
|---|---|---|---|---|---|---|---|
| Reflotron® Plus (Roche Diagnos-tics, Basel, Switzerland) | | Electrolytes, lipids, Hb, CK, liver enzymes, metabolites, creatinine | 30 | 2–3 min | 5.3 | 115–230V; AC | Test strips 2–34°C |
| Piccolo Express® (Abaxis) | | Electrolytes, lipids, liver enzymes, metabolites, creatinine | 9 | 8–9 min | 5.1 | 100–240V; AC | Rotor cassette 2–8°C |
| Dri-Chem NX500 IE/E (Fuji Film, Japan) | | Electrolytes, lipids, liver enzymes, metabolites, creatinine | 5–50 | 1–6 min | 24 | 100–240V; AC | Single slides 2–8°C |
| i-STAT® (Abbott Point of Care, USA) | | Electrolytes, Hb (calc), blood gases, base excess, sO2, lactate, glucose, creatinine | 65–95 | 2–17 min | 0.65 | 2 × 9V Lithium battery or rechargeable battery | Cartridges 2–8°C |
| i-Chroma™ (Boditech Med, South Korea) | | hsCRP, CRP, procalcitonin, testosterone, cortisol, CRP, PCT, ferritin, PSA, thyroid hormones, D-dimer, myoglobin | 5–150 | 3–15 min | 1.2 | 12V DC or AC | Cartridges 2–30°C |

| POCT device | Photo | Selected examples of test profiles measured | Sample volume (μL) | Time for result (mins) | Weight (kg) | Power source | Long-term reagent storage |
|---|---|---|---|---|---|---|---|
| Samsung LABGEO HC10 | | WBC, Hb, Hct, RBC, platelets, 13 additional parameters | 25 | 80 tests per hour | 12.8 | DC 12V, 5A, 60W | 15–30°C |
| Yumizen H500 (Horiba, France) | | Range of haematological markers including complete blood count and 5-part differential | 20 | 50 tests per hour | 23 | 100–240V; AC | Cuvettes 2–8°C |
| IPRO LFD reader (Oxon, UK) | | Salivary IgA, IgG, IL-6, cortisol, α amylase, testosterone, DHEA, CRP | 100 (saliva) | 0.3 min | 0.62 | AC or AA rechargeable batteries | Test strips 15–34°C |

include expansion of plasma volume, increased skin blood flow at a given Tc, decreased Tc threshold for cutaneous vasodilation and onset of sweating, and lower concentration of electrolytes in sweat following a period of conditioning (Chalmers *et al.* 2014). Because dehydration is deleterious to athletic performance and a serious health risk, and sweat concentration may indicate the degree of fluid loss and relative risk of heat stroke, electrolyte analysis of sweat is a potential field measure for athletes (Baker *et al.* 2014).

However, other than for research purposes, routine measures of sweat concentrations are currently rare in sports science. When sweat collection is made during exercise, it involves using absorbent patches that can be analysed for sweat concentrations of ions such as sodium ($Na^+$) and potassium ($K^+$) (Dziedzic *et al.* 2014). Portable analysers such as the Horiba B-722 and B-731 use ion-selective electrode technology to measure $Na^+$ and $K^+$ concentrations.

## TECHNICAL CONSIDERATIONS OF POCT IN SPORTS SCIENCE

Tables 33.1 and 33.2 provide an overview of some of the POCT devices that are available for use in the sports science field. Some of the more frequently measured biomarkers are listed.

Blood lactate concentration during and following acute exercise is one of the most common variables assessed in sports science. Up until the early 1990s, blood lactate was measured using the lactate dehydrogenase spectrophotometric method (LDH). Numerous handheld analysers, including those listed in Table 33.1, have since been developed that use the lactate oxidase method for lactate determination. POCT lactate analysers have shown high day-to-day reliability, moderate to high correlations with laboratory methods and low imprecision (coefficients of variation ~2%). However, several researchers have found relatively large differences between lactate concentrations determined by different analysers (Bishop *et al.* 1992; Buckley *et al.* 2003; Medbø *et al.* 2000; McNaughton *et al.* 2002; Pinnington and Dawson 2001; Pyne *et al.* 2000).

HemoCue® is a popular unit for measuring haemoglobin. It uses photometric measurement of whole (undiluted) blood after conversion of haemoglobin to azide methaemoglobin (Munoz *et al.* 2005). HemoCue values do not appear to be affected by alterations in plasma protein and electrolyte content in humans (McNulty *et al.* 1994). Comparisons between HemoCue POC test and laboratory studies have revealed good imprecision (CV% 0.9–1.3%), and accuracy ($r$ = 0. 99) (Munoz *et al.* 2005), although lower correlation coefficients ($r$ = 0.61–0.89) have been reported (Morris *et al.* 1999).

The i-STAT® analyser also measures Hb (calculated from the haematocrit) and corrects for electrolyte levels. However, the method may become less accurate when serum electrolytes and/or protein concentrations deviate from the norm (Morris *et al.* 1999).

Total creatine kinase levels in whole blood depend on factors such as age, gender, race, muscle mass and fibre-type composition, recent physical activity and climatic conditions (Brancaccio *et al.* 2007). It is therefore common to see large differences among individuals. CK activity that reflects muscle damage can be assessed from fingertip capillary samples. Systems such as the Reflotron use a colourimetric assay procedure. The reference interval for CK activity provided by the manufacturer is 24–195 IU/L, but it is possible to find players in professional sports with values in excess of 1500–2000 IU/L in the first 2 days following games (Coelho *et al.* 2011; Mougios 2007). In general, higher CK levels are found after exercise such as ironman events, collision-based sports, and resistance training or downhill running involving high-force eccentric muscular contractions.

## CONCLUSION

The use of various POCT devices in sports science will continue to grow for both biomarkers and other sensors. This will involve improvements in quality and accuracy of current measures, as well as new data collection methods. Developments continue in the areas of wearable and implantable biosensors, technologies incorporated into sports equipment and biochemical markers of exercise physiology and homeostasis. New technologies will emerge for tracking all training phases of sports conditioning and athlete monitoring. These developments are also being applied in sub-elite sports environments as costs are reduced, and this trend will continue. The challenge continues to be in establishing meaningful applications that are valid across individuals and that reliably track changes in physiological adaptation, performance and overtraining.

## REFERENCES

Anizan S, Huestis MA (2014) The potential role of oral fluid in antidoping testing. *Clinical Chemistry* **60**, 307–322. doi:10.1373/clinchem.2013.209676

Armstrong LE (2005) Hydration assessment techniques. *Nutrition Reviews* **63**, S40–S54. doi:10.1111/j.1753-4887.2005.tb00153.x

Armstrong LE, Soto J, Hacker FT, Casa D, Kavouras SA, Maresh CM (1998) Urinary indices during dehydration, exercise, and rehydration. *International Journal of Sport Nutrition* **8**, 345–355.

Baker LB, Ungaro CT, Barnes KA, Nuccio RP, Reimel AJ, Stofan JR (2014) Validity and reliability of a field technique for sweat Na+ and K+ analysis during exercise in a hot-humid environment. *Physiological Reports* **2**, e12007. doi:10.14814/phy2.12007

Bishop PA, Smith JF, Kime JC, Mayo JM, Tin YH (1992) Comparison of a manual and an automated enzymatic technique for determining blood lactate concentration. *International Journal of Sports Medicine* **13**, 36–39. doi:10.1055/s-2007-1021231

Brancaccio P, Maffulli N, Limongelli FM (2007) Creatine kinase monitoring in sport medicine. *British Medical Bulletin* **81**, 209–230. doi:10.1093/bmb/ldm014

Brolinson PG, Elliott D (2007) Exercise and the immune system. *Clinics in Sports Medicine* **26**, 311–319. doi:10.1016/j.csm.2007.04.011

Buckley JD, Bourdon PC, Woolford SM (2003) Effect of measuring blood lactate concentrations using different automated lactate analysers on blood lactate transition thresholds. *Journal of Science and Medicine in Sport* **6**, 408–421. doi:10.1016/S1440-2440(03)80267-0

Chalmers S, Esterman A, Eston R, Bowering KJ, Norton K (2014) Short-term heat acclimation training improves physical performance: a systematic review, and exploration of physiological adaptations and application for team sports. *Sports Medicine (Auckland, N.Z.)* **44**, 971–988. doi:10.1007/s40279-014-0178-6

Coad S, Mclellan C, Whitehouse T, Gray B (2015) Validity and reliability of a novel salivary immunoassay for individual profiling in applied sports science. *Research in Sports Medicine: An International Journal* **23**, 140–150. doi:10.1080/15438627.2015.1005300

Coelho DB, Morandi RF, de Melo MA, Silami-Garcia E (2011) Creatine kinase kinetics in professional soccer players during a competitive season. *Brazilian Journal of Kinanthropometry and Human Performance* **13**, 189–194.

Collomp K, Buisson C, Lasne F, Collomp R (2015) DHEA, physical exercise and doping. *The Journal of Steroid Biochemistry and Molecular Biology* **145**, 206–212. doi:10.1016/j.jsbmb.2014.03.005

Córdova A, Sureda A, Tur JA, Pons A (2010) Immune response to exercise in elite sportsmen during the competitive season. *Journal of Physiology and Biochemistry* **66**, 1–6. doi:10.1007/s13105-010-0001-2

Cormack SJ, Newton RU, McGuigan MR (2008) Neuromuscular and endocrine responses of elite players to an Australian rules football match. *International Journal of Sports Physiology and Performance* **3**, 359–374.

Coso JD, González-Millán C, Salinero JJ, Abián-Vicén J, Soriano L, Garde S, *et al.* (2012) Muscle damage and its relationship with muscle fatigue during a half-iron triathlon. *PLoS One* **7**, e43280. doi:10.1371/journal.pone.0043280

Coutts A, Duffield R (2010) Validity and reliability of GPS devices for measuring movement demands of team sports. *Journal of Science and Medicine in Sport* **13**, 133–135. doi:10.1016/j.jsams.2008.09.015

Crewther BT, Lowe TE, Ingram J, Weatherby RP (2010) Validating the salivary testosterone and cortisol concentration measures in response to short high-intensity exercise. *The Journal of Sports Medicine and Physical Fitness* **50**, 85–92.

Cummins C, Orr R, O'Connor H, West C (2013) Global positioning systems (GPS) and microtechnology sensors in team sports: a systematic review. *Sports Medicine (Auckland, N.Z.)* **43**, 1025–1042. doi:10.1007/s40279-013-0069-2

Demarle AP, Heugas AM, Slawinski JJ, Tricot VM, Koralsztein JP, Billat VL (2003) Whichever the initial training status, any increase in velocity at lactate threshold appears as a major factor in improved time to exhaustion at the same severe velocity after training. *Archives of Physiology and Biochemistry* **111**, 167–176. doi:10.1076/apab.111.2.167.14003

Dziedzic CE, Ross ML, Slater GJ, Burke LM (2014) Variability of measurements of sweat sodium using the regional absorbent patch method. *International Journal of Sports Physiology and Performance* **9**, 832–838. doi:10.1123/ijspp.2013-0480

Esser D, Alvare-Lamas G, de Vries MP, Weening D, Vonk RJ, Roelofsen H (2008) Sample stability and protein composition of saliva: implications for its use as a diagnostic fluid. *Biomarker Insights* **3**, 25–37.

Gatti R, De Palo EF (2011) An update: salivary hormones and physical exercise. *Scandinavian Journal of Medicine & Science in Sports* **21**, 157–169. doi:10.1111/j.1600-0838.2010.01252.x

Gleeson M (2007) Immune function in sport and exercise. *Journal of Applied Physiology* **103**, 693–699. doi:10.1152/japplphysiol.00008.2007

Gleeson M, Walsh NP (2012) The BASES expert statement on exercise, immunity, and infection. *Journal of Sports Sciences* **30**, 321–324. doi:10.1080/02640414.2011.627371

Guerriero RM, Giza CC, Rotenberg A (2015) Glutamate and GABA imbalance following traumatic brain injury. *Current Neurology and Neuroscience Reports* **15**, 27. doi:10.1007/s11910-015-0545-1

Halson S, Bridge MW, Meeusen R, Busschaert B, Gleeson M, Jones DA, *et al.* (2002) Time course of performance changes and fatigue markers during intensified training in trained cyclists. *Journal of Applied Physiology* **93**, 947–956. doi:10.1152/japplphysiol.01164.2001

Hoffman MD, Stuempfle KJ, Fogard K, Hew-Butler T, Winger J, Weiss RH (2013) Urine dipstick analysis for identification of runners susceptible to acute kidney injury following an ultramarathon. *Journal of Sports Sciences* **31**, 20–31. doi:10.1080/02640414.2012.720705

Hovda DA (2014) The neurophysiology of concussion. In *Concussion.* (Eds A Niranjan and LD Lunsford) pp. 28–37. Karger, Basel, Switzerland.

Kim J, Valdes-Ramirez G, Bandodkaretal AJ (2014) Non-invasive mouthguard biosensor for continuous salivary monitoring of metabolites. *Analyst (London)* **139**, 1632–1636. doi:10.1039/c3an02359a

Kratz A, Siegel AJ, Verbalis JG, Adner MM, Shirey T, Lee-Lewandrowski E, *et al.* (2005) Sodium status of collapsed marathon runners. *Archives of Pathology & Laboratory Medicine* **129**, 227–230.

Malon RSP, Sadir S, Balakrishnan M, Corcoles EP (2014) Saliva-based biosensors: noninvasive monitoring tool for clinical diagnostics. *BioMed Research International* **2014**, Article ID 962903. doi:10.1155/2014/962903

Martin DT, Ashenden M, Parisotto R, Pyne D, Hahn AG (1997) Blood testing for professional cyclists: what's a fair hematocrit limit? *Sportscience News*, <http://www.sportsci.org/news/news9703/AISblood.html>.

Mckune AJ, Bach CW, Semple SJ, Dyer BJ (2014) Salivary cortisol and α-amylase responses to repeated bouts of downhill running. *American Journal of Human Biology* **26**, 850–855. doi:10.1002/ajhb.22605

McLellan C, Lovell D, Gass G (2010) Creatine kinase and endocrine responses of elite players pre, during and post rugby league match play. *Journal of Strength and Conditioning Research* **24**, 2908–2919. doi:10.1519/JSC.0b013e3181c1fcb1

McNaughton LR, Thompson D, Philips G, Backx K, Crickmore L (2002) A comparison of the Lactate Pro, Accusport, Analox GM7 and Kodak Ektachem lactate analysers in normal, hot and humid conditions. *International Journal of Sports Medicine* **23**, 130–135. doi:10.1055/s-2002-20133

McNulty SE, Sharkey SJ, Schieren H (1994) Bedside hemoglobin measurements – sensitivity to changes in serum-protein and electrolytes. *Journal of Clinical Monitoring* **10**, 377–381. doi:10.1007/BF01618418

Medbø JI, Mamen A, Olsen OH, Evertsen F (2000) Examination of four different instruments for measuring blood lactate concentration. *Scandinavian Journal of Clinical and Laboratory Investigation* **60**, 367–380. doi:10.1080/00365510 0750019279

Meeusen R, Duclos M, Foster C, Fry A, Gleeson M, Nieman D, Raglin J, Rietjens G, *et al.* (2013) Prevention, diagnosis, and treatment of the overtraining syndrome: joint consensus statement of the European College of Sport Science and the American College of Sports Medicine. *Medicine and Science in Sports and Exercise* **45**, 186–205. doi:10.1249/MSS.0b013e 318279a10a

Mørkeberg JS, Belhage B, Damsgaard R (2009) Changes in blood values in elite cyclist. *International Journal of Sports Medicine* **30**, 130–138. doi:10.1055/s-2008-1038842

Morris SS, Ruel MT, Cohen RJ, Dewey KG, de la Briere B, Hassan MN (1999) Precision, accuracy, and reliability of hemoglobin assessment with use of capillary blood. *The American Journal of Clinical Nutrition* **69**, 1243–1248.

Mougios V (2007) Reference intervals for serum creatine kinase in athletes. *British Journal of Sports Medicine* **41**, 674–678. doi:10.1136/bjsm.2006.034041

Munoz M, Romero A, Gomez JF, Manteca A, Naveira E, Ramirez G (2005) Utility of point-of-care haemoglobin measurement in the HemoCue-B haemoglobin for the initial diagnosis of anaemia. *Clinical and Laboratory Haematology* **27**, 99–104. doi:10.1111/j.1365-2257.2005.00678.x

Nater UM, Rohleder N (2009) Salivary alpha-amylase as a non-invasive biomarker for the sympathetic nervous system: current state of research. *Psychoneuroendocrinology* **34**, 486–496. doi:10.1016/j.psyneuen.2009.01.014

Neville V, Gleeson M, Folland JP (2008) Salivary IgA as a risk factor for upper respiratory infections in elite professional athletes. *Medicine and Science in Sports and Exercise* **40**, 1228–1236. doi:10.1249/MSS.0b013e31816be9c3

Newsholme P, Lima MMR, Procopio J, Pithon-Curi TC, Doi SQ, Bazotte RB, *et al.* (2003) Glutamine and glutamate as vital metabolites. *Brazilian Journal of Medical and Biological Research* **36**, 153–163. doi:10.1590/S0100-879X2003000200002

Northoff H (2009) Editorial: exercise immunology review. *Exercise Immunology Review* **15**, 5.

Norton K, Norton L, Sadgrove D (2010) Position statement on physical activity and exercise intensity terminology. *Journal of Science and Medicine in Sport* **13**, 496–502. doi:10.1016/j.jsams.2009.09.008

Papa L, Ramia M, Edwards D, Johnson B, Slobounov S (2015) Systematic review of clinical studies examining biomarkers of brain injury in athletes after sports-related concussion. *Journal of Neurotrauma* **32**, 661–673. doi:10.1089/neu.2014.3655

Papacosta E, Nassis G (2011) Saliva as a tool for monitoring steroid, peptide and immune markers in sport and exercise science. *Journal of Science and Medicine in Sport* **14**, 424–434. doi:10.1016/j.jsams.2011.03.004

Pinnington H, Dawson B (2001) Examination of the validity and reliability of the Accusport blood lactate analyzer. *Journal of Science and Medicine in Sport* **4**, 129–138. doi:10.1016/S1440-2440(01)80014-1

Pyne DB, Boston T, Martin DT, Logan A (2000) Evaluation of the Lactate Pro blood lactate analyzer. *European Journal of Applied Physiology* **82**, 112–116. doi:10.1007/s004210050659

Reinke S, Taylor WR, Duda GN, von Haehling S, Reinke P, Volk HD, *et al.* (2012) Absolute and functional iron deficiency in professional athletes during training and recovery. *International Journal of Cardiology* **156**, 186–191. doi:10.1016/j.ijcard.2010.10.139

Rietjens GJ, Kuipers H, Adam JJ, Saris WHM, van Breda E, van Hamont D, *et al.* (2005) Physiological, biochemical and psychological markers of strenuous training induced fatigue. *International Journal of Sports Medicine* **26**, 16–26. doi:10.1055/s-2004-817914

Sawka MN, Burke LM, Eichner ER, Maughan RJ, Montain SJ, Stachenfeld NS (2007) American College of Sports Medicine position stand. Exercise and fluid replacement. *Medicine and Science in Sports and Exercise* **39**, 377–390.

Schabmueller CGJ, Loppow D, Piechotta G, Schutze B, Albers J, Hintsche R (2006) Micromachined sensor for lactate monitoring in saliva. *Biosensors & Bioelectronics* **21**, 1770–1776. doi:10.1016/j.bios.2005.09.015

Schroeder ET, Villanueva M, West DWD, Phillips SM (2013) Are acute post-resistance exercise increases in testosterone, growth hormone, and IGF-1 necessary to stimulate skeletal muscle anabolism and hypertrophy? *Medicine and Science in Sports and Exercise* **45**, 2044–2051. doi:10.1249/MSS.0000000000000147

Twist C, Highton J (2013) Monitoring fatigue and recovery in rugby league players. *International Journal of Sports Physiology and Performance* **8**, 467–474.

Vittek J, L'Hommedieu DG, Gordon GG, Rappaport SC, Southren AL (1985) Direct Radioimmunoassay (RIA) of salivary testosterone: correlation with free and total serum testosterone. *Life Sciences* **37**, 711–716. doi:10.1016/0024-3205(85)90540-5

Walsh NP, Gleeson M, Shephard RJ, Gleeson M, Woods JA, Bishop NC, *et al.* (2011) Position statement part one: immune function and exercise. *Exercise Immunology Review* **17**, 6–63.

WADA (World Anti-Doping Agency) (2013) *The World Anti-Doping Code, International Standard for Testing and Investigations.* World Anti-Doping Agency, Montreal, Canada.

World Anti-Doping Agency (2015) *The World Anti-Doping Code.* World Anti-Doping Agency, Montreal, Canada.

Wundersitz D, Josman C, Gupta R, Netto KJ, Gastin PB, Robertson S (2015) Classification of team sport activities using a single wearable tracking device. *Journal of Biomechanics* **48**, 3975–3981. doi:10.1016/j.jbiomech.2015.09.015

Wyatt F, Donaldson A, Brown E (2013) The overtraining syndrome: A meta-analytic review. *Journal of Exercise Physiology Online* **16**, 12–23.

Yasuda M, Honma S, Furuya K, Takashi Y, Yutaka K, Hisamitsu I, *et al.* (2008) Diagnostic significance of salivary testosterone measurement revisited: using liquid chromatography/mass spectrometry and enzyme-linked immunosorbent assay. *The Journal of Men's Health* **5**, 56–63. doi:10.1016/j.jomh.2007.12.004

# 34 Point-of-care testing in the pharmacy

*Geoff Herd*

**Summary**

Pharmacists are readily accessible in the community and now act as members of multidisciplinary teams for disease management programs and for health screening. Access to pathology test results is a key element of disease management and can potentially be improved by using point-of-care testing (POCT) devices in a pharmacy setting as part of daily routine. The most common conditions for which POCT is used in pharmacies include diabetes, hyperlipidaemia, anticoagulant control and infectious disease screening. The use of POCT devices enhances professional development for pharmacists, shows a high level of acceptance by patients and can help to reduce overall costs of health care. Nonetheless, issues of reimbursement of costs, licensing and registration, ongoing pathology support, and acceptance by other medical and health professionals may provide obstacles to the implementation of POCT in this setting.

## INTRODUCTION

This chapter will explore: (i) the types of POCT that are being used in pharmacy settings in different countries; (ii) the applications of POCT profiles that are most advantageous for patient management in this setting; (iii) the challenges facing pharmacies engaged in, or planning to develop, POCT services; and (iv) the quality management systems that should be used for POCT in pharmacies. A case study will also describe how POCT has been successfully implemented in the pharmacy setting in New Zealand. It is recommended that pharmacies seek the advice of medical laboratory professionals or specialist POCT providers with regard to the implementation of POCT programs. Pharmacies that plan to implement a POCT service are encouraged to review the practical guidelines for the implementation of POCT in the pharmacy outlined at the end of this chapter.

## OVERVIEW OF THE USE OF POCT IN THE PHARMACY SETTING

In the United Kingdom, community pharmacies have been identified as an easily accessible and cost-effective platform for delivering health care (Department of Health 2005). In Australia, over 90% of the population may visit a pharmacy at some point during the year (Benrimoj and Frommer 2004). Similarly, in both low- and middle-income countries, pharmacies are often seen as 'a first point of call' for advice on symptoms and for early diagnosis of illness. Pharmacies are often located within, or close to, neighbourhoods and enable access to over-the-counter (OTC) medications, traditional medication or prescribed medicines. Patients who visit pharmacies may

**Table 34.1.** Examples of 'over the counter' and POC tests available at pharmacies

| Tests or test profiles | Specific analytes |
|---|---|
| **'Over the counter' tests** | |
| Urinalysis | Glucose, ketones, blood, leucocytes, protein |
| Urine pregnancy testing | Beta-hCG |
| Ovulation detection and fertility (urine) | Luteinising Hormone (LH) and Follicle Stimulating Hormone (FSH) |
| Urine drug screening kits | Drugs of abuse: narcotics and tetrahydrocannabinol (THC) |
| Faecal occult blood | Blood and haemoglobin |
| Cholesterol | |
| Hepatitis C | |
| Human immunodeficiency virus (HIV) | |
| Prothrombin | |
| Vaginal pH | |
| Coeliac disease markers | Tissue transglutaminase (tTG) IgA and IgG; deamidated gliadin peptides (DGP) IgA and IgG |
| Tests for cardiovascular risk | Lipids (cholesterol, triglyceride and HDL-cholesterol) |
| **Diagnostic tests** | |
| Sexually transmitted infections | Hepatitis C (HCV) |
| | Human immunodeficiency virus (HIV) |
| **Monitoring tests** | |
| Tests for monitoring diabetes | Glucose and β-hydroxybutyrate |
| | Haemoglobin A1c (HbA1c) |
| | Lipids |
| Tests for patients on warfarin therapy | International normalised ratio (INR) |
| Tests for antipsychotic medication induced metabolic syndrome monitoring | HbA1c and lipids |
| Renal function | Creatinine |

purchase of a variety of POCT devices, such as home-use urine pregnancy and fertility tests kits or glucose meters and test strips. Pharmacists who advise on medications may also have an additional role in providing information on how to use some of these POCT devices and the interpretation of the test results. Some examples of OTC tests supplied by pharmacies and other tests provided in pharmacies are summarised in Table 34.1.

## EXAMPLES OF, OPPORTUNITIES AND EVIDENCE-BASE FOR, POCT APPLICATIONS IN PHARMACIES

POCT devices provide rapid on-site test results at the time of the consultation, which eliminate the delays encountered with conventional laboratory testing. The use of POCT devices in pharmacies can create opportunities for professional development, more involvement with patient care and education, disease management, expanded revenue streams and, at the same time, improve clinical decision making with regard to patient conditions. POCT in pharmacies has been used for screening and/or management of patients with both chronic and infectious diseases (Geerts *et al.* 2013; Gubbins *et al.* 2014; Gutierres and Welty 2004; Shaw *et al.* 2011). Table 34.2 lists a representative sample of published studies on the types of POCT and the technologies that have been used in pharmacies for disease management and screening.

### Screening for infectious diseases

Pharmacy-based POCT for infectious diseases has many benefits both for individual patients and the population because it can reduce the time between testing and diagnosis and at the same time help to reduce the possibility of disease transmission, improve time to treatment and also antibiotic stewardship (Gubbins *et al.* 2014; Klepser

**Table 34.2.** Examples of selected POCT studies undertaken in the pharmacy setting.

| Reference | Country | Point-of-care test | POCT device (manufacturer) |
|---|---|---|---|
| Armour *et al.* 2004 | Australia | Glucose | MediSense |
| Bluml *et al.* 2000 | USA | Total cholesterol | Cholestech LDX (Cholestech Corp) |
| Cranor *et al.* 2003 | USA | Glucose | Not specified |
| Davidson *et al.* 2000 | USA | Urine dipstick protein | Not specified |
| Geerts *et al.* 2013 | Netherlands | Creatinine and Potassium ion | i-STAT Analyser (Abbott Diagnostics) |
| Jaber *et al.* 1996 | USA | Glucose | One Touch Basic (Lifescan) |
| Jackson *et al.* 2004 | Australia | INR | CoaguChek S (Roche Diagnostics) |
| Jafari *et al.* 2001 | USA | Cholesterol and Triglycerides | Cholestech LDX (Cholestech Corp) |
| Jones 2008 | USA | INR | i-STAT Analyser (Abbott Diagnostics) |
| Darin *et al.* 2015a,b | United States | HIV | Uni-Gold Recombigen HIV 1/2 |
| Shaw *et al.* 2011 | New Zealand | INR | CoaguChek XS Plus (Roche Diagnostics) |
| Schneiderhan *et al.* 2014 | USA | HbA1c, Cholesterol and Triglycerides | A1c Now (PTS Diagnostics)<br>Cholestech LDX (Cholestech Corp) |
| Taylor *et al.* 2011 | United Kingdom | FBC for clozapine monitoring | Not specified |
| Tsuyuki *et al.* 2002 | Canada | Total cholesterol | Accutrend GC (Roche Diagnostics) |
| Yamada *et al.* 2005 | Canada | LDL-cholesterol | Cholestech LDX (Cholestech Corp) |

2015). A recent review by Weber *et al.* (2015) showed that Clinical Laboratory Improvement Amendments (CLIA)-waived rapid tests for influenza, group A streptococcus pharyngitis, *Helicobacter pylori*, human immunodeficiency virus (HIV) and hepatitis C virus (HCV) are available and could be used for pharmacy based infectious disease screening.

## HIV testing

Darin *et al.* (2015b) evaluated the acceptability and feasibility of pharmacist-provided rapid testing for HIV infection in two independent community pharmacies in Michigan, USA from October 2011 to March 2013. Pharmacists carried out 69 HIV tests and one (1.5%) client who returned a positive test was referred for confirmatory testing. The median time required for testing was 30 min (range 20–90). The project showed that pharmacist-provided HIV testing was feasible and acceptable in these two community pharmacies.

## HCV testing

A recent survey by Calderon *et al.* (2014) showed that a majority of patients would be receptive to the use of rapid POC HCV testing if this test was available in emergency departments and pharmacies. The convenience of saliva-based HCV antibody tests is a significant advantage over conventional blood, plasma or serum based tests. The performance of a USA Food and Drug Administration (FDA)-approved, CLIA-waived, rapid saliva test for HCV antibody has been reported by Cha *et al.* (2013), with the clinical sensitivity and specificity of the OraQuick HCV test being 97.8% (95% CI: 93.2–99.4%) and 100% (95% CI: 98.4–100%), respectively. These authors noted that the test would be suitable for both medical and non-medical settings such as pharmacies (Cha *et al.* 2013).

## Group A streptococcus testing

Pharmacies have also been involved in testing for influenza and group A streptococcus, which assists with notification during outbreaks and public health surveillance (Weber *et al.* 2015). Rapid POC tests for group A streptococcus pharyngitis have the advantage that patients who show positive results on throat swabs can be treated with antibiotics at the time of presentation and contacts traced in a timely fashion. Some pharmacies in the Hutt Valley and Northland, New Zealand, have been involved in the collection of throat swabs for patients with symptomatic sore throat. This is part of a national program called 'Sore throats matter' to increase the detection rates for group A streptococcus in order to help prevent the development of serious long-term complications including rheumatic fever (New Zealand Ministry of Health 2015).

## Screening for coeliac disease

Some pharmacies now offer a screening test for coeliac disease. Laboratory tests for markers of coeliac disease include antibodies to tissue transglutaminase (tTG) or antibodies to deamidated gliadin peptides (DGP). A 2014 report from the Coeliac Australia Medical Advisory Committee states that there were eight POCT methods on the market that test for a combination of markers including: tTG IgA, tTG IgA and IgG, tTG IgA, IgG and IgM and DGP IgA, IgG and tTotal IgA. Some of these POC tests require whole blood, others serum or plasma. The sensitivities of these qualitative POC tests for coeliac disease ranged from 70 to 97% but the specificities were better and ranged from 94 to 100%. Although the cost of these POC tests was relatively inexpensive (US$20–$40) per test, the interpretation of test results is subjective. In addition, up to 10% of results were false positive and 15–20% of results were false negative. These qualitative test kits are also not automated so tests results cannot be captured electronically (Coeliac Australia 2014). Their use in pharmacies therefore needs to be undertaken with caution, with the support of the local laboratory to verify the quality of the test method used, how the results compare with conventional assays and interpreted with expert clinical advice.

## Chronic disease risk and management – diabetes and hyperlipidaemia

In some pharmacy-led chronic disease management programs, POCT for glucose or cholesterol has been used as an intervention strategy in, or coordinated by, the pharmacy – with the primary outcome measures (e.g. HbA1c and lipids) being measured in the laboratory.

A randomised controlled trial to assess the effect of community pharmacist intervention on cholesterol risk management involving 54 pharmacies was implemented in Canada from 1998 to 2000 (Tsuyuki *et al.* 2002). In this trial, 344 patients with high risk for cardiovascular events, including atherosclerotic vascular disease, myocardial infarction, stable or unstable angina, coronary revascularisation or cerebral or peripheral vascular disease, were recruited for the intervention group. The study also included patients with diabetes and at least one other cardiovascular disease factor. The patients were randomised to pharmacist intervention, which included education, a brochure on risk factors, POC cholesterol testing, referral to their physician and regular follow-up at, 2, 4, 8, 12 and 16 weeks. The control group of 331 patients received the same brochure and general advice with limited follow-up and no POCT. The authors stated that the primary endpoint was a composite measure of improvement in the process of cholesterol risk management, defined as a complete fasting cholesterol measurement, or a new prescription of a cholesterol-lowering medication, or an increase in the dosage of cholesterol-lowering medication. This primary endpoint was achieved in 196 (57% of) intervention patients, whereas only 102 (31% of) patients accessing usual care achieved this goal ($P$ <0.001).

A 2-year, 'walk in' POC screening service for cholesterol showed that 150 of 301 participants required intervention and follow-up and that 52 (32% of) patients with high levels of cholesterol were previously undiagnosed (Jafari *et al.* 2001). This pharmacy-based program with self-referred patients, who paid US$20 for the service, was supported by a local clinical pathologist with follow-up lipid tests provided by a local laboratory. These authors also included some advice to pharmacies on how to establish a pharmacy-based POC lipid screening program and recommended that more pharmacists develop POC cholesterol screening programs.

In the USA, 26 pharmacies participated in a project termed Improve Persistence and Compliance with Therapy (ImPACT): Hyperlipidaemia (Bluml *et al.* 2000). The pharmacies used POC cholesterol testing to assist with hyperlipidaemia management. This observational study involved 397 dyslipidaemic patients, either newly diagnosed or poorly controlled, over an average of 24.6 months. At the end of the study, the rates for persistence and compliance with medication were 93.6% and 90.1%, respectively. The mean (±standard deviation) reduction in total cholesterol and triglycerides was 12.8% (±1.6%) and 10% (±6.5%), respectively. The mean increase in high density lipoprotein cholesterol (HDL-C) levels was 14.2% (±3.9%). The overall mean reduction in low density lipoprotein cholesterol (LDL-C) was 22.1% (±2.6%) measured using the POCT cholesterol device. The National Cholesterol Education Program (NCEP) Adult Treatment Panel guidelines recommend LDL-C goals of <4.1 mmol/L (160 mg/dL) for patients with less than two cardiac artery disease (CAD) risk factors, <3.4 mmol/L (130 mg/dL) for patients with two or more CAD risk factors and <2.6 mmol/L (100 mg/dL) for patients with a history of CAD. Based on these POCT cholesterol results, 62.5% of patients achieved the NCEP goals after 24.6 months. The authors did not mention any laboratory support for the project but concluded that collaboration between patients, health providers and pharmacists who have efficient access to POC test results can achieve improved outcomes in the management of dyslipidaemia.

The Asheville Project in North Carolina, USA involved 12 community pharmacies and included 194 patients with diabetes (Cranor *et al.* 2003). This quasi-experimental, longitudinal, pre- and post-cohort study ran from 1997 to 2001. The program enabled diabetes patients to access home glucose meter training, physical assessments and information on adherence to drug treatment, all of which was provided by the pharmacy. Patients were given incentives to participate with a free blood glucose meter and a waiver of co-payments for diabetes specific medication and supplies. Patients were followed up at 6-monthly intervals. In the first cohort of patients, followed up from the first to the seventh period, there was a lowering of mean laboratory HbA1c levels from 7.8% (±2.2%) to 6.8% (±1.3%). Similar reductions in mean HbA1c levels were reported for subsequent cohorts, but not all cohorts reached statistical significance. In terms of overall outcomes across all cohorts, 57.7–81.8% of patients showed improved HbA1c levels and the average medical cost decreased by US$1200 to US$1872 per patient per year compared with the baseline costs.

A multi-site intervention study to evaluate pharmacists' diabetes care services for type 2 diabetes patients was implemented in three regions in eastern and western Sydney and New South Wales (Armour *et al.* 2004). In the control and intervention groups, the pharmacists provided diabetes care in community pharmacies or a diabetes clinic attached to a teaching hospital. Blood glucose levels were only measured in the intervention group, who were provided with glucose meters by the pharmacists for home POC glucose monitoring. The pharmacists provided 1459 interventions during the study, including medical checks, self-care, lifestyle, medication adherence and diabetes education. In all, 106 patients in the intervention group and 82 patients in the control group completed the 9-month study. Patients in the intervention group ($n$ = 96) showed a linear reduction in mean glucose levels from visit 1 to visit 6, with an increase in the number of glucose readings between 4 and 8 mmol/L from 44 to 56% ($P$ <0.001) and a decrease in the number of glucose readings above 8 mmol/L from 54 to 42% ($P$ <0.001). The number of patients in the intervention group ($n$ = 53) with laboratory-measured HbA1c levels >7% decreased from 72% at baseline to 53% after 9 months; whereas in the control group ($n$ = 46), the percentage of patients whose HbA1c was >7% increased from 54 to 61%. The intervention group patients reported that they were 'extremely pleased with the service', wanted it to continue and felt that the input of the pharmacist had made significant changes to their diabetes control (Armour *et al.* 2004).

A 4-month, randomised controlled study in the USA was conducted on the effectiveness of a pharmacy-based care model for 39 non-insulin-dependent diabetes mellitus (NIDDM) patients (17 intervention and 22 control) (Jaber *et al.* 1996). The intervention group received training in the use of home based POCT blood glucose meters from the pharmacists. There was a reduction in mean HbA1c level from baseline (11.5 ±2.9%) to final (9.2 ±2.1%) in the intervention group, but there was no change in glycaemia in the control group whose mean baseline HbA1c level was 12.2 (±3.5%) and at the end of the study was 12.1% (±3.7%) ($P$ = 0.003). Interestingly, during the course of the study, there were 17 reported hypoglycaemic episodes in the intervention group, whereas there were only two reported hypoglycaemic reactions in the control group. The authors stated that this difference was because the intervention group were trained to recognise and document episodes of hypoglycaemia.

## Monitoring anticoagulation therapy

The benefits of in-pharmacy INR POCT for monitoring patients on warfarin therapy have been reported from rural Tasmania in Australia (Jackson *et al.* 2004), the United Kingdom (Thomas *et al.* 2009), the USA (Jones 2008) and New Zealand (Shaw *et al.* 2011).

A comparative study of pharmacist-performed fingerstick INR testing in an urban Coumadin Clinic program in Pennsylvania in the USA versus venepuncture and central laboratory testing, showed significant time savings and operational advantages (Jones 2008). Finger-stick blood collection, testing, review, dosing and future appointment scheduling services took 10 min versus a 'best case total process time' of 6 hours using conventional venepuncture and laboratory testing. The author noted that in this study anticoagulant monitoring using the conventional laboratory testing process was 'fragmented' and often required several phone calls, which may increase the possibility of ambiguous or poorly understood information being given to the patient, whereas the POCT pharmacy service eliminated the risk of misleading information being exchanged between the laboratory, the pharmacist and the patient (Jones 2008).

In New Zealand, a highly successful urban and rural Community Pharmacist Anticoagulant Management Service (CPAMS) is now in operation (Shaw *et al.* 2011). The CPAMS Program will be described in more detail later in this chapter and was covered in Chapter 13.

### Medication dosages and renal function

In elderly patients, appropriate medication dose is linked to adequate renal clearance of the drug prescribed. Pharmacists in the Netherlands described a feasibility study that used POC capillary blood creatinine testing to monitor renal function in elderly patients who were being treated with diabetes and cardiovascular drugs (Geerts *et al.* 2013). The service included comprehensive training for the pharmacists and a thorough quality assurance program supported by a central laboratory. The authors reported that 44 patients who had POC creatinine tests were found to have mild–moderate renal impairment, which indicated adjustment in therapy. The testing also included measurement of potassium ion to check for haemolysis during capillary blood sampling.

In a recent initiative, Kidney Health Australia and Sigma Pharmaceuticals have introduced an education initiative concerning kidney disease (called Kidney-Check™), which provides the opportunity for patients to perform a urine dipstick protein test as a screening test for kidney disease.

## ACCEPTABILITY OF POCT IN PHARMACIES

There is a body of evidence that patients find POCT in the pharmacy acceptable (Armour *et al.* 2004; Geerts *et al.* 2013; Jackson *et al.* 2004; Jafari *et al.* 2001; Jones 2008; Shaw *et al.* 2011). Jackson *et al.* (2004) described the convenience of POC INR testing for tourists in remote pharmacy settings of Australia. Geerts *et al.* (2013) surveyed 38 elderly patients with diabetes or cardiovascular disease who had POC capillary blood creatinine tests performed in a pharmacy. Patients were asked for their overall assessment of POCT and the advice they received. The mean satisfaction score for POCT was 4.50 (±0.51), using a 5-point Likert scale ranging from 1 = bad to 5 = very good. The views of five general practitioners (GPs) and five pharmacists were also explored. The mean Likert score for the question on usefulness of rapid availability of POC test results was 3.80 (±1.0) for the GPs and 4.60 (±0.55) for the pharmacists.

Pharmacy-based disease management programs can reduce morbidity and mortality and save on total health costs. For example, a community-pharmacy-based asthma management program using peak expiratory flow rate (PEFR) as a POC test was established in Indiana, USA (Rupp *et al.* 1997). This was part of an initiative to provide a 'living laboratory' to enable the development and marketing of clinical services in a community setting. The program included measurement of PEFR, drug treatment and quality of life measures. A review by the local Health Maintenance Organisation found that the paediatric patients who were enrolled in the asthma management program showed significant improvements in quality of life, including a 77% decrease in hospitalisation, a 78% decrease in emergency care visits and a 25% decrease in urgent care visits. These authors also provide valuable practical advice on the governance, management and implementation of the POCT service in the pharmacy.

Collectively, this overview illustrates that pharmacy-based or pharmacy-related POCT improved access to test results and there was a high level of acceptance by patients. Although they may not conclusively prove that use of POCT *per se* in the pharmacy improves outcomes, they demonstrate 'proof of concept' of the significant contribution that pharmacists working with GPs can have on disease management and monitoring medication and also that pharmacists can effectively use POCT devices in a pharmacy setting as part of daily routine.

## BARRIERS AND LIMITATIONS TO USING POCT IN PHARMACIES

Pharmacy-based POCT activities have many potential benefits, as just outlined, but there are limitations relating to regulatory, technical and cost issues. In addition, the list of OTC tests available in pharmacies also has limitations.

### Over-the-counter tests

OTC tests have the advantage that they are cost-effective, rapid and confidential. They are often used to detect specific conditions such as hypercholesterolaemia and early pregnancy or for monitoring (e.g. glucose or warfarin). In general, the tests correlate reasonably well with conventional laboratory tests but are not a substitute for clinical advice from a qualified health professional because the results of these tests need to be evaluated in the light of clinical history and examination with follow-up tests as required.

## Regulation of POCT devices

In the USA, most POC tests and devices are of low complexity and are classified as CLIA-waived (Gutierres and Welty 2004; Lippi *et al.* 2010). A 2013 review by Gubbins *et al.* (2014) showed that eight states in the USA have regulations that deal with POCT in the pharmacy and, in five of these states, the practice act specifies the POC tests a pharmacist may perform. As of late 2012, 44 states had collaborative drug therapy management (CDTM) provisions where 19 states allowed POC testing by pharmacists. According to Lippi *et al.* (2010), the 1998 European *in vitro* Diagnostics (IVDs) Medical Devices Directive (98/97/EC) was published and subsequently developed into law in the United Kingdom in 2002. Since 2003, all products placed on the market in the European Union and European Economic Area must comply with the directive and local member state laws. In 2001, France, Germany and Portugal had a formal process for registering some IVDs. In Australia, IVDs are regulated by the Therapeutic Goods Administration (Lippi *et al.* 2010). In New Zealand only pregnancy test kits are regulated under the Medicines Regulations 1984, but they are not medicines (Musaad and Herd 2013).

## Technical issues

POCT may be deceptively simple to use but is not without risk. POCT needs to be implemented in all primary care settings (including pharmacies) in a manner that safeguards the patient and, at the same time, provides rapid test results at a reasonable cost. Pharmacists who may not be professionally trained in medical diagnostic testing require appropriate on-site training and certification to ensure clinical safety. Training programs should include the requirements for the pre-analytical, analytical and post-analytical phases of testing (Lippi *et al.* 2010; NZPOCTAG 2014) and the potential sources and amplifiers of error (Plebani 2008) associated with each of these test phases.

Pharmacists need to interpret POCT results, be aware of the test limitations, the causes of false negative and false positive results and how the results correlate with conventional laboratory testing. Ideally, tests such as glucose and triglycerides should be performed on fasting patients. Some glucose meter test strips may produce falsely high glucose results in ambulant patients with low haematocrits or those who may be receiving Icodextrin or Intragam P due to the presence of maltose. INR results may be affected by other medication, such as macrolide antibiotics and antifungal agents.

Most of the published reports describing the use of POCT devices in pharmacies for the management of diabetes and hyperlipidaemia do not include data on quality control testing on the POCT devices used or how the results correlated with laboratory tests performed at the local laboratory. This information is important because most of these reports describe relatively long-term programs where there is potential for deterioration in the performance of reagents and equipment, changes in reagent lot numbers and changes in personnel.

Other potential barriers to the use of POCT in pharmacies include reimbursement of costs, licensing and registration, personnel requirements, lack of ongoing laboratory support and acceptance by other medical personnel. Regarding reimbursement, in the USA, pharmacists can charge patients or be reimbursed by third-party insurers for CLIA-waived POC tests for infectious diseases, but the legislative and regulatory oversight varies between states, is confusing and a significant barrier to providing POCT services (Gubbins *et al.* 2014).

Ongoing funding for some programs can be challenging. For example, a pharmacist-run diabetes management program was established in a free medical clinic for a high-needs African-American community. The experimental group were managed using detailed algorithms for glycaemic and lipid control. The initial algorithms required laboratory-based albumin:creatinine ratio (ACR) tests on patient samples with negative urine dipstick test results. However, due to financial constraints, the option for urine ACR testing was later withdrawn (Davidson *et al.* 2000). Another pharmacy-based POCT program for the management of metabolic syndrome was affected by financial constraints, where POC lipid and HbA1c testing became unsustainable because community mental health centres were unable to submit and collect claims for CLIA-waived tests (Schneiderhan *et al.* 2014).

Personnel constraints can also adversely affect programs. One study in Canada described important barriers where some of the investigators in a lipid management program were unable to participate with follow-up of patients and also staff shortages meant that 13 out of 39 pharmacists could not be involved in the program (Yamada *et al.* 2005).

From a practical perspective, pharmacies also need to have adequate on-site facilities for conducting POCT (Jaber *et al.* 1996; Rupp *et al.* 1997).

## EXAMPLE OF A SUCCESSFUL POCT MODEL IN THE PHARMACY SETTING

### Community Pharmacist Anticoagulant Management Service (CPAMS) in New Zealand

A pilot program involving 16 pharmacies funded by Health Workforce New Zealand was established as a Community Pharmacy Anticoagulant Management Service (CPAMS) in 2010. The service is now funded by local District Health Boards (DHBs) and provided free of charge to the patient. Pharmacies enrolled in CPAMS measure INR for patients on warfarin using the Roche CoaguChek XS Plus POCT device and an online clinical decision support system. These technologies help to improve access to health care (Price and Kricka 2007) and the model is consistent with the New Zealand Ministry of Health concept of 'better, sooner, more convenient' health care (New Zealand Ministry of Health 2011).

A 2011 review of the CPAMS pilot showed that the mean time in therapeutic range (TTR) for all 671 patients whose results were evaluated was 78.6%, rising slightly to 79.4% and 80.2% for patients who had been in the CPAMS for 16 weeks or 26 weeks, respectively. All pharmacies achieved a mean TTR for their respective patients of >70% (range 71.4–84.1%), well above the recommended target of 60% (Shaw *et al.* 2011).

Since 2012, the CPAMS program has been funded by District Health Boards throughout New Zealand and is well regulated. There is a formal application process and, if successful, the pharmacy must have private consulting facilities, with high-speed internet access for the INROnline clinical decision support system used in the program (www.inronline.net) (see also Chapter 13). Pharmacists must undergo full training involving the theoretical and practical aspects of anti-coagulation, patient consultation and the use of INROnline. There must be at least two pharmacists certified to carry out the testing in order to cover leave and unplanned absences. DHBs require that GPs who refer patients are required to sign off standing orders for each patient and that the pharmacist must request GP review for INRs <1.5 or >4.0. The warfarin dose adjustments are made using INROnline.

New providers are entitled to claim a US$1072 establishment fee and are responsible for purchasing the equipment and consumables. The ongoing funding to the pharmacy is US$30 per month per patient, or US$363 per year per patient.

Under normal circumstances, a minimum of 45 patients need to be recruited by a participating pharmacy and patients must not have anti-phospholipid syndrome, the lupus anticoagulant or be on chemotherapy. Enrolled pharmacies are required to carry out internal quality control tests and participate in an external proficiency testing (PT) program. CPAMS is supported by quality management systems based on ISO 22870:2006 and the NZPOCTAG Best Practice Guidelines for Point of Care Testing (ISO 2006; NZPOCTAG 2014). Pharmacies enrolled in the CPAMS program within the Canterbury District Health Board catchment are also included in the Canterbury Health Laboratories scope of accreditation for POCT by International Accreditation New Zealand (IANZ 2015).

Patient satisfaction questionnaires were completed by 430 of the 693 (62%) enrolled patients (Shaw *et al.* 2011). The survey results showed that 98.1% preferred capillary blood testing over venepuncture, 96.9% of patients found the service more convenient and 93.6% stated that it saved time. Some patients felt that the INR monitoring process was less fragmented, there was less likelihood of miscommunication and they felt more involved in their treatment. In the same report, 35 of 41 participating pharmacists (85%) were surveyed. All reported the CoaguChek XS Plus was easy to use and that they would continue to offer the service for patients on warfarin; 97% were confident the CoaguChek XS Plus results were reliable, while 94% felt that, through access to INR POC testing, they could assist patients with other aspects of their health care. Questionnaires were also completed by 28 out of 115 (24% of) GPs associated with CPAMS: 89% were confident that pharmacists could manage patient's treatment safely and the test results were reliable (Shaw *et al.* 2011).

## SOME PRACTICAL GUIDELINES FOR THE IMPLEMENTATION OF POCT IN THE PHARMACY

A brief concluding outline of the requirements for POCT services in pharmacies is provided in the following checklist.

### Clinical governance

- Governance by a multidisciplinary group comprised of pharmacists, GPs, pathologists and medical scientists should be considered.
- Develop cultural and clinical oversight on test selection for the setting and local population.

- Where practicable, accreditation for POCT services in accordance with ISO 22870:2006 should be considered.
- Development of program processes, communication systems and procedures is required.
- Therapeutic protocols and endpoints in consultation with patient care providers should be developed.
- Standing orders may be required for patients on medications for ongoing treatment.
- Incorporate clinical audit, review, continuous quality improvement and incident management.

### Use of laboratory validated POCT assays and quality control in the pharmacy

- Seek advice from local accredited pathology laboratories on devices and tests, bias and interferences and how the results correlate with conventional methods.
- Standardise reference intervals and units of measurement for each analyte with those reported by the local accredited medical laboratories.
- Performance of QC tests and participation in PT programs is highly desirable where practicable.

### Training and certification

- Collaborate with suppliers to ensure that staff are adequately trained to use POCT.
- Procedure documentation and quick reference guides need to be readily accessible.
- Ensure that there are sufficient numbers of trained staff to cover leave.

### Safety

- Devices such as glucose meters should be disinfected after use between patients.
- Staff should be aware of biohazards and wear personal protective equipment.

### Integration of POCT between providers and patient medical records

- Devices that incorporate connectivity and can be interfaced with patient management systems should be used where possible.

### Facilities and accommodation requirements for POCT equipment and consumables

- a private consulting area
- blood and other specimen collection equipment
- accessibility for elderly or disabled patients
- a hand basin and sink, in or near the consulting area
- approved facilities for the disposal of bio-hazardous materials
- high-speed internet access and printer in the consulting area for data entry
- adequate space and storage for test reagents, both at ambient temperature and refrigerated.

The following list of references also provide advice on governance and management of POCT services in pharmacies: AACB (2010); Geerts *et al.* (2013); Gubbins *et al.* (2014); Gutierres and Welty (2004); Herd and Musaad (2015); Jafari *et al.* (2001); Kost (2001); Lippi *et al.* (2010); NZPOCTAG (2014); Pearson (2006); Rupp *et al.* (1997); Shaw *et al.* (2011).

## REFERENCES


AACB (Australasian Association of Clinical Biochemists) (2008) *Point of Care Testing Implementation Guide*. AACB, Mount Lawley, Western Australia, <http://www.aacb.asn.au/documents/item/155>.

AACB (2010) *Guidelines for Conducting Quality Control and Quality Assurance for POCT*. AACB, Sydney, <http://www.aacb.asn.au/documents/item/243>.

Armour CL, Taylor SJ, Hourihan F, Smith C, Krass I (2004) Implementation and evaluation of Australian pharmacists' diabetes care services. *Journal of the American Pharmacists Association* **44**, 455–466. doi:10.1331/1544345041475625

Benrimoj SI, Frommer MS (2004) Community pharmacy in Australia. *Australian Health Review* **28**, 238–246. doi:10.1071/AH040238

Bluml BM, McKenny JM, Cziraky MJ (2000) Pharmaceutical care services and results in Project ImPACT: hyperlipidaemia. *Journal of the American Pharmaceutical Association* **40**, 157–165.

Calderon Y, Cowan E, Schramm C, Stern S, Brusalis C, Iscoe M, *et al.* (2014) HCV and HBV testing acceptability and knowledge among urban emergency department patients and pharmacy clients. *Preventive Medicine* **61**, 29–33. doi:10.1016/j.ypmed.2013.12.026

Cha YJ, Park Q, Kang FS, Yoo BC, Park KU, Kim JW, *et al.* (2013) Performance evaluation of the OraQuick hepatitis C virus rapid antibody test. *Annals of Laboratory Medicine* **33**, 184–189. doi:10.3343/alm.2013.33.3.184

Coeliac Australia (2014) *Position Statement on Point of Care Testing for coeliac antibodies*. The Coeliac Society of Australia, Medical Advisory Committee, <http://www.coeliac.org.au/uploads/65701/ufiles/Position_Statements/CAP-SPoCTCD.pdf>.

Cranor CW, Bunting BA, Christensen DB (2003) The Asheville Project: long-term clinical and economic outcomes of a community pharmacy diabetes care program. *Journal of the*

*American Pharmaceutical Association* **43**, 173–184. doi:10.1331/108658003321480713

Darin KM, Scarsi KK, Klepser DG, Klepser SA, Reeves A, Young M, *et al.* (2015a) Consumer interest in community pharmacy HIV screening services. *Journal of the American Pharmacists Association* **55**, 67–72. doi:10.1331/JAPhA.2015.14069

Darin KM, Klepser ME, Klepser DE, Klepser SA, Reeves A, Young M, *et al.* (2015b) Pharmacist-provided rapid HIV testing in two community pharmacies. *Journal of the American Pharmacists Association* **55**, 81–88. doi:10.1331/JAPhA.2015.14070

Davidson MB, Karlan VJ, Hair TL (2000) Effect of a pharmacist-managed diabetes care program in a free medical clinic. *American Journal of Quality* **15**, 137–142. doi:10.1177/106286060001500403

Department of Health (2005) *Implementing the New Community Pharmacy Contractual Framework.* Department of Health, London, UK, <webarchive.nationalarchives.gov.uk/+/www.dh.gov.uk/en/PublicationsandStatistics/Publications/ PublicationsPolicyAndGuidance/DH_4109256>.

Geerts AF, de Koning FH, de Vooght KM, Egberts AC, de Smet PA, van Solinge WW (2013) Feasibility of point-of-care creatinine testing in a community pharmacy to monitor drug therapy in ambulatory elderly patients. *Journal of Clinical Pharmacy and Therapeutics* **38**, 416–422. doi:10.1111/jcpt.12081

Gubbins PO, Klepser ME, Dering-Anderson AM, Bauer KA, Darin KM, Klepser S, *et al.* (2014) Point-of-care testing for infectious diseases: opportunities, barriers and considerations in the community pharmacy. *Journal of the American Pharmacists Association* **54**, 163–171. doi:10.1331/JAPhA.2014.13167

Gutierres SL, Welty TE (2004) Point-of-care testing: an introduction. *The Annals of Pharmacotherapy* **38**, 119–125. doi:10.1345/aph.1D212

Herd GCE, Musaad SMA (2015) Clinical governance for point-of-care testing at health provider level. *The New Zealand Medical Journal* **128**, 41–46.

IANZ (International Accreditation New Zealand) (2015) IANZ website, <www.ianz.govt.nz>.

ISO (International Organization for Standardization) (2006) *ISO 22870:2006. Point-of-care testing (POCT) – Requirements for Quality and Competence.* ISO, Geneva, Switzerland.

Jaber LA, Halapy H, Fernet M, Tummalapalli S, Diwakaran H (1996) Evaluation of a pharmaceutical care model on diabetes management. *The Annals of Pharmacotherapy* **30**, 238–243.

Jackson SL, Peterson GM, House M, Bartlett T (2004) Point-of-care monitoring of anticoagulant therapy by rural community pharmacists: description of successful outcomes. *The Australian Journal of Rural Health* **12**, 197–200. doi:10.1111/j.1440-1854.2004.00604.x

Jafari M, Masih M, Emerson JF (2001) The value of pharmacist involvement in a point-of-care service, walk-in lipid screening program. *Pharmacotherapy* **21**, 1403–1406. doi:10.1592/phco.21.17.1403.34416

Jones JB (2008) Side-by-side "lean" process mapping of fingerstick i-STAT PT-INR versus venipuncture Stago PT-INR. *Point of Care* **7**, 181–182. doi:10.1097/01.POC.0000335890.29594.9e

Klepser ME, Adams AJ, Klepser DG (2015) Antimicrobial stewardship in outpatient settings: leveraging innovative physician-pharmacist collaborations to reduce antibiotic resistance. *Health Security* **13**, 166–173. doi:10.1089/hs.2014.0083

Kost G (2001) Preventing medical errors in point-of-care testing: security, validation, performance, safeguards and connectivity. *Archives of Pathology & Laboratory Medicine* **125**, 1307–1315.

Lippi G, Plebani M, Favaloro EJ, Trenti T (2010) Laboratory testing in pharmacies. *Clinical Chemistry and Laboratory Medicine* **48**, 943–953. doi:10.1515/CCLM.2010.184

Musaad SMA, Herd GCE (2013) Point-of-care testing governance in New Zealand: a national framework. *The New Zealand Medical Journal* **126**, 72–79.

New Zealand Ministry of Health (2011) *Better, Sooner, More Convenient Primary Health Care in the Community.* New Zealand Ministry of Health, <www.health.govt.nz/our-work/primary-health-care>.

New Zealand Ministry of Health (2015) *Sore Throat Clinics in the Hutt Valley,* <http://www.health.govt.nz/search/results/pharmacy?page=1>.

NZPOCTAG (New Zealand Point of Care Testing Advisory Group) (2014) *Best Practice Guidelines for Point-of-Care Testing.* New Zealand Point-of-Care Testing Advisory Group, New Zealand.

Pearson J (2006) Point-of-care testing and clinical governance. *Clinical Chemistry and Laboratory Medicine* **44**, 765–767. doi:10.1515/CCLM.2006.129

Plebani M (2008) Laboratory errors and patient safety: the case of POCT. *Point of Care* **7**, 122. doi:10.1097/01.POC.0000335885.91475.f2

Price CP, Kricka LJ (2007) Improving healthcare accessibility through point of care technologies. *Clinical Chemistry* **53**, 1665–1675. doi:10.1373/clinchem.2006.084707

Rupp MT, McCallian DJ, Sheth KK (1997) Developing and marketing a community-pharmacy based asthma management program. *Journal of the American Pharmaceutical Association* **NS37**, 649–699.

Schneiderhan ME, Schuster SM, Davey CS (2014) Twelve-month prospective randomized study of pharmacists utilizing point-of-care testing for metabolic syndrome and related conditions in subjects prescribed antipsychotics. *The Primary Care Companion for CNS Disorders* **16**(5). doi:10.4088/PCC.14m01669

Shaw J, Harrison J, Harrison J (2011) 'Community pharmacist-led anticoagulation management service: final report'. School of Pharmacy, Faculty of Medical and Health Sciences, University of Auckland, Auckland, New Zealand.

Taylor D, Sutton J, Hannah Family (2011) *Evaluating the Pharmacist Provision of Clozapine Services.* Department of Pharmacy and Pharmacology, University of Bath, Bath, UK.

Thomas MA, Sall A, Perkins M, Blount N, Ducroq DH (2009) An external quality assessment scheme for point of care testing in high street pharmacies – the UK model. *Clinical Chemistry and Laboratory Medicine* **47** (Supplement), S324.

Tsuyuki RT, Johnson JA, Teo KK, Simpson SH, Ackman ML, Biggs RS, *et al.* for the Study of Cardiovascular Risk Intervention by Pharmacists (SCRIP) Investigators (2002) A randomized trial of the effect of community pharmacist intervention on cholesterol risk management. *Archives of Internal Medicine* **162**, 1149–1155.

Weber NC, Klepser ME, Akers JM, Klepser DG, Adams AJ (2015) Use of CLIA-waived point-of-care tests for infectious diseases in community pharmacies in the United States. *Expert Review of Molecular Diagnostics* **11**, 1–12.

Yamada C, Johnson JA, Robertson P, Pearson G, Tsuyuki RT (2005) Long-term impact of a community pharmacist intervention on cholesterol levels in patients at high risk for cardiovascular events: extended follow-up of the second study of cardiovascular risk intervention by pharmacists (SCRIP-plus). *Pharmacotherapy* **25**, 110–115. doi:10.1592/phco.25.1.110.55619

# 35 Point-of-care testing with ultrasound

*Michael Jong, Margo Wilson, Tia Renouf and Michael Parsons*

**Summary**

Ultrasound has become portable and even handheld. It is a very useful tool in rural and remote practices, especially where there is limited access to other diagnostic imaging services and where the primary health-care providers have to manage patients themselves without specialty backup. As an extension of the physical examination, point-of-care ultrasound (POCUS) allows clinicians to visualise selected anatomy and functions of the body in real time and enhances the accuracy of the clinical examination. It has become indispensable for physicians caring for patients in critical, emergency and urgent care settings. POCUS is especially valuable in rural practices.

## SETTING THE SCENE FOR POCUS

### Health-care setting 1

A car went off the road. One passenger was pronounced dead on the scene and another is critically injured, in shock and has a Glasgow Coma Scale of 4. You are in a rural community with an emergency department staffed by two nurses. There is just one surgeon and one anaesthetist on call. You have a computed tomography (CT) service and the on-call technologist is at home.

*Consider how POCUS can help you with the management of this patient.*

### Health-care setting 2

You are in a remote community with no access to imaging except a portable ultrasound. The nearest location for imaging is a 4-h drive or a 20-min plane trip away, at great expense. Your 30-year-old female patient has a 1-day history of a spontaneously swollen and painful leg.

*Consider how POCUS can help with the diagnosis of the painful swollen leg.*

### Health-care setting 3

You are in a remote community where there is a basic X-ray service. An elderly man presents with a 1-day history of persistent non-productive cough and acute shortness of breath. He is known to have chronic pulmonary disease (COPD) and is a smoker. He has pitting leg oedema and you wonder if he has acute exacerbation of COPD complicated by congestive cardiac failure, pneumonia, atelectasis or pneumothorax.

*Consider how POCUS can help in the diagnosis and management.*

In each of these cases, POCUS in the hands of the treating clinician can facilitate prompt diagnosis and guide the definitive assessment of treatment responses.

## BASICS OF ULTRASONOGRAPHY

Fig. 35.1 shows the basic components of an ultrasound system and how ultrasound works in simple terms.

### Physics of ultrasound

Piezo-electric crystals in the ultrasound transducer emit pulses of ultrasound. This produces echoes from underlying structures that are received by the transducer and used to generate images on the ultrasound screen.

The following are the basic principles of ultrasound:

- The more perpendicular the ultrasound beam hits a structure, the greater the returning echo. Deviation from the perpendicular probe position results in less return of the echo and produces lower quality images.
- Interfaces with different acoustic impedance provide clear images. Acoustic impedance is the stiffness in molecular movement. Interfaces are produced when two tissues with different acoustic impedance sit next to each other. Optimal visualisation of the interface can be achieved through slow methodical manipulation of the probe.
- Air in the lungs and bowel conduct sound poorly and structures behind them cannot be seen.
- Bone reflects ultrasound very well and nothing can be seen behind a bone.
- Fatty tissue increases sound absorption and scatter. This leads to progressive attenuation and decreased ability to visualise deeper structures. Images will appear granular.

### Transducers

Depending on their application, there are several different types of transducers that are used with ultrasound systems – curvilinear, cardiac, linear and endocavity (Fig. 35.2). Frequency is directly related to image resolution and inversely related to tissue penetration. This means the low frequency curvilinear probe is better for imaging deep structures, such as the aorta. Conversely, higher frequency probes function best when visualising more superficial structures, for applications such as musculoskeletal (MSK), vascular access and lung views. Five to 7.5 MHz transducers are generally used for children and for superficial structures. Two or 2.5 MHz transducers are usually used for the obese abdomen. For superficial tissues, such as the thyroid, breast and scrotum, 7 to 15 MHz is appropriate. For the heart, abdomen and second and third trimester obstetrics, 3 to 7 MHz is optimal.

### Controls

Most bedside ultrasound machines will have a wide variety of features and capabilities beyond those needed by most

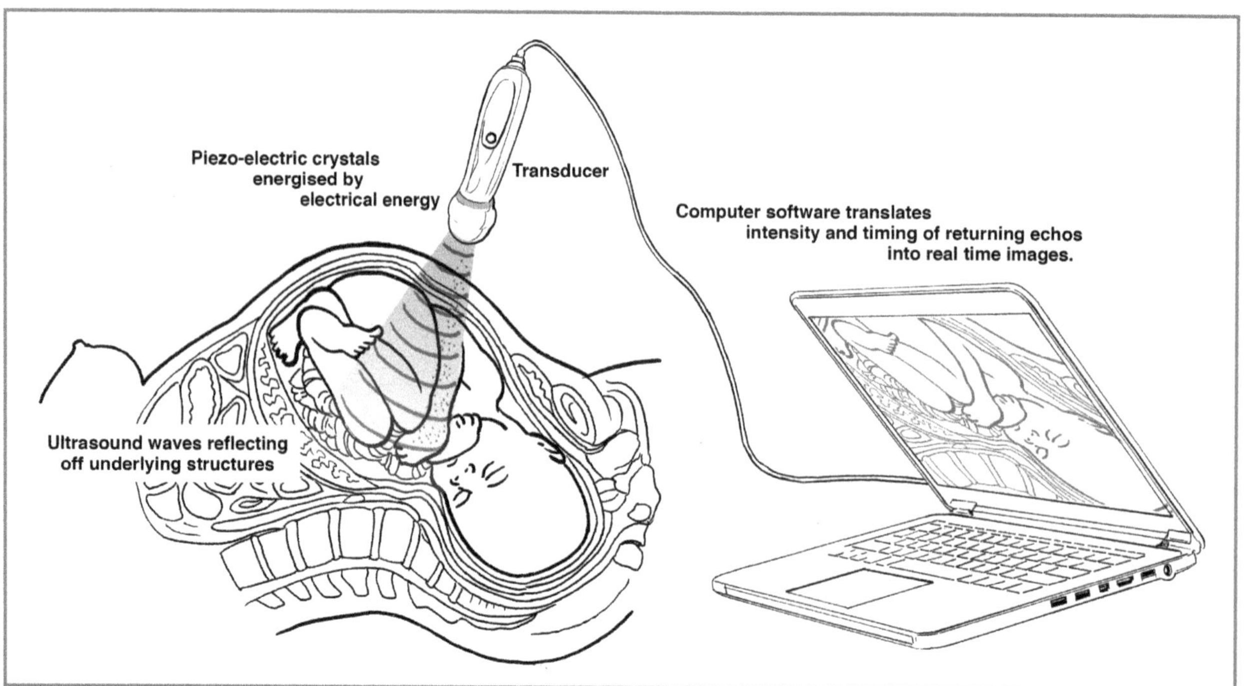


Fig. 35.1. Ultrasound – the basic principles.

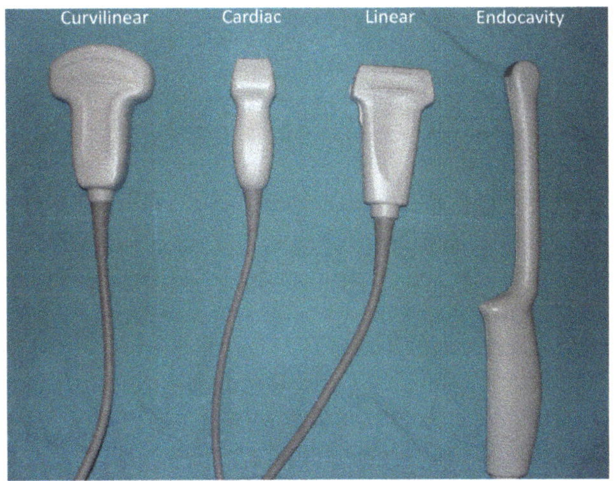


**Fig. 35.2.** Examples of different types of transducers.

practitioners. A good understanding of a few basic functions will help optimise image generation and allow safe application of POCUS to patient care. Knowledge of depth and gain (amplification) control is a good place to start.

After choosing the best probe, apply knowledge of superficial anatomy and landmarks to generate and centre an initial image. Once the area of interest is identified, begin optimising the image appearance by adjusting depth and gain. Depth adjustment will adjust the field of view and enable magnification of key image features. Gain increases signal strength. Increasing the gain increases the brightness of the image but reduces the ability to differentiate the interfaces. The use of minimal gain will increase the ability to visualise the interface, or area of interest. Visibility may be improved by darkening the room, but this may not be practical in a trauma room. Some machines have programmed default settings that apply to specific probes and the region being scanned (abdomen, obstetrics, cardiac or small parts).

Additional controls may be useful in specific circumstances. The freeze function makes it easier to obtain measurements and calculate volume. Colour Doppler can help quantify flow in vascular structures and can be set to show red towards and blue away from the transducer. The M-mode (motion mode) feature can be useful in cardiac and lung scanning. Most machines will have the capability to save still images and short videos to use for later review, quality initiatives or teaching purposes.

## BENEFITS OF POCUS

POCUS facilitates rapid acquisition of relevant clinical information, thereby reducing the time to consultation or discharge, and improving patient satisfaction (Sohoni *et al.* 2014). When performed by skilled clinicians, it is an excellent risk-reducing tool, shortening the time to definitive therapy, and decreasing the rate of complications from blind invasive procedures (Arienti and Camaggi 2011).

POCUS provides rapid, repeatable, and multisystem assessment to guide diagnosis and management of critically ill patients in the emergency department. Emergency department echocardiography offers anatomic and haemodynamic information at the point of care (POC). In addition, POCUS can match or exceed the speed and utility of existing tests such as chest radiograph with thoracic ultrasonography or central venous pressure determination with measurement of the inferior vena cava via ultrasonography (Peterson and Arntfield 2014). POCUS significantly decreases time to operative care in patients with suspected torso trauma. It has reduced the use of other resources such as computed tomography (CT), and resulted in fewer days in hospital and fewer complications (Melniker *et al.* 2006).

Ultrasound was found to be a useful and reliable diagnostic tool in prehospital emergency transportation (Heegaard *et al.* 2010; Hoyer *et al.* 2010). Non-physician health providers in remote settings successfully perform ultrasound when direction and interpretation of findings is provided by physicians through telehealth (Jong 2012).

## PITFALLS/LIMITATIONS

As with any clinical examination, the accuracy of the POCUS depends on the skill of the practitioner. Adding POCUS to the traditional examination enhances the practitioner's level of comfort and confidence in their assessment. The potential for false negative investigations always exists and can stem from patient, operator and equipment factors. A major advantage of POCUS is the opportunity for repeat bedside assessment in the monitored setting. This is particularly important for the trauma patient with a clinical suspicion of free intra-abdominal fluid. Performance of serial POCUS examinations allows the clinician to overcome pitfalls related to patient body habitus, bowel gas and subtle positive findings. Practitioners, however, need to know their limitations and be guided primarily by good clinical judgment.

Like any diagnostic imaging studies, POCUS can discover incidental findings (Tewari *et al.* 2015). This may lead to other tests or interventions that may not be of benefit to the patient.

Doppler studies (for investigation of blood flow) in the first trimester are not within the domain of most rural health practitioners and should be avoided because this carries the potential risk of heat generation and negative outcomes in the developing embryo.

## STRATEGIES IN LEARNING HOW TO USE ULTRASOUND

To gain skills in the use of ultrasound technology, start by attending a basic course on ultrasound and gradually build a repertoire with experience. Initially use ultrasound for something simple such as looking for a foetal head or determining whether a lump is cystic or solid. Remember not to rely totally on the limited ultrasound imaging but use it to add another dimension to the total assessment of the patient. With increasing use, it is possible to work towards improved competency and to broaden applications for the use of ultrasound from basic to more advanced scanning.

Blended learning models can combine the use of learning management systems for pre-course online review of materials, followed by face-to-face hands-on instruction and practice (Lewiss *et al.* 2014).

Medical students with minimal training were able to successfully use pocket-sized POCUS as a supplement to standard physical examination and acquire acceptable relevant anatomical recordings for presentation and review. They were able to correctly interpret their images with great accuracy (Andersen *et al.* 2014). Peer mentoring by senior medical students is a useful method for teaching sonography to preclinical medical students (Jeppesen and Bahner 2012).

Simulators can be used to allow learners to practice image generation and interpretation. Low-fidelity simulators are usually static, meaning that they lack the real-time variability provided with hands-on scanning. High-fidelity simulators are usually high-tech and often high cost. They frequently use computer-generated cases of virtual sonographic anatomy that can be visualised with a mock probe.

Objective Structured Assessment of Ultrasound Skills using 1 assessor and 5 cases would result in similar reliability with a high (0.81) generalisability coefficient when comparing novices, intermediates and experts (Todsen *et al.* 2015).

Brief ultrasound instruction followed by just-in-time training with in-person or remote expert tele-ultrasound guidance is another way of gaining expertise.

## FUNCTIONALITIES/USES

POCUS applications continue to broaden as it becomes ever more functional in the hands of clinicians (Connell and Wu 2014). This section will describe what is feasible in a rural setting.

### Ultrasound in major trauma

In the multiply injured patient, ultrasound is used as part of the primary survey to look for intra-abdominal bleed and for pericardial effusion. This should not interfere with resuscitation. The ultrasound should ideally be located in the trauma room in the emergency department. The indications for the use of ultrasound in trauma are:

- patients with history of abdominal trauma
- trauma patients who are hypotensive
- trauma patients who have impaired consciousness because of head injury or drugs.

A 3–5 MHz curvilinear or a cardiac transducer (Fig. 35.2) is the best for a quick, <5 min, scan to look for an intraperitoneal bleed and ultrasound signs of cardiac tamponade.

In a supine position, intraperitoneal fluid will first accumulate in the pelvis and later be visible in the hepatorenal space, in the right upper quadrant. The minimum volume of fluid detectable by ultrasound in the intraperitoneal cavity ranges from ~250 to 600 mL (Branney *et al.* 1995; Gracias *et al.* 2001). By the time an intra-abdominal bleed has resulted in hypotension, fluid should be easily seen with POCUS. Nonetheless, pitfalls must always be taken into consideration. Clinical gestalt should take precedence and direct the resuscitation; ultrasound should be used as a tool to answer specific questions. Worsening vital signs should prompt a return to the A of ABCDE in advanced trauma life support (ATLS) and also to a repeat scan for free fluid during the assessment of C (circulation).

Fluid is most likely to be present at the anterior aspect of the hepatorenal space and as it increases it may be seen in the subdiaphragmatic region, above the liver.

### Scanning for deep vein thrombosis

POCUS can be used to look for deep vein thrombosis (DVT) in the vessels of the lower limb. Once images of relevant anatomy are seen, the presence of venous compressibility can be assessed.

False negative scans for DVT must always be considered. About 2% of patients with a negative initial ultrasound have a positive repeat ultrasound 1 week later (Kearon *et al.* 1998). Isolated thrombi in the iliac veins or superficial femoral veins within the abductor canal are not picked up by ultrasonography. False positive scans may be associated with pelvic tumours or abscesses because they can lead to non-compressibility of the femoral vein even in the absence of thrombosis (Birdwell *et al.* 2000).

### Lumps and bumps

Ultrasonography is useful to evaluate soft tissue pathology such as haematoma, abscess and foreign bodies. It can show where to best place a needle to drain a haematoma or abscess, and help judge the likelihood of the intervention's success before starting the procedure. It also helps to identify nerves and vascular structures in order to avoid preventable complications associated with bedside procedures.

Breast lump ultrasound is useful to determine if the lump is solid or cystic, and to localise a cystic area for aspiration.

### Central venous access under ultrasound guidance

Ultrasound guided central venous access is becoming standard practice. In 2008, the College of Physicians and Surgeons of Ontario suggested that consideration be given to ultrasound-guided central catheter insertion (CPSO 2008). The Institute of Medicine, Agency for Health Care Research and Quality, and the National Institute for Health and Clinical Excellence recommend ultrasound guided central venous access (Rothschild 2001; NIHCE 2002).

The main advantage of ultrasound is that it generates an image of the central vein and the adjacent artery. Looking at the images reduces the operator's reliance on anatomical landmarks that may be indistinct, and takes into account anatomic variations. This makes it easier for rural doctors who do occasional central lines to successfully cannulate the central vein. Ultrasound reduces complications such as inadvertently needling the adjacent artery and nerve. That said, strong knowledge of relevant surface anatomy is still essential to safely place a central line. Ultrasound is a valuable adjunct to this knowledge.

### Limited echocardiography

Limited echocardiography can be a very useful tool to look for pericardial effusion, estimate ventricular function and determine the presence of cardiac standstill. Images are generated based on the reflection of ultrasound from acoustic interfaces, such as the boundary between the blood in the left ventricle and the myocardium.

In the rural setting, limited echocardiography can help the clinician to make critical decisions in management. Using echocardiography regularly to augment the stethoscope, ECG, chest X-rays and other investigations will help rural physicians to become more proficient in the use of echocardiography and will help with the management of critically ill patients. Formal echocardiography, if available, can be done when patients are more stable.

### Lung

Using CT as a gold standard, ultrasonography is more sensitive than chest X-ray in picking up pneumothorax (90.9% *v.* 50.2%, respectively) (Alrajhi *et al.* 2012). The normal respiratory movement of the opposing visceral and parietal pleura produces ultrasound image features such as lung sliding and comet tail. The absence of these features indicates that a pneumothorax is present.

Ultrasonography is useful to diagnose pathology involving the lung parenchyma or surrounding structures. Alveolar air is reduced in pneumonia and interstitial fluids are increased in congestive heart failure (CHF), but also when air or fluids are collected in the pleural space (Volpicelli 2014). Pleural effusion and haemothorax look like hypoechoic, black areas in the dependent part of the thorax. A large fluid collection is often seen in association with an atelectatic lung segment.

With respiration, an ultrasound of a normal 'dry' lung creates horizontal line artefacts known as A-lines. With wet lungs, the artefacts are vertical and are known as B-lines. B-lines look like comet tails. Increasing numbers and confluence of these B-lines are associated with increasing fluid in the interstitium and alveoli from pulmonary oedema or from respiratory distress syndrome.

With consolidation and atelectasis the lung looks like a solid organ. This is sometimes called hepatisation of the lung. Ultrasononography can help differentiate between consolidation, where the dark air bronchogram changes with respiration, and atelectasis, where the image looks the same with respiration.

### Musculoskeletal POCUS

Traditionally, plain radiographs identify fractures. POCUS has recently been used to diagnose musculoskeletal injuries, and has been shown to be as sensitive as radiography in the detection of many types of fractures

(Griffith *et al.* 1999; Lyon and Blaivas 2003). Given that the bony cortex is brightly echogenic on ultrasound, any disruption is readily identified. Not only does POCUS aid in the identification of fractures, it also directs subsequent attempts at reduction (Chinnock *et al.* 2011). The use of POCUS allows physicians to correctly identify and treat many fractures while minimising the patient's length of stay in the emergency department.

Joint effusions are often readily apparent with POCUS, even when only subtle physical exam findings exist. Ultrasound-guided aspiration can help facilitate the diagnosis of the suspected septic joint. Potential tendon injuries, such as Achilles tendon rupture, can also be assessed with POCUS.

### Urology

POCUS of the kidney and bladder is an emerging option for the evaluation of patients presenting with urinary issues. Measurement of vertical, horizontal and longitudinal dimensions of the bladder can be combined to calculate residual volume (Chan 1993) and to assess urinary retention.

Bedside ultrasound is being adopted as part of the clinical pathway for the evaluation of renal colic without ionising radiation (Dalziel and Noble 2013). It can detect hydronephrosis, a marker of presumed obstructive uropathy, and stratify patients who may need to have further imaging (Dalziel and Noble 2013).

### Intravascular volume

Inferior vena cava volume measurement can estimate intravascular volume and right atrial pressure. In children, a transverse scan of the aorta at its maximum diameter during systole and inferior vena cava during expiration at the sub-xiphoid abdomen is useful for determining dehydration. A 27% collapse of the diameter of the inferior vena cava from inspiration to expiration has a sensitivity of 93% (95% CI = 81–100%) and a specificity of 35% (95% CI = 20–51%) in determining severe dehydration (Levine *et al.* 2010).

### Aorta

Abdominal pain is a very common clinical presentation. POCUS helps to rule out life threatening diagnoses, of which abdominal aortic aneurysm (AAA) is an important consideration (Sue 2014). To rule out AAA, it is essential to visualise the entire length of the aorta from the epigastric region to its bifurcation, near the level of the umbilicus. Care should be taken to visualise the suprarenal aorta: a less common site of AAA. Frequent pitfalls include obesity, bowel gas and abdominal pain. Manoeuvres such as probe pressure, serial scanning and having the patient take deep breaths may help to overcome these imaging challenges.

### Early pregnancy

Unlike many POCUS scans in which imaging is used to 'rule out pathology', the goal in early pregnancy is to 'rule in' an intrauterine pregnancy (IUP), and thereby exclude ectopic pregnancy. As with any clinical assessment, all data points such as history, risk factors, physical examination and laboratory results must be taken into consideration when faced with a potential diagnosis of ectopic pregnancy. The absence of classical features such as risk factors, β hCG above a particular cut-off and even vaginal bleeding should not prompt exclusion of this potentially life-threatening diagnosis in the pregnant patient (Micks and Sue 2015).

Transvaginal or transabdominal POCUS can be used to detect ectopic pregnancy. A transvaginal probe, which can be placed closer to the uterus than a transabdominal probe, is better able to visualise an IUP. It also picks up key findings at an earlier gestational age.

As always, and particularly in the presence of an indeterminate POCUS scan, practitioners must follow their clinical impression and obtain further investigation as necessary and as patient stability dictates.

Other functionalities of POCUS that are useful in rural practice include intubation, abdominal, nerve blocks, thyroid, intracranial, and spinal ultrasound.

## CONCLUSION

Ultrasonography is a very useful tool in rural practice. It has to be portable or easily available to use in rural practices that include ambulatory clinics, emergency departments, inpatients, maternity units and operating rooms.

## REFERENCES

Alrajhi K, Woo MY, Vaillancourt C (2012) Test characteristics of ultrasonography for the detection of pneumothorax: a systematic review and meta-analysis. *Chest* **141**, 703–708. doi:10.1378/chest.11-0131

Andersen GN, Viset A, Mjolstad O, Salvesen O, Dalen H, Haugen B (2014) Feasibility and accuracy of point-of-care pocket-size ultrasonography performed by medical students. *BMC Medical Education* **14**, 156. doi:10.1186/1472-6920-14-156

Arienti V, Camaggi V (2011) Clinical applications of bedside ultrasonography in internal and emergency medicine. *Internal and Emergency Medicine* **6**, 195–201. doi:10.1007/s11739-010-0424-3

Birdwell BG, Raskob GE, Whitsett TL, Durica SS, Comp PC, *et al.* (2000) Predictive value of compression ultrasonography for deep vein thrombosis in symptomatic outpatients: clinical implications of the site of vein noncompressibility. *Archives of Internal Medicine* **160**, 309–313. doi:10.1001/archinte.160.3.309

Branney SW, Wolfe RE, Moore EE, Albert NP, Heinig M, Mestek M, *et al.* (1995) Quantitative sensitivity of ultrasound in detecting free intraperitoneal fluid. *The Journal of Trauma and Acute Care Surgery* **39**, 375–380. doi:10.1097/00005373-199508000-00032

Chan H (1993) Noninvasive bladder volume measurement. *Journal of Neuroscience Nursing* **25**, 309–312.

Chinnock B, Khaletskiy A, Kuo K, Hendey GW (2011) Ultrasound-guided reduction of distal radius fractures. *The Journal of Emergency Medicine* **40**, 308–312. doi:10.1016/j.jemermed.2009.09.018

CPSO (College of Physicians and Surgeons of Ontario) (2008) Use of ultrasound-guided central venous catheter insertion urged. *Dialogue* **4**, 24–25.

Connell MJ, Wu TS (2014) Bedside musculoskeletal ultrasonography. *Critical Care Clinics* **30**, 243–273. doi:10.1016/j.ccc.2013.10.003

Dalziel PJ, Noble VE (2013) Bedside ultrasound and the assessment of renal colic: a review. *Emergency Medicine Journal* **30**, 3–8. doi:10.1136/emermed-2012-201375

Gracias VH, Frankel HL, Gupta R, Malcynski J, Gandhi R, Collazzo L, *et al.* (2001) Defining the learning curve for the Focused Abdominal Sonogram for Trauma (FAST) examination: implications for credentialing. *American Journal of Surgery* **67**, 364–368.

Griffith JF, Rainer TH, Ching AS, Law KL, Cocks RA, Metreweli C (1999) Sonography compared with radiography in revealing acute rib fracture. *AJR. American Journal of Roentgenology* **173**, 1603–1609. doi:10.2214/ajr.173.6.10584808

Heegaard W, Hildebrandt D, Spear D, Chason K, Nelson B, Ho J (2010) Prehospital ultrasound by paramedics: results of field trial. *Academic Emergency Medicine* **17**, 624–630. doi:10.1111/j.1553-2712.2010.00755.x

Hoyer HX, Vogl S, Schiemann U, Haug A, Stolpe E, Michalski T (2010) Prehospital ultrasound in emergency medicine: incidence, feasibility, indications and diagnoses. *European Journal of Emergency Medicine* **17**, 254–259. doi:10.1097/MEJ.0b013e328336ae9e

Jeppesen KM, Bahner DP (2012) Teaching bedside sonography using peer mentoring: a prospective randomized trial. *Journal of Ultrasound in Medicine* **31**, 455–459.

Jong M (2012) Resuscitation by video in northern communities. *International Journal of Circumpolar Health* **69**, 519–527.

Kearon C, Ginsberg JS, Hirsh J (1998) The role of venous ultrasonography in the diagnosis of suspected deep venous thrombosis and pulmonary embolism. *Annals of Internal Medicine* **129**, 1044–1049. doi:10.7326/0003-4819-129-12-199812150-00009

Levine AC, Shah SP, Umulisa I, Munyaneza RBM, Dushimiyimana JM, Stegmann K, *et al.* (2010) Ultrasound assessment of severe dehydration in children with diarrhea and vomiting. *Academic Emergency Medicine* **17**, 1035–1041. doi:10.1111/j.1553-2712.2010.00830.x

Lewiss RE, Hoffmann B, Beaulieu Y, Phelan MB (2014) Point-of-care ultrasound education: the increasing role of simulation and multimedia resources. *Journal of Ultrasound in Medicine* **33**, 27–32. doi:10.7863/ultra.33.1.27

Lyon M, Blaivas M (2003) Evaluation of extremity trauma with sonography. *Journal of Ultrasound in Medicine* **22**, 625–630.

Melniker LA, Leibner E, Mckenney MG, Lopez P, Briggs WM, Mancuso CA (2006) Randomized controlled clinical trial of point-of-care, limited ultrasonography for trauma in the emergency department: the first sonography outcomes assessment program trial. *Annals of Emergency Medicine* **48**, 227–235. doi:10.1016/j.annemergmed.2006.01.008

Micks T, Sue K (2015) The occasional ectopic pregnancy. *Canadian Journal of Rural Medicine* **20**, 139–144.

NIHCE (National Institute for Health and Care Excellence) (2002) *Guidance on the Use of Ultrasound Locating Devices for Placing Central Venous Catheters*. NIHCE, <www.nice.org.uk/pdf/ultrasound_49_GUIDANCE.pdf>.

Peterson D, Arntfield RT (2014) Critical care ultrasonography. *Emergency Medicine Clinics of North America* **32**, 907–926. doi:10.1016/j.emc.2014.07.011

Rothschild JM (2001) Ultrasound guidance of central vein catheterization. In *Making healthcare safer: a critical analysis of patient safety practices*. AHRQ Publication 1. (Eds AJ Markowitz and RM Wachter) pp. 245–253. Agency for Healthcare Research and Quality, Rockwell MD, USA.

Sohoni A, Bosley J, Miss JC (2014) Bedside ultrasonography for obstetric and gynecologic emergencies. *Critical Care Clinics* **30**, 207–226. doi:10.1016/j.ccc.2013.10.002

Sue K (2014) The occsional ED ultrasound: abdominal aorta. *Canadian Journal of Rural Medicine* **19**, 103–106.

Tewari A, Shuaib W, Maddu KK, Salastekar N, Beck S, Johnson J-O, *et al.* (2015) Incidental findings on bedside ultrasonography: detection rate and accuracy of resident-performed examinations in the acute setting. *Canadian Association of Radiologists Journal* **66**, 153–157. doi:10.1016/j.carj.2014.04.004

Todsen T, Tolsgaard MG, Olsen BH, Henriksen BM, Hillingsø JG, Konge L, *et al.* (2015) Reliable and valid assessment of point-of-care ultrasonography. *Annals of Surgery* **261**, 309–315. doi:10.1097/SLA.0000000000000552

Volpicelli G (2014) Point-of-care lung ultrasound. *Praxis (Bern)* **103**, 711–716. doi:10.1024/1661-8157/a001690

# 36 Stakeholder perspectives on point-of-care testing

*Wilton Braund, Brooke Spaeth, Malcolm Auld, Justin Busbridge, Lauren Foohey and Connie Mardis*

**Summary**

There are a number of key stakeholders involved in the day-to-day operation of point-of-care testing (POCT) in primary care and hospital settings. Depending on the size/scope of the POCT program, stakeholders may include: the doctor actively managing the patient based on the POCT result; the POCT Coordinator or Regional Supervisor responsible for the organisation and management of POCT services at the network/regional level; the POCT operator who performs the POC test *in situ*; the patient, who is the consumer of the POCT service; and the industry partner who provided the POCT device and consumables for testing. This chapter provides a brief personal perspective from a representative of each of these stakeholders.

## A CLINICAL PERSPECTIVE (DR WILTON BRAUND)

I write as a physician/internal medicine specialist who has practiced in endocrinology, diabetes and as a general internal medicine specialist in acute hospital practice and office practice for 35 years. The last 15 years have been with the benefit of POCT.

What are the day-to-day experiences that make me want to have POCT available in my rooms? Let me give a scenario: a 32 year old woman who has had Type 1 diabetes since her early teen years arrives, saying: 'I don't think you will be pleased with my HbA1c: I haven't really been taking care of myself well enough.' Naturally, she has not remembered to attend the laboratory a few days before the appointment to use the HbA1c request form with which I supplied her at the last appointment.

Why have I used the word 'naturally'? It is very common and very natural for a patient to forget to have the blood test in advance. It requires two episodes of leave from work: one to have the test and one to visit my office to discuss the result. People with diabetes have increased 'sick' leave from work – not because they are actually ill, but because they have many appointments to go to. Attending a laboratory can come a long way down the agenda for a busy or a financially straitened person. Omitting to have laboratory tests can also be a feature of being fed up with the whole nuisance and rigmarole of having diabetes.

After that opening sentence of her conversation, 'I don't think you will be pleased with my HbA1c; I haven't really been taking care of myself well enough', it is all too easy to devote the remaining minutes of my consultation to ways in which her diabetes control might be made tighter. But what if she has had a POC test for HbA1c? A high result (e.g. 9.8%) might confirm the intended thrust of the consultation; but a tight-control result (e.g. 6.8%) would mean the consultation can be completely redirected. It might create time and opportunity to re-examine her for any emerging complications. Or the consultation might be directed towards why she made such a remark, why her self-esteem is low and whether she has depression. This 'change of frame' effect of a POCT result has been a common scenario in my diabetes practice.

It is these aspects of POCT that are so important. The diagnosis or assessment of the patient's current need is so rapidly clarified or altered that maximum value can be extracted from the consultation – a consultation that has already been paid for. And, in addition, the patient makes savings in time, effort and absence from work.

POCT is a 'disruptive' technology. But does it cause a disruption in the doctor's offices? It does indeed require staff time for the tests to be performed – most POC tests take 5–10 min. Most patients, however, have a few minutes to spare in the waiting room and prefer this small delay to the idea of a separate trip to the laboratory.

What is the downside? Firstly, POCT is expensive. Laboratories need have no fear of a tsunami of POCT that will destroy their revenues. Secondly, a clinician needs to identify a small group of POC tests that suit his or her practice. In a remote area, this might include tests that are usually the province of emergency departments, such as troponin. To have an unlimited number of POCT devices is expensive and exhausting. Finally, results are only clinically useful if they are analytically reliable. Someone in the practice must perform quality control (QC) testing and/or proficiency testing (PT) testing. Indeed, if POCT is to be reimbursed by anyone other than the patient, QC and PT are essential steps to obtain accreditation and, in turn, should the reimbursement come from insurers or from government?

Has POCT's moment arrived for general and specialised clinicians? In those countries where these tests are reimbursed, there has been rapid adoption of POCT. This is not only by general practitioners, but also by domiciliary nursing services and by aged care centres.

Further evidence of the value of POCT lies in the predictive algorithms that are now in use in haematology and cardiology (with for example D-dimer and troponin). Finally, the adaptation of molecular testing to POCT platforms means that infectious disease can now be diagnosed accurately at the POC, while antibiotic stewardship can now be supported by POCT in sexual health clinics. Because there is a strong chance that the patient will not return for the results of their tests, immediate results, within around 1 hour, assume great importance in the decision whether to treat with antibiotic. If the latter decision is made empirically, without the benefit of POCT, the majority of those treated will not actually need antibiotic.

## A POCT COORDINATOR PERSPECTIVE (BROOKE SPAETH AND MALCOLM AULD)

Brooke Spaeth is POCT Coordinator for the Northern Territory POCT Program operating in a very challenging environment in remote Australia (see Chapter 28). Malcolm Auld supports the program as on-ground Regional POCT Supervisor, based in Alice Springs.

What I enjoy as a POCT Coordinator working with remotely located health services and staff is knowing that I am assisting with providing a service to patients with both acute and chronic illnesses that was not accessible previously to these patients. The contact I have as a POCT Coordinator with the remote health centre staff is something I really enjoy and it makes me want to ensure their POCT work is as streamlined and easy as possible, because I know that the staff are already dealing with a huge workload of usually very sick patients with multiple co-morbidities. As part of my role, I have developed a deep respect for the remote staff who work in some of the most isolated areas in Australia where the appropriate resources to assist patient care are often not available or difficult to access.

As a POCT Coordinator for 7 years now, some of the most rewarding comments I have received from remote staff/operators have been along the following lines:

From remote nurse 1: 'Thank you for helping us to get our POCT device and providing all of the support, we were just now able to perform our first troponin test on a patient with chest pain and rule out a heart attack and the patient was able to remain in the community. Normally we would have to evacuate any patients presenting with chest pain.'

From remote doctor 1: 'The ability to get the HbA1c test result immediately on the DCA device allows me to fully engage the patient in discussing how best to treat their diabetes and help them make healthier lifestyle choices. The golden 6 min to the result popping up on the screen is the best opportunity to fully grasp the patient's attention and discuss their diabetes care.'

From remote doctor 2: 'Before we were able to perform electrolyte testing on-site we had a patient with chronically low potassium (due to the medication he was taking) who had to be evacuated by air every time he presented unwell and needed a laboratory potassium test as we could not confirm his status on-site. This evacuation cost approximately $20 000 each time and was a 2000 km return journey for the patient. Now we can perform the test and get his potassium result in 2 min'.

The most satisfying component of being a regional POC Supervisor in the Northern Territory POCT Program is being able to work cooperatively and collaboratively with health service managers, clinicians, remote area nurses, administrators, technicians and other health professionals across multiple agencies to ensure the POCT program runs successfully. This has included: many conversations in-person, by phone and email around training sessions; dissemination of reagents and consumables and establishing reliable systems/processes; and finally seeing clinicians at the point-of-health-care delivery being able to use and manage the POCT device effectively as an adjunct in providing clinical care in the most cost-efficient manner for the health of patients we serve.

## A POCT OPERATOR PERSPECTIVE (JUSTIN BUSBRIDGE)

For over two decades I have worked in remote health-care settings in both Scotland (Outer Hebrides) and Australia (Northern Territory) and have seen how POCT has completely transformed the patient and clinician experience.

Many blood pathology tests require rapid analysis and need to be performed frequently, but the logistics of getting these samples to the laboratory is often difficult. In such cases, the only option is to move the patient closer to the testing laboratory, or move the testing closer to the patient, this latter option facilitated by POCT. A good example is the INR test for monitoring warfarin therapy.

Before the introduction of POCT to our remote general practice clinic in the Outer Hebrides, Scotland, we could only test those patients with relatively stable INR results. The venous sample was taken by the nurse and then transported by road to the nearest laboratory once or twice per week, along with the groceries and parcels going to town. Test results took at least another 2 days before being reported to the treating GP (making the time between blood collection and return of results approximately a week). Such a time-lag was too long for patients requiring frequent monitoring (twice per week); so those patients would have to travel to the main hospital, a return journey that could be up to 200 km. There the patient would attend a warfarin clinic where venous blood samples were tested immediately in the laboratory and drug doses titrated on the spot. However, the journey on slow rural roads might take 4 hours of a patient's time. This was impractical for many patients and to initiate warfarin we would have to admit patients to hospital, perhaps for many weeks until stable INR results were achieved. This time commitment meant some patients refused to accept warfarin medication, thus increasing their risk of a heart attack or stroke.

In remote Australia, pathology laboratory handling requirements made our INR samples unreliable. For example, sample tubes needed to be completely filled, then centrifuged to separate the serum before being frozen and packed in insulated boxes ready for transport by the local bus to the nearest laboratory, a process which involved many hours and hundreds of kilometres in transit often in temperatures reaching 48°C. Attempting to transport Indigenous patients closer to a pathology laboratory was not possible due to cultural and economic barriers, because traditional Indigenous people often refuse to go to urban hospitals. They would prefer no medication at all rather than leave their desert communities.

POCT has dramatically changed the human and logistic faces of those Scottish and Australian experiences. In remote Scotland, what was a long drive or extended hospital stay has become an approximately 10 minute encounter at the local GP clinic. In remote Australia I am now able to get an almost instant INR result based on a simple finger-prick POC test. After relaying the INR result to the doctor I can then immediately adjust the warfarin dose as required. In very remote Australia, POCT has meant that what was not possible at all is becoming increasingly common place and the use of warfarin in cardiac patients is now a viable option.

Apart from INR, POCT is providing a whole raft of new blood tests that we can use to manage both chronic diseases and critically ill patients. As a remote area nurse working in these areas there is only so much I can diagnose with simple assessment tools such as blood pressure, oxygen saturation, temperature, perhaps ECGs as well as my own clinical skills. The POC tests now available in remote Australia have proved invaluable, and include troponin, blood gases, white cell and differential count, electrolytes and renal function tests plus HbA1c. Tests such as cardiac markers and blood gases can assist in avoiding an unnecessary air evacuation (a risky undertaking, let alone extremely expensive), as well as buying valuable time in an acute emergency, and I have seen POCT save lives. Creatinine and potassium can help us evaluate the deterioration of an Indigenous renal patient who has stayed overlong in the remote homeland and missed their dialysis session. A POC HbA1c result is available from a finger-prick of blood in the consultation room, giving it immediate impact and relevance, and enabling me to negotiate future management plans with the patient. It has been invaluable in facilitating real improvements in diabetes control.

For a nurse or doctor working in remote desert Australia, it is easy to see how POCT is valuable. The isolation of remote clinics and harsh climate make laboratory samples unreliable, and the time lag in receiving results devalues their relevance. In contrast, I can use POCT results immediately to help manage both emergency treatments and chronic diseases, plus it is a mode of testing that overcomes the cultural barriers faced by Indigenous people accessing urban-based services.

## A PATIENT'S PERSPECTIVE (PATIENT WITH DIABETES)

From a personal perspective, I was diagnosed with diabetes some 25 years ago now as a result of follow-up for a high cholesterol result that was performed opportunistically on a POCT device; this is somewhat ironic as POCT was very much in its infancy in our country at that time. The diagnosis of diabetes was made following an oral glucose tolerance test (OGTT), an experience I found most uncomfortable and 'unpalatable'. This was my first encounter with laboratory pathology testing and I'd like to make several points regarding this form of testing. The laboratory-based person may often view the patient as 'just another blood sample for analysis', with their main concern being, for example, 'has the request form been filled in appropriately and is the sample suitable for analysis? I'd ask the laboratory person to stop and think for a moment that there is indeed a real person, with feelings and worries, at the 'front end' of that sample.

I am undoubtedly one of the world's worst patients. The actual act of venipuncture every 3 months for my management review holds no fears, but (like I'm sure is the case for many others with diabetes) I endure considerable stress and worry in the days leading up to the blood taking and then in the days after the event before I visit my specialist to get my results. Will my HbA1c level be good or has it shifted upwards, as it inevitably seems to do? Are my kidneys OK? Will I have protein in my urine this time? Has something changed for the worse in my biochemical profile? My biggest long-term concern about living with diabetes is the perhaps inevitable onset of complications – especially kidney disease and retinopathy. I've always thought that life without sight would be the worst possible thing to experience and so my regular visit to the eye specialist is just as traumatic as the 3-monthly blood-taking episode.

After progressing through oral medication and now onto insulin, finger-prick blood glucose testing has become part of my daily routine. Yes, it is a chore and an imposition in the morning and at meal time, but these POCT results gives me instant awareness of my diabetes status, with a sense of immediate gratification if the results indicate my glucose levels are within 'good' limits. POCT provides me with strong messages of positive reinforcement that my diet and exercise regimes are working well and makes me want to be compliant with my medication taking because I know my POCT results will be good if I do the right thing. I've particularly noted when I stick most rigidly to my exercise regime (which includes the gym, tennis and cycling), then my HbA1c results are always very good. Now my doctor has access to a POCT device for HbA1c too, and it is just so simple and convenient to have the test done while you are at your appointment.

So living with diabetes is not all doom and gloom. You can definitely live comfortably and happily with diabetes, as I have done for many years and POCT is a critical factor in daily life for me but I do acknowledge that the diabetes patient does have a never-ending uphill battle to keep ahead of the disease (and I'll need my POCT and medications for the rest of my life)!

## AN INDUSTRY PERSPECTIVE (LAUREN FOOHEY AND CONNIE MARDIS)

With POCT at the forefront of health-care delivery, our industry acknowledges that POC solutions can immediately impact the lives of patients who may be suffering from a chronic disease or a life-threatening critical illness. We believe that, whether a patient is dealing with the day-to-day challenges of a chronic disease or facing a life-threatening situation, every moment counts. Getting test results quickly and accurately – in the doctor's office, at the hospital bedside, or in the emergency department – is vital, because less time spent on tests means more time focussed on patient care. For millions of chronically or critically ill patients around the world who depend on the right results at the right time, POCT matters.

With the ultimate goal of improving patient care, adoption of POCT continues to grow at a high rate and industry needs to be at the forefront of diagnostic innovation and opportunity. Emerging markets need to focus on cost-effectiveness and scalability to meet high patient volumes.

Efficiently managing all aspects of a POCT program requires close collaboration among health-care institutions, device manufacturers and information technology vendors. Although the present growth of POCT is strong, further adoption of POCT depends on how well the industry manages to overcome the challenges POCT Coordinators face in managing their programs.

# CONCLUSION

# 37 A 2020 vision for point-of-care testing

*Mark Shephard*

**Summary**

This brief concluding chapter consolidates and reflects upon many of the common themes presented throughout the book and provides an insight to the possible future of point-of-care testing (POCT) as we move towards the year 2020. Opportunities for technological innovation, new markets for POCT (with an emphasis on meeting the needs of resource-limited settings), prospects for new POCT research, and more streamlined integration of POCT in health systems will be explored.

## THE EVER-EVOLVING DEFINITION OF POINT-OF-CARE TESTING

POCT has been one of the fastest growing sectors of the diagnostic pathology industry over the past two decades. As we move towards the year 2020, there seems little chance of this growth abating, with global market sales of POCT products predicted to reach US$27.5 billion by 2018 (Isbell 2015) and US$34.6 billion by 2021 (Gomez 2013).

As discussed in the opening chapter of this book, many definitions for POCT have been proposed over the past 20 years based on functional, technological, operational or even geographical contexts of this mode of testing (Drain *et al.* 2014), with most definitions emphasising that POCT is performed rapidly near the patient and should lead expeditiously to clinical benefit for the patient. Definitions continue to evolve with Pai *et al.* (2015) challenging current thinking and arguing that POCT should become more 'goal oriented' rather than 'product oriented'; with the goal being to complete the 'test and treat' cycle within the same clinical encounter. They argue correctly that: 'systems for rapid reporting of test results to care providers, and a mechanism to link test results to appropriate counselling and treatment are as important as the technology itself. If systems for reporting the results and follow-up care are not in place, then POC testing is unlikely to have an impact on clinical or public health outcomes.' There is merit in their reasoning because a recurring theme throughout this book has been that, where POCT has failed to deliver an 'improved outcome', factors outside the conduct of the POC test itself have been the causative agents. Also implicit in their definition is that 'size (or weight or *perhaps* cost) doesn't matter'; indeed, they contend that restricting POCT to small, portable (or *cheap*) devices for example can impose barriers for use of new technologies: technologies that may in fact prove to be 'very impactful and cost effective in the right context'.

Certainly, in my experience, POCT will not work effectively in isolation and, in my teaching to university students, I always emphasise that the 'P' in 'POCT' stands for people and partnerships and I encourage health professionals working in POCT to embrace this concept of partnership and collaboration. Gomez (2013) reinforces this view: 'tomorrow's health care delivery will be less specialised in nature and emphasise patient-centred approaches and coordinated care teams, promoting wellness and effective team management … there will be a need for … medical devices and information-sharing tools that provide timely health status information at the POC.' Clearly, POCT is perfectly positioned to be embedded in 'tomorrow's health care'.

Perhaps by the year 2020, we may reach a global consensus on 'what POCT is', but then again, as technological innovation and new market opportunities continue to evolve, so may the definition of POCT be driven to continually change.

## CONTINUING TECHNOLOGICAL INNOVATION

State-of-the art advances in POCT technology have now resulted in devices that: (i) are capable of performing a wide range of test profiles; (ii) require very small sample volumes; (iii) have sophisticated sensing and detection systems that can produce results of high analytical quality; and (iv) have the capacity to electronically transmit those results to a clinical or laboratory information system that can be managed remotely from the site of test origin. Over the past decade in particular, device manufacturers have been responsive to the trend towards POCT being conducted by non-laboratory-trained health professionals in primary care environments and are now producing devices that have minimal manual steps and are as simple as possible to use with appropriate training.

Where to now for technological innovation? Certainly, interest from the commercial world in novel diagnostic POC technologies that have application for diseases of global impact (such as HIV, malaria and TB) has never been stronger, with the likes of the Bill and Melinda Gates Foundation and Grand Challenges, Canada generously funding large-scale grants for the development of new POC diagnostics for global health.

*In vitro* technologies that most practising scientists/health professionals are not currently familiar with will become common place; some have been discussed in the book, such as paper-based microfluidics (with postage-stamp sized, two-or three-dimensional microPADS for measuring proteins/enzymes), microwave-accelerated metal-enhanced fluorescence (MAMEF) and new types of amplification technology (e.g. recombinase polymerase/helicase dependent amplification). Many others, such as magnetoresistive sensor technology, field-effect transistor technology (based on nanotubes, nanowires and nanoribbons) and optical immunosensor systems are 'real possibilities' for next generation technologies (Gordon and Michel 2012).

Diagnostic devices will increasingly be linked to smartphones or tablets with web- or cloud-based connectivity (including Wi-Fi and Bluetooth) that will, in real-time:

- allow automatic data capture, graphing and web-or cloud-based storage
- provide decision support for test interpretation, follow-up action using clinical algorithms and/or calculation of drug dosage
- deliver additional clinical information such as nutritional or other lifestyle advice
- transmit photographs of tests strips from handheld devices for visual reading/interpretation by a clinician at an external location
- act as an interface for viewing ultrasound images or ECG readings (Blick 2015; Kiechle 2015).

Papali (2016) describes how NASA is mitigating the risk of medical emergencies on its international space station by training crew members to conduct on-board POC ultrasound and transmitting results for Earth-based telemedicine consultation. They argue the lessons learnt from this experience are applicable to providing health care in rural and remote health services on Earth. Kiechle (2015) describes a pocket mobile ECG device where wireless electrodes transmit a signal that is captured by the smartphone and displayed on the screen as an ECG graph. Gomez (2013) argues that the combination of light-weight, biocompatible paper-based microfluidic devices with smartphones equipped with high-resolution cameras may become the tool of choice to perform several POC diagnostic tests in the developing world.

Chin *et al.* (2013) provide a practical example of the synergy between microfluidics and smartphones in the developing world. They developed a microfluidic device called mChip (a mobile microfluidic chip for immunoassay of protein markers) together with a low-cost mobile device with cell-phone and satellite communication technologies. These were used to perform and transmit results of HIV POCT conducted in two different clinical settings in Rwanda (167 patients presenting to a remote clinic and

40 patients presenting to a clinic at a local hospital). The analytical performance of the mChip in both settings yielded close to 100% sensitivity and 100% specificity. The mobile device successfully transmitted all test results from the clinics to a medical records database stored in the cloud. They concluded: 'it is likely that mobile health devices with increased functionalities can deliver an expanded range of healthcare services right to patients, no matter how remote their location'.

As a way of the future, Kricka *et al.* (2015) describes 'personal health networks' as a network of devices including weight scales, blood pressure monitors, blood glucose monitors, caloric intake monitors and step counters that all have wireless capability and can transmit health information to a database overseen by a treating doctor/other health professional.

Another growth area of POCT is 'minimally invasive' wearable or implantable sensors, which can also be linked to medical 'apps' on smartphones, tablets or smartwatches with wireless connectivity (Kricka *et al.* 2015). Implanted continuous glucose monitoring systems (CGMS) have been described in Chapter 9. A recent iteration of CGMS uses fluorescent microbeads implanted transdermally to wirelessly transmit glucose readings when exposed to UV light. Other wearable applications include smart clothing, patches and wearable tattoos for monitoring temperature, respiration, blood pressure, heart rate, oxygen saturation and glucose (Kiechle 2015). Perhaps the future will also hold a place for *in vivo* POCT devices; Holloway (2015) describes near-infrared laser probes that can differentiate non-invasively and in real-time between normal and abnormal tissue during surgery.

Further development and refinement of specimen types suitable for use at the POC are likely as we move towards 2020; these include breath, saliva and fingerprints. Breath analysis for exhaled volatile organic compounds (VOC) may be useful in certain cancers and lung infections, while the detection of transmissible viruses such as influenza and Ebola (Chapter 24) in exhaled breath may become a reality using POCT platforms. Samples collected from latent fingerprints may have a role in detecting excreted metabolites of drugs of abuse (Kiechle 2015).

## NEW NICHE MARKETS FOR POINT-OF-CARE TESTING

There are a multitude of potential new and growth markets for POCT.

Retail health outlets (such as pharmacies and supermarkets) provide ever-expanding opportunity for POCT. Kricka *et al.* (2015) reports that, in the USA, an estimated 3000 such outlets are now offering POC tests including HbA1c, adenovirus, blood glucose, influenza A/B, lipid profile, mononucleosis, pregnancy, group A streptococcus and urine dipstick testing. In Japan, a traditionally conservative consumer of POCT, pharmacies are now able to conduct HbA1c POC testing under a US$10 self-pay test, with more than 10 other basic clinical chemistry tests under consideration for this sector (Abel 2015).

Other future settings for POCT that have been largely unexplored or have just 'scratched the surface' include defence, disaster events, security/quarantine/bioterrorism, mining, space and other extreme environments. Mention must be made of direct-to-consumer testing over the internet, where there is no clinical, analytical or technical oversight; this testing is fraught with risk and the potential for error and/or serious misinterpretation of results and should be strongly discouraged. As Tolan and Karon (2015) state: 'even if a (direct-to-consumer) result (for an infectious disease test) is negative, a counselling opportunity to advise on reducing risk of infection is lost.'

Although not a new market, there is no doubt the use of POCT in resource-limited settings for infectious disease will be a major area of continuing growth for POCT as we head towards 2020.

## POINT-OF-CARE TESTING IN RESOURCE-LIMITED SETTINGS

Mazzola and Pérez-Casas (2015) describe health delivery services (including pathology services) in resource-limited settings as having a tiered system comprising four levels (Table 37.1). In practice, health service delivery including access to timely medical care and the quality of laboratory services can be poor in many such settings (Pai *et al.* 2012). This is not intended to reflect negatively on the many committed and dedicated health professionals who work in the health sector, but rather is a symptom of an often dysfunctional health system and/or lack of resources or funds to support the system. Drain *et al.* (2014) argue that limited availability of laboratory-based tests is harmful for resource-limited settings because it drives syndromic management (management based on clinical history, unsupported by laboratory testing), which can in turn lead to under-diagnosis, over-treatment or both.

**Table 37.1.** An example of the model of health-care delivery (including pathology services) that has been used in resource-limited settings (Source: adapted from Mazzola and Pérez-Casas 2015)

| Health-care delivery level | Example of pathology service | Human resources |
|---|---|---|
| 4. National | Antibiotic resistance testing in a reference laboratory | Senior laboratory specialist |
| 3. Regional/provincial | High throughput molecular testing (NAAT) | Laboratory scientists or senior technician |
| 2. District | Low throughput molecular testing (NAAT) | Laboratory technicians and assistants |
| 1. Primary care or community-based outreach | Rapid diagnostic testing (RDT) using lateral flow devices | Primary care health professionals (e.g. GPs, nurses and/or community health workers) |

The greatest need for pathology testing is at Level 1, where most patients present but where testing capabilities via laboratory services are extremely limited or non-existent. Herein lays a major opportunity for POCT for the present and for the future – particularly in relation to infectious diseases (Peeling and McNerney 2014).

Certainly there are many significant challenges for the programmatic implementation and scale-up of POCT in resource-limited settings, as well as many unmet clinical needs (Pai *et al.* 2012; Peeling and Mabey 2010). Some of these challenges are listed in Table 37.2; however, POCT protagonists should be buoyed by the many examples provided throughout this book that show that POCT can be used sustainably at Level 1 primary care sites by locally trained health workers in resource-poor environments. Existing POCT programs are now challenging the model presented in Table 37.1, with sophisticated molecular POC test systems successfully being used in some Level 1 settings with appropriate infrastructure.

Peeling and Mabey (2010) have set a charter for the way forward to deliver streamlined and effective POCT services in low resource settings (Table 37.3).

## POINT-OF-CARE TESTING FOR INFECTIOUS DISEASES

A significant body of evidence has been presented throughout the book highlighting that molecular-based

**Table 37.2.** Barriers to the implementation and scale-up of POCT (Source: adapted from Pai *et al.* 2012)

| Barrier | Commentary |
|---|---|
| Awareness | Some health workers may not be aware of available POC tests. |
| Cultural/societal | Perceived lack of confidentiality and stigma may reduce acceptance of POCT in tight-knit communities. |
| Economic | Some POC tests may be priced at a level that is unaffordable in many countries. |
| Fit for purpose | Many tests are single disease focussed, whereas many patients have multiple co-morbidities. |
| Health-system related | Negative sentiment of some laboratory health professionals to POCT, fearing loss of control and finances. |
| Infection risk | Clinics may be unwilling to perform tests that may expose health workers to risk of infection. |
| Infrastructure | Clinics may lack regular power, refrigeration, storage, waste disposal units, for example. |
| Operational | Difficulty in seeking reimbursement for POCT conducted without laboratory support/linkage. |
| Policy-related | Lack of evidence-base on POC tests can result in uncertain policy direction/clinical algorithms. |
| Quality testing | Primary care staff must be trained to conduct quality testing before performing patient tests. |
| Regulatory | Poor regulation of POCT can lead to easy availability of suboptimal/poor quality tests. |
| Supply chain | Supply chain deficiencies may lead to suboptimal or poor quality POCT and significant wastage of consumables. |
| Technical/medical | Some clinical staff prefer syndromic management over diagnostic certainty. |
| Training | If unqualified staff perform POCT and errors result, confidence in POCT can be undermined. |
| Work flow balance | Staff shortages/turnover and high workload may reduce the uptake of POCT. |

**Table 37.3.** A checklist for the delivery of effective POCT in low-resource settings (Source: adapted from Peeling and Mabey 2010)

| Checklist |
| --- |
| ✓ Advocacy for appropriate POC diagnostics that are 'fit for purpose' |
| ✓ Product partnership developments |
| ✓ A drive for innovation in the developing world |
| ✓ Development of harmonised regulatory standards |
| ✓ Bridging the gap between research and policy |
| ✓ Capacity building for uptake and delivery of POC tests |
| ✓ Provision of proficiency testing panels to monitor quality |
| ✓ Education for health-care providers |

POC tests for infectious disease have revolutionised the future direction of this sector of the POCT market (Nichols 2015; Peeling and McNerney 2014; St John and Price 2014). Using nucleic acid amplification technology (NAAT), infectious disease POCT can now be performed with a clinical sensitivity and specificity matching that of the laboratory. At present, NAAT-based devices and reagent systems are expensive, while turnaround time for POCT results are often much longer (often in the order of 'hours' rather than 'minutes') than most clinical biochemistry or haematology POCT applications. My wish for the future would be that industry scale down this technology – from a footprint, turnaround time and cost perspective – to enable its even wider application in the developing world where infectious disease burdens and the need for POCT is greatest. This trend has already begun with, for example, the impending release of the Cepheid GeneXpert® Omni. Leveraging its existing Xpert cartridge technology, the Omni is a single module device with an integrated rechargeable battery (and supplemental power supply), full cloud-based connectivity and a small footprint (weighing 1 kg and standing 23 × 7 × 11 cm). It is designed specifically for use in low-resource settings and clinics.

There is also significant need for NAAT technology (and other technologies under development) to be multiplexed (i.e. use a single platform to detect multiple related infectious diseases); for example, respiratory viral panels, STI panels and panels for diseases arising from outbreaks/catastrophic events such as Ebola, Lassa and Dengue viruses in sub-Saharan Africa (Abel 2015). Multiplexing has the added advantage of simplifying, to an extent, the training requirements of POCT operators for these devices. Finally, as we move towards 2020, there will be an increasing need for the rapid diagnosis of antibiotic- or drug-resistant organisms in hospitals and long-term-care facilities (Nichols 2015). As described in Chapter 23, molecular-based POCT is already available for the detection of *Mycobacterium tuberculosis* DNA and resistance to rifampicin with a turnaround time of <2 h. How long before it will be possible to have a similar test available for antibiotic resistant strains of gonorrhoea for example?

## PRIORITIES FOR GROWING THE EVIDENCE-BASE FOR POINT-OF-CARE TESTING

The growth of POCT will only continue if there is parallel growth in the evidence-base to support its efficacy. In the 1990s/early 2000s, most studies on POCT focussed on analytical quality of testing. This period coincided with an era of scepticism that POCT could not possibly be 'as good as the laboratory'. However, there is now strong evidence that modern POCT devices can deliver results of equivalent quality to the laboratory. Future studies of analytical quality should be focussed at the intended site of field implementation, with testing conducted by its intended field operators rather than be conducted under controlled laboratory conditions.

The need for qualitative and quantitative studies of the clinical and operational effectiveness of POCT remain important, particularly in resource-limited settings, and studies of these types should continue to be of significance for POCT researchers. Chapter 8 is intended to help researchers with the choice and application of appropriate study designs, with well-constructed intervention trials most needed.

Looking forward, the main priority for POCT research should unquestionably be studies of cost-effectiveness. High-quality cost-effectiveness studies are needed to convince governments that POCT can deliver fiscal benefits to the health system and encourage them to support the uptake of POCT programs, but these studies are severely lacking at present. The reason is simple. Most scientists/researchers are not trained in this area and therefore, to achieve success in this field, researchers must engage with health economists, who do have the necessary skills to design, implement and analyse cost-effectiveness studies. Again, here is a new partnership opportunity for POCT.

Studies of cultural effectiveness can be a growth area for POCT, particularly for resource-limited settings where Indigenous people represent the bulk of the population. There is considerable opportunity for innovation here but the researcher must first be equipped with cultural awareness/cultural safety training and skills. In my experience, working in partnership with Indigenous people can be a rich and highly rewarding endeavour.

## INTEGRATING POINT-OF-CARE TESTING WITHIN THE HEALTH SYSTEM

Perhaps the greatest challenges for POCT moving forward to the year 2020 are to establish its 'place', exert its collective voice, seize opportunity and embed itself within the global health system.

POCT needs leadership, advocacy and a strong voice at the political level. Lobbying should ensure governments clearly recognise the benefits of POCT for patient care in primary care settings and, as a result, develop funding policies to support the dissemination of POCT to localities where it is most needed clinically. In Australia, the government will not reimburse or promote POCT unless the clinical or economic benefit is clearly established and the quality of testing is assured (Abel 2015). As Pai *et al.* (2012) assert: 'at the country level, POCT diagnostics need to be integrated within health systems, supported by financing [reimbursement], incentives, training and information and communication technology … the best POCT, without a business model, is unlikely to be scaled up.'

## IMPROVEMENTS TO POCT NETWORKS AND SYSTEMS

This book has focussed strongly on the key elements required to establish and maintain a POCT program and the need for stakeholder engagement. As we move towards 2020, we need to be constantly mindful of how we can improve these test systems/networks.

### Better management support

In some parts of the world, laboratory health professionals remain resistant to the uptake of POCT for reasons including: (i) lack of control or oversight for POCT conducted outside their laboratory network; (ii) lack of clarity regarding which agency will accept ownership of a POCT program; (iii) uncertainty about who will provide overall management of a decentralised POCT Program; and (iv) lack of staff time/resources to support field POCT (Pai *et al.* 2012). Rather than resisting change, I would challenge laboratories to embrace change and be flexible and supportive of POCT in primary care settings.

I also see significant opportunity for the proliferation of specialist POCT providers. The specialist POCT provider's 'core business' involves implementing and managing POCT programs and networks through ongoing training, competency assessment, quality management, technical support and ideally evidence-based research. The specialist POCT provider should include health professionals with the collective experience and expertise to deliver the intensive level of support that is required to ensure quality-assured and sustainable POCT programs at the primary care level.

### More engagement with industry and product developers

Industry should aspire to provide optimised services in relation to stock management, support for device maintenance/repair, provision of single lot numbers of QC material for long-term monitoring of quality, and support for training. Product developers and manufacturers need to be more cognisant of the real-world context (e.g. conditions, settings, users, resources [or lack of]) in which their products will be used and/or the need for the product to be scaled-up (Pai *et al.* 2012). Only with this understanding can developers deliver a product that will match and target the needs of specific public health programs. Garcia *et al.* (2015) took a party of 22 diagnostic developers, global health researchers and project funders on a 6-day expedition to the Peruvian jungle, desert and highlands to see first-hand the challenges of providing health care in resource-limited settings and to assess the appropriateness of their POC tests currently under development. Most developers indicated they would now change their current or future device designs as a result of their experience and acknowledged there was no 'one size fits all' solution. Fertile opportunities exist for partnerships between POCT Coordinators with knowledge of POCT systems, researchers (public and private) with disease expertise and those with science and engineering backgrounds to develop a new wave of POCT diagnostics that meet targeted product profiles (TPPs).

### Smarter, more practical quality monitoring solutions for POCT

By 2020, my wish is that we have a global consensus regarding what constitutes an acceptable quality framework for conducting POCT; a consensus that is scalable according to clinical need and complexity of device and flexible in terms of being adaptable, practical, relevant, innovative and cost-effective in primary care settings while at all times assuring patient safety and minimising risk of harm.

In the next 5 years, it would be desirable for proficiency testing (PT) providers to develop low-cost, simple-to-prepare PT products with a matrix that matches the sample type required for the POC test. There is also an immediate need for expert guidelines and recommendations on the use of parallel patient testing as a PT solution.

### Linking POC test results to clinical pathways/algorithms

To emphasise again, POC test results alone are of limited value unless they are integrated into clinical algorithms/treatment pathways, which will in turn facilitate timeliness of clinical action (with POCT then delivering a goal-oriented, rather than product-oriented, outcome).

### Continuing improvements to connectivity

There will be a continuing need for the development of IT systems that can keep pace with advancing POCT technologies. Optimising the connectivity capabilities of POCT devices will facilitate their integration into healthcare systems by streamlining data management and eliminating manual data transcription.

### Flexible accreditation frameworks

Peeling and Mabey (2010) advocate for harmonised regulatory standards at regional or international levels. This is a laudable goal because lack of regulation can unquestionably lead to proliferation of sub-standard POCT. Certainly, accreditation bodies need to consider the diversity and complexity of POCT networks and allow flexibility in their assessment of such models. Imposing a laboratory-style accreditation framework on a network operating in a remote low resource setting will be doomed to fail.

## COURTING THE NEXT GENERATION OF POCT FUTURE LEADERS

The next generation of potential POCT leaders is currently sitting in lecture theatres or studying online at universities (or higher education institutions) around the world. I am a firm believer that POCT should be taught widely across the university sector at a course or topic level in undergraduate or postgraduate degrees covering, for example, medical science, health science, paramedic science, forensic science, medicine, nursing, public health, Indigenous health, rural and remote health and pharmacy. Today's students seem to 'get' POCT and they want to help make a difference to people's lives in the community setting. Here is the genesis of the future leaders of POCT, and we need to encourage and mentor students selectively recruited from these health disciplines for long and rewarding careers in POCT (Shephard *et al.* 2015).

## CONCLUSION

Future opportunities for POCT are only limited by the narrowness of our collective vision for it. Although it is impossible to say with certainty where POCT will be by the year 2020, whichever way you look at it, the future of POCT looks bright. POCT is available for all health professionals of varying backgrounds from across the globe to embrace. I encourage you to take up the challenge and become a POCT champion.

## REFERENCES

Abel G (2015) Current status and future prospects of point-of-care testing around the globe. *Expert Review of Molecular Diagnostics* **15**, 853–855. doi:10.1586/14737159.2015.1060126

Blick KE (2015) An editorial on point-of-care testing: past, present and future trends. *Point of Care* **14**, 143–145. doi:10.1097/POC.0000000000000068

Chin CD, Cheung YK, Laksanasopin T, Modena MM, Chin SY, Sridhara AA, *et al.* (2013) Mobile device for disease diagnosis and data tracking in resource-limited settings. *Clinical Chemistry* **59**, 629–640. doi:10.1373/clinchem.2012.199596

Drain PK, Hyle EP, Noubary F, Freedberg KA, Wilson D, Bishai WR, *et al.* (2014) Diagnostic point-of-care tests in resource-limited settings. *The Lancet Infectious Diseases* **14**, 239–249. doi:10.1016/S1473-3099(13)70250-0

Garcia PJ, You P, Fridley G, Mabey D, Peeling R (2015) Point-of-care diagnostic tests for low-resource settings. *Lancet* **3**, 257–258.

Gomez FA (2013) The future of microfluidic point-of-care diagnostic devices. *Bioanalysis* **5**, 1–3. doi:10.4155/bio.12.307

Gordon J, Michel G (2012) Discerning trends in multiplex immunoassay technology with potential for resource-limited settings. *Clinical Chemistry* **58**, 690–698. doi:10.1373/clinchem.2011.176503

Holloway PAH (2015) Point-of-care testing in the United Kingdom. *Point of Care* **14**, 121–123. doi:10.1097/POC.0000000000000075

Isbell TS (2015) Point-of-care testing: a look inside the crystal ball. *Point of Care* **14**, 167–168. doi:10.1097/POC.0000000000000074

Kiechle FL (2015) Point-of-care testing: One view of past, present and future challenges. *Point of Care* **14**, 157–164. doi:10.1097/POC.0000000000000069

Kricka LJ, Park JY, Reiprish A, Polsky TG, Nardiello MH (2015) The evolution and future of point-of-care testing. *Point of Care* **14**, 110–115. doi:10.1097/POC.0000000000000067

Mazzola LT, Pérez-Casas C (2015) *HIV/AIDS Diagnostics Technology Landscape*. UNITAID Secretariat, World Health Organization, Geneva, Switzerland.

Nichols JH (2015) Point-of-care testing: past experience and future challenges. *Point of Care* **14**, 103–105. doi:10.1097/POC.0000000000000079

Pai NP, Vadnais C, Denkinger C, Engel N, Pai M (2012) Point-of-care testing for infectious diseases: diversity, complexity and barriers in low- and middle-income countries. *PLoS Medicine* **9**, e1001306. doi:10.1371/journal.pmed.1001306

Pai M, Ghiasi M, Pant Pai N (2015) Point-of-care diagnostic testing in global health: what is the point? *Microbe* **10**, 103–107.

Papali A (2016) Providing health care in rural and remote areas: lessons from the international space station. *Bulletin of the World Health Organization* **94**, 73–74. doi:10.2471/BLT.15.162628

Peeling RW, Mabey D (2010) Point-of-care tests for diagnosing infections in the developing world. *Clinical Microbiology and Infectious Diseases* **16**, 1062–1069. doi:10.1111/j.1469-0691.2010.03279.x

Peeling RW, McNerney R (2014) Emerging technologies in point-of-care molecular diagnostics for resource-limited settings. *Expert Review of Molecular Diagnostics* **14**, 525–534. doi:10.1586/14737159.2014.915748

Shephard MDS, Halls HJ, Motta LA (2015) Online Point-of-Care Coordinator Graduate Certificate Program for global point-of-care testing. In *Global Point-of-Care – Strategies for Disaster, Emergencies, and Public Health Resilience*. (Eds GJ Kost and CM Curtis) pp. 341–346. AACC Press, Washington DC, USA.

St John A, Price CP (2014) Existing and emerging technologies for point-of-care testing. *The Clinical Biochemist Reviews* **35**, 155–167.

Tolan NV, Karon BS (2015) The evolution of point-of-care testing: can we improve our future knowing our past? *Point of Care* **14**, 146–150. doi:10.1097/POC.0000000000000071

# Index

www.ingramcontent.com/pod-product-compliance
Lightning Source LLC
LaVergne TN
LVHW060615110826
845154LV00003B/90
*9781486305186*